ALLE ZEIT WACH 1842

Neuropsychopharmacology 2

Proceedings of the XVIth C.I.N.P. Congress,
Munich, August 15–19, 1988

Edited by
W. E. Bunney, Jr., H. Hippius, G. Laakmann
and M. Schmauß

Springer-Verlag
Berlin Heidelberg New York
London Paris Tokyo
Hong Kong Barcelona

W. E. Bunney, Jr., M. D.
Professor of Psychiatry
College of Medicine
University of California at Irvine
Irvine, CA 92717, USA

Professor Dr. Hanns Hippius
Professor Dr. Gregor Laakmann
Psychiatrische Klinik und Poliklinik
der Universität München
Nußbaumstraße 7
8000 München 2, FRG

Priv. Doz. Dr. Max Schmauss
Bezirkskrankenhaus Augsburg
Dr.-Mack-Straße 1
8900 Augsburg, FRG

With 106 Figures

ISBN 3-540-50252-1 (in 2 Volumes) Springer-Verlag Berlin Heidelberg New York
ISBN 0-387-50252-1 (in 2 Volumes) Springer-Verlag New York Berlin Heidelberg

Library of Congress Cataloging-in-Publication Data. Collegium Internationale Neuro-psychopharmacologicum. Congress (16th : 1988 : Munich, Germany) Neuropsychopharmacology : proceedings of the XVIth C.I.N.P. Congress, Munich, August 15–19, 1988 / edited by W. E. Bunney ... [et al.]. p.cm. Includes index. ISBN 0-387-50252-1 (U.S. : alk. paper) 1. Neuropsychopharmacology-Congresses. I. Bunney, William E., II. Title. [DNLM: 1. Mental Disorders-drug therapy-congresses. 2. Nervous System-drug effects-congresses. 3. Psychopharmacology-congresses. 4. Psychotropic Drugspharmacology-congresses. QV 77C6975n] RM315.C58 1988 615′.78-dc20 DNLM/DLC for Library of Congress.

Typesetting: Fotosatz-Service Köhler, D-8700 Würzburg
2125/3130-543210 – Printed on acid-free paper

Contents

12 Neuropeptides: Basic Research

13 Clinical Aspects of Neuropeptide Research

14 Postmarketing Surveillance of Psychotropic Drugs

Contents of Companion Volume 1

List of Contributors (Volumes 1 + 2)

Adresses are given at the beginning of the respective contribution

10 PET Imaging in Neurosciences and Psychiatry

Strategies for In Vivo Quantification of Human Neuroreceptors by Positron Emission Tomography *

D. F. WONG and L. T. YOUNG [1]

Introduction

At the present time, a number of groups of investigators are studying neuroreceptors and neurotransmitter systems with positron emission tomography (PET). In vivo quantification of neuroreceptors has been accomplished only in the past decade, and techniques are therefore still undergoing modification and validation. One of the earliest findings suggested a decline in the density of central dopamine D_2 neuroreceptors with age and different slopes of density versus age for men and women (Wong et al. 1984). Although there has been a steady improvement in imaging methods, controversy has surrounded many of the findings obtained with these techniques. Nevertheless, potential findings in neuropsychiatric illnesses at least stimulate future investigation and may, more optimistically, provide real insight into pathophysiology.

Abnormalities in neuroreceptor binding (and in some cases neuroreceptor densities) have been demonstrated in a number of neuropsychiatric disorders including schizophrenia (Wong et al. 1986c; Farde et al. 1987), temporal lobe epilepsy (Frost et al. 1988), poststroke depression (Mayberg et al. 1988), bipolar affective disorder (Wong et al. 1988), and Tourette's syndrome (Wong et al. 1988). The complexity and novelty of PET neuroreceptor imaging procedures indicate that improvements are still needed, and that the reliability of results obtained with such techniques may be questioned.

Very recently, two studies of drug-naive schizophrenics using different radiologands, PET techniques, and patient populations had markedly different results. One study completed in 1986 at the Johns Hopkins Medical Institutions in Baltimore (Wong et al. 1986c) demonstrated an approximately twofold elevation in D_2 receptor density (B_{max}) in ten drug-naive schizophrenics and five drug-free schizophrenics as compared to 11 normal controls (Fig. 1) using the ligand [^{11}C]*N*-methylspiperone (NMSP). These elevated densities continue to be demonstrated in our sample, which has since been expanded to 20 drug-

* This work was supported in part by NIMH Contract R01 MH42821 (to D.F.W) and the Medical Council of Canada (to L.T.Y.).

[1] Department of Radiology and Nuclear Medicine, The Johns Hopkins Medical Institutions, Baltimore, MD, USA.

Neuropsychopharmacology
Edited by Bunney/Hippius/Laakmann/Schmauß

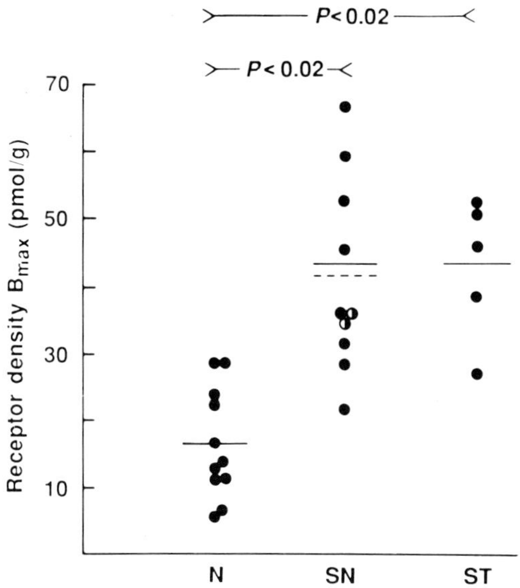

Fig. 1. Dopamine D_2 receptor density (B_{max}) in the caudate nucleus in normal volunteers (*N*) and in drugnaive (*SN*) and drug-treated (*ST*) schizophrenics. *Solid horizontal lines*, mean values in each group. For the drug-naive group this line is the value for the eight subjects who had only a single 7.5-mg dose of haloperidol before their second PET scan (43.3 ± 5.7 pmol/g). *Dotted line*, mean of all ten subjects, including the two who received more than a single dose of haloperidol before their second PET scan (average receptor density in this group, 41.7 ± 4.6 pmol/g). Mean receptor densities for the normal volunteers and the drug-treated group were 16.6 ± 2.5 and 43.3 ± 4.7 pmol/g, respectively. There was a significant difference (*t* test with Bonferroni correction for multiple inference) between either the eight or ten drug-naive or the drug-treated schizophrenics and the normal subjects. (From Wong et al. 1986c)

naive schizophrenics, with a continuation in these elevations (Tune et al. 1989; Wong et al. 1989a, c). In 1987, a Swedish group at the Karolinska Institute using PET with the radioligand [^{11}C]raclopride did not demonstrate significant differences in D_2 receptor density or affinity between 15 drug-naive schizophrenics and normal controls (Farde et al. 1987). It has become clear that there are many factors which might contribute to such markedly different findings (Table 1). For present purposes, these divergent results between two studies of the same neuroreceptor in the same disorder serve as an example to illustrate some important considerations regarding PET neuroreceptor imaging in living human brain.

It is of interest that a similar problem occurred in the study of patients at risk to develop Huntington's disease using the [^{18}F]2-deoxyglucose (FDG) technique to measure cerebral glucose metabolism. Although two studies showed reductions in caudate glucose metabolism in subjects at risk for Huntington's disease (Mazziotta et al. 1987; Hayden et al. 1987), a later study did not (Young et al. 1987). These results are surprising since patients in all

Table 1. Comparison of Johns Hopkins University (JHU) and Karolinska Institute PET D_2 dopamine receptor studies

	JHU [a]	Karolinska [b]
n	10	15
Age		
Patients	31.2±3.6	24.0±3.7
Controls	24.3±2.0	29.1±4.6
Duration of illness	4.7 years	1.9 years [c]
Ligand	[^{11}C]NMSP	[^{11}C]Raclopride
B_{max} determination	Two PET scans with Wolfe plot and model comparison	Two PET scans with Scatchard plot

[a] Wong et al. (1986a, c).
[b] Farde et al. (1987).
[c] At the time of the scan, one-half of the subjects had been ill for less than 6 months.

three studies met the same diagnostic criteria and were all studied in the same country. Significant differences are present in the methods of image analysis which may in part account for divergent findings. These results are of particular concern since measurement of cerebral glucose metabolism with FDG is probably the most well-established PET technique. Following a number of important methodological issues in the development and interpretation of PET, neuroreceptor studies are considered.

Methodological Issues

Patient and Control Population

Perhaps partly due to the complex technology associated with PET scanning, an important issue in interpreting studies which attempt to quantify neuroreceptors is often neglected: the patient and control populations. Diagnostic criteria and clinical characteristics of patients are fundamental in designing and interpreting clinical investigations, particularly in psychiatry which has few disease markers or definitive diagnostic tests. Schizophrenia is a chronic debilitating neuropsychiatric disease which usually begins in adolescence or early adulthood (Lehmann and Cancro 1985). There are widely varying clinical presentations, in addition to variable symptoms occurring at different stages of illness. There appears to be a heterogeneous population of patients as well as differences in the acute versus chronic stages of this disorder. It is plausible that neurochemical findings in schizophrenia may become more prominent at later stages of illness rather than at the onset of symptoms. This situation would be consistent with computed tomography scan abnormalities which were found to be more apparent in chronic versus acute schizophrenia (Luchins 1982).

Regarding the controversy over D_2 receptor findings in the Hopkins versus Karolinska studies (Table 1), patients in the study from Johns Hopkins were older (mean age 31 ± 4 years, $n = 10$) and had been ill for a longer time (4.7 years) compared with the Swedish patients (mean age 24 ± 4, $n = 15$; mean duration of illness, 1.9 years). If D_2 receptor changes occur at a later stage of illness, such clinical issues may be relevant. The duration of illness, time of scanning relative to the first episode, the presence or absence of psychotic features, premorbid personality traits, and predominant positive or negative symptoms are just some examples of potentially relevant factors which may be important in interpreting PET neuroreceptor imaging in schizophrenia. Generally, it can be stated that there are relevant issues which relate to typical clinical manifestations of a particular neuropsychiatric disorder which must be carefully considered in the design and interpretation of a PET study.

In addition to clinical issues in the patient group, attention must be directed towards selecting appropriate control groups. Matching on the basis of age sex is extremely important in the case of D_2 receptor imaging, in which a fall with age (Wong et al. 1984) in addition to sex differences was suggested and continues to be found with more sophisticated models (Wong et al. 1986a, c, 1988, 1989a, c). Moreover, socioeconomic status and level of education need also be considered. In practice, it is difficult to recruit subject groups matched on these variables for such complex procedures as PET neuroreceptor studies. Since an essential feature of schizophrenia is the presence of impairment in social functioning (American Psychiatric Association 1987), matching on socioeconomic status and level of education may not be an appropriate. It is not clear, however, how important these variables are in the design or interpretation of PET studies. Indeed, there are many other variables which may potentially confound experimental design. All need to be considered and subject groups matched on important variables.

Radioligand Pharmacology

Important initial considerations in choosing a PET strategy to quantify a neuroreceptor in vivo in human brain include pharmacologic parameters of the proposed radioligand, such as the kinetics and affinity of binding, selectivity, and specificity. In general, PET radioligands can be divided into two types, those which reach a quasi-equilibrium during the PET scan and those which do not. The first type of ligand, for example raclopride, is rapidly reversible and displays considerable dissociation during the time interval of the PET scan. In the latter group, because of the time frame of the PET scan which is based on the short half-life of typical radioisotopes (^{11}C, $t_{1/2} = 20$ min; ^{18}F, $t_{1/2} = 110$ min), these nonequilibrating ligands, such as NMSP, can be considered to bind "irreversibly" because of minimal dissociation from brain regions. Perhaps this binding parameter is the most important factor in the design and development of a model to quantify neuroreceptors with the particular PET radioligand. Specific modelling issues are addressed below.

Table 2. In vitro binding constants for three D_2 ligands. (From Andreasen et al. 1988)

Variable	^{3}H-Labeled ligands		
	Haloperidol[a]	Methylspiperone[a]	Raclopride[b]
k_{off} (min^{-1})	0.122	0.022	0.023
k_{on} (min^{-1})	0.085	0.086	0.084
K_D (nM) calculated	1.44	0.25	0.3
K_D (nM) measured in vitro	1.3	0.10	1.2
K_I' or K_D (nM) measured in vivo (PET)	1.4[c]	–	7.3[d]

[a] P. Seeman, personal communication; human data.
[b] Kohler et al. (1985); animal data.
[c] Wong et al. (1986a, b); K_I', human data.
[d] Farde et al. (1987); K_D, human data.

The affinity of a PET radioligand for neuroreceptors of interest is also extremely important. In most cases, in vitro estimates of such binding parameters obtained in animals or postmortem human brain are valuable in choosing a ligand. Differences in the affinity of a ligand for the D_2 receptor are relevant to the controversy around PET D_2 receptor measurements in schizophrenia. For example [^{11}C]NMSP used by the Hopkins group has about a five- to ten-fold higher affinity (Table 2) than that of the published values for [^{11}C]raclopride or [^{3}H]raclopride (Kohler et al. 1985; Lyon et al. 1987). Reversible ligands with lower affinity lead to potentially greater susceptibility to competition from endogenous neurotransmitters. Recently, Seeman et al. (1989) found in animal studies a reduction in apparent B_{max} in the presence of 100 nM dopamine with [^{3}H]raclopride but not with [^{3}H]NMSP (Fig. 2). They suggest that this is an important factor which might explain the discrepancies between the Hopkins and Swedish findings, as intrasynaptic dopamine levels may interfere with B_{max} estimates obtained with raclopride. Furthermore, we have recently found that amphetamine (10 mg/kg i.v.) administered to mice prior to injection reduces the striatal to cerebellar ratios of both [^{3}H]NMSP and [^{3}H]raclopride binding at 30 min by approximately 30%, but at 2 h postinjection such decreases only occur with raclopride binding (unpublished data).

High-affinity ligands that do not reach equilibrium may also be subject to complex receptor-ligand interactions. Chugani et al. (1988) suggested that the [^{3}H]spiperone-receptor complex was internalized into intracytoplasmic vesicles, in addition to remaining at the synaptic membrane. Such a mechanism, if onfirmed, would increase our understanding of the functional and dynamic re of these receptors being measured by some PET ligands (Fig. 3). We are ly axamining such synaptic and cellular events which may influence T quantitative measures of D_2 receptor in human brain.

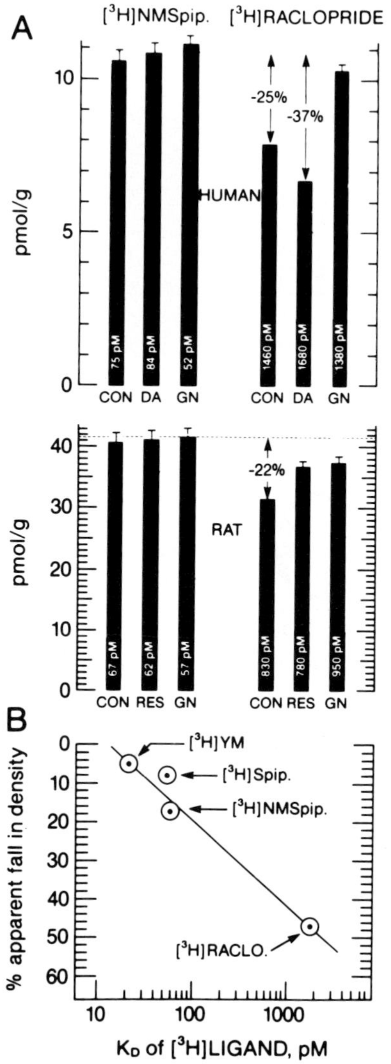

Fig. 2. **A** Dopamine D_2 receptor densities using [^{3}H]methylspiperone ([^{3}H]*NMSpip*) and [^{3}H]raclopride. Densities were unaffected by exogenous dopamine (*DA*; 100 n*M*), by 100 μ*M* guanilylimidodiphosphate (*GN*), or by reserpine (*RES*; 3 mg/kg i.p., 24 h prior to death). The density of [^{3}H]raclopride binding sites, however, was lower than that of [^{3}H]methylspiperone here by 22%–25% and by 37% in the presence of 100 n*M* dopamine. Human data are for the same human caudate nucleus (brain T 181) done three times, and data are averaged. *Error bars* indicate SEM. Rat data for $n = 4$. Centrifugation method throughout (Seeman et al. 1987). The mean K_D value (SEM was ±8%) is shown at the bottom of each bar. *CON*, control values. **B** *Ordinate* indicates the apparent fall (percentage of control) in the density of binding sites for each of four [^{3}H]-labeled neuroleptic ligands (*YM*, YM-09151-2; *Spip.*, spiperone; *Raclo.*, raclopride) upon the addition of 2000 n*M* exogenous dopamine (in 0.1% ascorbic acid in buffered medium, pH 7.4). The K_D of each [^{3}H]-labeled ligand was obtained by saturation analysis on human brain striata. Centrifugation method. (From Seeman et al. 1989)

Modeling Issues

As mentioned in the previous section, modeling approaches with NMSP, which binds irreversibly, and raclopride, which binds reversibly, are distinctly different (Table 2). In general, there are two types of models in PET receptor studies, dynamic nonequilibrium and equilibrium, which have been used with the radioligands NMSP and raclopride, respectively.

The Hopkins study used a dynamic model in which two PET scans with [^{11}C]NMSP were performed, unblocked and blocked (haloperidol 7.5 mg p.o.

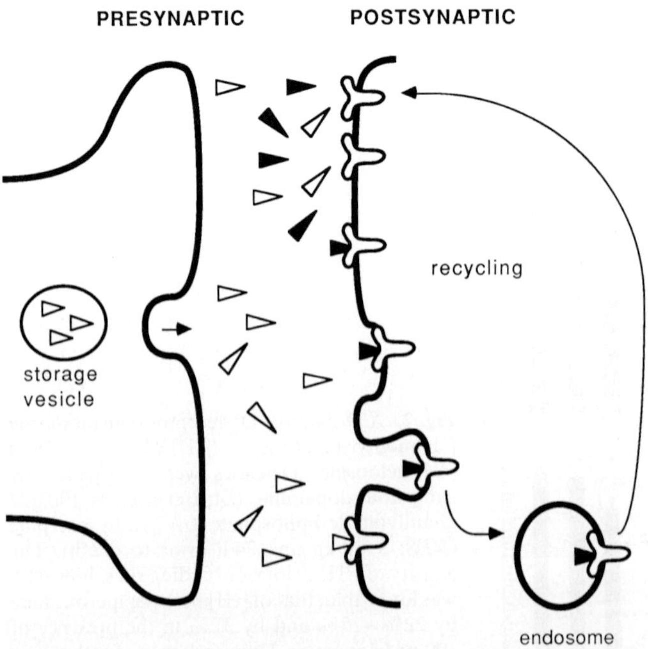

Fig. 3. Schematic representation of a striatal synaptic junction illustrating some of the complexities associated with PET radioligands binding to dopamine D_2 receptors. *Clear triangles*, endogenous dopamine released from the pre-synaptic vesicles; *dark triangles*, radiolabeled ligand imaged with PET. Two potential pharmacologic parameters which influence PET radioligand binding are shown: competition for binding with endogenous dopamine and internalization of the radioligand-surface receptor complex into the postsynaptic nerve terminal. In the first case, high levels of this endogenous dopamine could compete with their lower affinity ligand, e.g., [^{11}C]raclopride. In the latter case, internalization of the radioligand-surface receptor complex suggests that PET imaging may reflect functional turnover of surface receptors. Although Chugani et al. (1988) suggested that spiperone may be internalized, this has not yet been replicated by other groups

4 h before scan) in each subject. The B_{max} estimates derive from the brain haloperidol concentration divided by the difference in the reciprocal of blocked and unblocked rate constants (Wong et al. 1986 a). The first type of model, the dynamic nonequilibrium, requires the appropriate input function analysis of blood radioactivity, which in some cases is crucial to demonstrate differences in patient groups. For example, the initial use of tissue ratios of caudate to cerebellum binding, traditionally used as a measure of specific to nonspecific binding in rodent in vivo studies (Kuhar et al. 1978), failed to demonstrate differences in several disseases, such as Tourette's, schizophrenia and bipolar disorder (Wong et al. 1985). This is probably due to confounding blood flow changes that are not taken into consideration by simple tissue ratios but are accounted for by kinetic models (Wong et al. 1986 a, b; Mintun et al. 1984). This potential problem of flow limitation has occurred with a number of ligands under development. Kinetic modeling procedures attempt to distin-

guish receptor binding components of interest to allow separate estimation of density (B_{max}) and affinity (K_d). In some cases, a steady-state condition may be reached between some of the compartments, for instance, nonspecific binding and unmetabolized radioligand in the case of [^{11}C]NMSP for D_2 dopamine receptor quantification (Wong et al. 1986a, b). Such conditions can also be used in the model calculations to estimate factors such as the labeled metabolites or partition coefficient for [^{11}C]NMSP. Indeed, analogous steady-state conditions are assumed in the Sokoloff-Phelps-Huang glucose metabolism model (Sokoloff et al. 1977; Huang et al. 1980).

On the other hand, in an equilibrium model (actually quasi-equilibrium after a bolus injection since equilibrium requires a constant infusion), the use of simple tissue ratios in a Scatchard-type analysis has both historical and theoretical precedent. Thus the use of tissue ratios for estimating receptor density and affinity with PET radioligands, as was done with [^{11}C]raclopride by Farde et al. (1986, 1987), may be an acceptable simplification. However, proof of meeting these assumptions of a quasi-equilibrium are important factors which need to be validated in this model with its simplification. In the case of [^{11}C]raclopride, the initial studies of Farde et al. (1986, 1987) did not measure the input function or labeled metabolites or analyze rate constants with a kinetic model. These studies are currently being carried out with raclopride (L. Farde, personal communication). It is important to note that both of these rather different modeling approaches are variants of analysis of the same three- or four-compartment model. Furthermore, both models require validation of assumptions which are examined below.

Validation of Assumptions in Quantitative Models

All quantitative models used in PET make a number of assumptions. Such assumptions must be tested for their validity. For example, partition coefficients for oxygen in ^{15}O methods (Frackowiak et al. 1980) and the lump constants for glucose metabolism determined with FDG (Phelps et al. 1979) have been assumed for many PET studies. Especially in the latter case, problems have occurred with these assumptions, as evidenced by the variation in lump constants in neoplasia or in stroke (Hawkins et al. 1981, 1986). The complexity of quantitative receptor modeling is illustrated by examining some of the assumptions made in these models and validation experiments which are currently underway.

The amount of available D_2 receptor ligands, haloperidol, and NMSP are important in our multicompartmental model (Wong et al. 1986a). It has been suggested that differences in binding to plasma protein of such ligands may be different in patients and controls (Farde et al. 1988). We examined the degree of binding of [11C]NMSP to plasma proteins in normal subjects ($95.7 \pm 0.36\%$ bound, mean $\pm$ SEM; $n = 12$) and patients with schizophrenia, bipolar disorder, and other neuropsychiatric illnesses ($95.6 \pm 0.4\%$ bound; $n = 21$). These recent results indicate that the amount of NMSP which is available for binding to brain D_2 receptors is very similar in patients and normals. It follows that the same should be true for another butyrophenone, haloperidol, which has very similar structure and pharmacology to NMSP. We are currently testing the binding of haloperidol to plasma proteins directly with [^{18}F]haloperidol in patients and controls. The fact that patients reported in Wong et al. (1986c) and those studied since (Wong et al. 1989a, c) had normal serum protein and albumin measures and were well nourished by history at the time of the scan (L. E. Tune, personal communication) also argues against differences in protein binding across patient groups. Such studies are crucial since an accurate estimation of available haloperidol in brain is necessary in our calculation of D_2 receptor density.

A related assumption involves the partition coefficient for haloperidol between brain and plasma. In studies with [^{3}H]haloperidol (Wong et al. 1986c), partition coefficients for haloperidol were found to be approximately 3 (gram brain tissue per milliliter plasma), which is compatible with previous assumptions. These partition coefficients require special attention since they represent partitioning relative to plasma, whereas total serum haloperidol levels are used in our calculations. Additional experiments are being carried out with [^{18}F]haloperidol to measure the partition coefficient in postmortem brain from controls and subjects with various neuropsychiatric disorders.

It is assumed that binding reaches equilibrium in PET studies with reversibly bound radioligands (i.e., equilibrium model). Farde et al. (1986, 1987) measured total binding in D_2 receptors in striatum divided by their estimate of free concentration derived from cerebellar brain values of [^{11}C]raclopride assumed to be at equilibrium. In these studies they did not employ a dynamic model to demonstrate binding equilibrium. We have demonstrated how this can be accomplished (Wong et al. 1986b) with equilibrium binding of [^{11}C]NMSP to cortical 5-HT_2 (serotonin type 2) receptors (quasi-equilibrium is reached since the binding to 5-HT_2, in contrast with that to D_2 receptors, is reversible). Such analyses require that the complete blood and brain time activity curves (radioactivity plotted against time) are known up until the time that binding ratios are examined. The assumption that equilibrium has been reached, when in fact it has not yet been achieved, may unfavorably alter measurements of receptor density and affinity.

Another important model assumption to consider is the treatment of labeled radioligand metabolites. Knowledge of the concentration of labeled metabolites is necessary to determine the true input function from the arterial capillary side to the brain region containing the neuroreceptors. We previously employed a model correction for metabolites involving the relationship between the volume of distribution of the tracer in cerebellum as it falls relative to total plasma radioactivity (Wong et al. 1986a). Although, at that time, HPLC metabolite analysis of the actual blood samples showed good correlation with our model, we have since improved the specificity and sensitivity of HPLC metabolite methods (adapted from Eddington and Young 1988). We have recently examined a large number of patient studies and demonstrated a close relationship between the metabolite and model corrections (Wong et al.

1989a, c). Furthermore, receptor densities calculated with both modeled metabolite corrections and HPLC measured metabolite corrections, using both blocked (with haloperidol) and unblocked scans, are closely correlated in a number of subjects (Wong et al. 1989b). The equilibrium model of Farde et al. (1986) measures brain tissue ratios without blood sampling. They assume a quasi-equilibrium among compartments so that metabolite corrections are unnecessary. However, this is another assumption which needs to be proven by kinetic analysis before simplification to measuring brain ratios can be safely employed. Violation of such model assumptions may contribute to the differences in results obtained from different centers, such as those between the Hopkins and Karolinska studies. The assumptions made in any quantitative model must ultimately be validated to ensure the appropriateness of such models.

PET Instrumentation

There are currently a number of different PET scanners available. Newer systems have more rings of detectors and other modifications which can improve the in plane spatial resolution of structures to less than 5 mm. Such precision is particularly important when very small structures are of interest to the investigator. In the two studies examining D_2 receptors in schizophrenia, different PET systems were employed although both systems had similar spatial resolution. Equipment differences are unlikely to account for discrepant findings in the absence of gross pathology in a structure, for example, the striatum in schizophrenia. On the other hand, in a neuropsychiatric disorder with marked atrophy, such as Alzheimer's disease, or with striatal degeneration, such as Huntington's disease, PET camera differences may be very relevant. As interest is focused on smaller structures and as the spatial resolution reaches theoretical limits of PET (in the order of a few millimeters), issues such as scatter attenuation correction, will become important factors in the determination of abnormalities in disorders as well as variability between research centers.

Anatomical Alignment and Localization

Since neuroreceptor binding determined with PET yields functional images, they must be based on an appropriate anatomical scheme. In both the Hopkins and Karolinska studies, X-ray CT was employed prior to the PET procedure for alignment purposes. At present, both centers have the ability to overlay magnetic resonance imaging or CT scans with PET images with appropriate registration procedures which improve the placement of regions of interest. In these particular studies of drug-naive schizophrenics, regions of interest were determined in different manners; in the Hopkins study investigators identified peak values in a 2×2 pixel area on PET images whereas a CT overlay was used in the Karolinska study. It is unlikely that differences in the placement of regions of interest was a significant confounding factor because of the modest resolution of both scanners and the fact that brain structures were relatively easy to examine. Although unlikely to account for the discrepancies between the two studies, these procedures may contribute to the considerable variance in measures of receptor B_{max}. Recent developments in the anatomic localization and placement of regions of interest will diminish this source of variance in future PET neuroreceptor studies.

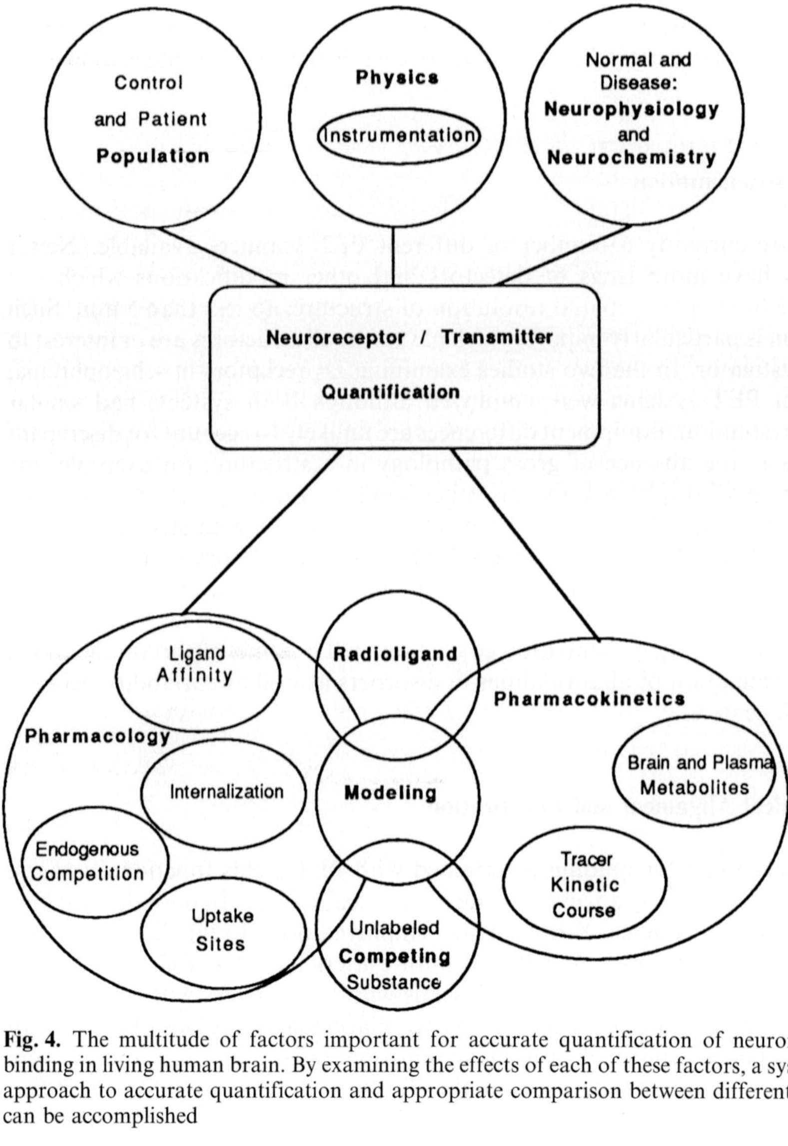

Fig. 4. The multitude of factors important for accurate quantification of neuroreceptor binding in living human brain. By examining the effects of each of these factors, a systematic approach to accurate quantification and appropriate comparison between different studies can be accomplished

Discussion

In the present review, a number of important considerations for the design and interpretation of PET neuroreceptor studies are presented (Fig. 4). Different methodological and clinical issues in various PET centers around the world may result in discrepant findings in the same neuropsychiatric disorder. An example of divergent findings in two PET neuroreceptor studies examining D_2 dopamine receptors in schizophrenia illustrates the importance of addressing such issues. The ongoing work of validating model assumptions in both these centers will improve PET neuroreceptor quantification methodology. Patient and control population factors require further study. Differences between experimental approaches could be examined directly and controlled by studying the same patients groups with both ligands, as suggested in a recent review (Andreason et al. 1988). Probably the most compelling current explanation for this discrepancy is that NMSP and raclopride may be subject to different pharmacologic factors, such as competition with endogenous dopamine, or that these ligands may bind to different sites. The recent findings of Seeman et al. (1989) and our ongoing studies support potentially important pharmacologic factors. Such an explanation would allow for consistency in both approaches but emphasizes the importance of basic pharmacologic differences, rather than modeling considerations, as major factors in the quantification of neuroreceptors in living human brain. Such a discussion surrounding the apparent D_2 dopamine receptor controversy has important implications for future PET studies of neuropsychiatric disorders.

Acknowledgements. Special acknowledgement is due to clinical collaborators Drs. L. E. Tune, G. D. Pearlson, and C. Ross, who were responsible for the recruitment and characterization of patients, in addition to sharing in hypothesis testing in schizophrenic and bipolar patients; to Drs. R. F. Dannals, H. Ravert, and A. Wilson, who were responsible for radioligand production and development; to Drs. M. Kuhar and H. N. Wagner Jr. for helpful discussions; to Dr. D. Young for HPLC method development; to Drs. A. Gjedde, P. D. Wilson, and R. D. Parker for modeling and statistical considerations; to Dr. S. Resnick for comments on the manuscript; and thanks to D. Burkhardt, E. Balcavage, E. Minkin, and B. Chan for technical assistance.

References

American Psychiatric Association (1987) Diagnostic and statistical manual of mental disorders, 3rd edn. American Psychiatric Association, Washington

Andreasen NC, Carson R, Diksic M, Evans A, Farde L, Gjedde A, Hakim A, Lal S, Nair N, Sedvall G, Tune L, Wong D (1988) Workshop on schizophrenia, PET, and dopamine D_2 receptors in the human neostriatum. Schizophr Bull 14(3):471–484

Chugani DC, Ackermann RF, Phelps ME (1988) In vivo [^{3}H]spiperone binding: evidence for accumulation in corpus striatum by agonist-mediated receptor internalization. J Cereb Blood Flow Metab 8:291–303

Eddington ND, Young D (1988) Sensitive electrochemical high performance liquid chromatography assay for the simultaneous determination of haloperidol and reduced haloperidol. J Pharm Sci 77:541–543

Farde L, Hall H, Ehrin E, Sedvall G (1986) Quantitative analysis of D_2 dopamine receptor binding in the living human brain by PET. Science 231:258–261

Farde L, Wiesel F-A, Hall H, Halldin C, Stone-Elander S, Sedvall G (1987) Letter to the editor: No D_2 receptor increase in PET study of schizophrenia. Arch Gen Psychiatry 44:671–672

Farde L, Sedvall G, Wiesel F-A, Hall H, Halldin C, Stone-Elander S (1988) Letter to the editor: brain dopamine receptors in schizophrenia: PET problems. Arch Gen Psychiatry 45:599–600

Frackowiak RS, Lenzi G, Jones T, Heather JD (1980) Quantitative measurement of regional cerebral blood flow and oxygen metabolism in man using ^{15}O and positron emission tomography: theory, procedure, and normal values. J Comput Assist Tomogr 4:727–736

Frost JJ, Mayberg HS, Fisher RS, Douglass KH, Dannals RF, Links JM, Wilson AA, Ravert HT, Rosenbaum AE, Snyder SH, Wagner HN Jr (1988) Mu-opiate receptors measured by positron emission tomography are increased in temporal lobe epilepsy. Ann Neurol 23:231–237

Hawkins RA, Phelps ME, Huang SC, Kuhl DE (1981) Effect of ischemia on quantification of local cerebral glucose metabolic rate in man. J Cereb Blood Flow Metab 1:37–51

Hawkins RA, Phelps ME, Huang SC (1986) Effects of temporal sampling, glucose metabolic rates, and disruptions of the blood-brain barrier on the FDG model with and without a vascular compartment: studies in human brain tumors with PET. J Cereb Blood Flow Metab 6:170–183

Hayden MR, Hewitt J, Stossl AJ, Clark G, Ammann W, Martin WRW (1987) The combined use of positron emission tomography and DNA polymorphysms for preclinical detection of Huntington's disease. Neurology 37:1441–1447

Huang SC, Phelps ME, Hoffman EJ, Sideris K, Selin CJ, Kuhl DE (1980) Noninvasive determination of local cerebral metabolic rate of glucose in man. Am J Physiol 238:E69–E82

Johnstone EC, Crow TJ, Frith CD, Owens DGC (1988) The Northwick Park "functional" psychosis study: diagnosis and treatment response. Lancet 8603:119–125

Kohler C, Hall H, Ogren S-O, Gawell L (1985) Specific in vitro and in vivo binding of ^3H-raclopride. Biochem Pharmacol 34:2251–2259

Kuhar MJ, Murrin LC, Malouf AT, Klemm N (1978) Dopamine binding in vivo: the feasibility of autoradiographic studies. Life Sci 22:203–210

Lehmann HE, Cancro R (1985) Schizophrenia: clinical features. In: Kaplan HI, Sadock BJ (eds) Comprehensive textbook of psychiatry, 4th edn. Williams and Wilkins, Baltimore, pp 680–712

Luchins DJ (1982) Computed tomography in schizophrenia disparities in the prevalence of abnormalities. Arch Gen Psychiatry 39:859–860

Lyon RA, Titeler M, Frost JJ, Whitehouse PJ, Wong DF, Wagner HN Jr, Dannals RF, Links JM, Kuhar MJ (1986) ^3H-3-*N*-methylspiperone labels D_2 dopamine receptors in basal ganglia and S_2 serotonin receptors in cerebral cortex. J Neurosci 6:2941–2949

Mayberg HS, Robinson RG, Wong DF et al. (1988) PET assessment of cortical S_2-serotonin receptor binding: lateralized changes following stroke and their relationship to depression. Am J Psychiatry 145(8):937–943

Mazziotta JC, Phelps ME, Dahl JJ, Huang SC, Baxter LR, Riege WH, Hoffman JM, Kuhl DE, Canto AB, Wapenski JA, Markham CH (1987) Reduced cerebral glucose metabolism in asymptomatic subjects at risk for Huntington's disease. N Engl J Med 316:357–362

Mintun MJ, Raichle ME, Kilbourn MR, Wooten GF, Welch MJ (1984) A quantitative model for the in vivo assessment of drug binding sites with positron emission tomography. Ann Neurol 15:217–227

Phelps ME, Huang SC, Hoffman EJ, Selin C, Sokoloff L, Kuhl DE (1979) Tomographic measurement of local cerebral glucose metabolic rate in humans with (F-18)2-fluoro-2-deoxy-D-glucose: validation of method. Ann Neurol 6(5):371–388

Seeman P, Bzowej NH, Guan HC, Bergeron C, Reynolds GP, Bird ER, Riederer P, Jellinger K, Tourtellotte WW (1987) Human brain D_1 and D_2 dopamine receptors in schizophrenia, Alzheimer's, Parkinson's and Huntington's diseases. Neuropsychopharmacology 1:5–15

Seeman P, Guan HC, Niznik HB (1989) Endogenous dopamine lowers the dopamine D_2 receptor density as measured by [^{3}H]raclopride: Implications for positron emission tomography of the human brain. Synapse 3:96–97

Sokoloff L, Reivich M, Kennedy C, des Rosiers MH, Patlak CS, Pettigrew KD, Sakurada O, Shinohara M (1977) The [^{14}C]deoxyglucose method for the measurement of local cerebral glucose utilization: theory, procedure, and normal values in the conscious and anesthetized albino rat. J Neurochem 28:897–916

Tune LE, Wong DF, Pearlson GD, Young LT, Villemagne V, Dannals RF, Young D, Wilson AA, Ravert HT, Links JM, Midha K, Wagner HN Jr (1989) D_2 dopamine receptors in drug naive schizophrenics: update on 20 subjects. Schizophr Res 2:114

Wong DF, Wagner HN Jr, Dannals RF, Links JM, Frost JJ, Ravert HT, Wilson AA, Rosenbaum AE, Gjedde A, Douglass KH, Petronis JD, Folstein MF, Toung JKT, Burns HD, Kuhar MJ (1984) Effects of age on dopamine and serotonin receptors measured by positron tomography in the living human brain. Science 226:1393–1396

Wong DF, Wagner HN Jr, Pearlson G, Dannals RF, Links JM, Ravert H, Wilson AA, Suneja S, Bjorvvinssen E, Kuhar MJ, Tune L (1985) Dopamine receptor binding of C-11 3-*N*-methylspiperone in the caudate in schizophrenia and bipolar disorder: a preliminary report. Psychopharmacol Bull 21:595–598

Wong DF, Gjedde A, Wagner HN (1986a) Quantification of neuroreceptors in living human brain. I. Irreversible binding of ligands. J Cereb Blood Flow Metab 6:137–146

Wong DF, Gjedde A, Wagner HN Jr, Dannals RF, Douglass KH, Links JM, Kuhar MJ (1986b) Quantification of neuroreceptors in living human brain. II. Inhibition studies of receptor density and affinity. J Cereb Blood Flow Metab 6:147–153

Wong DF, Wagner HN Jr, Tune LE, Dannals RF, Pearlson GD, Links JM, Tamminga CA, Broussolle EP, Ravert HT, Wilson AA, Toung JK, Malat J, Williams JA, O'Tuama LA, Snyder SH, Wagner HN (1986c) Positron emission tomography reveals elevated D_2 dopamine receptors in drug naive schizophrenics. Science 234:1558–1563

Wong DF, Singer H, Pearlson G, Tune L, Ross C, Villemagne V, Dannals RF, Links JM, Wilson A, Ravert H, Wagner HN, Gjedde A (1988) D_2 dopamine receptors in Tourette's syndrome and manic depressive illness. J Nucl Med 29:820

Wong DF, Pearlson GD, Tune LE, Young LT, Ross C, Villemagne V, Dannals RF, Young D, Singer H, Wilson AA, Ravert HT, Links JM, Midha K, Wagner HN Jr (1989a) Update on PET methods for D2 dopamine receptors in schizophrenia and bipolar disorder. Schizophr Res 2:115

Wong DF, Young D, Young LT, Tune LE, Minkin E, Chan B, Midha K, Dannals RF, Parker RD, Wilson PD, Wilson AA, Ravert HT, Natarajan TK, Wagner HN Jr, Gjedde A (1989b) Validation studies of PET D_2 dopamine receptor quantification in schizophrenia using [C-11] NMSP. J Nucl Med 30:731

Wong DF, Young LT, Pearlson G, Singer H, Tune L, Ross C, Dannals RF, Wilson AA, Ravert HT, Links J, Wagner HN Jr, Gjedde A (1989c) D_2 dopamine receptor densities measured by PET are elevated in several neuropsychiatric disorders. J Nucl Med 30:731

Young AB, Penney JB, Starosta-Rubinstein S, Markel D, Berent S, Rothley J, Betley A, Hichwa R (1987) Normal caudate glucose metabolism in persons at risk for Huntington's disease. Arch Neurol 44:254–257

Positron Emission Tomography with [^{18}F]Deoxyglucose and Topographic EEG in Schizophrenia

M. S. Buchsbaum, J. Wu, K. Nuechterlein, S. Guich, S. Potkin, M, Lagunas-Solar, and W. E. Bunney, Jr. [1]

Introduction

Cerebral Blood Flow. Regional metabolic information was first obtained by Ingvar and Franzen (1974), who imaged human cerebral blood flow with xenon 133 in patients with schizophrenia and controls. A normal cerebral landscape was described in the resting subject, with relatively high flows in the frontal lobes and relatively lower flows in temporal and occipital regions; schizophrenics tended to lose this normal hyperfrontal pattern. Statistical analyses revealed that neither frontal nor occipital flow rates in themselves showed significant differences between groups, but that a frontal/occipital ratio did reach significance (1.10 in normals, 1.04 in younger patients, 0.95 in older patients). Ingvar and Franzen (1974) introduced the term hypofrontality to describe this pattern. Such ratio comparisons are a standard feature of much research in the psychophysiology of schizophrenia. Since individual baseline cerebral blood flows differ greatly, like EEG, heart rate, or other autonomic measures, ratios between data obtained at two different scalp locations were used to reveal this effect. Cerebral blood flow studies are reviewed elsewhere (Buchsbaum and Haier 1987; Weinberger et al. 1988).

Positron Emission Tomography. The first research in positron emission tomography (PET) has focused on the frontal lobes, because cerebral blood flow studies a decade ago found patients to have diminished flow in this area, and because this area is known to be important in attention, motivation, and the planning and organizing of behavior. Our earlier studies (Buchsbaum et al. 1982b, 1984a, c, 1987a) and many of those of others (see Buchsbaum and Haier 1987 for review) have resembled the cerebral blood flow data with patients showing a relatively diminished frontal/occipital ratio.

Electroencephalography. Increased delta activity in schizophrenia was one of the earliest EEG findings. Patients never medicated with neuroleptics and untreated revealed a higher delta index (Hoagland 1937) and greater percent age of frontal slow activity (Jasper et al. 1939). Although no specific EEG patterns have as yet been established as pathognomonic for schizophrenia (e.g., Itil 1977), several recent quantitative topographic studies have indicated an

[1] Department of Psychiatry, University of California, Irvine, CA 92717, USA.

Neuropsychopharmacology
Edited by Bunney/Hippius/Laakmann/Schmauß

increase in delta activity in the frontal regions (Buchsbaum et al. 1982c; Morihisa et al. 1983; Morstyn et al. 1983; Guenther and Breitling 1985). We have suggested that these results parallel the findings of reduced frontal lobe function as assessed by PET and cerebral blood flow (see review by Buchsbaum and Haier 1987). Delta activity over regions of low flow is well known clinically and has been linked directly to blood flow change in EEG/xenon flow studies by Ingvar et al. (1976) and Tolonen and Sulg (1981). In PET studies, we found that a group of patients with relatively lower metabolic rates in the frontal lobe had increased frontal delta (Buchsbaum et al. 1982a) and assessed PET/EEG correlations (Buchsbaum et al. 1984b).

Methodological Issues. However, these imaging studies with blood flow, PET, and EEG have not been uniform in demonstrating frontal dysfunction (Buchsbaum and Haier 1987) or increased delta (Buchsbaum et al. 1987b). Neuroleptics may not influence the cortex as much as the basal ganglia (Buchsbaum et al. 1987a) and so may not be an important artifact; however controlled neuroleptic studies with randomized design have not yet been carried out. Lack of an activating task has been suggested to be important in the negative PET studies (Weinberger et al. 1988; Buchsbaum and Haier 1987). A critical uncontrolled variable in many studies has been the activity of the patient during the functional study. PET, EEG, and cerebral blood flow are extremely sensitive to the mental activity of the subject. Recent studies have indicated that deficits of attentional and information-processing tasks are among the most consistent abnormalities found to characterize schizophrenia, and that the diminished function of the frontal lobes is most prominent in patients performing a task which activates the frontal lobe (Weinberger et al. 1988; Cohen et al. 1987). We chose for this purpose the Continuous Performance test (CPT) because this task has shown particular sensitivity to schizophrenic performance deficit (Nuechterlein and Dawson 1984), and because it showed reduced frontal metabolic rates on PET scans (Cohen et al. 1987).

EEG studies have been criticized for having eye movement artifacts which had not been fully deleted (Karson et al. 1987), and which therefore lead to spuriously elevated delta. This we addressed with careful visual inspection of records and with the simultaneous examination of metabolic rate with PET. Since eye movements might appear as increased metabolic rates in active frontal eye fields (area 8) this would not be expected to be associated with reduced metabolism in schizophrenia. An examination of the correlation between frontal delta and the extent of frontal hypometabolism thus would address the artifact issue.

Methods

Patients. The patient group comprised 15 patients with schizophrenia (14 men 1 women; mean age, 27 $\pm$ 6.4 years). These patients were recruited from the clinical and research programs of the University of California at Irvine (UCI) and Los Angeles (UCLA) and do not overlap with earlier samples. Thirteen of the 15 patients were right-handed; two were left-handed. PET data on 13 of these patients is presented elsewhere (Buchsbaum et al. 1990). Patients were off all psychoactive medication for a minimum of 31 days and a mean of 30 weeks. For long-acting injectable antipsychotic medication the minimum period of medication was 8 weeks. All patients were in good physical health, and none had noteworthy abnormalities on physical examination or as found on laboratory tests. Patients with history of seizure disorder, major head trauma, or substance abuse were excluded. Psychiatric interviews and assessments of the patients were carried out at UCLA independently of PET laboratory procedures in the week before the scan. The diagnostic work-up included the Present State Exam (PSE; Wing et al. 1974) modified to allow use of DSM-III criteria, the expanded version of the Brief Psychiatric Rating Scale (BPRS; Overall and Gorham 1962; Lukoff et al. 1986). The mean BPRS score (sum of first 18 items) was 31.7 $\pm$ 12. Mean educational level was 12.8 years. Patients received the CPT at the interview as well as during the glucose uptake period.

The normal control group for this study consisted of 18 subjects (14 men, 4 women; mean age 26.2 $\pm$ 8.1). Of these, nine right-handed volunteers (mean age 27.8 $\pm$ 8.9) had both eyes closed, resting EEG, and EEG recorded during the CPT. PET was obtained on all 18. Subjects were screened for health, as were the patients, by physical exam, medical history, laboratory measures, and psychiatric interview at UCI. The BPRS was not done.

Experimental Procedure and Task. Subjects had two intravenous lines inserted for [^{18}F]deoxyglucose (FDG) infusion and blood sampling 30–50 min before data collection. They were then seated in a darkened room and instructed to rest with their eyes closed. Two to four 30-s epochs of EEG were then recorded. Next, they were instructed in the CPT and performed 20–40 practic trials. This task involves viewing a series of single digits presented at 2-s intervals and pressing a button each time the digit 0 appears. Targets are presented irregularly with by a slide projector fitted with an electronic shutter and controlled by a microcomputer. Details of the procedure are presented elsewhere (Nuechterlein et al. 1983; Buchsbaum et al. 1987b). The task was then begun and FDG injected 1–2 min later. EEG was then recorded a second time.

Positron Emission Tomography. Glucose metabolic rate was imaged using sterile, pyrogen-free FDG, prepared at the Crocker Nuclear Laboratory, University of California at Davis. Before PET scanning, an individually molded, thermosetting plastic mask was made for each subject to minimize head movement. For the PET procedure, subjects were seated in a darkened isolation room, and intravenous lines were placed for FDG administration and for blood sampling. The left arm was wrapped in a heated pad for arterialization of venous blood. The task was then begun, and 2–3 min later 4–

5 mCi FDG was injected. Task performance continued for 32–36 min, and then the patient was moved to the scanner. Nine planes (CTI NeuroECAT) at 10-mm intervals and parallel to the canthomeatal line were scanned between 45 and 100 min after FDG injection. Scan details are described elsewhere (Buchsbaum et al. 1987b).

Computerized Topographic Electroencephalography (CTE). A set of 32 Grass gold disc electrodes were placed with Grass electrode paste on subjects' scalps using 19 standard International 10–20 System leads, three additional midline leads (FF and FC at 10% steps and Oz), two additional temporal leads (TT1, 2) between T3–T5 and T4–T6 at 5% steps and eight additional leads (FTC1, 2; CP1, 2; TCP1, 2; and PO1, 2) at the centers of squares formed by other electrodes. Recordings were referenced to linked ears. Two to four 30-s epochs were recorded for each condition.

EEG Data Collection and Processing. The EEG was recorded using a 32-channel amplifier system designed at the NIMH by Drs. Coppola and Morgan. The amplifier uses a Burr Brown INA-101 direct coupled (0.5 Hz 3 dB single-pole RC) to a following stage of amplification at gain 2000. The output is high-pass filtered with a corner at 50 Hz using a linear phase Reticon 5613 with roll-off approximately 24 dB per octave. EEG activity was digitized on-line (with a PDP-11/34) at 200 buffer points per second, and low-frequency subharmonics were removed by an autoregressive filter (Coppola 1979). The amplifiers were calibrated by recording a 10-Hz standard signal through all channels and determining the calibration factor for each channel; each channel was the proportionally adjusted before analysis. A window function consisting of a

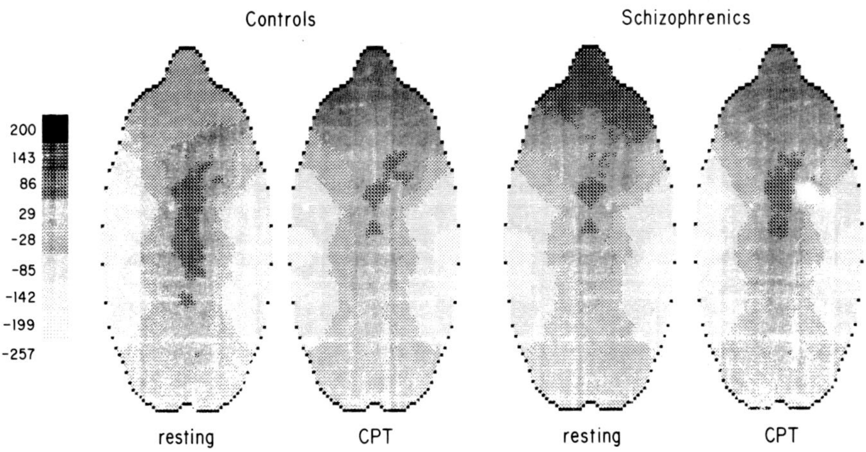

Fig. 1. Comparison of normalized delta in controls and patients with schizophrenia while resting and during CPT performance and PET FDG uptake. Scale shows z values (×100); *black* indicates values of 2.00 and above. Note darker (greater relative delta) in frontal region of patients

10% cosine taper was obtained by weighing the 50 buffer points at either end of each 2.56-s epoch by a cosine bell. A standard fast Fourier transform was applied to the 2.56-s epochs, and the power spectrum estimates were computed at 0.39-Hz steps. For smoothing, four adjacent estimates were summed to yield 1.56-Hz resolution, with the final estimates expressed as magnitude values in microvolts (square root of power). The activity estimated for the following bands was computed by summing adjacent values: delta, 0.78–4.30 cps; theta, 4.34–7.80 cps; alpha, 8.20–12.90 cps; and beta I, 13.30–19.90 cps.

Each 2.56-s epoch was visually inspected for artifacts, and any epoch containing artifacts was eliminated. The power spectral values for the artifact-free 2.56-s epochs were then averaged to yield one representative 2.56-s epoch of power spectral values for each subject in each condition.

MAP Technique. Topographic maps were computed by linear interpolation from the four nearest electrodes (Buchsbaum et al. 1985c). For each of the pixel elements in the map four corresponding weights were multiplied by the appropriate four spectral power values. Interpolation values were displayed on an approximately equal area map of the cortical surface using dot density representation of power value. The map was developed from sagittal sections of the brain. The maps are scaled in nine shades of gray with a 4 × 4 dot matrix in a 1–16 dot range.

Statistical Analysis. For PET, we matched the method of our previous two earlier studies (Buchsbaum et al. 1982b, 1984a, b, c). The PET image was processed with computer alogrithms to isolate the frontal and occipital cortex at three levels above the canthomeatal line. A four-way ANOVA was used to analyze the data as in earlier studies and a frontal/occipital ratio calculated. To compare the patient and control groups *t* tests were used.

For EEG, statistical analyses were performed using three-way ANOVA with the BMDP2V program (Dixon 1981) with a design of one grouping factor

Table 1. Normalized delta activity in normals and in schizophrenic patients for anteroposterior lead array

	Rest	CPT
Normals		
F7-F3-F4-F8	−0.22	0.07
T3-C3-C4-T4	−0.50	−0.58
TT1-TCP1-TCP2-TT2	−0.64	−0.74
T5-P3-P4-O2	−0.07	−0.24
O1-PO1-PO2-O2	0.29	0.11
Schizophrenics		
F7-F3-F4-F8	0.11	−0.19
T3-C3-C4-T4	−0.64	−0.57
TT1-TCP1-TCP2-TT2	−0.91	−0.86
T5-P3-P4-T6	−0.30	−0.18
O1-PO1-PO2-O2	0.29	0.38

and two within factors: group (normal, schizophrenic) by lead (32 channels) by condition (rest, CPT) for each of four frequencies: delta, theta, alpha, and beta 1. This design was employed on both microvolt and normalized values. Normalization (z transformation) was done by calculating the mean and standard deviation across the 32 leads for each condition in each subject and then expressing the 32 lead values as the value minus the mean divided by the standard deviation. To test more specifically for anterior/posterior and lateral gradient differences, 20 leads were selected to comprise a 4×5 electrode matrix (Table 1). A four-way ANOVA was then performed on a design of group by row (five rows of four leads for anterior/posterior gradient) by column (four columns of five leads for left/right gradient) by condition. This analysis was also done for both microvolt and normalized power spectral values. Post hoc t test maps are presented only if lead by condition or lead by group interactions are significant.

Results

Frontal Lobe Metabolism in Schizophrenics. Frontal lobe metabolism was lower relative to the occipital lobe in patients with schizophrenia than in normal controls. We calculated the frontal/occipital ratio exactly as in our previous reports for the supraventricular slice, right hemisphere, as this index had best separated the groups (Buchsbaum et al. 1984a, b, c). The resulting ratios were 0.95 (SD, 0.07) in patients and 1.00 (SD, 0.06) in normals ($t = 2.04$; $p < 0.05$). The effect was more marked at the midventricular level (1.05 versus 1.15) and the infraventricular level (1.18 versus 1.09; $p < 0.01$). Additional analyses on glucose metabolic rate in the frontal cortex are reported elsewhere (Buchsbaum et al. in press).

Delta Distribution in Normals and Schizophrenics. The frontal delta excess in schizophrenics that we observed earlier (Buchsbaum et al. 1982a) was statistically confirmed in this new sample with the critical interaction of group by anteroposterior position by condition ($F = 6.97$, df = 2.4, 43.2; $p = 0.001$; Fig. 1). The four-way interaction (group by condition by anteroposterior by mediolateral) was also significant ($F = 2.01$, df = 8.1, 145.0; $p = 0.048$). Using all 32 leads in a three-way (group by condition by lead) ANOVA also yielded significant group by condition by lead interaction ($F = 3.30$, df = 2.91, 52.4; $p = 0.028$). Since the ANOVA revealed significant interactions, follow-up t tests were done revealing delta differences in frontal areas, apparently stemming from resting EEG.

Correlations Between Delta and Glucose Metabolic Rate. We have previously reported that these patients with schizophrenia showed relative hypofrontality, more marked on the right side (Buchsbaum et al. 1984a). This has been tested both in our recent report (Buchsbaum et al. 1990) and in the original blood flow study (Ingvar and Franzen 1974) by computing the frontal/occipital ratio. To examine whether the patients with elevated frontal delta were the same ones with metabolic hypofrontality, we correlated delta amplitude at Fp 1 and Fp 2 during the CPT with the frontal/occipital ratios obtained from the supraventricular slice. These correlations were −0.58 ($p < 0.02$; one-tailed) for the right side and −0.49 ($p < 0.05$; one-tailed). The correlations at other frontal leads were: F 4, −0.59; F 8, −0.54; FF, −0.57 (all, $p < 0.025$). Correlations for occipital delta were all nonsignificant (0.40 at Oz, 0.43 at O 1, 0.36 at O 2). During rest, the frontal correlations were not significant, but posterior leads showed significant positive correlations: Oz = 0.59; O 1 = 0.55, O 2 = 0.67 (all, $p < 0.02$).

Discussion

Positron Emission Tomography and Hypofrontality. The first goal of this study was to replicate our earlier findings of a relative reduction in frontal lobe metabolic rate in a new, unmedicated group of patients with schizophrenia. Examination of the frontal/occipital ratio for the right frontal region revealed a significant decrease among patients with schizophrenia. This decrease was of approximately the same proportions as in the earlier studies and matches in magnitude the frontal/posterior ratios in the original Ingvar and Franzen (1974) study.

Computerized Electroencephalographic Topography. In this study as in our previous report (Buchsbaum et al. 1982 a) we found greater levels of delta activity in the frontal lobes of patients with schizophrenia than in normal controls. This is consistent with the quantitative topographic reports of Morstyn et al. (1983), Morihisa et al. (1983), and Guenther and Breitling (1985). It is also consistent with the data presented in two other studies. Williamson and Mamelak (1987) studied 12 acutely ill schizophrenics, 6 unmedicated and 12 normal volunteers; frontal but not temporal or occipital delta was significantly elevated in the patients while ill (tested, as appropriate in replication, with a one-tailed *t* test) but not after all patients were treated. Karson et al. (1987) similarly found frontal delta significantly higher in schizophrenics than normals using a MANOVA on sets of four or five leads. They did not report on the critical group by electrode position interaction effect however.

Karson et al. (1987) suggest that our results as well as those of Morihisa et al. and of Guenther and Breitling are flawed due to inclusion of EEG artifacts. The current data are not consistent with this interpretation. While our records are individually inspected for eye movement artifacts, it is often argued that the process was not sufficiently selective. But the correlation between measured cortical metabolic rate and delta cannot so easily be explained as an artifact. If our delta were only due to eye movements, we might have expected a positive correlation between electrical activity and increased metabolism in the frontal lobe eye fields (e.g., area 8) or no correlation at all. The negative correlation observed between delta and metabolism is consistent with the hypothesis of reduced activity in the frontal lobes being nonartifactually reflected in increased delta.

In this study, our first analyses were done to replicate our earlier findings of reduced frontal metabolism in unmedicated patients with schizophrenia and of increased delta activity in the EEG over this same area. We therefore limited our measures to the same ones previously used, the frontal/occipital ratio to assess metabolic hypofrontality and the normalized delta to similarly assess relative frontal activity. The next steps will be an examination of the clinical correlates of these measures and the application of increasingly detailed analysis of the separate regions within the frontal lobes. The concurrent use of multiple forms of imaging, PET and computerized electroencephalographic tomography in this study, allows new physiological information to be learned about EEG from the spatially accurate PET but also the evaluation of artifacts not common to the two modalities.

References

Buchsbaum MS, Haier RJ (1987) Functional and anatomical brain imaging: impact on schizophrenia research. Schizophr Bull 13:115–132

Buchsbaum MS, Cappelletti J, Coppola R, Rigal F, King AC, van Kammen DP (1982a) New methods to determine the CNS effects of antigeriatric compounds: EEG topography and glucose use. Drug Dev Res 2:489–496

Buchsbaum MS, Ingvar DH, Kessler R, Waters RN, Cappelletti J, van Kammen DP, King AC, Johnson JL, Manning RG, Flynn RW, Mann LS, Bunney WE, Sokoloff L (1982b) Cerebral glucography with positron tomography. Arch Gen Psychiatry 39:251–259

Buchsbaum MS, Rigal F, Coppola R, Cappelletti R, King C, Johnson J (1982c) A new system for gray-level surface distribution maps of electrical activity. EEG Clin Neurophysiol 53:237–242

Buchsbaum MS, DeLisi LE, Holcomb HH, Cappelletti J, King AC, Johnson J, Hazlett E, Dowling-Zimmerman S, Post EM, Morihisa J, Carpenter W, Cohen R, Pickar D, Weinberger DR, Margolin R, Kessler RM (1984a) Anteroposterior gradients in cerebral glucose use in schizophrenia and affective disorders. Arch Gen Psychiatry 41:1159–1166

Buchsbaum MS, Kessler R, King A, Johnson J, Cappelletti J (1984b) Simultaneous cerebral glucography with positron emission tomography and topographic electroencephalography. In: Pfurtscheller G, Jonkman EJ, Lopes de Silva FH (eds) Brain ischemia: quantitative EEG and imaging techniques. Progress in brain research, vol 62. Elsevier Scientific, Amsterdam

Buchsbaum MS, Mirsky AF, DeLisi LE, Morihisa J, Karson CN, Mendelson WB, King AC, Johnson J, Kessler R (1984c) The Genain quadruplets: electrophysiological, positron emission, and X-ray tomographic studies. Psychiatry Res 13:95–108

Buchsbaum MS, Hazlett E, Sicotte N, Stein M, Wu J, Zetin M (1985) Topographic EEG changes with benzodiazepine administration in generalized anxiety disorder. Biol Psychiatry 20:832–842

Buchsbaum MS, Wu JC, DeLisi LE, Holcomb HH, Hazlett E, Cooper-Langston K, Kessler R (1987a) Positron emission tomography studies of basal ganglia and somatosensory cortex neuroleptic drug effects: differences between normal controls and schizophrenic patients. Biol Psychiatry 22:479–494

Buchsbaum MS, Wu J, Haier R, Hazlett E, Ball R, Katz M, Sokolski K, Lagunas-Solar M, Langer D (1987b) Positron emission tomography assessment of effects of benzodiazepines on regional glucose metabolic rate in patients with anxiety disorder. Life Sci 40:2393–2400

Buchsbaum MS, Nuechterlein KH, Haier RJ, Wu J, Sicotte N, Hazlett E, Asarnow R, Potkin S, Guich S, Lagunas-Solar M (1990) Glucose metabolic rate in normals and schizophrenics during the continuous performance test assessed by positron emission tomography. Br. J Psychiatry 156:216–227

Cohen RM, Semple WE, Gross M, Nordahl TE, DeLisi LE, Holcomb HH, King CA, Morihisa JM, Pickar D (1987) Dysfunction in a prefrontal substrate of sustained attention in schizophrenia. Life Sci 40:2031–2039

Comar D, Zarifian E, Verhas M, Soussaline F, Maziere M, Berger G, Loo H, Cuche C, Kellershohn C, Deniker P (1979) Brain distribution and kinetics of 11 C-chloropromazine in schizophrenics: positron emission tomography studies. Psychiatry Res 1:23–29

Coppola R (1979) Isolating low frequency activity in EEG spectrum analysis. Electroencephalogr Clin Neurophysiol 46:224–226

Dixon WJ (1981) BMDP statistical software. University of California Press, Berkeley, pp 388–412

Guenther W, Breitling D (1985) Predominant sensorimotor area left hemisphere dysfunction in schizophrenia measured by brain electrical activity mapping. Biol Psychiatry 20:515–532

Hoagland H (1938) Electro-encephalograms in schizophrenia. Am J Psychiatry 95:

Ingvar DH, Franzen G (1974) Abnormalities of cerebral blood flow distribution in patients with chronic schizophrenia. Acta Psychiatry Scand 50:425–462

Ingvar DH, Sjolund B, Ardo A (1976) Correlation between dominant EEG frequency, cerebral oxygen uptake and blood flow. EEG Clin Neurophysiol 41:268–276

Itil TM (1977) Qualitative and quantitative EEG findings in schizophrenia. Schizophr Bull 3:61–79

Jasper HH, Fitzpatrick CP, Solomon P (1939) Analogies and opposites in schizophrenia and epilepsy. Electroencephalographic and clinical studies. Am J Psychiatry 95:835–851

Karson CN, Coppola R, Morihisa JM, Weinberger DR (1987) Computed electroencephalographic activity mapping in schizophrenia. The resting state reconsidered. Arch Gen Psychiatry 44:514–517

Lukoff D, Nuechterlein KH, Ventura J (1986) Manual for expanded Brief Psychiatric Rating Scale (BPRS). Schizophr Bull 12:594–602

Morihisa JM, Duffy FH, Wyatt RJ (1983) Brain electrical activity mapping (BEAM) in schizophrenic patients. Arch Gen Psychiatry 40:719–728

Morstyn R, Duffy FH, McCarley (1983) Altered topography of EEG spectral content in schizophrenia. EEG Clin Neurophysiol 56:263–271

Nuechterlein KH, Dawson ME (1984) Information processing and attentional functioning in the developmental course of schizophrenic disorders. Schizophr Bull 10:160–203

Nuechterlein KH, Parasuraman R, Jiang Q (1983) Visual sustained attention: image degradation produces rapid decrement over time. Science 220:327–329

Overall JE, Gorham DR (1962) The Brief Psychiatrc Rating Scale. Psychol Rep 10:799–812

Tolonen U, Sulg IA (1981) Comparison of quantitative EEG parameters from four different analysis techniques in evaluation of relationships between EEG and CBF in brain infarction. EEG Clin Neurophysiol 51:177–185

Weinberger DR, Berman KF, Illowsky BP (1988) Physiological dysfunction of dorsolateral prefrontal cortex in schizophrenia. III. A new cohort and evidence for a monoaminergic mechanism. Arch Gen Psychiatry 45:609–615

Williamson P, Mamelak M (1987) Frontal spectral EEG findings in acutely ill schizophrenics. Biol Psychiatry 22:1021–1024

Wing JK, Cooper JE, Sartorius N (1974) Measurement and classification of psychiatric symptoms. Cambridge University Press, London

PET Imaging of D_2 Receptors in the Living Baboon and Human Brain in Normal and Pathological Conditions Using $[^{76}Br]$Bromolisuride

B. Mazière, C. Loch, P. Hantraye, O. Stulzaft, J. L. Martinot, A. Syrota, and M. Mazière[1]

Introduction

In the early 1970s, brain imaging was revolutionized by the combination of computer and external detection systems for electromagnetic waves resulting in three-dimensional imaging techniques such as magnetic resonance imaging and X-ray computed tomography, which measure structures, and single photon or positron emission tomography (PET), which measure functions. PET, which noninvasively monitors the time course of a regional tissue tracer concentration following the administration of a molecule labeled with a positron-emitting radionuclide, allows the study of the brain at work by measuring either metabolic or neurotransmission activities. Thus, when the tracer is known to interact selectively with a receptor, it can be used as a ligand to probe in vivo the regional distribution and affinity of the binding sites involved.

For the in vivo mapping of dopamine receptors, most of the radioligands used are dopamine antagonists belonging to the neuroleptic pharmacological family. This selectivity of neuroleptics was discovered when it was demonstrated, soon after they were introduced in general psychiatry, that their therapeutic potencies paralleled their in vitro affinity for blocking D_2 receptors. The first two neuroleptics to be labeled with positron emitters were chlorpromazine (Mazière et al. 1975) and pimozide (Crouzel et al. 1980), but the possibility of visualizing in animals dopamine-enriched structures in vivo was first demonstrated using spiperone labeled with the gamma emitter ^{77}Br (Friedman et al. 1982). This experiment revealed the interest of butyrophenones. Later on spiperone and its *N*-alkyl, *N*-fluoroalkyl or *p*-bromo derivatives, were labeled with the positron emitters ^{11}C (Wagner et al. 1983; Arnett et al. 1984), ^{18}F (Kilbourn et al. 1984; Arnett et al. 1986; Barrio et al. 1987; Welch et al. 1988), and ^{76}Br (Mazière et al. 1984).

However, spiperone and its derivatives, as all the butyrophenones, also have in vivo high affinity for central serotonin receptors (Frost et al. 1987). Research on the development of more specific D_2 radioligands has shown the interest of other series of dopamine antagonists, benzamide and ergolene analogues. The prominent interest of benzamides such as raclopride, a

[1] Service Hospitalier Frédéric Joliot, CEA, 91406 Orsay, France.

Neuropsychopharmacology
Edited by Bunney/Hippius/Laakmann/Schmauß

sulpiride analogue, labeled with ^{11}C is well documented (Farde et al. 1985). This paper describes some of the interesting properties of an ergolene derivative, 2-bromo-lisuride (BLIS), and its utilization, after labeling with ^{76}Br for PET imaging of D_2 receptor enriched structures.

Bromolisuride

Semisynthetic ergolene derivatives such as lergotrile (Clémens et al. 1975), pergolide (Fuller et al. 1979), bromocryptine (Thorner et al. 1980), and lisuride (Horowski and Wachtel 1976) are dopamine agonists used in clinical practice for their potent dopaminomimetic properties. However, the brominated

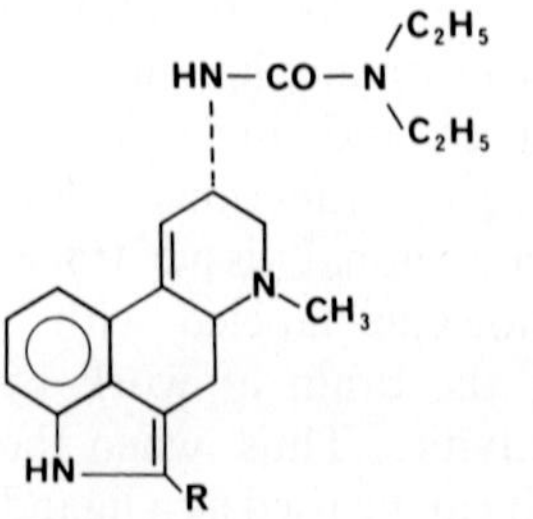

R=H LISURIDE

R=Br 2-BROMOLISURIDE

Fig. 1. Chemical structure of lisuride and 2-bromolisuride

derivative of lisuride, BLIS (Fig. 1), possesses definite antidopaminergic properties, as was recently demonstrated in neuropharmacological and neurobiochemical investigations (Wachtel et al. 1983). Therefore, bromolisuride labeled with the 16-h half-life positron-emitting radionuclide [^{76}Br]BLIS may be considered a potential candidate for PET clinical investigations of D_2 receptors. Consequently, its affinity and selectivity for dopamine receptors were, first of all, investigated in vitro and in vivo in rats and baboons.

Animal Experiments

The in vitro binding parameters of this new radioligand were evaluated on homogenates of rat striatal membranes, nonspecific binding being defined as the activity remaining bound in the presence of 1 μ*M* spiperone. Analysis of saturation data using a nonlinear least-squares regression program revealed a single population of binding sites with an apparent dissociation constant of 0.54 n*M* (SD, 0.1) and a maximal density (55.5 pmol/g; SD, 6.1) consistent with that found for the reference ligand spiperone.

The pharmacological selectivity of this binding was assessed in vitro in competition experiments carried out with various drugs having specific antagonist properties for D_1, D_2 dopaminergic (SCH 23390, spiperone, thioproperazine), serotoninergic (ketanserin), and adrenergic (prazosin, yohimbine, propranolol) receptors. The binding of [^{76}Br]BLIS to rat striatal membranes was inhibited only by the known dopamine D_2 antagonists spiperone and thioproperazine. Their inhibition constants (K_i), determined using five concentrations of compounds according to a modified Cheng-Prussof equation (Hartley and Seeman 1978), were, respectively, 0.38 and 10 nM. Compounds known to interact with other receptors did not possess any appreciable potency for preventing [^{76}Br]BLIS binding.

In vivo the same selectivity of [^{76}Br]BLIS for D_2 receptors was demonstrated when increasing doses of various specific drugs were coinjected intravenously in rats with the radioligand. Prevention of [^{76}Br]BLIS uptake by various brain structures was analyzed postmortem 3 h after the administration of the radioligand when the striatal radioactive concentration was maximum. In these in vivo competition experiments only D_2 antagonists, such as spiperone (ID_{50} = 12 nmol/kg) or thioproperazine (ID_{50} = 18 nmol/kg) were able to prevent, selectively and in a dose-dependent manner, the striatal accumulation of [^{76}Br]BLIS. In the other brain structures, including cortex and cerebellum, no competition was apparent, regardless of which cold drugs were used (Fig. 2).

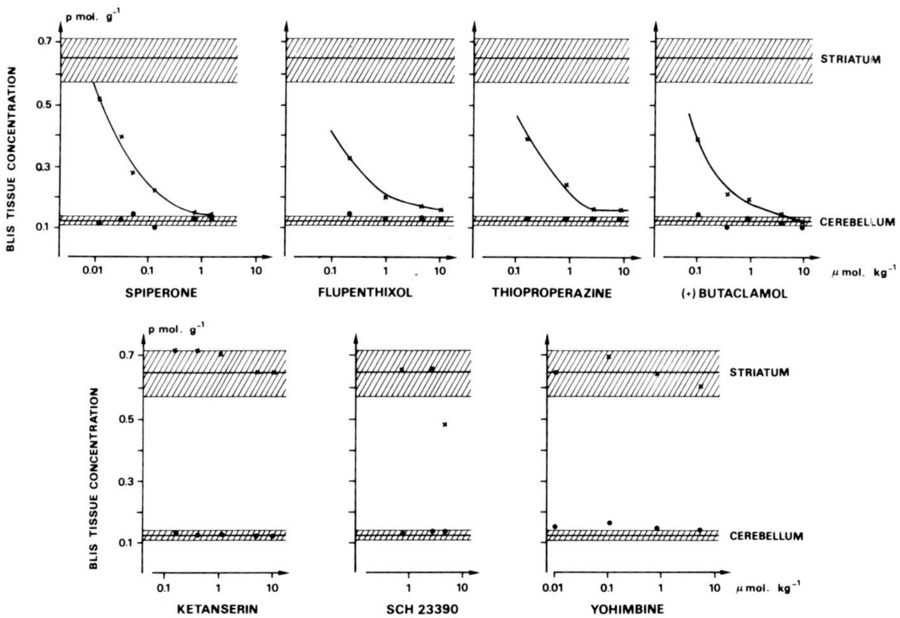

Fig. 2. Prevention of [^{76}Br]BLIS binding in different rat brain structures by various intravenously coinjected drugs. *Shaded areas* correspond to control [^{76}Br]BLIS concentrations (mean ± SD; $n = 20$) in the striatum and the cerebellum

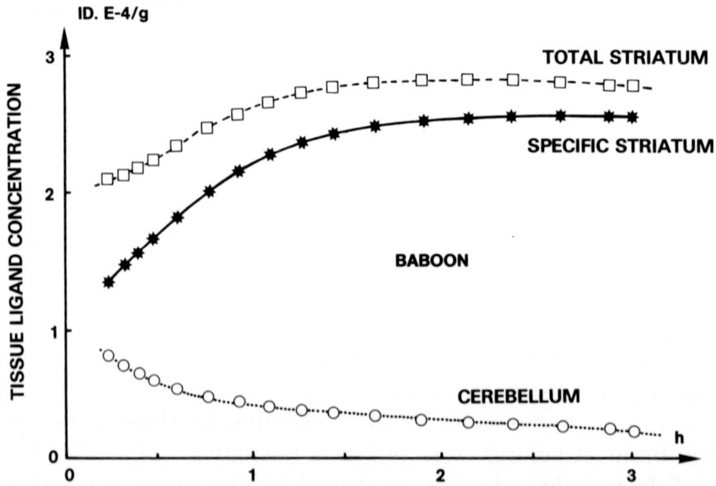

Fig. 3. Time course of BLIS accumulation in striatum and cerebellum in a baboon injected with 1 nmol [^{76}Br]BLIS. Specific striatal binding is defined as the difference between the ligand concentration in the striatum and that in the cerebellum

After these preliminary in vitro and in vivo experiments, 1–2 mCi [^{76}Br]BLIS were administered intravenously to baboons (*Papio papio;* 12–15 kg) for PET investigations. The animals were anesthetized with ketamine, curarized with alloferine, and positioned in a nonpainful position in a four-ring, seven-slice PET camera (time of flight, LETI) so that the orbitomeatal line was parallel to the planes of detectors. Brain radioactivity was then registered for 5 h with imaging times of 5–15 min. Preferential localization of the radioactivity in the basal ganglia was observable as early as 10 min after the administration of the radioligand (Fig. 3). The data on radioactivity uptake per unit volume measured as a function of time in various brain structures showed a rapid accumulation in the striatum (maximum, 90 min postinjection).

The radioactivity concentrations in the cortical and cerebellar regions decreased throughout the experiment, and from 30 min postinjection the activity levels were identical in both structures. The greatest contrast between the basal ganglia and the other parts of the brain (striatum to cerebellum ligand concentration ratio, 11.5) was observed 2 h after [^{76}Br]BLIS injection. This uptake was saturable and could then be displaced by administrating, 30 min after the radioligand, a dose (2 mg/kg) of haloperidol, which induced a selective decrease in the radioactivity measured in the striatum while leaving the cerebellar radioactivity uptake curve unchanged.

For measuring the actual parameters of in vivo binding, different biomathematical models (dynamic or equilibrium models) have been proposed. As the specific striatal [^{76}Br]BLIS concentration reached an equilibrium state within 2 h, a saturation model identical to that described by Farde et al. (1985) for

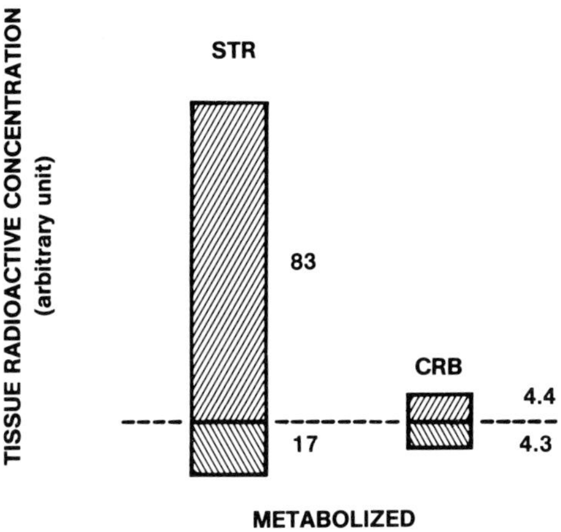

Fig. 4. Metabolic analysis of radioactivity in baboon striatum (*STR*) and cerebellum (*CRB*) performed 3 h after the intravenous administration of [^{76}Br]BLIS

raclopride was used. Before performing any calculations, the radioactivity measured in each structure had to be corrected for the radioligand metabolism. For this correction we used the results of postmortem biochemical analysis of baboon brains performed 3 h after the intravenous administration of the radioligand (Mazière et al. 1988), which showed that 83% of the radioactivity in the striatum and 52% in the cerebellum still represented unchanged bromolisuride (Fig. 4).

Then in a series of experiments we analyzed the saturation of [^{76}Br]BLIS specific binding in baboon striatum by increasing the mass of injected ligand from 0.8 to 45 nmol/kg. For the determination of B_{max} and K_d, the specific binding and free radioligand concentrations had to be determined for each experiment. Specific binding was defined as the difference between the ligand concentration in the striatum and that in the cerebellum. Free striatal ligand concentration was assessed in preliminary experiments. Biochemical analysis of baboon brains performed after intravenous injection of the radiotracer show that the free [^{76}Br]BLIS concentration was equal to 43% of the total cerebellar activity. Using this coefficient, this free activity was computed, for each experiment, from the cerebellar activity measured by PET. Nonlinear fitting of the experimental free and specifically bound radioligand concentrations (Fig. 5) allowed us to estimate the in vivo B_{max} (30–40 pmol/g) and K_d (0.62–0.71 n*M*).

To check the validity of these data, the animals were sacrificed at the end of the last PET experiments. B_{max} and K_d values were then measured in vitro on striatal membrane homogenates. The values found for B_{max} (40 pmol/g structure) and K_d (0.1 n*M*) were correlated closely with the previous values obtained in vivo. An estimation of the sensitivity of such an in vivo determination of the density of receptors was obtained during the study of a

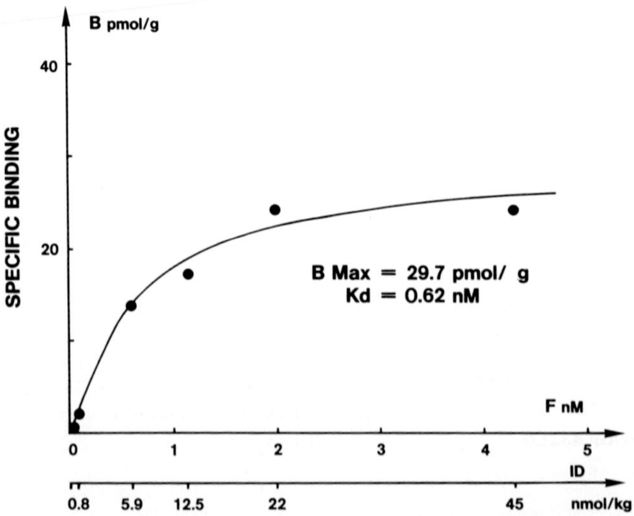

Fig. 5. Saturation curve for in vivo specific [^{76}Br]BLIS binding to a baboon striatum. The curve was obtained by nonlinear regression analysis with six experimental data points obtained with different doses (*ID*) of [^{76}Br]BLIS

primate model of Huntington's chorea resulting from unilateral excitotoxic striatal lesions. A similar in vivo analysis demonstrated a 10% decrease in the density of D_2 receptors in the lesioned striatum. This low decrease was later correlated with postmortem histological results (Hantraye et al. 1989).

Clinical Investigations

From these animal studies it appeared that [^{76}Br]BLIS is suitable for the characterization of striatal D_2 receptors in humans by PET, and before using it in pathological investigations the characteristics of its in vivo binding in control subjects needed to be measured. For this purpose, 1 mCi [^{76}Br]BLIS was injected intravenously in controls. Due to the high specific activity of the radioligand (higher than 1 mCi/nmol) the mass of injected drug was lower than 1 nmol. Under these conditions it could be easily calculated that less than 0.1% of the striatal receptors were occupied by the ligand.

The time course activity curves computed from the sequential images obtained at the levels of basal ganglia and cerebellum show a selective accumulation of the radioligand in the striata and, on the contrary, a rapid clearance from the cerebellum (Fig. 6). Two hours postinjection most of the activity was found in the striata while the cerebellar and cortical uptakes remained very low (Fig. 7). This selective striatal uptake should be saturable, and in tomographic images registered under the same conditions in patients treated with high doses of haloperidol no specific striatal accumulation was observed.

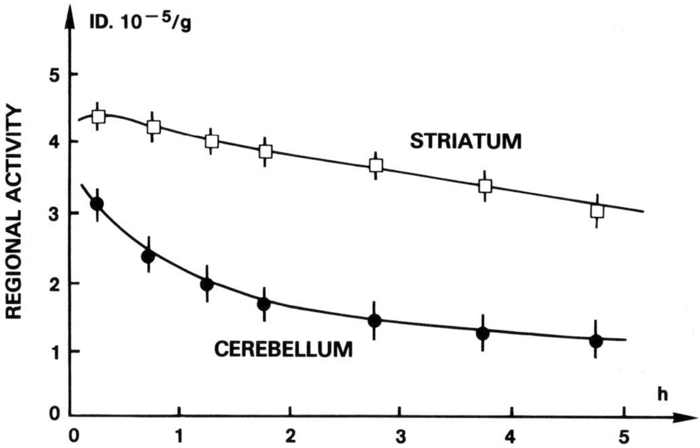

Fig. 6. Radioactivity in the *striatum* and *cerebellum* in a human volunteer as a function of time after intravenous injection of 1 mCi [^{76}Br]BLIS

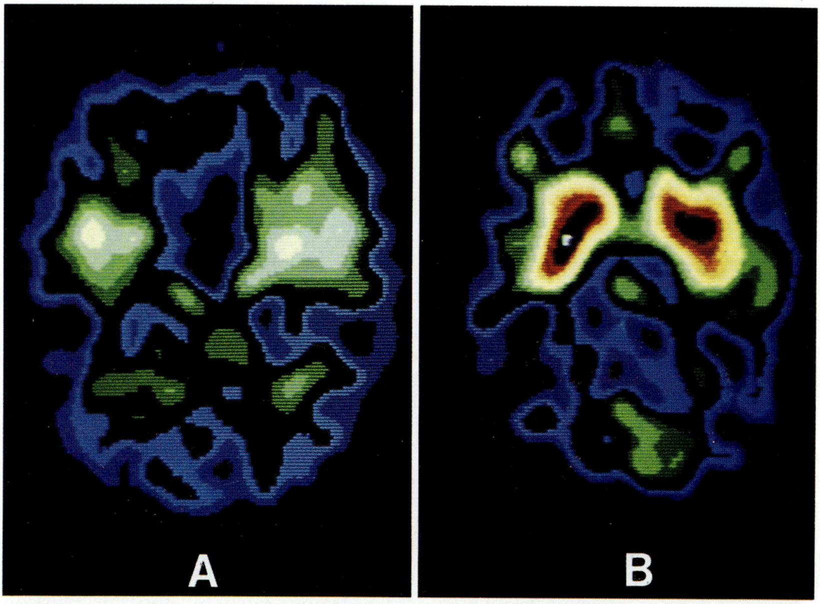

Fig. 7. PET scans through the cerebellum (**A**) and the striatum (**B**) of one healthy volunteer registered 2 h after the intravenous administration of 1 mCi [^{76}Br]BLIS. The color scale shows the highest concentration of the ligand as red and the least as blue

In the clinical situation, a classical way to quantify the striatal specific binding consists in the calculation of a striatum-to-cerebellum radioactive concentration ratio (S/C). Compared to the modeling techniques, this determination is much more rapid (a single PET examination is needed) and, moreover, does not require the administration of doses of cold drug partially to occupy the receptors. This ratio, which can be considered a satisfactory reflection of specific binding (i.e., a composite of affinity and receptor; Baron et al. 1986), was found to be at maximum 2 h postinjection and to remain constant at least for 2 h. In a group of 11 young control adults, this specific binding index was 3.8, with a standard deviation of 10%.

Concluding Remarks

In schizophrenia, the in vivo studies of D_2 receptors using PET have led to conflicting results (Wong et al. 1986; Crawley et al. 1986; Farde et al. 1990), and using [^{76}Br]BLIS we conducted a new investigation and compared the S/C ratios measured in controls and in age-matched untreated schizophrenics (Martinot et al. 1988). The preliminary results obtained with a group of 16 patients of both sexes gave a mean S/C ratio of 4.04, which is not significantly different from that measured in controls.

The various results obtained in these animal experiments and preliminary human investigations show that bromolisuride labeled with ^{76}Br possesses sufficient affinity, selectivity, and stability for in vivo studies and is thus suitable for PET clinical investigations of D_2 receptor neurological or mental pathologies.

Acknowledgements. We would like to thank Schering AG and Dr. R. Horowski for the gift of the various unlabeled lismide derivatives.

References

Arnett CD, Fowler J, Wolf AP, Logan J, MacGregor R (1984) Mapping brain neuroleptic receptors in the live baboon. Biol Psychiatry 19:1365–1375

Arnett CD, Wolf AP, Shiue CY, Fowler JS, MacGregor RR, Christman DR, Smith MR (1986) Improve delineation of human dopamine receptors using (18 F)-*N*-methylspiroperidol and PET. J Nucl Med 27:1878–1882

Barrio JR, Satyamurthy N, Hoffman JM, Huang SC, Mazziotta JC, Bida GT, Keen RE, Hawkins RA, Ninnenson CH, Phelps ME (1987) In vivo binding of 3-(2′(18 F)fluoroethyl)spiperone (FESP) to dopamine D2 receptors: from rodents to humans. J Cereb Blood Flow Metab 7:S357

Baron JC, Mazière B, Loc'h C, Cambon H, Sgouropoulos P, Bonnet AM, Agid Y (1986) Loss of striatal (76 Br)bromospiperone binding sites demonstrated by positron emission tomography in progressive supranuclear palsy. J Cereb Blood Flow Metab 6:131–136

Clémens JA, Smalstig EB, Schaar CJ (1975) Inhibition of prolactin secretion by lergotrile mesylate: mechanism of action. Acta Endocrinol (Copenh) 79:230–237

Crawley JC, Crow TJ, Johnstone EC, Oldland SRD, Owen F, Owen DGC, Poulter M, Smith T, Veall N, Zanelli GD (1986) Dopamine D2 receptors in schizophrenia studied in-vivo. Lancet, 224

Crouzel C, Mestelan G, Kraus E, Lecomte JM, Comar D (1980) Synthesis of 11 C-labelled neuroleptic drug: pimozide. Int J Appl Radiat Isot 31:544–548

Farde L, Ehrin E, Eriksson L, Greitz T, Hall H, Hedstrom CG, Litton JE, Sedvall G (1985) Substituted benzamides as ligands for visualization of dopamine receptor binding in the human brain by positron emission tomography. Proc Natl Acad Sci USA 82:3863–3867

Farde L, Wiesel FA, Stone-Elander S, Halldin C, Nordström A-L, Hall H, Sedvall G (1990) D2 dopamine receptors in neuroleptic-naive schizophrenic patients. Arch Gen Psychiatry 47:213–219

Friedman AM, Huang CC, Kulmala HA, Dinerstein R, Navone J, Brundsen B, Gawlas D, Cooper M (1982) The use of radiobrominated *p*-bromospiroperidol for gamma-ray imaging of dopamine receptors. Int J Nucl Med Biol 9:57–61

Frost JJ, Smith AC, Kuhar MJ, Dannals RF, Wagner HN (1987) In vivo binding of 3H-*N*-methylspiperone to dopamine and serotonin receptors. Life Sci 40:987–995

Fuller RH, Clémens JA, Kornfeld EC, Snoddy HR, Smalstig EB, Bach NJ (1979) Effects of (8-β)-8-methylthiomethyl-6-propylergoline on dopaminergic function and brain dopamine turnover in rats. Life Sci 24:375

Hantraye P, Riche D, Mazière M, Mazière B, Loc'h C, Isacson O (1989) Anatomical, behavioral and positron emission tomography studies of unilateral excitotoxin lesions of the baboon caudate-putamen as a Primate model of Huntington's disease. In: Neural mechanisms in disorders of movement, AR Crossman and MA Sambrook eds, J Libbey, 183–193

Hartley EJ, Seeman P (1978) the effect of varying (3H)spiperone concentration on its binding parameters. Life Sci 23:513

Horowski R, Wachtel H (1976) Direct dopaminergic action of lisuride hydrogenomaleate, an ergot derivative, in mice. Eur J Pharmacol 36:373–383

Kilbourn MR, Welch MJ, Dence D, Tewson TJ, Saji H, Maeda M (1984) Carrier-added and no-carrier-added synthesis of (18F)spiroperidol and (18F)haloperidol. Int J Appl Radiat Isot 35:591–598

Martinot JL, Huret JD, Peron-Magnan P, Baron JC, Boulenger JP, Mazière B, Syrota A, Loo H (1990) Striatal D2 dopaminergic receptors ascertained in vivo by positron emission tomography and 76Br-bromospiperone in untreated schizophrenics. Brit J Psychiat (to be published)

Mazière M, Sainte-Laudy JL, Crouzel C, Comar D (1975) Synthesis and distribution kinetics of 11C-chlorpromazine in animals. In: Subramanian G, Rhodes B, Cooper J, Sodd V (eds) Radiopharmaceuticals. Society of Nuclear Medicine, New York, pp 189–195

Mazière B, Loc'h C, Hantraye P, Guillon R, Duquesnoy N, Soussaline F, Naquet R, Comar D, Mazière M (1984) 76Br-bromospiroperidol: a new tool for quantitative in vivo imaging of neuroleptic receptors. Life Sci 35:1349–1356

Mazière B, Loc'h C, Stulzaft O (1988) A new and rapid analytical procedure for measuring unchanged radiopharmaceuticals in blood and tissue samples. J Label Comp Radiopharm 26:490–491

Thorner MO, Fluckiger E, Calne DEB (1980) Bromocryptine: a clinical and pharmacological review. Raven, New York

Wachtel HW, Kehr W, Sauer G (1983) Central antidopaminergic properties of 2-bromolisuride, an analogue of the ergot dopamine agonist lisuride. Life Sci 33:2583–2597

Wagner HN, Burns HD, Dannals RF, Wong DF, Langstrom B, Duelfer T, Frost JJ, Ravert HT, Links JM, Rosenbloom SB, Lukas SE, Kramer AV, Kuhar MJ (1983) Imaging dopamine receptors in the human brain by positron emission tomography. Science 221:1264–1266

Welch MJ, Katznellenbogen JA, Mathias J, Brodack JW, Carlson KE, Chi DY, Dence CS, Kilbourn MR, Perlmutter SJ, Raichle ME, Ter-Pogossian MM (1988) *N*-3-(18F) Fluoropropylspiperone: the preferred 18F labelled spiperone analog for positron emission tomographic studies of the dopamine receptor. Int J Rad Appl Instrum [B] 15:83–97

Wong DF, Wagner HN, Tune LE, Dannals RF, Pearlson GD, Links JM, Tamminga CA, Broussole EP, Ravert HT, Wilson AA, Toung JKT, Malat J, Williams JA, O'Tuama LA, Snyder SH, Kuhar MJ, Gjedde A (1986) Positron emission tomography revealed elevated D2 dopamine receptors in drug-naive schizophrenics. Science, 234:1558–1563

Dopamine Metabolism in Brain Studied with PET*

K. L. LEENDERS[1]

Introduction

In recent years it has become possible to measure in vivo certain aspects of human striatal dopaminergic function using radiolabeled tracers and positron emission tomography (PET). Further validation and expansion of this method may lead to elucidation of the pathophysiology of brain disorders in which a disturbance of one or more neurotransmitter systems has been demonstrated. Through PET studies it will now be possible to relate changes in neurotransmitter function to clinical features. Particularly, longitudinal studies starting in an early phase of the disease and using various types of tracers seem to be promising. Cross-sectional cohort studies are less suitable due to the rather small number of patients which currently can be scanned. This is caused not only by the relatively long duration of the scanning procedures; the radiochemistry is often complicated and needs to be performed immediately before a scan due to the short radioactive half-life of the radionuclides incorporated in the tracer molecules. However, data handling and analysis are the most time-consuming aspects of measuring tissue function with PET. Reduction of count measurements into manageable units and conversion of time-activity curves into meaningful pharmacological or biochemical entities is a formidable task. It seems that developments in this field are still in an early stage. The inevitably low number of patients treated per scan laboratory, in combination with the small number of PET centers worldwide, makes the accumulation of biological or clinical results with PET a slow process.

Positron Emission Tomography

The compounds (ligands) used with PET are administered in trace amounts. A PET scanner is able to detect the uptake of these tracers into tissue such as brain or heart since a special type of radionuclide is incorporated as a label in the

* Part of the text of this chapter has appeared in *Parkinsonism and Aging* (eds. Calne DB et al.), Raven Press, New York, 1989.

[1] Paul Scherrer Institut, 5234 Villigen, Switzerland.

Neuropsychopharmacology
Edited by Bunney/Hippius/Laakmann/Schmauß

tracer molecules. These radionuclides (e.g., oxygen 15, carbon 11, or fluorine 18) decay by emitting a positron a particle with the same mass as an electron but positively charged. There are three main reasons for choosing this type of radionuclide. First, they are nuclides of physiological atoms, which means that their incorporation into the required tracer molecules does not change, or only slightly changes, the chemical properties of the tracer. Secondly, the short radioactive half-life (minutes to a few hours) allows administration of tracer in a dose sufficient to obtain measurable signals while keeping the radiation dose low enough for human use. Thirdly, the characteristic physical features accompanying positron emission are the basis of tomographical measurement of regional radioactivity.

Shortly after emission from a decaying nucleus a positron collides with an electron. This results in conversion of the masses of the positron and electron into two simultaneous high-energy gamma rays (511 keV) traveling in opposite directions. The construction of most PET tomographs is such that a ring of detectors surrounds the body. Simultanuous stimulation of two opposite detectors (coincidence event) by the two gamma rays resulting from emission of a positron allows exact determination of the direction from which the event took place. After collection of sufficient coincidence events (counts) within a certain time frame (seconds to minutes), the distribution of local radioactivity in the scanned cross-section (plane) can be calculated by standard tomographical reconstruction techniques. Thus for each region in the brain a time-activity curve can be determined in absolute units of radioactivity (microcurie per milliliter tissue). The build up and wash out of tracer in a brain tissue region become more meaningful when compared with the dose delivered to the brain via the arterial system. To obtain this information a series of blood samples is usually taken from a small indwelling radial artery cannula after administration of the tracer. From this a so-called arterial input curve is then derived. Whether the next step, calculation of a pharmacological or biochemical entity related to the tracer molecule. The mathematical models which are used for this purpose vary widely in complexity, and various assumptions are a waiting validation.

Dopaminergic PET Tracers

Presynaptic Tracers

L-[^{18}F]Fluoro-3,4-Dihydroxyphenylalanine (*[^{18}F]Dopa*). This analogue of L-dopa can be used as a tracer for L-dopa transport from blood to brain, dopamine formation, and subsequent conversion into metabolites (in striatum mainly HVA and DOPAC; Garnett et al. 1983; Firnau et al. 1987; Leenders et al. 1986a, b, c, 1988b). Figures 1 and 2 illustrate the radioactivity distribution throughout the brain after [^{18}F]dopa administration in a healthy volunteer and a patient with Parkinson's disease, respectively. Table 1 summarizes the findings to date in movement disorders using [^{18}F]dopa and other tracers.

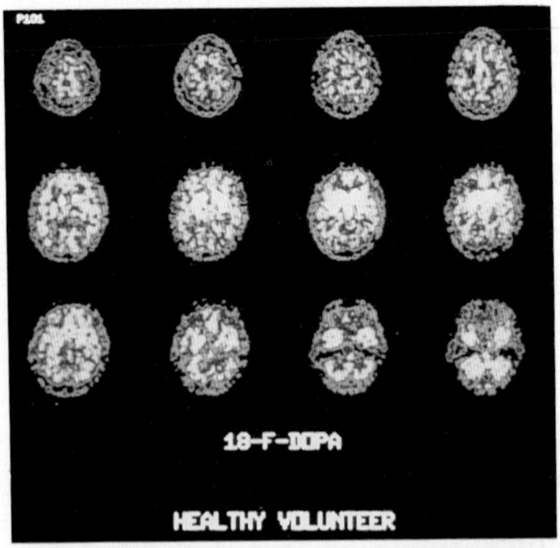

Fig. 1. L-[^{18}F]6-fluorodopa uptake measured in a healthy volunteer's brain 1–2 h after tracer administration. The images "cut" the brain from top to bottom by 12 simultaneously measured transaxial planes. The measurements were performed by the author using the PET tomography at the MRC Cyclotron Unit, Hammersmith Hospital, London, UK

After intravenous administration only a small fraction is taken up by the brain because of the slow passage through the blood-brain barrier (Fig. 3). L-Dopa transport across the blood-brain barrier is an active, energy-dependent, and strictly stereoselective process in competition with other large neutral amino acids (Leenders et al. 1986c). [^{18}F]Dopa is decarboxylated to [^{18}F]dopamine in the endothelial cells of brain capillaries and in the brain tissue itself, particularly in decarboxylase-rich regions such as striatum. [^{18}F]Dopamine is further metabolized into [^{18}F]HVA and [^{18}F]DOPAC, but Firnau and colleagues (1987) showed that in monkey brain the first 1–1.5 h

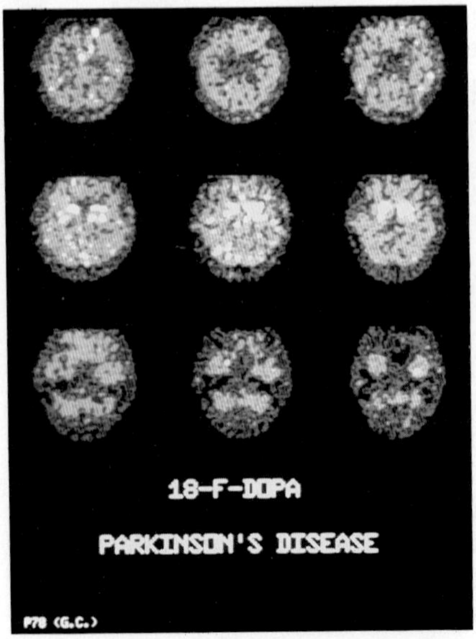

Fig. 2. The same as Fig. 1, but now nine images of a patient with Parkinson's disease. Note the diminished uptake in the striatal regions, particularly the putamen

Table 1. Summary of PET results using various tracers in patients with movement disorders

	Energy metabolism	Presynaptic dopaminergic system	Postsynaptic dopaminergic system
	CBF, oxygen and glucose utilization	Fluorodopa, Nomifensine	Spiperones, Raclopride
Parkinson's disease	Decreased (globally), increased (focally?)	Decreased	Normal, (sometimes increased?)
Huntington's disease	Decreased (globally, focally)	Normal	Decreased
Multiple system atrophy	Decreased? (probably)	Decreased	Decreased (?)
Progressive supranuclear palsy	Decreased (globally, focally)	Decreased	Decreased
Dystonia	Normal	Normal or decreased	Normal (sometimes increased?)

CBF, Cerebral blood flow.

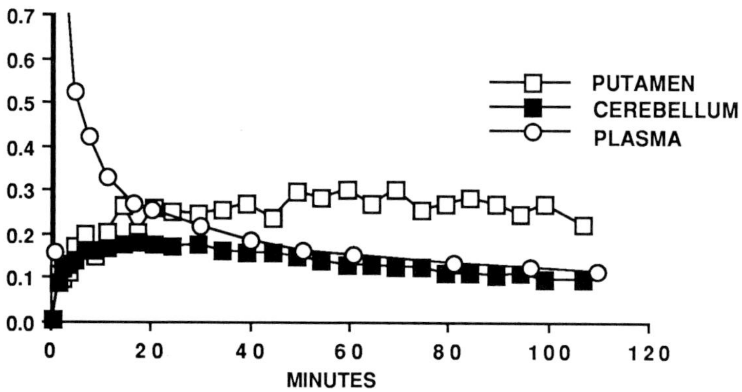

Fig. 3. Time-activity curve of L-[^{18}F]6-fluorodopa uptake in putamen, cerebellum, and arterial plasma in a healthy volunteer

after [^{18}F]dopa administration the radioactivity in striatum was predominantly [^{18}F]dopamine. Since this metabolic pathway runs only in one direction, the sum of [^{18}F]dopamine, [^{18}F]HVA, and [^{18}F]DOPAC formation must thus be determined by the regional dopadecarboxylation rate. In cerebral tissues other than the striatum the O-methylated derivative was the principal labeled compound; in arterial plasma of with carbidopa-pretreated subjects the main metabolite after [^{18}F]dopa administration was found to be the O-methylated derivative (Boyes et al. 1986).

Recently, the author and colleagues performed paired PET scans on five healthy volunteers using L-[^{18}F]6-fluorodopa without and with oral carbidopa (150 mg) pretreatment. Radioactivity uptake in brain was increased by about 30% in both striatal and nondopaminergic regions relative to arterial radioactivity. The five pairs of PET scans showed similar results. (A detailed report is in preparation.) An explanation for the findings could be that carbidopa inhibits decarboxylation of the tracer in the endothelial cells of brain capillaries. On the other hand, a change in metabolite formation in blood by carbidopa might give rise to increased bioavailability of [^{18}F]dopa to the brain. Results of the determination of plasma metabolites in these studies are needed before a firm statement can be made as to which of the two above-mentioned mechanisms is the more likely.

Further advances in [^{18}F]dopa uptake measurements with PET may be made using catechol-*O*-methyltransferase (COMT) inhibitors suitable for human use. Blocking of methylation in the periphery would improve the arterial input curve; total radioactivity in the plasma may possibly be equivalent to [^{18}F]dopa itself. Blocking of tissue methylation would result in all the activity being derived from [^{18}F]dopa or a metabolite beyond the decarboxylation step. The kinetic modeling of cerebral [^{18}F]dopa uptake to estimate regional dopamine formation would certainly become easier if such blocking measures could be implemented. The positive effect of a COMT inhibitor on [^{18}F]dopa uptake in rats has been demonstrated by Cumming and colleagues (1987).

[^{18}F]Dopa uptake into brain can be expressed as a regional unidirectional influx constant K_i (Fig. 4). As expected, this index for presynaptic striatal dopa decarboxylation activity is markedly decreased in patients with Parkinson's disease (Figs. 4, 5). No overlap with control is seen for putaminal values, but some patients' caudate nucleus values are in the normal range (Fig. 5). Mean

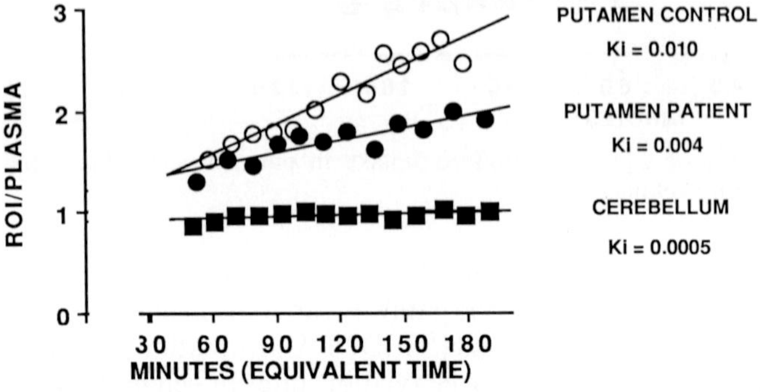

Fig. 4. Multiple time graphical plot analysis of L-[^{18}F]6-fluorodopa uptake in putamen and cerebellum using arterial plasma as reference in a healthy volunteer and a patient with Parkinson's disease. The slope of the linear regression line represents the unidirectional influx constant (K_i). In healthy striatal regions this influx constant is highest and in non-dopaminergic regions approaches zero

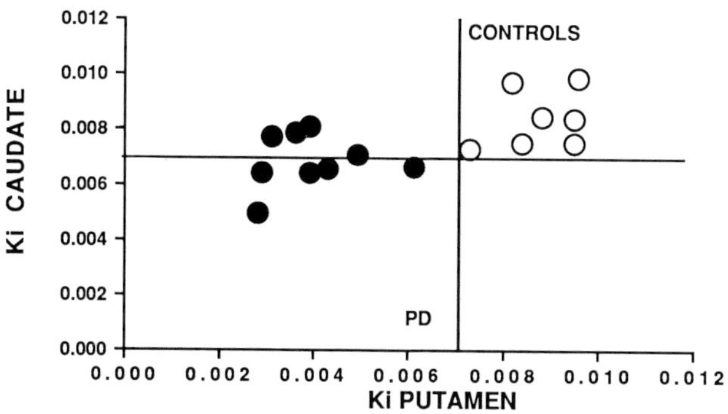

Fig. 5. L-[^{18}F]6-Fluorodopa uptake (K_i values; see Fig. 4) in putamen and caudate nucleus in a group of controls ($n = 7$) and patients with Parkinson's disease (*PD*; $n = 9$)

values for putamen are ±40% of control and for caudate nucleus ±85% of control. The same percentage decreases in dopa decarboxylase activity in postmortem brain of parkinsonian patients were found by Nagatsu and colleagues (1980).

[^{11}C]Nomifensine (*[^{11}C]NMF*). NMF binds specifically to catecholamine uptake sites on nerve terminals (Slater and Crossman 1984; Scatton et al. 1984). In striatum specific nomifensine binding is related virtually only to binding to dopaminergic nerve terminals. Unilateral lesions of the nigrostriatal dopaminergic pathway in rats produced a marked (±80%) decrease in specific striatal binding of [^{3}H]NMF (Scatton et al. 1984). This decrease was of the same magnitude as the reduction in endogenous striatal dopamine. A unilateral lesion of the locus ceruleus did not change tracer uptake.

NMF labeled with the positron emitting radionuclide carbon 11 ([^{11}C]NMF) has been used in PET studies (Aquilonius et al. 1987; Leenders et al. 1988a). A similar experiment as that reported by Scatton and colleagues (1984) in rats using autoradiography and [^{3}H]NMF was performed on a rhesus monkey using PET and [^{11}C]NMF (Leenders et al. 1988a). PET scans were performed before and after administration of MPTP, a neurotoxin specifically damaging or destroying dopaminergic neurones. MPTP was slowly infused as a solution (1.2 mg in total) through a catheter positioned to the right internal carotid artery via the femoral artery. Within 2 days left-sided akinesia developed, occasionally accompanied by marked dystonic postures of left upper or lower limb. After apomorphine or levodopa the akinesia disappeared, and normal use of the limbs was observed. In addition, over about 45 min rotation to the left occurred.

Striatal [^{11}C]NMF uptake 2 days after the lesion was normal on both sides. However, 9 days after the lesion the difference between striatal and non-dopaminergic brain tissue activity was reduced between 80% and 90% in the right striatum but was normal on the left side. Apparently MPTP had been taken up by the nerve terminals in the right hemisphere and resulted in rapid

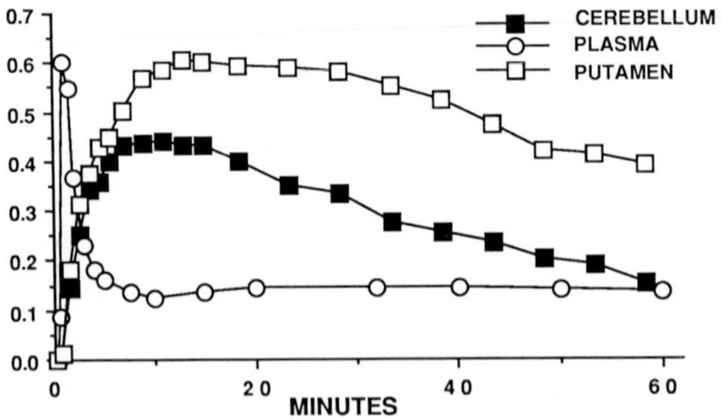

Fig. 6. Time-activity curve of [^{11}C]nomifensine uptake in putamen, cerebellum, and arterial plasma in a healthy volunteer

functional but slower structural damage to the dopaminergic nigrostriatal pathway. Six weeks after the lesion the same [^{11}C]NMF uptake reduction was seen in the right striatum, but after 5 months and after 1 year the uptake had recovered to about 50%. Clinically only mild left-sided hypokinesia was noticeable from several months after the lesion onwards.

Human studies using [^{11}C]NMF and PET have also been performed. Figure 6 illustrates the distribution of radioactivity in a healthy subject's brain. The tracer is seen to concentrate in striatum, but [^{11}C]NMF is also accumulated in thalamic regions.

It is proposed here that striatal [^{11}C]NMF activity is determined by dopaminergic and thalamic [^{11}C]NMF activity by adrenergic uptake sites. An abundance of adrenergic innervation of the rat thalamus has been shown by Lindvall and colleagues (Lindvall 1974).

As with [^{18}F]dopa (see above) striatal uptake of [^{11}C]NMF is likewise diminished in patients with Parkinson's disease (Fig. 7). Both putaminal and caudate nucleus values are now outside the normal range. Mean values for putamen are ± 40% of control and for caudate nucleus ± 60% of control. This

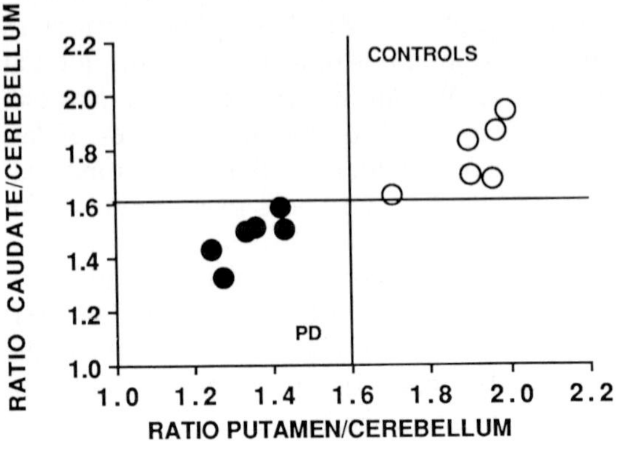

Fig. 7. Ratio of putamen or caudate nucleus over cerebellum values of [^{11}C]nomifensine uptake in controls ($n = 6$) and patients with Parkinson's disease (*PD*; $n = 6$)

is not far from the values (30% and 50%, respectively) of [^{3}H]GBR 12935 (another substance binding to monaminergic uptake sites) binding in putamen and caudate nucleus in postmortem parkinsonian brain presented by Maloteaux and colleagues (1988).

Both [^{18}F]dopa and [^{11}C]nomifensine are thus found to be only $\pm 40\%$ decreased in putamen of parkinsonian patients. This is markedly less than the decreases in endogenous dopamine concentrations usually reported (5%–15% of control values). These findings suggest that, although in Parkinson's disease most of the dopaminergic nerve cells of the nigrostriatal system may be defective in producing endogenous dopamine, still a considerable number of cells (and thus striatal nerve terminals) may survive structurally. This would explain why at initial stages of the disease exogenously administered dopa is clinically so effective: dopa can be decarboxylated and handled (retained) as dopamine in the still sizable number of nerve terminals. When the disease progresses, possibly accelerated by the influence of the regular flooding of the system by exogenous dopa, more nerve terminals are lost, and therapeutic responses become more erratic, following more directly plasma dopa levels. Careful longitudinal studies comparing clinical progression with PET binding measures may provide confirmation of this.

Postsynaptic Tracers

The use of postsynaptic PET tracers in psychiatric diseases in man is extensively dealt with in other chapters of this volume. Here only some additional comments concerning movement disorders are made.

[^{11}C]Methylspiperone (*[^{11}C]MSP*). Spiperone is a neuroleptic drug (butyrophenone) and is essentially a dopamine D_2 receptor antagonist. The radiolabeled analogue [^{11}C]MSP therefore binds predominantly to D_2 receptors in striatum where these receptors are highest in concentration (Fowler et al. 1986). However, binding to serotonin receptors also occurs (Frost et al. 1987), which particularly dominates binding in cortical regions.

[^{11}C]MSP has been used in man (Wagner et al. 1983; Wong et al. 1984), and Eckernäs and colleagues (1987) discuss the mathematical modeling associated with quantification of [^{11}C]MSP uptake. Reports about its use in Parkinson's disease have been scarce so far (Leenders et al. 1985; Hägglund et al. 1987). Untreated parkinsonian patients showed similar striatal [^{11}C]MSP uptake compared to healthy controls. Levodopa drug treatment seemed to reduce [^{11}C]MSP uptake to some extent (Leenders et al. 1985), but the number of patients studied was small. These findings are in agreement with postmortem results showing virtually no change in dopamine D_2 receptor densities in parkinsonian patients (Bokobza et al. 1984). The apparently intact postsynaptic dopaminergic system in this chronic disease, in the presence of a severe presynaptic lesion, explains why dopaminergic drug treatment is effective at all in Parkinson's disease. Patients with other chronic neurodegenerative disease associated with parkinsonian features such as Steele-Richardson-Olszewski syndrome do not respond or do so only slightly on levodopa therapy. In this condition impaired presynaptic dopaminergic function (Boyes et al. 1986) is accompanied by striatal dopamine D_2 receptor decreases (Baron et al. 1985), probably due to striatal neuronal cell loss.

[^{11}C]Raclopride. Raclopride is a neuroleptic drug (substituted benzamide) that can also be radiolabeled to visualize dopamine receptor binding in human brain with PET (Farde et al. 1985). This compound is specific for dopamine D_2 receptors, and quantitative analysis of these receptors is possible (Farde et al. 1986). [^{11}C]Raclopride has not yet been used extensively in patients with Parkinson's disease, but a recent report (Lindvall et al.1987) on two patients showed normal striatal values before and after engraftment of homologous adrenal medulla tissue. The above-mentioned unilaterally lesioned (right internal carotid artery MPTP infusion) rhesus monkey was studied using [^{11}C]raclopride (Aquilorius et al. 1987). Two days after the lesion an increased ($\pm$50%) specific tracer uptake was found in the lesioned striatum in the presence of a clinically impaired presynaptic dopaminergic function. Six weeks after the lesion increased [^{11}C]raclopride and marked decreased [^{11}C]NMF (see above) was found in the lesioned striatum but normal values on the unlesioned side. After 5 months and after 1 year [^{11}C]raclopride uptake was normal again, while the presynaptic function was still impaired. This suggests that acute lesions of the nigrostriatal system can provoke a temporary increase in striatal dopamine D_2 receptor density, however a chronic lesion of this system seems compatible with normal postsynaptic receptor density, at least in the absence of postsynaptic neuronal cell loss (see discussion of [^{11}C-MSP]).

References

Aquilonius SM, Bergström K, Eckernäs SA, Hartvig P, Leenders KL, Lundqvist H, Antoni G, Gee A, Rimland A, Uhlin J, Långström (1987) In vivo evaluation of striatal dopamine reuptake sites using ^{11}C-nomifensine and positron emission tomography. Acta Neurol Scand 76:283–287

Baron JC, Maziere B, Loc'h C, Sgouropoulos P, Bonnet AM, Agid Y (1985) Progressive supranuclear palsy: loss of striatal dopamine receptors demonstrated in vivo by positron tomography. Lancet ii:1163–1164

Bokobza B, Ruberg M, Scatton B, Javoy-Agid F, Agid Y (1984) (3-H)-spiperone binding, dopamine and HVA concentrations in Parkinson's disease and supranuclear palsy. Eur J Pharmacol 99:167–175

Boyes RE, Cumming P, Martin WRW, McGeer EG (1986) Determination of plasma [^{18}F]-6-fluorodopa during positron emission tomography: elimination and metabolism in carbidopa treated subjects. Life Sci 39:2243–2252

Cumming P, Boyes BE, Martin WRW, Adam M, Ruth T, McGeer EG (1987) Altered metabolism of [^{18}F]-6-fluorodopa in the hooded rat following inhibition of catechol-*O*-methyltransferase with U-0521. Biochem Pharmacol 36:2527–2531

Eckernäs SA, Aquilonius SM, Hartvig P et al. (1987) Positron emission tomography (PET) in the study of dopamine receptors in the primate brain: evaluation of a kinetic model using ^{11}C-*N*-methyl-spiperone. Acta Neurol Scand 75:168–178

Farde L, Ehrin E, Eriksson L, Greitz T, Hall H, Hedstrom CG, Litton JE, Sedvall G (1985) Substituted benzamides as ligands for visualisation of dopamine receptor binding in the human brain by positron emission tomography. Proc Natl Acad Sci USA 82:3863–3867

Farde L, Hall H, Ehrin E, Sedvall G (1986) Quantitative analysis of D_2 dopamine receptor binding in the living human brain by PET. Science 231:258–261

Firnau G, Sood S, Chirakal R, Nahmias C, Garnett ES (1987) Cerebral metabolism of 6-[F-18]fluoro-L-dopa in the primate. J Neurochem 48:1077–1082

Fowler JS, Arnett CD, Wolf AP, Shiue C-Y, MacGregor RR, Halldin C, Långström B, Wagner Jr HN (1986) A direct comparison of the brain uptake and plasma clearance of *N*-(^{11}C)methylspiroperiod and (^{18}F)*N*-methylsprioperidol in baboon using PET. Nucl Med Biol 13 (3):281–284

Frost JJ, Smith AC, Kuhar MJ, Dannals RF, Wagner Jr HN (1987) In vivo binding of ^{3}H-*N*-methylspiperone to dopamine and serotonin receptors. Life Sci 40:987–995

Garnett ES, Firnau G, Nahmias C (1983) Dopamine visualised in the basal ganglia of living man. Nature 305:137–138

Hägglund J, Aquilonius S-M, Eckernäs S-Å, Hartvig P, Lundquist H, Gullberg P, Långström B (1987) Dopamine receptor properties in Parkinson's disease and Huntington's chorea evaluated by positron emission tomography using ^{11}C-*N*-methyl-spiperone. Acta Neurol Scand 75:87–94

Leenders KL, Herold S, Palmer AJ, Turton D, Quinn N, Jones T, Frackowiak RSJ, Marsden CD (1985) Human cerebral dopamine system measured in vivo using PET. J Cereb Blood Flow Metabol 5 [Suppl]:517–518

Leenders KL, Frackowiak RJS, Quinn N, Marsden CD (1986 a) Brain energy metabolism and dopaminergic function in Huntington's disease measured in vivo using positron emission tomography. Movement disorders 1:69–77

Leenders KL, Palmer AJ, Quinn N, Clark JC, Firnau G, Garnett ES, Nahmias C, Jones T, Marsden CD (1986 b) Brain dopamine metabolism in patients with Parkinson's disease measured with positron emission tomography. J Neurol Neurosurg Psychiat 49:853–856

Leenders KL, Poewe WH, Palmer AJ, Brenton DP, Frackowiak RSJ (1986 c) Inhibition of L-[^{18}F]fluorodopa uptake into human brain by amino acids demonstrated by positron emission tomography. Ann Neurol 20:258–262

Leenders KL, Aquilonius SM, Bergström K, Bjurling P, Crossman AR, Eckernäs SA, Gee AG, Hartvig P, Lundqvist H, Långström B, Rimland A, Tedroff J (1988 a) Unilateral MPTP lesion in a rhesus monkey: effects on the striatal dopaminergic system measured in vivo with PET using various novel tracers. Brain Res 445:61–67

Leenders KL, Frackowiak RJS, Lees AJ (1988 b) Steele-Richardson-Olszewski syndrome. Brain energy metabolism, blood flow and fluorodopa uptake measured by positron emission tomography. Brain 111:615–630

Lindvall O, Björklund A, Nobin A, Stenevi U (1974) The adrenergic innervation of the rat thalamus as revealed by the glyoxylic acid fluorescence method. J Comp Neurol 154:317–348

Lindvall O, Backlund EO, Farde L, Sedvall G, Freedman R, Hoffer B, Nobin A, Seiger Å, Olson L (1987) Transplantation in Parkinson's disease: two cases of adrenal medullary grafts to the putamen. Ann Neurol 22:457–468

Maloteaux JM, Vanisberg MA, Laterre C, Agid FJ, Agid Y, Laduron PM (1988) [^{3}H]GBR 12935 binding to dopamine uptake sites: subcellular localization and reduction in Parkinson's disease and progressive supranuclear palsy. Eur J Pharmacol 156:331–340

Nagatsu T, Oka K, Yamamoto T, Matusu H, Kato T, Yamamoto C, Nagatsu I, Iizuka R, Narabayashi H (1980) Catecholaminergic enzymes in Parkinson's disease and related extrapyramidal diseases. In: Riederer P, Ursdin E (eds) Transmitter biochemistry of human brain tissue. Macmillan, London

Scatton B, Dubois A, Dubocovitch ML, Zahniser NR, Fage D (1984) Quantitative autoradiography of 3H-nomifensine binding sites in rat brain. Life Sci 36:815–822

Slater P, Crossman AR (1984) Autoradiographic distribution of [^{3}H]-nomifensine in brain. In: Linford-Rees W, Priest RG (eds) Nomifensine. A pharmacological and clinical profile. Royal Society of Medicine, London, pp 15–19

Wagner HN, Burns HD, Dannals RF, Wong DF, Långström B, Duelfer T, Frost JJ, Ravert HT, Links JM, Rosenbloom SB, Lukas SE, Kramer AV, Kuhar MJ (1983) Imaging dopamine receptors in the human brain by positron tomography. Science 221:1264–1266
Wong DF, Wagner Jr HN, Dannals RF, Links JM, Frost JJ, Ravert HT, Wilson AA, Rosenbaum AE, Gjedde A, Douglass KH, Petronis JD, Folstein MF, Toung JKT, Burns HD, Kuhar MJ (1984) Effects of age on dopamine and serotonin receptors measured by positron tomography in the living human brain. Science 226:1393–1396

11 The Brain–Immune System Interactions

Activation of Human Monocytes by the Neuropeptide Substance P and by Immune Interferon-γ: Evidence of Different Mechanisms *

F. J. WIEDERMANN [1], C. J. WIEDERMANN [1], M. HEROLD [2], D. GEISSLER [3], G. KONWALINKA [3], and H. BRAUNSTEINER [4]

Introduction

The sources of inflammatory and immunomodulatory mediators are remarkably diverse. Of interest with regard to the pathophysiology of several inflammatory diseases is evidence that the peripheral terminals of primary afferent nociceptors are activated by noxious stimuli not only to produce pain but also to release proinflammatory mediators (Holzer 1988). One such mediator is substance P (SP), an undecapeptide from the tachykinin family of peptides. The significance of the antidromic release of SP from peripheral terminals into surrounding tissues is supported by the detection of increased levels of SP in inflammed tissues in patients (Pernow 1987).

SP acts on vascular smooth muscle and endothelium to increase blood flow and vascular permeability (Holzer 1988). SP also enhances the proliferation of connective tissue cells, and it stimulates the production of prostaglandins and collagenase (Lotz et al. 1987; Hartung et al. 1986). Target cells involved in the inflammatory response and affected by SP include mast cells, polymorphonuclear leukocytes, and mononuclear phagocytes (Mø; for review, see Wiedermann et al. 1989). SP has been shown specifically to modulate in vitro functions of eosinophils, lymphocytes, and natural killer cells (Payan and Goetzl 1987). The concept that SP modulates immunological responses has been supported by the identification of receptors on some of these leukocytes (for review, see Payan and Goetzl 1987; Wiedermann et al. 1986).

Mø influence host defense responses through their capacity to present antigens and to release several types of soluble mediators (Unanue and Allen

* This work was supported by a grant from the Österreichische Industriellen-Vereinigung, Landesgruppe Tirol, 1987.

[1] Laboratory of Neuroimmunology, Department of Internal Medicine, University of Innsbruck School of Medicine, 6020 Innsbruck, Austria.

[2] Laboratory of Rheumatology, Department of Internal Medicine, University of Innsbruck School of Medicine, 6020 Innsbruck, Austria.

[3] Laboratory of Experimental Hematology, Department of Internal Medicine, University of Innsbruck School of Medicine, 6020 Innsbruck, Austria.

[4] Laboratories of Neuroimmunology, Rheumatology, and Experimental Hematology, Department of Internal Medicine, University of Innsbruck School of Medicine, 6020 Innsbruck, Austria.

Neuropsychopharmacology
Edited by Bunney/Hippius/Laakmann/Schmauß

1987). The significance of neuronal SP in host defense responses by modulating functions of Mø was recently substantiated by the finding that Mø are induced to produce the cytokines interleukin-1, interleukin-6, and tumor necrosis factor-α by SP (Lotz et al. 1988). In order to understand better the mechanisms of inflammatory and immunomodulatory actions of SP, we investigated possible interactions of SP with immune interferon-γ (IFN-γ) in Mø activation using induction of neopterin release as an indirect indicator (Anonymous 1988).

Materials and Methods

Preparation of Cells. Mononuclear cells (MNC) from normal adult human peripheral blood were obtained as previously described (Wiedermann et al. 1989) by Lymphoprep (Nyegaard, Oslo, Norway) density gradient centrifugation, washed twice in Hank's balanced salt solution without Ca^{2+} and Mg^{2+} (HBSS; Heilmittelwerke, Vienna, Austria), resuspended in RPMI-1640 medium containing 2 m*M* L-glutamine, 25 m*M* HEPES buffer (all from Sigma, Munich, FRG), 50 U/ml penicillin, 50 µg/ml streptomycin (both from Biochemie, Kundl, Austria) and 10% heat-inactivated human pool serum, and enumerated. Cell preparations were greater than 95% viable by trypan blue exclusion. For some experiments, MNC (1×10^6) were allowed to adhere for 90 min at 37 °C in 1 ml medium per well of plastic Nunc four-well tissue culture trays. Nonadherent cells were removed by washing four times with HBSS, and fresh medium containing test substances was added. Adherent monolayers were more than 90% monocytes by representative staining for nonspecific esterase.

Culture of Cells. MNC (10^6/ml) and adherent MNC were stimulated with either 100 U/ml IFN-γ (human recombinant, Genentech, South San Francisco, CA, USA) and/or with 10^{-7} *M* SP, SP (1–9), or SP (3–11; all from Peninsula, Belmont, CA, USA) in culture at a 37°, fully humidified atmosphere with 5% CO_2 for 1–5 days. SP at the given concentration was previously shown maximally to induce in vitro chemotaxis of human monocytes (Wiedermann et al. 1989). Medium was harvested from adherent MNC cultures and from spun MNC culture supernatants after incubation with the above mediators, and neopterin was detected by means of a specific radioimmunoassay (Hellige, West Berlin) (Anonymous 1988).

Results and Discussion

As described previously (Huber et al. 1984), IFN-γ specifically induces adherent MNC to release neopterin into culture media (Fig. 1). In vivo, increased concentrations of neopterin have been reported in urine and other biological fluids after administration of IFNs α and β as well as γ and are seen in patients with conditions causing a stimulation of cellular immunity with increased Mø activity, such as viral and other infections, graft-versus-host disease, and malignancy (Anonymous 1988). In vitro, Mø release neopterins into the culture media primarily under the influence of IFN-γ produced by T-lymphocytes and is accompanied by a rise in intracellular concentration of

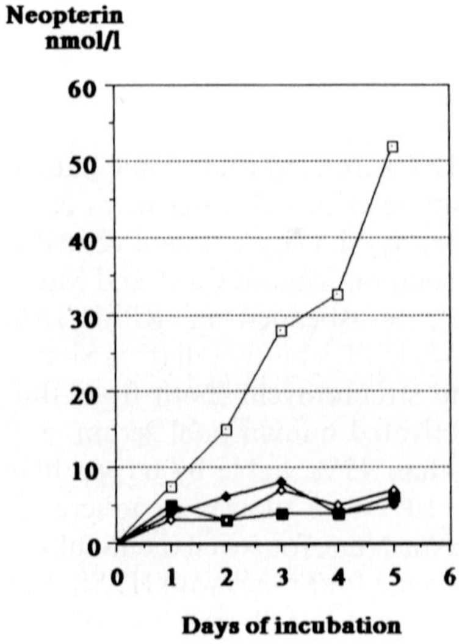

Fig. 1. Effects of 100 U/ml IFN-γ (□) and 10^{-7} *M* SP (◆), SP (1–9) (◇), or SP (3–11) (■) on release of neopterin in culture of human peripheral blood MNC (1×10^6/ml). Results are the mean of three separate experiments performed in duplicate

guanosine triphosphate and in guanosine triphosphate cyclohydrolase activity (reviewed in Anonymous 1988). Even though some diseases, for example, rheumatoid arthritis (Lotz et al. 1987) where elevated levels of SP are thought to play a pathogenetic role, also show elevated levels of neopterin (Reibenegger et al. 1986), SP and its fragments fail to induce neopterin release from MNC-containing T-lymphocytes or from adherent MNC that lack IFN-γ producing T-lymphocytes (Fig. 1). Therefore, indirectly these data also suggest that SP does not induce release of IFN-γ from T-lymphocytes. Neopterin increases in culture media are normally already seen at low concentrations of IFN-γ activating Mø (Huber et al. 1984).

Addition of SP to adherent MNC that are exposed to IFN-γ has no influence on the amounts of neopterin released (Table 1). Thus, SP activation of these cells does not involve at least part of the metabolic pathway classically elicited by IFN-γ, nor does it modulate this IFN-γ response.

Substance P and IFN-γ share several actions. As, for example, shown for IFN-γ (Nathan et al. 1983), SP stimulates phagocytic activities of Mø (Bar-Shavit et al. 1980; Hartung et al. 1986). Differences between IFN-γ and SP also exist. SP induces release of cytokines from Mø directly (Lotz et al. 1988),

Table 1. Effect of substance P on interferon-γ induced release of neopterin from adherent cells of human peripheral blood mononuclear cells (1×10^6/ml)

	Control	SP (10^{-7} M)	IFN-γ (100 U/ml)	SP + IFN-γ (10^{-7} M + 100 U/ml)
Neopterin (nmol/l)	1.43 (0.27)	1.53 (0.41)	3.28 (0.97)	3.18 (0.93)

Media were harvested after 24 h of culture, and neopterin was determined by radioimmunoassay. Mean (SEM) of three separate experiments, each performed in duplicate. Differences between control and SP and between IFN-γ and SP + IFN-γ both $p > 0.1$.

whereas IFN-γ only primes Mø to show an enhanced cytokine release to exogenous endotoxin (Pace et al. 1983). Whether this difference is directly related to differences in the neopterin response is currently unknown. The functional role of neopterin in the immune response has not yet been discovered (Anonymous 1988).

Relatively high levels of neopterin are found in tumor patients (Anonymous 1988). As SP in vitro failed to induce neopterin release from Mø, as shown here, and to activate tumoricidal Mø functions, as shown by Koff and Dunegan (1985), it is tempting to speculate that SP in vivo also has no direct bearing on Mø antitumor activities. Indirectly, however, SP may still play modulatory roles in T-lymphocyte dependent Mø functions, as Mø recruit other immune cells and modulate their activity by producing and releasing a vast array of potent mediators that promote immunological, inflammatory, and reparative process, a mechanism most recently shown to be affected by SP (Lotz et al. 1988).

Acknowledgement. Our thanks to Mrs. M. Niedermühlbichler for expert technical assistance.

References

Anonymous (1988) Neopterins in clinical medicine (Editorial). Lancet i:509–511

Bar-Shavit Z, Goldman R, Stabinsky Y, Gottlieb P, Fridkin M, Teichberg VI, Blumberg S (1980) Enhancement of phagocytosis – a newly found activity of substance P residing in its N-terminal tetrapeptide sequence. Biochem Biophys Res Commun 94:1445–1451

Hartung H-P, Wolters K, Toyka KV (1986) Substance P: binding properties and studies on cellular responses in guinea-pig macrophages. J Immunol 136:3856–3863

Holzer P (1988) Local effector functions of capsaicin-sensitive sensory nerve endings: involvement of tachykinins, calcitonin gene-related peptide and other neuropeptides. Neuroscience 24:739–768

Huber C, Batchelor JR, Fuchs D, Hausen A, Lang A, Niederwieser D, Reibenegger G, Swetly P, Troppmair J, Wachter H (1984) Immune response-associated production of neopterin: release of macrophages primarily under the control of interferon-gamma. J Exp Med 160:310–316

Koff WC, Dunegan MA (1985) Modulation of macrophage-mediated tumoricidal activity by neuropeptides and neurohormones. J Immunol 135:350–354

Lotz M, Carson DA, Vaughan JH (1987) Substance P activation of rheumatoid synoviocytes: neural pathway in pathogenesis of arthritis. Science 235:893–895

Lotz M, Vaughan JH, Carson DA (1988) Effect of neuropeptides on production of inflammatory cytokines by human monocytes. Science 241:1218–1221

Nathan CF, Murray HW, Wiebe ME, Rubin BY (1983) Identification of interferon-gamma as the lymphokine that activates human macrophage oxidative metabolism and antimicrobial activity. J Exp Med 158:670–689

Pace JL, Russell SW, Schreiber RD, Altman A, Katz DA (1983) Macrophage activation: priming activity from a T-cell hybridoma is attributable to interferon-gamma. Proc Natl Acad Sci USA 80:3782–3786

Payan DG, Goetzl EJ (1987) Substance P receptor-dependent responses of leukocytes in pulmonary inflammation. Am Rev Respir Dis 136:s39–s43

Pernow B (1987) Research on tachykinins: clinical trends. In: Henry JL, Couture R, Cuello AC, Pelletier G, Quirion R, Regoli D (eds) Substance P and neurokinins. Substance P and neurokinins. A satelite symposium of the 30th international congress of the international union of physiological sciences, Montreal. Springer, Berlin Heidelberg New York, pp 372–379

Reibenegger G, Egg D, Fuchs D, Günther R, Hausen A, Werner ER, Wachter H (1986) Urinary neopterin reflects disease activity in patients with rheumatoid arthritis. Arthritis Rheum 29:1063–1070

Unanue ER, Allen PM (1987) The basis for the immunoregulatory role of macrophages and other accessory cells. Science 236:551–557

Wiedermann CJ, Sertl K, Pert CB (1986) Substance P receptors in rat spleen: characterization and autoradiographic distribution. Blood 68:1398–1401

Wiedermann CJ, Apperl A, Niedermühlbichler M, Geissler D, Kieselbach G, Konwalinka G, Braunsteiner H (1989) Cellular mechanisms in neurogenic inflammation by substance P. In: Hadden JW, Masek K, Nistico G (eds) Interactions between central nervous system, endocrine system and immune system. Pythagora, Rome

Neuroimmunomodulation: Electrophysiological Patterns in Brain During the Course of Immune Responses *

H. OVADIA and D. SAPHIER [1]

Introduction

The discipline of neuroimmunomodulation is concerned with the mutual interaction between the immune system and the central nervous system (CNS; Cohn 1985). A great deal of evidence has accumulated indicating that the CNS exerts an immunomodulatory effect on peripheral immune reactions, and that the immune system sends signals, as yet unidentified, which cause brain arousal and modulation of neuroendocrine responses. This communication, whereby the CNS provides fine tuning of immune function, is crucial to host defense in both health and disease.

The immune system is probably fully autonomous in its self-nonself discrimination. The identification of antigens and the propagation of the immune effector mechanisms are determined mainly by the genome and can be carried out in vitro in cloned cell lines. CNS intervention of the immune system most likely occurs primarily during those processes categorized as antigen independent, such as ontogeny, cell turnover, migration, and sensitivity to signals (Cohn 1985). These antigen-independent processes are very important in determining the intensity and duration of the immune response, enabling defense mechanisms of the host to be fully geared.

Stress is a major biological phenomenon which links the CNS with immune function. Acute exposure of experimental animals to stressors results in suppression of both humoral and cellular immune responses (Solomon 1969; Monjan and Collector 1977). On the other hand, repeated exposure to the same stressor results in adaptation and in some cases to enhanced immune response (Monjan and Collector 1977; Gisler 1974). Several studies have shown that various perturbations of the CNS, such as electrolytic lesions and electrical stimulation, induce changes in the peripheral immune system. Lesions of the anterior hypothalamus caused a marked decrease in the blastogenic response to mitogens (Rosjman et al. 1985), and inhibition of neural autoimmune diseases (Wertman et al. 1985). Biziere et al. (1985) demonstrated the importance of cerebral lateralization on immune responses. Lesions of the left cerebral

* This work was supported by grants from the Israeli National Council for Research and Development, and European Community, and the Jacob and Hilda Blaustein Foundation.
[1] Department of Neurology, Neuroimmunology Research Unit, Hadassah University Hospital, Eim Karem, POB 12000, 91120 Jerusalem, Israel.

Neuropsychopharmacology
Edited by Bunney/Hippius/Laakmann/Schmauß

neocortex in mice depressed cell-mediated responses without affecting B-cell response. A parallel finding was observed by Geschwind and Behan (1982) who found that immune disorders, such as atopic diseases, autoimmune thyroiditis, and migraine, were more frequent in left-handers and their relatives than in right-handers.

The routes of communication between the CNS and the immune system have been partially delineated by morphological studies done by Felten et al. (1985) and Bulloch (1985). These authors demonstrated the extensive innervation of germinal centers in lymphoid tissues, thereby introducing the notion of direct innervation and contact between the CNS and the immune system.

A number of studies have demonstrated electrophysiological responses within the central nervous system following the administration of antigenic agents (Griogoriev 1981; Besedovsky et al. 1977; Korneva 1987) and that such changes occur during the entire course of the immune response (Saphier et al. 1987). The role of adrenal glucocorticoid hormones in the suppression of immune responses is well documented, and it is probable that this neuroendocrine axis is of great importance in the feedback interaction between the immune and nervous systems (MacLean and Reichlin 1981). Thus in our studies, these responses were recorded within the endocrine hypothalamus in sites known to be of particular importance in the regulation of hypothalamo-hypophyseal-adrenocortical activity (Saphier and Feldman 1986) and also known to influence the course of immune responses and experimental autoimmune diseases (Jankovic and Isakovic 1973; Wertman et al. 1985).

Experimental Findings

In our first experiments, we used a conscious rat model bearing chronically implanted recording electrodes in the preoptic area/anterior hypothalamus (POA/AH) and hypothalamic paraventricular nucleus (PVN), the primary site of corticotropin-releasing factor and vasopressin-secreting neurones regulating pituitary secretion of adrenocorticotropic hormone (Swanson et al. 1983). Rats were sensitized using a 10% suspension of sheep red blood cells (SRBC) injected intraperitoneally on the second and third days after recording baseline POA/AH and PVN multiunit activity (MUA). POA/AH MUA increased from a basal level of 14.65 ± 2.07 Hz to a maximum level of 33.06 ± 6.93 Hz ($p < 0.005$) 5 days following SRBC injection. This increase correlated with the initial appearance of serum anti-SRBC antibodies. Basal POA/AH was achieved again by the 9th day, and significant decreases were recorded on days 3 and 8 following the sensitization (Fig. 1). Significant increases in PVN MUA were also recorded and appeared to be delayed with respect to those in the POA/AH, occurring on the 6th day (Fig. 2). Furthermore, we were able to demonstrate increases in plasma corticosterone levels on day 8 following SRBC insection (Weidenfeld et al., unpublished observations), in accordance with the previous works of Besedovsky et al. (1977) and others (Shek and Sabiston

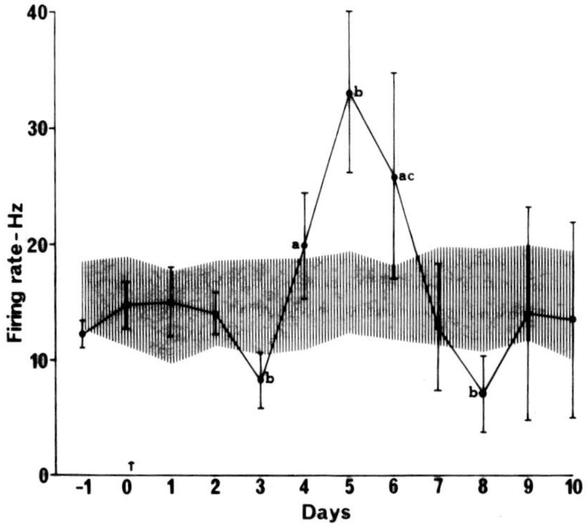

Fig. 1. Preoptic area/anterior hypothalamus MUA recorded before and after SRBC sensitization (*arrow*). Significance levels: *a*, $p < 0.05$ compared with day 0; *b*, $p < 0.005$, compared with day 0; *c*, $p < 0.05$ compared with day 5. (From Saphier et al. 1987)

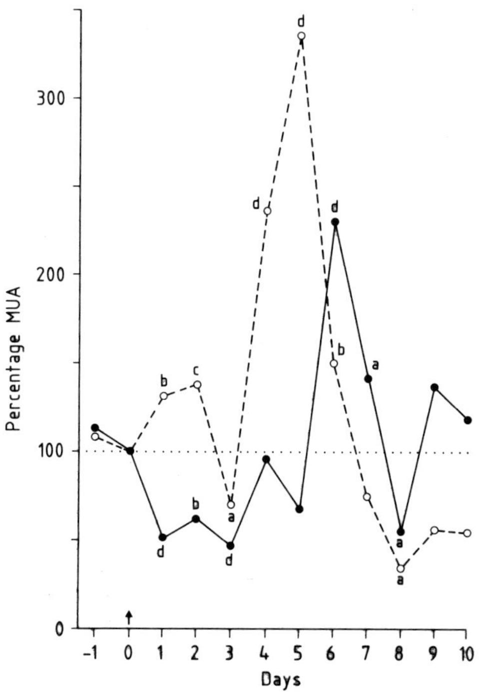

Fig. 2. POA/AH MUA (*broken line*) and PVN MUA (*solid line*) recorded before and after SRBC sensitization (*arrow*). Data transformed into percentages from original values obtained from conscious rats. Significance levels obtained by comparison with the mean MUA recorded on day 0; *a*, $p < 0.05$; *b*, $p < 0.025$; *c*, $p < 0.01$; *d*, $p < 0.005$. (From Saphier et al. 1987)

1983). We believe that the recorded changes in PVN MUA and also possibly those in the POA/AH are associated in a complex manner with the alterations in circulating corticosterone levels (Saphier et al. 1987).

In another group of rats, also sensitized with 10% SRBC 3 weeks before initiation of the same protocol as desribed above, we recorded POA/AH MUA changes during induction of the secondary immune response to SRBC. MUA

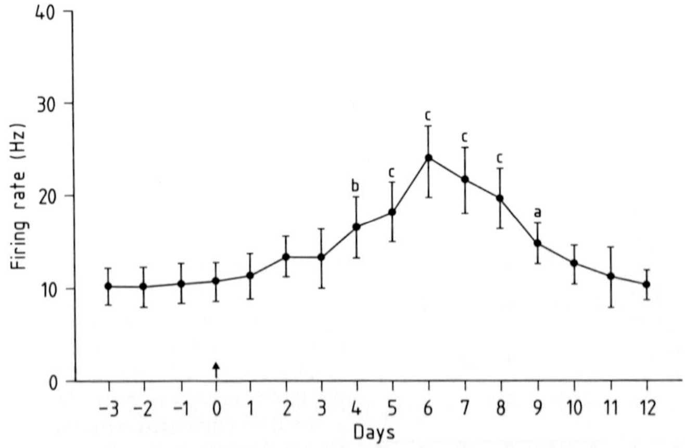

Fig. 3. The effect of secondary immune response to SRBC on POA/AH MUA. SRBC were injected 2 weeks after the first antigenic challenge. Significance levels obtained by comparison with the mean MUA recorded at day -3; *a*, $p < 0.05$; *b*, $p < 0.01$; *c*, $p < 0.01$. (From Saphier et al. 1987)

increased significantly between days 4 and 9 following the challenge, with maximal increases recorded on day 6 (Fig. 3). The profile of this response was different from that of the first response in that there were no recorded decreases, the maximal increase appeared later and was smaller, and there were more days of significantly increased activity.

Treatment of a group of rats with the immunosuppressive drug cyclophosphamide (25 mg/kg daily intraperitoneal injection, after each recording period) was able to prevent both the production of serum antibodies to the SRBC challenge and increases in POA/AH. This was true for the majority of animals (5/6). In the one remaining animal, a low titer of anti-SRBC antibodies were detected on the 10th day, and this animal also exhibited a small increase in POA/AH MUA on day 5 following the SRBC challenge (Table 1).

The current consensus of opinion favors the concept of soluble products elaborated by the immune system during the course of immune responses as the factors responsible for the above-reported changes in neural and neuroendocrine activity. Several laboratories have begun investigating the effects of neuroimmunomodulatory factors upon these parameters, and effects of interferon-α (IFN-α) and interleukin 1 (IL-1) have been demonstrated (Dafny et al. 1985; Besedovsky et al. 1986; Blatteis 1985).

In our laboratory, we have also investigated the effects of IFN, IL-1, thymic humoral factor (THF; Trainin et al. 1985), and histamine (HIS) upon cortical EEG, POA/AH MUA, and corticosterone secretion following intracerebroventricular administration in conscious rats (Saphier et al. 1988). Saline administration was shown not to alter POA/AH MUA but increased the total time and duration of synchronized EEG periods for up to 45 min after injection. Both IFN-α and THF significantly reduced POA/AH activity and increased

Table 1. POA/AH MUA recorded following SRBC immunization and cyclophosphamide-immunosuppressed rats

Experimental group	% MUA change (day 5/6)	Anti-SRBC titer (day 10)
SRBC	+305	1:128
SRBC + CY (5/6 rats)	−1	ND
SRBC + CY (1/6 rats)[a]	+36	1:32

Rats were immunized with 10% SRBC and MUA was recorded every day. Values of the peak activity of each experimental group are illustrated for comparison. Antibodies against SRBC were detected by hemagglutination test in sera obtained at day 10 post immunization. ND, not detected; CY, cyclophosphamide.

[a] One rat treated with cyclophosphamide showed a significant change in POA/AH MUA and later developed serum antibodies to SRBC.

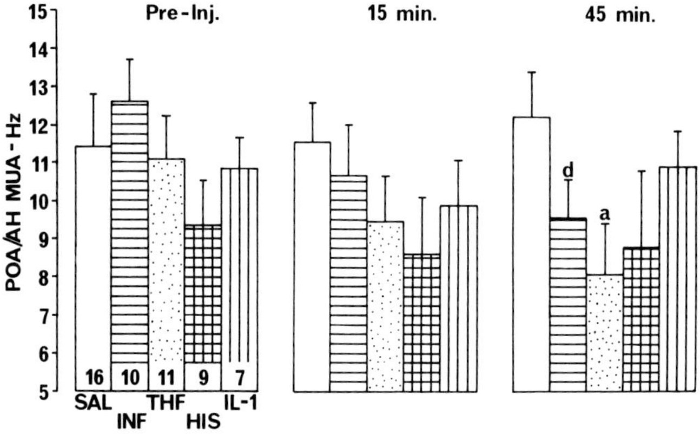

Fig. 4. POA/AH MUA recorded following intracerebroventricular injection of immunomodulatory reagents as indicated. The number of tests made for each substance are shown in the bars. Significance levels were obtained by comparison with preinjection discharge rate: *a*, $p < 0.05$; *d*, $p < 0.005$

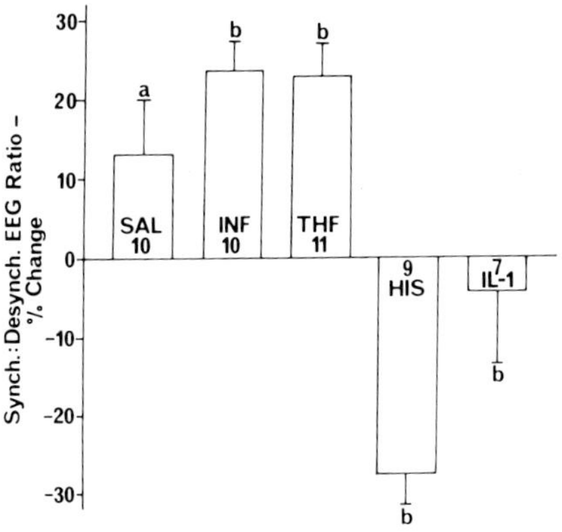

Fig. 5. Histogram describing the effect of immunomodulatory reagents upon cortical EEG synchronization/desynchronization ratio. Significance levels: *a*, $p < 0.025$; *b*, $p < 0.005$ compared with ratios prior to injection

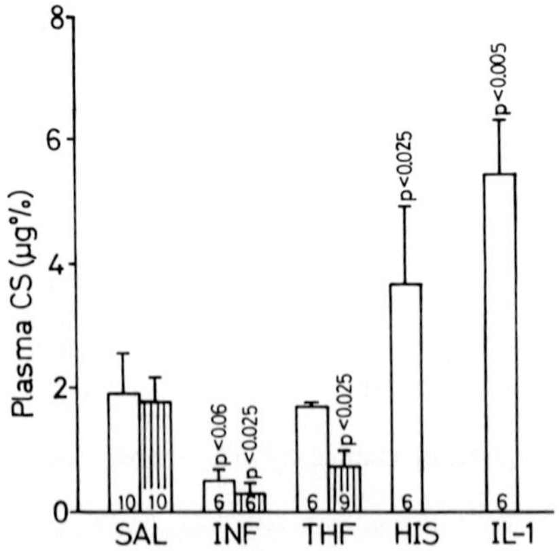

Fig. 6. Histogram showing the effects upon basal plasma corticosterone levels of intracerebroventricular administration of the reagents indicated. Corticosterone levels were measured following acute (*open bars*) or chronic (*shaded bars*) administration of the reagents. Significance levels obtained by comparison to saline treated animals

EEG synchronization while decreasing plasma corticosterone levels. HIS and IL-1 did not affect POA/AH MUA but decreased EEG synchronization and increased plasma corticosterone levels. These results (summarized in Figs. 4–6) demonstrate that several factors elaborated by the immune system are able to alter EEG discharge, adrenocortical secretory activity, and neural activity in an area of the brain known to be influenced during the course of immune responses and known to modulate both immune and neuroendocrine secretory activity.

Concluding Remark

Although the above studies have demonstrated extensive influences of immune activity upon the central nervous system, the sites, mechanisms, and physiological significance of the recorded effects require considerable clarification. In particular, the elucidation of factors involved in the neurophysiological responses await identification, as do the responsive neural elements and their efferent targets.

References

Besedovsky H, Sorkin E, Felix D, Haas H (1977) Hypothalamic changes during the immune response. Eur J Immunol 7:325–328

Besedovsky HO, del Rey A, Sorkin E, Dinarello CA (1986) Immunoregulatory feedback between interleukin 1 and glucocorticoid hormones. Science 233:652–654

Biziere K, Guillaumin JM, Degenne D, Bardos P, Renoux M, Renoux G (1985) Lateralized neocortical modulation of the T-cell lineage. In: Guillemin R, Cohn M, Melnechuk T (eds) Neural modulation of immunity. Raven, New York, p 81

Blateis CM (1985) Central nervous system effects of interleukin 1. In: Klueger MJ, Oppenheim JJ, Towanda MC (eds) The physiologic metabolic and immunologic actions of IL-1. Liss, New York, p 107

Bulloch K (1985) Neuroanatomy of lymphoid tissue: a review. In: Guillemin R, Cohn M, Melnechuk T (eds) Neural modulation of immunity. Raven, New York, p 111
Cohn M (1985) What are the must elements of immune responsiveness? In: Guillemin R, Cohn M, Melnechuk T (eds) Neural modulation of immunity. Raven, New York, p 3
Dafny N, Prieto-Gomez B, Reyes-Vazquez C (1985) Does the immune system communicate with the central nervous system? Interferon modifies central nervous activity. J Neuroimmunol 9:1–12
Felten DL, Felten SY, Carlson SL, Olschowka JA, Livnat S (1985) Noradrenergic and peptidergic innervation of lymphoid tissue. J Immunol 135:755s–765s
Geschwind N, Behan P (1982) Left-handedness: association with immune disease, migraine and development learning disorder. Proc Natl Acad Sci USA 79:5097–5100
Gisler RH (1974) Stress and the hormonal regulation of the immune response in mice. Psychother Psychosom 23:192–208
Grigoriev VA (1981) Dynamics of DC potential of hypothalamic structures in early terms of immune reaction development. Physiol J USSR 67:463–467
Jankovic BD, Isakovic K (1973) Neuro-endocrine correlates of immune response. I. Effects of brain lesions on antibody production, Arthus reactivity and delayed hypersensitivity in the rat. Int Arch Allergy Appl Immunol 45:360–372
Korneva EA (1987) Electrophysiological analysis of brain reactions to antigen. Ann NY Acad Sci 496:318–337
MacLean D, Reichlin S (1981) Neuroendocrinology and the immune system. In: Ader R (ed) Psychoneuroimmunology. Academic, New York, p 475
Monjan AA, Collector MI (1977) Stress-induced modulation of the immune response. Science 196:307–308
Rosjman TL, Cross RJ, Brooks WH, Marksbery WR (1985) Neuroimmunomodulation. Effects of neural lesions on cellular immunity. In: Guillemin R, Cohn M, Melnechuk T (eds) Neural modulation of immunity. Raven, New York, p 95
Saphier D, Feldman S (1986) Effects of stimulation of the preoptic area on paraventricular nucleus unit activity and corticosterone secretion in freely moving rats. Neuroendocrinology 42:167–173
Saphier D, Abramsky O, Mor G, Ovadia H (1987) Multiunit electrical activity in conscious rats during an immune response. Brain Behav Immun 1:40–51
Saphier D, Kidron D, Abramsky O, Trainin N, Pecht M, Burstein Y, Ovadia H (1988) Neurophysiological changes in the brain following central administration of immunomodulatory factors. Isr J Med Sci 24:261–263
Shek PV, Sabiston BH (1983) Neuro-endocrine regulation of immune processes – change in circulating corticosterone levels induced by the primary antibody response in mice. Int J Immunopharmacol 5:23–33
Solomon GF (1969) Stress and antibody response in rats. Int Arch Allergy 35:97–104
Swanson LW, Sawchenko PE, Rivier J, Vale W (1983) Organization of ovine corticotropin-releasing factor immunoreactive cells and fibers in the rat brain: an immunohistochemical study. Neuroendocrinology 36:165–186
Trainin N, Handzel ZT, Pecht M (1985) Biological and clinical properties of THF. Thymus 7:137–150
Wertman E, Ovadia H, Feldman S, Abramsky O (1985) Prevention of EAE by anterior hypothalamic lesions in rats. Neurology 35:1468–1470

Sympathetic Noradrenergic Neural Contacts with Lymphocytes and Macrophages in the Splenic White Pulp of the Rat: Site of Possible Bidirectional Communication and Local Regulation Between the Nervous and Immune Systems *

S. Y. FELTEN and D. L. FELTEN [1]

Sympathetic Noradrenergic Nerve Terminals Contact Lymphocytes in the Splenic White Pulp of the Rat

Primary and Secondary Immune Organs Are Innervated by Postganglionic Noradrenergic Nerve Fibers

Evidence from many fields of investigation points toward communication between the nervous and immune systems in both directions (Ader 1981; Goetzl 1985; Guillemin et al. 1985; Jankovic et al. 1987). Numerous psychosocial factors can influence immune responses. Specific stressors in rodents are associated with altered immune responses and sometimes with altered resistance to tumors or pathogens. Discrete lesions in hypothalamic and limbic regions of the central nervous system (CNS) can result in transient or long-lasting changes in specific measures of immune reactivity (see Felten and Felten 1987 for discussion). Although these studies indicate the existence of communication between the nervous system and the immune system, they do not reveal the pathways or the mechanisms by which this is accomplished.

The two major routes by which the nervous system can signal visceral structures in the body are the neuroendocrine system and the autonomic nervous system. A massive body of evidence substantiates neuroendocrine modulation of immune responses and the activities of individual cells of the immune system (see Berczi 1986, 1987 for a summary). Virtually every hormone in the hypothalamic-pituitary-target organ axis exerts some influence on specific activities of the immune system. It also is evident that some hormones of the anterior pituitary are produced by lymphocytes, and that releasing factors can act on lymphocytes as well as pituicytes (Weigent and Blalock 1987). Nerves are found in both primary and secondary immune organs. Although the sympathetic postganglionic noradrenergic innervation of

---

* This research was supported by grants N00014-84-K-0488 from the Office of Naval Research, RO1 NS25223 from NIH, RO1 MH42073 from NIMH, and a John D. and Catherine T. MacArthur Foundation Prize Fellowship to D.L.F.

[1] Department of Neurobiology and Anatomy, University of Rochester School of Medicine, 601 Elmwood Ave., Rochester, NY 14642, USA.

Neuropsychopharmacology
Edited by Bunney/Hippius/Laakmann/Schmauß

immune organs is extensive and has been studied in greater detail than other innervation, peptidergic nerve fibers also are present in both primary and secondary immune organs (see Felten et al. 1988 for review).

Sympathetic noradrenergic (NA) nerve fibers supply smooth muscle compartments (vasculature, capsules, trabeculae) and the lymphoid parenchyma of both primary and secondary immune organs (Felten et al. 1981, 1984, 1985, 1987b, 1988, 1989; Felten and Felten 1989). NA nerve fibers are distributed in specific compartments of these immune organs. In the bone marrow, NA fibers branch from the vasculature into the parenchyma (Calvo 1968; Felten et al. 1985). In the thymus, NA fibers distribute mainly in the cortex, along the vasculature and among thymocytes, although some fibers are present in the medulla (Williams et al. 1981; Bellinger et al. 1988). In secondary immune organs, the NA nerve fibers are associated particularly with compartments containing T-lymphocytes and macrophages. In the spleen, NA fibers distribute with the central arteriolar system of the white pulp, are present among T-lymphocytes in the periarteriolar lymphatic sheath (PALS) and alongside macrophages at the marginal sinus, and also distribute in parafollicular sites and more sparsely in the marginal zone (Ackerman et al. 1987a, b; Felten et al. 1987a, 1988; Williams and Felten 1981; Williams et al. 1981). In lymph nodes, NA fibers distribute in the medullary cords and in the paracortical and cortical zones (Williams et al. 1981; Felten et al. 1985, 1984; Livnat et al. 1985). In gut-associated lymphoid tissue, NA fibers traverse the T-dependent zones and distribute in the lamina propria (Felten et al. 1981).

Noradrenergic TH + Nerve Fibers Are Distributed in Specific Compartments of the Splenic White Pulp

We have carried out detailed examination of the splenic white pulp at the light microscopic level to localize the NA sympathetic nerve fibers within specific compartments (Ackerman et al. 1987a, b; Felten et al. 1987a). Our initial studies with histofluorescence for the localization of catecholamine-containing nerve fibers were accompanied by neurochemical analysis with high-performance liquid chromatography with electrochemical detection to identify the catecholamine present in the spleen (Williams and Felten 1981; Williams et al. 1981). The vast majority of the catecholamine content was norepinephrine (NE), not dopamine or epinephrine. In more recent investigation of the source of the NA innervation (Bellinger et al. 1989), we traced the connections with retrograde transport to the superior mesenteric/celiac ganglion in the rat, and then carried out ganglionectomy studies and 6-hydroxydopamine (6-OHDA) denervation studies to further explore the source and identity of this innervation. The innervation clearly is a classical postganglionic noradrenergic sympathetic supply. Tyrosine-hydroxylase (TH) immunocytochemistry then was developed as an additional aid for localization of these fibers. Similar ganglionectomy and 6-OHDA denervation also eliminated TH+ profiles. Careful mapping of profiles with histofluorescence and TH immunocytochemistry indicated the direct overlap of these markers, with the TH immunocytochemistry providing a slightly greater sensitivity and providing much better resolution of background compartmentation and structural identification. Thus, we have established the use of TH+ nerve profiles in the splenic white pulp as an excellent marker for NA sympathetic nerve fibers. TH immunocytochemistry offers the opportunity for double labeling; we have used nickel enhancement of TH profiles (black) and used a second label for identification of surface markers of subsets of lymphocytes and macrophages (brown), providing excellent resolution of the compartmentation of the TH+ fibers (Felten et al. 1987a).

TH+ fibers enter the spleen with the vasculature and form particularly dense bundles of fibers at the hilar region. The fibers then distribute with the capsular and trabecular system throughout the spleen. Abundant innervation also continues with the vasculature along the central arteriolar system of the white pulp and distributes extensively within the white pulp. Only sparse fibers are distributed in nontrabecular regions of the red pulp. The first impression of the distribution of TH+ nerve fibers in the white pulp is that they branch away from the central arteries and distribute through the PALS, along the marginal sinus, and into the marginal zone. However, this impression has been called into question by the developmental studies of Ackerman et al. (1989); at day 1 of postnatal age, TH+ profiles were present along the outside of the developing PALS, at the site of the presumptive marginal sinus, at a time when the vasculature did not possess smooth muscle cells and clearly was not innervated by TH+ fibers. Only later, at approximately 1 week of age, were fibers found along the vasculature in addition to their compartmentation in the PALS and along the marginal sinus.

The TH+ fibers along the central arteriolar system appeared to be present in adults in a compartment strictly associated with the smooth muscle of the vessels. However, this adventitial zone forms the border between the central artery and the PALS, suggesting that NE released from these terminals may diffuse sufficiently to interact with both smooth muscle cells of the vasculature and lymphocytes in the PALS, a possibility even more strongly supported by electron microscopic (EM) evidence, described below. TH+ nerve fibers also were distributed among T-lymphocytes (both T helper and T cytotoxic/suppressor subsets) throughout the PALS. Linear profiles of NA varicosities were distributed along the marginal sinus, adjacent to ED3+ macrophages. Additional TH+ profiles were scattered among lymphocytes and macrophages in the marginal zone. The follicles appeared to lack innervation except along the outside (parafollicular) edge, where linear profiles coursed. More detailed examination of the follicular areas suggests that some fine TH+ nerve fibers extend into the follicles among the B-lymphocytes and adjacent to the small, scattered clusters of T-lymphocytes. Thus, the density and distribution of TH+ nerve fibers is not uniform and show specific patterns of developmental maturation.

TH+ Nerve Terminals End Adjacent to Lymphocytes and Macrophages in the Periarteriolar Lymphatic Sheath and at the Marginal Sinus of the Spleen

We have extended our analysis of TH+ nerve profiles in the splenic white pulp to the EM level (Felten and Olschowka 1987; Felten et al. 1988, 1987b). Observations at the light microscopic level in 1 μm thick sections permit a direct comparison with adjacent thin sections observed at the EM level. We have used TH immunocytochemistry in unstained sections (Figs. 1, 2) to visualize the nerve terminals and their associations with immunocytes; the TH+ profiles show a dense reaction product that can be visualized readily. In sections stained with uranyl acetate and lead citrate, more detail of cytoplasmic inclusions in the TH+ profiles can be seen, but the sections are much darker, and scanning grids to find these profiles is more difficult and time consuming. In TH+ profiles with heavy metal staining, both mitochondria and clusters of vesicles can be seen, particularly if the TH+ immunocytochemical reaction product (diaminobenzidine) is not overwhelmingly dense. These observations, along with the absence of TH+ staining in the spleen of ganglionectomized rats or rats treated with 6-OHDA, provide strong evidence that the TH+ profiles are indeed the NA nerve terminals. We do not have confidence in the identification of nerve profiles in the spleen at the EM level unless a specific marker, such as TH immunocytochemistry, is used. Although we see bundles of nerve fibers, some of which are TH+ and some of which are not, and we see profiles of 0.2–1.5 μm that contain vesicles and mitochondria, we cannot demonstrate unequivocally that these actually are nerve terminals without a specific marker. Many cell types in the PALS have long processes whose cross-sections could resemble nerve profiles, and many cells have very dense cytoplasmic inclusions that include vesicles. For these reasons, we have carried out extensive controls to be certain that the profiles that we have observed with TH immunocytochemistry are indeed neural profiles.

We began our observations at the adventitia of the central arterioles because of the very clear landmarks and division of cell types, even at the EM level. The TH+ nerve profiles were abundant along the central arterioles, consistent with our observations at the light microscopic level. The TH+ terminals were separated from the smooth muscle cells by the usual basement membrane, typical of peripheral NA "synapses" that often are quite distant from their target cells, separated by at least a basement membrane. Many of these terminals also were invested by what appeared to be Schwann cells. However, at the outer edge of the adventitia, at its junction with lymphocytes at the beginning of the PALS, surprisingly close contacts were observed between the TH+ nerve terminals and lymphocytes (Fig. 1). There was a direct association of nerve terminal membrane and lymphocyte membrane, separated by approximately 6 nm in cases where the smooth appositions could be seen clearly for long distances. There was not an intervening basement membrane; these contacts were far closer than the "contacts" with smooth muscle that routinely are called peripheral synapses or neuroeffector junctions. Thus, in the adventitia of the central arterioles, a site where abundant TH+ profiles had

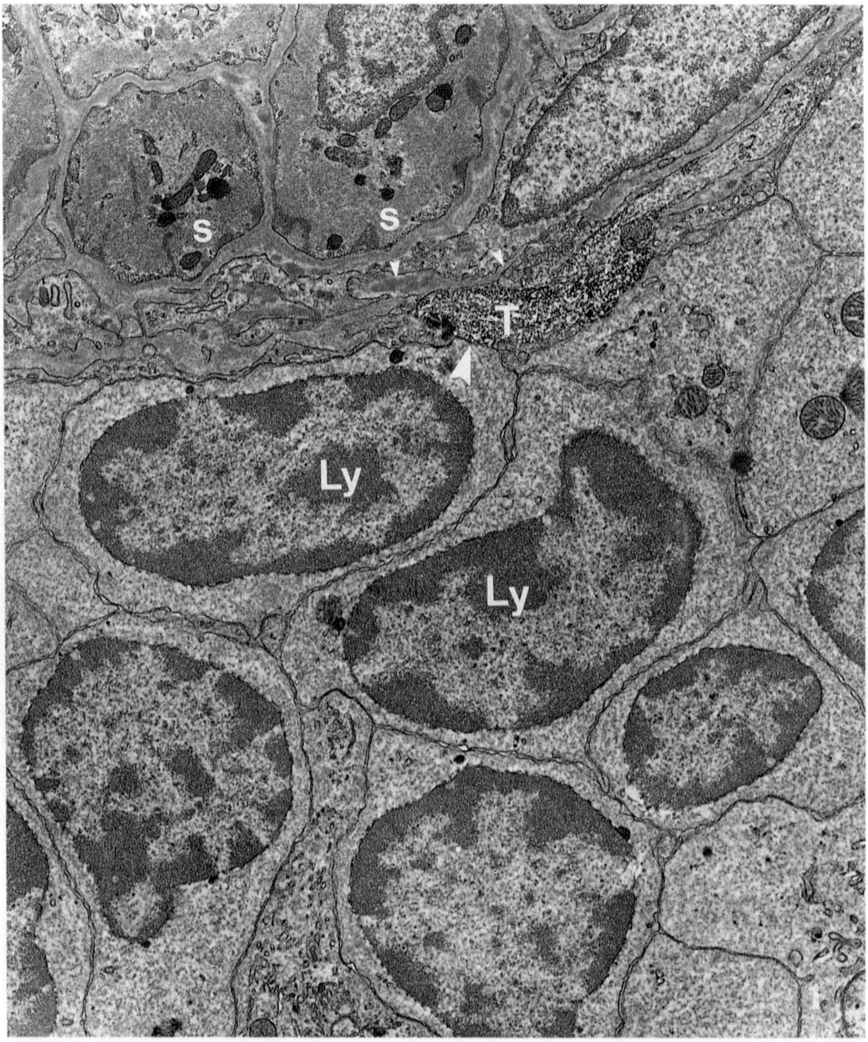

Fig. 1. A TH+ nerve terminal (*T*) in the adventitia separating the smooth muscle cells (*s*) of a central arteriole of the white pulp from the adjacent lymphocytes (*Ly*) and other cells of the PALS. This nerve terminal is separated from the smooth muscle cells by a basement membrane (*small arrowheads*) but is in direct contact with a lymphocyte (*large arrowhead*) and an adjacent cell in the PALS. EM immunocytochemistry for tyrosine hydroxylase (TH). Adult Fischer 344 rat. (×10600)

been observed and were considered to be unequivocally associated with the smooth muscle of the vasculature, the junctional contacts with lymphocytes were closer than with smooth muscle cells.

These TH+ nerve terminals also were present in deeper regions of the PALS, distant from the adventitia. Some bundles of NA nerve fibers coursed through the PALS, often invested with Schwann cell processess; however, some

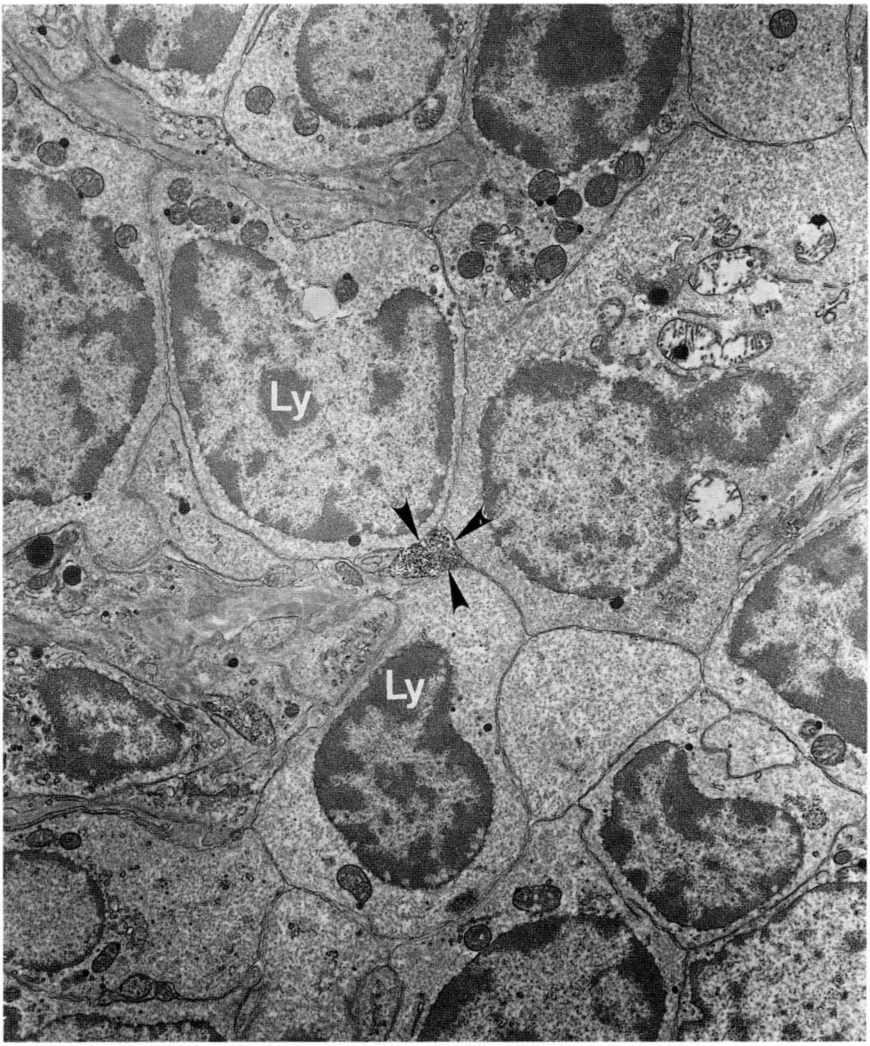

Fig. 2. A TH+ nerve terminal directly contacting (*arrowheads*) three lymphocytes (*Ly*) within the PALS, distant from the central arteriolar system. EM immunocytochemistry for tyrosine hydroxylase (TH). Adult Fischer 344 rat. (×10600)

TH+ profiles contacted lymphocytes directly, with the Schwann cell process moving aside. TH+ nerve terminals also were found abutting one more lymphocytes (Fig. 2) at all levels of the PALS. In thin sections through the marginal sinus, similar TH+ nerve terminals were found adjacent to lymphocytes and macrophages.

The site of apposition of these TH+ nerve terminals with lymphocytes showed a smooth region of close membrane apposition, sometimes with slight thickening of the membranes. No postjunctional specializations were found, consistent with sympathetic NA contacts elsewhere in the periphery, both with smooth muscle cells and with parenchymal cells of target organs. Neuroeffector junctions in the periphery usually do not demonstrate postsynaptic specializations that are characteristic of many CNS synapses between nerve terminals and other neurons. We have concluded that lymphocytes and macrophages are likely targets of TH+ nerve terminals in the splenic white pulp. On strictly anatomical characteristics, had we not begun these studies with the usual bias that NA sympathetic nerve terminals have their principal contacts with smooth muscle of the vasculature, we would be inclined to consider the lymphocytes as an even more likely target than the smooth muscle cells, even at the PALS–central arteriolar junctions.

Evidence for Directional Communication from Nerve Terminals to Lymphocytes

Criteria for Noradrenergic Neurotransmission with Lymphocytes as Targets

The anatomical findings of abundant NA innervation of the parenchyma of the spleen and other immune organs and the demonstration of direct neuroeffector junctions between TH+ nerve terminals and lymphocytes in the splenic white pulp raised the possibility that sympathetic NA neurotransmission might be influencing immune functions directly, providing a direct anatomical link between the brain and cells of the immune system. However, for such neurotransmission to be demonstrated, four criteria must be met: (a) presence and compartmentation of the neurotransmitter in nerves near the site of communication; (b) release of the neurotransmitter; (c) appropriate receptors on the target cells, with a second messenger system to provide intracellular recognition of ligand-receptor interaction; and (c) a pharmacologically predictable functional effect of the neurotransmitter involving the target cells. The novel part of substantiating these criteria in the immune system is the mobile nature of the target cells, a phenomenon not encountered previously in the more traditional sympathetic NA target tissues of cardiac muscle, smooth muscle, and secretory glands.

The first criterion of presence of NE in nerves in the splenic white pulp, and the specific compartmentation of those nerves, has been addressed in detail above and clearly is fulfilled.

The second criterion of release of NE from splenic nerves has been demonstrated from classical observations (von Euler 1946) and by recent neurochemical observations in our laboratories. Measurements of NE with in vivo dialysis techniques has shown the availability of free NE in the extracellular fluid of the spleen (Felten et al. 1986). Ganglionectomy reduced splenic content by more than 90% (Bellinger et al. 1989), and 6-OHDA treatment had a similar effect (Williams et al. 1981; Felten et al. 1985). Preliminary observations from micropunched regions of white pulp and red pulp in the rat spleen suggest that neurally derived NE percolates through the spleen and is present as a paracrine secretion.

The third criterion of appropriate adrenoceptors on the target cells has been documented in great detail. Adrenoceptors, particularly of the β_2 subclass, have been found on lymphocytes (both B- and T-lymphocytes, including T subsets), monocytes and macrophages, and granulocytes (Bishopric et al. 1980; Coffey and Hadden 1985; Hadden et al. 1970; Landmann et al. 1981, 1985) (see Felten et al. 1987b for summary). We have found β-adrenoceptors on both T- and B-lymphocytes in adult rat spleen, with greater numbers on B-lymphocytes, perhaps reflecting an enhanced expression on cells a greater distance from the source of NA nerve terminals. We also have found β-adrenoceptors on lymphocytes in the developing rat spleen at postnatal day 1. The β-adrenoceptor appears to be linked with a adenylate cyclase mechanism, with cyclic AMP as the second messenger. Pharmacological studies have suggested the presence of α-adrenoceptors on lymphocytes as well (Sanders et al. 1985a; Sanders and Munson 1985; Coffey et al. 1975).

The fourth criterion of a pharmacologically predictable functional effect of NE on lymphocyte responses has been studied in detail, but this is complicated by the fact that lymphocytes are involved in complex interactions in vivo and do not demonstrate simplistic unidirectional responses that provide an equivalent of a postsynaptic potential in a neuron. Initial studies in thymocytes indicated that NE stimulates cyclic AMP and diminishes proliferation while enhancing differentiation (Singh 1979, 1985; Singh and Owen 1976), an observation which we have confirmed (Felten et al. 1987b). This has led to the often-cited simplistic notion that NE is inhibitory to immune function. However, Sanders and Munson demonstrated that in vitro antibody responses are enhanced by NE by a β-adrenoceptor mediated mechanism (Sanders and Munson, 1984a, b; Sanders and Munson 1985b), suggesting that an observation of a specific proliferation of a specific cell type in the immune system may not be applicable to a complex process such as an in vitro antibody response. It is even more difficult to draw conclusions from somewhat artificial in vitro observations such as mitogen responses to the in vivo physiological role for NE in a fully functioning system with a complex local microenvironment and continuous lymphocyte trafficking.

We have approached the question of a functional role for the NA innervation through specific denervation studies, particularly employing the neurotoxic agent 6-OHDA, with controls for direct toxic effects or temporary NE release during nerve terminal death (Felten et al. 1984, 1985, 1987b; Livnat et al. 1985, 1987). Our studies have demonstrated that specific NA denervation of the spleen is followed by greatly diminished primary antibody responses (80% decrease in spleen to systemic antigen challenge, 97% decrease in popliteal lymph node response to foot pad antigen challenge), approximately 50% decrease in delayed hypersensitivity response to a contact sensitizing agent, approximately 50% decrease in cytotoxic T-lymphocyte response and interleukin 2 (IL-2) secretion, and enhanced natural killer cell activity, both baseline and poly I:C stimulated. Thus, specific immune reactivity is affected differentially by denervation, depending upon the response, the cell types involved, the age and sex of the animal, and the extent of the denervation. Our observations of proliferative responses have shown complex alterations; in some cases, B-lymphocyte proliferation is enhanced by denervation, such as the inguinal lymph nodes of the mouse, but in other cases, both T- and B-lymphocyte proliferation is diminished by denervation. The spleen does not react in a similar fashion to lymph nodes when denervated, and specific lymph nodes respond differently in lymphocyte proliferative responses when denervated. It therefore appears likely that NE is a potent modulator of many specific responses of immunocytes and may have as complex a role in the modulation of in vivo responses as do the interleukins. From a classical perspective, it appears that NE fulfills the major criteria for neurotransmission with lymphocytes and other immunocytes as targets. However, the response of the target cells to this NA neurotransmission may be transient while the lymphocyte is present in an appropriate site.

Possible Modes of Communication Between Norepinephrine Derived from Nerve Terminals and Lymphocytes

Our neurochemical observations suggest that NE is present in sufficient concentrations throughout the spleen to exert a paracrine effect on immunocytes with adrenoceptors; the availability of NE depends upon the integrity of the NA nerves, from which a vast majority of the NE is derived. Even hormonally derived NE and epinephrine may depend upon the integrity of the NA sympathetic nerves for the greatest extent of their effects since they are avidly taken up by a high-affinity uptake carrier, stored in the nerve terminals, and subsequently released (Berecek and Brody 1982). If NE is present in the spleen as a paracrine secretion from NA nerves (perhaps even more prominent in spleen than in other less abundantly innervated immune organs), then the question of the direct neuroeffector junctions must be addressed. These junctions may provide a local region where apposing lymphocytes may be exposed to even higher concentrations of NE that the paracrine environment provides. However, an alternativ hypothesis also is possible, that these junctions are sites where cytokines secreted by immune cells regulate NA secretion from the nerve terminals (discussed below).

The most obvious mode of communication between neurally derived NE and immunocytes is a direct ligand-receptor interaction, in keeping with the evidence that NE fulfills the criteria for neurotransmission with cells of the immune system as targets. This would be a common mechanism for NE available as both a paracrine secretion throughout the spleen or in very high concentration in the immediate vicinity of the NA terminals in contact with lymphocytes and macrophages. However, several other possibilities must also be considered. NE released from nerve terminals may act on accessory cells, such as mast cells, altering the secretion of other signal molecules, such as histamine or serotonin. Such secondary effects of NE could be very complex.

A further possibility is that NE may itself bind directly to peptides of neural or immune origin, thereby altering the effects of the peptide (see Root-Bernstein and Westfall 1984 for discussion of this possible mechanism). Recent studies suggest that NE or other neurotransmitters may act synergistically with cytokines or may counteract synergistic effects (Frohman et al. 1988; Boyle et al. 1988; Beckner and Farrar 1988), a role consistent with neuromodulation.

The mode of action of NE also may depend upon colocalized peptides found in those nerve terminals. Recent evidence from Olschowka's laboratory (Olschowka et al. 1988) has shown the presence of neuropeptide Y in nerve fibers in the spleen; double-staining observations suggest that neuropeptide Y may be colocalized with NE in the sympathetic NA nerve fibers. The action of NE may depend upon the extent of corelease of the colocalized peptides, adding further to possible synergistic or counteracting effects. It is clear that the mode of action of NE may not be simple, in keeping with the very complex functional effects of NE on immune response and other immune parameters.

Evidence for Directional Communication from Immunocytes to Noradrenergic Nerve Terminals

Immunization in rodents results in alterations of electrical activity in specific hypothalamic nuclei (Besedovsky et al. 1977; Saphier et al. 1987), elevation in adrenocorticotropic hormone (ACTH) secretion and glucocorticoid secretion (Besedovsky et al. 1981, 1985), and a decrease in NE levels in the hypothalamus (Besedovsky et al. 1983; Carlson et al. 1987a). Within the hypothalamus, this decrease in NE was measured in microdissected paraventricular nucleus at the peak of the immune response (Carlson et al. 1987), suggesting a possible link between the NE changes, elevated activity in the CRF-ACTH-glucocorticoid axis, and increased electrical activity in these same circuits. Besedovsky and colleagues found that systemic IL-1 administration resulted in a rise in ACTH and glucocorticoids similar to that seen in immunized rodents (Besedovsky et al. 1986). IL-1 has been reported to evoke release of ACTH from primary cultures of pituitary cells (Bernton et al. 1987) or pituitary-derived AtT-20 cells (Woloski et al. 1985), although some contradictory data also have been reported (Uehara et al. 1987). Systemic administration of IL-1 results in release of CRF from the brain, enhancing secretion of ACTH and glucocorticoids (Berkenbosch et al. 1987; Sapolsky et al. 1987). However, since IL-1 probably does not cross the blood-brain barrier in appreciable quantities, even at the circumventricular organs such as the organum vasculosum of the lamina terminals, peripheral IL-1 may evoke release of a second signal molecule that in turn acts on the CRF neurons directly or through IL-1 producing neurons of the hypothalamus (Breder et al. 1988). IL-1 also produces a drop in NE content in specific central sites, including hypothalamic nuclei such as the paraventricular nucleus, and an increase in 3-methoxy-4-hydroxyphenylglycol, a major metabolite of NE, suggesting an increased turnover (Dunn 1988). Since this increase in hypothalamic NE turnover correlated with increased corticosterone levels, a reasonable hypothesis for the combined interactions of IL-1 and hypothalamic NE with the CRF neurons of the hypothalamus is that IL-1 acts on the NE terminals in the paraventricular nucleus to enhance CRF release. It is also possible that IL-1 acts directly on the CRF neurons. However, these findings suggest that the cytokine IL-1 can act directly on the NE terminals in the paraventricular nucleus of the hypothalamus and increase turnover.

Studies of NE in the spleen suggest a parallel influence of cytokines on NE in this organ. During the peak response to immunization, NE levels decrease in the spleen but not in other peripheral organs (del Rey et al. 1981, 1982; Carlson et al. 1987c). Rats raised in a germ-free environment demonstrated higher NE levels than those raised in a barrier facility or a normal vivarium environment, suggesting that the level of antigenic exposure influences NE content and turnover of the spleen. This is a remarkable finding in view of the high degree of stability of splenic NE in other experimental circumstances; drug-induced depletion of lymphocytes from the spleen did not alter NE content or turnover despite a major alteration in the size and cellularity of the white pulp (Carlson et al. 1987b). Although it is possible that this alteration in splenic NE occurred due to CNS effects evoked by immunization, with subsequent activation of specific central autonomic circuits, this effect would have to be precise and viscerotopically limited, since such an alteration in NE was not found in other peripheral organs. A more likely explanation is a direct interaction of a cytokine secreted during the peak of the immune response that acts locally, within the splenic microenvironment, to alter NE release from terminals in that organ only. IL-1 certainly is a potential mediator of this response, although other cytokines cannot be ruled out at this time.

A Model for Bidirectional Neural-Immune Interactions: Local Communication and Regulation Between Sympathetic Nerve Terminals and Immunocytes in the Spleen

A large body of evidence from our laboratory and others points strongly to sympathetic NA innervation of lymphocytes and other cells of the immune system. The criteria for NA neurotransmission with immunocytes as targets have been fulfilled. However, the relative role of direct ligand-receptor interactions, secondary effects on other signal molecules, and synergistic or counteractive effects with cytokines or neuropeptides acting on cells of the immune system has not been determined for NE at present. Recent studies also demonstrate that IL-1 can alter central NE metabolism, perhaps influencing CRF secretion as a consequence, providing a possible mechanism for the effects of immunization on central NE metabolism and glucocorticoid elevation. A parallel phenomenon has been suggested for splenic NE following immunization.

We are drawn back to the direct contacts between NA nerve terminals and lymphocytes in the splenic white, and ask what role they might play in such bidirectional communication. It is possible that these terminals both release NE in response to central signals and respond to cytokines in the local microenvironment as a feedback control on that release. If NE is acting directly to influence second messenger systems in lymphocytes and other immune cells, as the evidence strongly supports, or is acting to enhance signal-to-noise ratio of other biological signal molecules of immune or neural derivation, as is the case in some CNS circuits and may occur with NE modulation of cytokine effect on lymphocytes, then feedback from the affected lymphocytes to the NA neurons innervating the spleen would be expected. Such feedback loops may be long loops, through the hypothalamus, as described above for the IL-1–NE–CRF interactions, or may be short feedback loops at a local level. We hypothesize that the direct contacts between NA nerve terminals and lymphocytes may function as both neuroeffector junctions and effector-neural junctions. The alteration of splenic NE during immunization, but not during major compartmental alterations induced by immunosuppressive drug administration, suggests that cytokines can influence local NE secretion. The direct contacts may provide the anatomical site for responding immune cells to release cytokines that regulate NE release. We hypothesize that these contacts are sites of bidirectional regulation and local communication between the nervous and immune systems within the microenvironment of the splenic white pulp.

Acknowledgement. We thank John Housel for excellent technical assistance.

References

Ackerman KD, Felten SY, Bellinger DL, Felten DL (1987a) Noradrenergic sympathetic innervation of the spleen. III. Development of innervation in the rat spleen. J Neurosci Res 18:49–54

Ackerman KD, Felten SY, Bellinger DL, Livnat S, Felten DL (1987b) Noradrenergic sympathetic innervation of spleen and lymph nodes in relation to specific cellular compartments. Prog Immunol 6:588–600

Ackerman KD, Felten SY, Dijkstra CD, Livnat S, Felten DL (1989) Parallel development of noradrenergic innervation and cellular compartmentation in the rat spleen. Exp Neurol 103:239–255

Ader R (1981) Psychoneuroimmunology. Academic, New York

Beckner SK, Farrar WL (1988) Potentiation of lymphokine-activated killer cell differentiation and lymphocyte proliferation by stimulation of protein kinase C or inhibition of adenylate cyclase. J Immunol 140:208–214

Bellinger DL, Felten SY, Felten DL (1988) Maintenance of noradrenergic sympathetic innervation in the involuted thymus of the aged Fischer 344 rat. Brain Behav Immun 2:133–150

Bellinger DL, Felten SY, Lorton D, Felten DL (1989) Origin of noradrenergic innervation of the spleen in rats. Brain Behav Immun 3:291–311

Berczi I (1986) Pituitary function and immunity. CRC, Boca Raton

Berczi I (1987) Hormones and immunity. MTP, Lancaster

Berecek KH, Brody MJ (1982) Evidence for a neurotransmitter role for epinephrine derived from the adrenal medulla. Am J Physiol 242:H593–H601

Berkenbosch J, van Oers J, del Rey A, Tilders J, Besedovsky H (1987) Corticotropin-releasing factor-producing neurons in the rat activated by interleukin-1. Science 238:524–526

Bernton EW, Beach JE, Holaday JW, Smallridge RC, Fein HB (1987) Release of multiple hormones by a direct action of interleukin-1 on pituitary cells. Science 238:519–521

Besedovsky HO, Sorkin E, Felix D, Haas H (1977) Hypothalamic changes during the immune response. Eur J Immunol 7:325–328

Besedovsky HO, del Rey AE, Sorkin E (1981) Lymphokine-containing supernatants from Con A-stimulated cells increase corticosterone blood levels. J Immunol 126:385–387

Besedovsky HO, del Rey AE, Sorkin E, Da Prada M, Burri R, Honegger C (1983) The immune response evokes changes in brain noradrenergic neurons. Science 221:564–565

Besedovsky HO, del Rey A, Sorkin E, Lotz W, Schwulera U (1985) Lymphoid cells produce an immunoregulatory glucocorticoid increasing factor (GIF) acting through the pituitary gland. Clin Exp Immunol 59:622–628

Besedovsky H, del Rey AE, Sorkin E, Dinarello CA (1986) Immunoregulatory feedback between interleukin-1 and glucocorticoid hormones. Science 233:652–654

Bishopric NH, Cohen HJ, Lefkowitz RJ (1980) Beta adrenergic receptors in lymphocyte subpopulations. J Allergy Clin Immunol 65:29–33

Boyle M, Yamamoto G, Chen M, Rivier J, Vale W (1988) Interleukin 1 prevents loss of corticotropic responsiveness to β-adrenergic stimulation in vitro. Proc Natl Acad Sci USA 85:5556–5560

Breder CD, Dinarello CA, Saper CB (1988) Interleukin-1 immunoreactive innervation of the human hypothalamus. Science 240:321–324

Calvo W (1968) The innervation of the bone marrow in laboratory animals. Am J Anat 123:315–328

Carlson SL, Felten DL, Livnat S, Felten SY (1987a) Alterations of monoamines in specific central autonomic nuclei following immunization in mice. Brain Behav Immun 1:52–63

Carlson SL, Felten DL, Livnat S, Felten SY (1987b) Noradrenergic sympathetic innervation of the spleen. V. Acute drug-induced depletion of lymphocytes in the target fields of innervation results in redistribution of noradrenergic fibers but maintenance of compartmentation. J Neurosci Res 18:64–69

Carlson SL, Felten SY, Livnat S, Felten DL (1987c) Splenic norepinephrine turnover is increased during an immune response in mice (Abstract). Soc Neurosci Abstr 13:380.13

Coffey RG, Hadden JW (1985) Neurotransmitters, hormones, and cyclic nucleotides in lymphocyte regulation. Fed Proc 44:112–117

Coffey RG, Hadden EM, Hadden JW (1975) Norepinephrine stimulation of lymphocyte ATPase by an alpha adrenergic receptor mechanism. Endocr Res Commun 2:179–198

del Rey AE, Besedovsky HO, Sorkin E, Da Prada M, Arrenbrechts S (1981) Immunoregulation mediated by the sympathetic nervous system. Cell Immunol 63:329–334

del Rey AE, Besedovsky HO, Sorkin E, Da Prada M, Bondiolotti GP (1982) Sympathetic immunoregulation: difference between high- and low-responder animals. Am J Physiol 242:R30–R33

Dunn A (1988) Systemic interleukin-1 administration stimulates hypothalamic norepinephrine metabolism paralleling the increased plasma corticosterone. Life Sci 43:429–435

Felten DL, Felten SY (1987) Immune interactions with specific neural structures. Brain Behav Immun 1:279–283

Felten DL, Felten SY (1989) Innervation of the thymus. In: Kendall MD (ed) Thymus update. Harwood Academic, London, pp 73–88

Felten SY, Olschowka JA (1987) Noradrenergic sympathetic innervation of the spleen. II. Tyrosine hydroxylase (TH)-positive nerve terminals form synaptic-like contacts on lymphocytes in the splenic white pulp. J Neurosci Res 18:37–48

Felten DL, Overhage JM, Felten SY, Schmedtje JF (1981) Noradrenergic sympathetic innervation of lymphoid tissue in the rabbit appendix: further evidence for a link between the nervous and immune systems. Brain Res Bull 7:595–612

Felten DL, Livnat S, Felten SY, Carlson SL, Bellinger DL, Yeh P (1984) Sympathetic innervation of lymph nodes in mice. Brain Res Bull 13:693–699

Felten DL, Felten SY, Carlson SL, Olschowka JA, Livnat S (1985) Noradrenergic and peptidergic innervation of lymphoid tissue. J Immunol 135:755s–765s

Felten SY, Housel J, Felten DL (1986) Use of in vivo dialysis for evaluation of splenic norepinephrine and serotonin. Soc Neurosci Abstr 12:1065

Felten DL, Ackerman KD, Wiegand SJ, Felten SY (1987a) Noradrenergic sympathetic innervation of the spleen. I. Nerve fibers associate with lymphocytes and macrophages in specific compartments of the splenic white pulp. J Neurosci Res 18:28–36

Felten DL, Felten SY, Bellinger DL, Carlson SL, Ackerman KD, Madden KS, Olschowka JA, Livnat S (1987b) Noradrenergic sympathetic neural interactions with the immune system: structure and function. Immunol Rev 100:225–260

Felten SY, Felten DL, Bellinger DL, Carlson SL, Ackerman KD, Madden KS, Olschowka JA, Livnat S (1988) Noradrenergic sympathetic innervation of lymphoid organs. Prog Allergy 43:14–36

Felten DL, Felten SY, Madden KS, Ackerman KD, Bellinger DL (1989) Development, maturation and sensecence of sympathetic innervation of secondary immune organs. In: Schreibman MP, Scanes CG (eds) Development, maturation and senescence of neuro-endocrine systems. Academic, New York, pp 381–396

Frohman EM, Vayuvegula B, van den Noort S, Gupta S (1988) Norepinephrine inhibits gamma-interferon-induced MHC class II (Ia) antigen expression on cultured brain astrocytes. J Neuroimmunol 17:89–101

Goetzl EJ (ed) (1985) Neuromodulation of immunity and hypersensitivity. J Immunol [Suppl] 135

Guillemin R, Cohn M, Melnechuk T (1985) Neural modulation of immunity. Raven, New York

Hadden JW, Hadden EM, Middleton E (1970) Lymphocyte blast transformation. I. Demonstration of adrenergic receptors in human peripheral lymphocytes. Cell Immunol 1:583–595

Jankovic BD, Markovic BM, Spector NH (1987) Neuroimmune interactions. Ann NY Acad Sci 496:

Landmann R, Bittiger H, Buhler FR (1981) High affinity beta-2-adrenergic receptors in mononuclear leucocytes: similar density in young and old subjects. Life Sci 29:1761–1771

Landmann R, Burgisser E, West M, Buhler FR (1985) Beta adrenergic receptors are different in subpopulations of human circulating lymphocytes. J Recept Res 4:37–50

Livnat S, Felten SY, Carlson SL, Bellinger DL, Felten DL (1985) Involvement of peripheral and central catecholamine systems in neural-immune interactions. J Neuroimmunol 10:5–30

Livnat S, Madden KS, Felten DL, Felten SY (1987) Regulation of the immune system by sympathetic neural mechanisms. Prog Neuropsychopharmacol Biol Psychiatry 11:145–152

Olschowka JA, Felten SY, Bellinger DL, Lorton D, Felten DL (1988) NPY-positive nerve terminals contact lymphocytes in the periarteriolar lymphatic sheath of the rat splenic white pulp (Abstract). Soc Neurosci Abstr 14:1280

Root-Bernstein RS, Westfall FC (1984) Serotonin binding sites. I. Structure sites on myelin basic protein. LHRH, MSH, ACTH, interferon, serum albumin, ovalbumin, and red pigment concentrating hormone. Brain Res Bull 12:425–436

Sanders VM, Munson AE (1984a) Beta-adrenoceptor mediation of the enhancing effect of norepinephrine on the murine primary antibody response in vitro. J Pharmacol Exp Ther 230:183–192

Sanders VM, Munson AE (1984b) Kinetics of the enhancing effect produced by norepinephrine and terbutaline on the murine primary antibody response in vitro. J Pharmacol Exp Ther 231:527–531

Sanders VM, Munson AE (1985a) Norepinephrine and the antibody response. Pharmacol Rev 37:229–248

Sanders VM, Munson AE (1985b) Role of alpha adrenoceptor activation in modulating the murine primary antibody response in vitro. J Pharmacol Exp Ther 232:395–400
Sanders VM, McCall CO, Horsman DA (1985) Kinetics of the alpha-2 adrenoceptor-induced inhibition of the primary antibody response in vitro. Fed Proc 44:1488
Saphier D, Abramsky O, Mor G, Ovadia H (1987) Multiunit electrical activity in conscious rats during an immune response. Brain Behav Immun 1:40–51
Sapolsky R, Rivier C, Yamamoto G, Plotsky P, Vale W (1987) Interleukin-1 stimulates the secretion of hypothalamic corticotropin-releasing factor. Science 238:522–524
Singh U (1979) Effect of catecholamines on lymphopoiesis in fetal mouse thymic explants. Eur J Immunol 14:757–759
Singh U (1985) Effect of sympathectomy on the maturation of fetal thymocytes grown within the anterior eye chambers in mice. Adv. Exp Biol Med 186:349–356
Singh U, Owen JJT (1976) Studies on the maturation of thymus stem cells – the effects of catecholamines, histamine, and peptide hormones on the expression of T alloantigens. Eur J Immunol 6:59–62
Uehara A, Gottschall PE, Dalh RR, Arimura A (1987) Stimulation of ACTH release by human interleukin-1β but not by interleukin-1α in conscious, freely-moving rats. Biochem Biophys Res Commun 146:1286–1290
von Euler US (1946) The presence of a substance with sympathin E properties in spleen extracts. Acta Physiol Scand 11:168
Weigent DA, Blalock JE (1987) Interactions between the neuroendocrine and immune systems: common hormones and receptors. Immunol Rev 100:79–108
Williams JM, Felten DL (1981) Sympathetic innervation of murine thymus and spleen: a comparative histofluorescence study. Anat Rec 199:531–542
Williams JM, Peterson RG, Shea PA, Schmedtje JF, Bauer DC, Felten DL (1981) Sympathetic innervation of murine thymus and spleen: evidence for a functional link between the nervous and immune systems. Brain Res Bull 6:83–94
Woloski BMRNJ, Smith EM, Meyer WJ, Fuller GM, Blalock JE (1985) Corticotropin-releasing activity of monokines. Science 230:1035–1037

12 Neuropeptides: Basic Research

Gene Expression of Opioid Peptides is Regulated by Electrical Activity

V. Höllt[1], K. Feasey[1], N. Kley[2], I. Moneta[1], and B. Morris[2]

A fundamental question in neurobiology is how the level of gene expression within neurones is regulated by the electrical and neurochemical signals that they receive. In the simplest model, depolarization of the cell membrane may lead not only to neurotransmitter release but also to an altered rate of transmitter synthesis. In this paper we summarize our recent data showing that depolarization of neuronal, sympathetic, and endocrine cells alter the levels of mRNA coding for the opioid peptide precursors proopiomelanocortin (POMC), proenkephalin, and prodynorphin in vitro or in vivo.

Methods

Cell Cultures. Proenkephalin gene regulation was studied in cultures of bovine chromaffin cells in vitro, as described recently (Kley et al. 1986). Regulation of the POMC gene was investigated in AtT-20/D-16v cells – a tumor cell line derived from a mouse pituitary tumor – as reported previously (von Dreden et al. 1988). Briefly, the cells were plated on 24-well dishes and maintained in Dulbecco's modified Eagle medium. The cells were allowed to attach for 2 days. Thereafter the medium was changed, the drugs added, and the cells cultered for a further 24–48 h.

In Vivo Experiments. In vivo electrical stimulation of the dentate gyrus of the hippocampus was performed in male Sprague-Dawley rats (250–300 g). A bipolar concentric electrode was stereotaxically placed in the dentate gyrus of the left hippocampus. The acute stimulation procedure consisted of five high-frequency trains (250 Hz; 250 ms; 50 V) delivered at 20-min intervals. Animals were killed 4, 7, or 22 h after stimulation (Morris et al. 1988). In the chronic stimulation procedure ("kindling") the left hippocampi were stimulated three times a day with high-frequency trains (52 Hz; 1000 ms; 0.2-ms pulses; 300–600 μA). One day after development of stage 4 kindling the rats were killed, along with corresponding sham-operated controls (Morris et al. 1987).

[1] Physiologisches Institut der Universität München, Pettenkoferstraße 12, 8000 München 2, FRG.
[2] Max-Planck-Institut für Psychiatrie, Am Klopferspitz 18a, 8033 Martinsried, FRG.

Neuropsychopharmacology
Edited by Bunney/Hippius/Laakmann/Schmauß

RNA Measurements. Total RNA was extracted from hippocampal tissue using the lithium chloride technique (Auffray and Rougeon 1980). Total RNA from cultured cells was isolated using the acid thiocyanate phenolchloroform extraction (Chomczynski and Sacchi 1987). Aliquots of the RNA extracts were subjected either to dot blot analysis (White and Bancroft 1982) or to Northern blot analysis after separation by gel electrophoresis and transfer to nylon filters (Nytran; Schleicher and Schuell). The filters were hybridized with ^{32}P-labeled probes complementary to mouse POMC, rat and bovine proenkephalin, and rat prodynorphin mRNAs. Preparation of the cRNA probes has recently been described (von Dreden et al. 1988; Morris et al. 1988). After hybridization the filters were apposed to X-ray film, and the autoradiograms were scanned by a densitometer. In addition to Northern blot analysis, RNA samples isolated from the bovine chromaffin cells were measured by solution hybridization as described (Pittius et al. 1985).

In Situ Hybridization. Cryostat sections (10 μm) of rat brains were mounted onto slides. Fixation, denaturation, and hybridization conditions were as described by Morris et al. (1986). For determination of proenkephalin mRNA, in situ hybridization was carried out using a nick-translated ^{32}P-proenkephalin probe; in case of prodynorhpin mRNA a 100-base radiolabeled oligonucleotide was used. After hybridization the sections were apposed to X-ray film. Densitometric measurements were conducted using a Leitz-Texture Analysis System with microscope-linked densitometer.

Results

Effect of Membrane-Depolarizing Agents on Proenkephalin mRNA Levels in Cultured Bovine Chromaffin Cells. Figure 1 shows the effect of various membrane-depolarizing agents on mRNA levels coding for proenkephalin in cultured bovine adrenal chromaffin cells after treatment for 48 h. Depolarization with 20 m*M* K^+ increased the levels of proenkephalin mRNA to 85% above control. After treatment with veratridine – a substance which depolarizes cells by activating voltage-sensitive Na channels – a particularly high increase in proenkephalin mRNA (fourfold) was observed. The effects of veratridine and of K^+ were antagonized by the specific Na^+ channel blocker tetrodotoxin (TTX). TTX itself did not inhibit the basal levels of proenkephalin mRNA. The involvement of Ca^{2+} channels in the effect of K^+ and veratridine is also shown in Fig. 1. The Ca^{2+} blocker D 600 markedly reduced the stimulatory effect of high K^+ and of veratridine. In contrast, BAY K 8644 – a compound which increases the opening time of the voltage-sensitive Ca^{2+} channels – potentiated the K^+-induced increase in cellular levels of proenkephalin mRNA. However, D 600 and BAY K 8644 did not alter the basal levels of proenkephalin mRNA in the chromaffin cells.

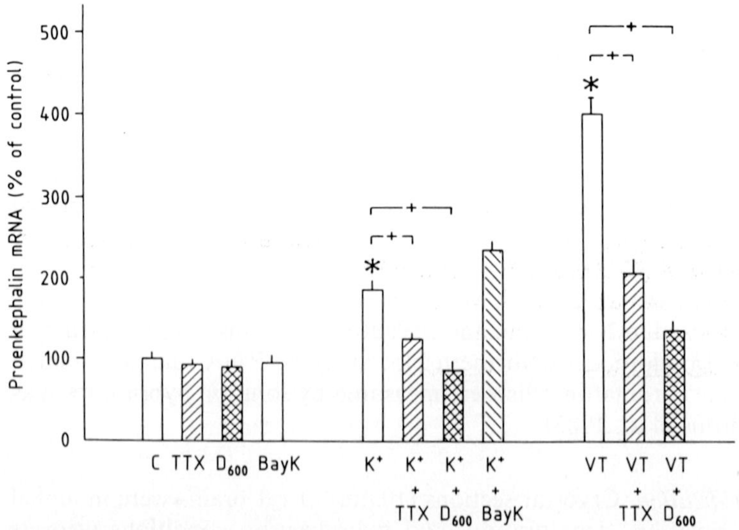

Fig. 1. Effect of depolarizing agents K^+ (20 m*M*) and veratridine (*VT*; 10 μ*M*) on the proenkephalin mRNA levels in primary cultures of bovine chromaffin cells and its modulation by tetrodotoxin (*TTX*; 1 μ*M*), D 600 (50 μ*M*), and BAY K 8644 (*BayK*; 0.1 μ*M*). Cells were treated for 48 h as described in text. Values represent means ±SEM from six cultures. *Asterisks*, $p < 0.01$ compared with control; *pluses*, $p < 0.05$ compared with respective stimulated condition (one-way analysis of variance, Newman Keul's test)

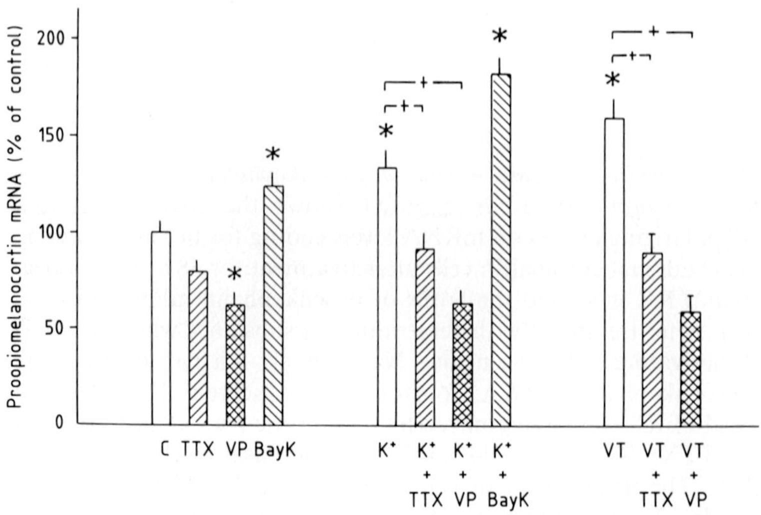

Fig. 2. Effect of depolarizing agents K^+ (20 μ*M*) and veratridine (*VT*; 10 μ*M*) on the levels of POMC mRNAS in mouse AtT-20 pituitary tumor cells and its modulation by tetrodotoxin (*TTX*; 1 μ*M*), verapamil (*VP*; 50 μ*M*), and BAY K 8644 (*BayK*; 0.1 μ*M*). Cells were treated for 48 h as described in text. Values represent means ±SEM of six cultures. *Asterisks*, $p < 0.05$ compared with control; *pluses*, $p < 0.05$ with respective stimulated condition (one-way analysis of variance, Scheffe's test)

Effect of Membrane Depolarization on the Levels of POMC mRNA in Cultured Pituitary Tumor Cells In Vitro. Figure 2 shows that 20 mM K^+ and 10 μM veratridine increase the levels of POMC mRNA in mouse AtT-20 pituitary tumor cells. This effect was antagonized by the Na^+ channel blocker TTX and by the Ca^{2+} channel blocker verapamil. In addition, the Ca^{2+} agonist BAY K 8644 potentiated the stimulatory effect of K^+ on POMC mRNA levels in the pituitary cells. In contrast to the chromaffin cells, the Ca^{2+} channel modulating drugs (verapamil, BAY K 8644) altered the POMC mRNA levels in the AtT-20 cells also under basal conditions.

Effect of Electrical Stimulation of the Dentate Gyrus on the Levels of Proenkephalin and Prodynorphin mRNA in the Hippocampus In Vivo. Figure 3 shows sections of rat brain after in situ hybridization with prodynorphin or proenkephalin cDNA probes. Within the hippocampus, mRNA coding for prodynorphin is localized within the granule cell layer of the dentate gyrus, as indicated by the high grain density in this structure (Fig. 3 A, D). Electrical stimulation of the left gyrus dentatus with five high-frequency pulses caused a decrease in the level of prodynorphin mRNA (Fig. 3 B) and an increase in the level of proenkephalin mRNA (Fig. 3 C) at the site ipsilateral to the stimulation. Continuous stimulation of the left hippocampus three times daily, which

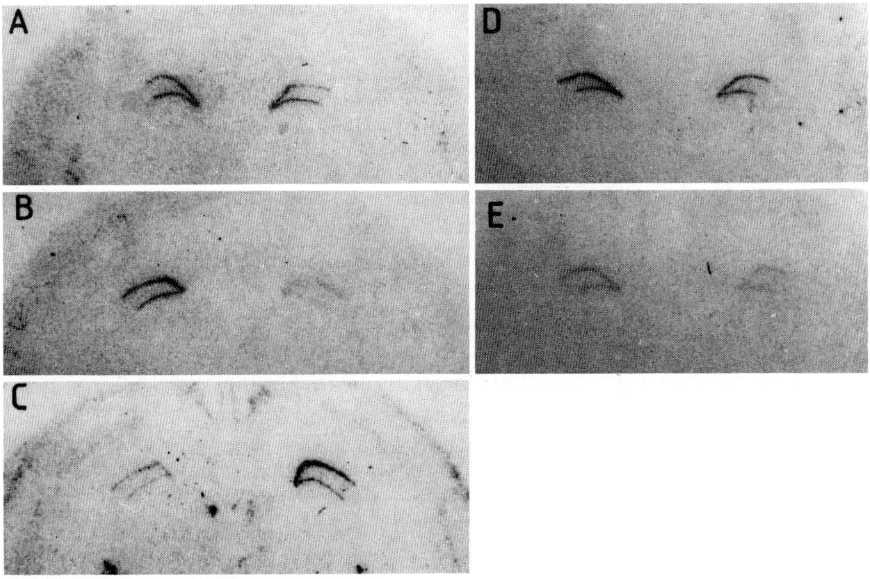

Fig. 3 A–E. Effect of unilateral electrical stimulation on levels of prodynorphin and proenkephalin mRNA in rat hippocampus. Sections were taken from sham-stimulated animals (**A, D**) and from animals 22 h after stimulation of the left dentate gyrus (*right side;* **B, C** and rats in which the left dentate gyrus was chronically stimulated to induce stage 4 kindled rats (**E**). Sections were hybridized with prodynorphin (**A, B, D, E**) or proenkephalin (**C**) cDNA probes. Exposure time was 28 days

results in stage 4 kindling, caused a disappearance of the grain densities overlaying the granule cell layers not only at the ipsilateral but also at the contralateral site (Fig. 3 E versus Fig. 3 D).

Discussion

The present paper summarizes results showing that opioid peptide mRNAs are modulated by depolarizing stimuli in vitro and by direct electrical stimulation of cells in vivo. An increase in the levels of mRNA coding for proenkephalin and POMC was observed after treatment of bovine chromaffin cells and of anterior pituitary cells after depolarization with high K^+ and with veratridine. These effects were completely prevented by the specific Na^+ channel blocker TTX, indicating that membrane depolarization increased POMC mRNA by an activation of voltage-dependent Na^+ channels. On the other hand, TTX did not alter proenkephalin or POMC mRNA levels under basal (nonstimulated) conditions. This suggests that Na^+ channels play no major role in maintaining basal levels of opioid peptide gene expression.

The stimulatory effect of veratridine and K^+ was completely abolished by the Ca^{2+} channel blocker verapamil or D600. In contrast, BAY K 8644 – a drug which holds Ca^{2+} channels in an open state – augmented the effect of high K^+.

These results indicate that membrane depolarization which activates voltage-dependent Na^+ and Ca^{2+} channels initiates an entry of calcium ions which trigger the gene expression of proenkephalin in chromaffin and of POMC mRNA in AtT-20 pituitary cells. In the AtT-20 cells an entry of Ca^{2+} ions may exert a tonic stimulatory effect on POMC gene expression under basal conditions which can be inhibited by Ca^{2+} channel blockers. In contrast, an influx of Ca^{2+} ions does not regulate the expression of the proenkephalin gene in non-stimulated chromaffin cells. There is now an increasing amount of data showing that Ca^{2+} influx plays a critical role not only in excitation-secretion coupling but also in the mechanisms linking excitation of neuronal or endocrine cells to long-term adaptive changes in the biosynthesis of neuropeptides. For instance, Ca^{2+} ions have been implicated in the control of prolactin gene expression in pituitary cells (Bancroft et al. 1985).

In contrast to the observation on cultured bovine chromaffin cells (Kley et al. 1986; Naranjo et al. 1986), depolarization with K^+ has been shown to decrease the proenkephalin mRNA in organ cultures of intact rat adrenal medullae (Black et al. 1984; LaGamma et al. 1985). Although this discrepancy may reflect species differences, pilot experiments in our laboratory clearly showed that high K^+ increases proenkephalin mRNA also in cultured adrenal medullary chromaffin cells of the rat. This finding indicates that the regulation of the proenkephalin gene in cultured chromaffin cells is different from that in whole adrenal medullary tissue. In fact, there appears to exist a tonic inhibitory control of proenkephalin gene expression by neural activity in vivo, since denervation of the splanchnic nerve in rats results in an increase in the level of proenkephalin mRNA in the adrenal medullae (Kilpatrick et al. 1984). On the other hand, an increase in the impulse activity of the splanchnic nerve by stress or insulin treatment of rats in vivo causes an increase in the expression of the proenkephalin gene in the adrenal medulla (Kanamatsu et al. 1986; Fischer-Colbrie et al. 1988). The reasons for these discrepant observations are unknown.

Interestingly, direct electrical stimulation of the dentate gyrus in vivo also causes an increase in the proenkephalin mRNA levels in the granule cells of the hippocampus. Moreover, preliminary studies with primary cultures of fetal brain tissue indicated that depolarization with K^+ or veratridine increases proenkephalin mRNA levels in rat forebrain cultures (Simantov and Höllt, unpublished data). Taken together, our results indicate that an increase in the electrical activity of neuronal and sympathetic cells results in an increase in the gene expression of proenkephalin. Similarly, electrical activation of pituitary cells results in an increase in the expression of the POMC gene. In contrast, electrical stimulation of the hippocampus results in a decrease in the level of mRNA coding for prodynorphin. This result suggests that the prodynorphin gene is negatively regulated by electrical activity. Whereas the decrease in the prodynorphin mRNA levels in the dentate gyrus is observed initially only at the site of stimulation, chronic stimulation results in a decrease in the prodynorphin mRNA also in the contralateral hippocampus. This indicates that long-term stimulation may result in plasticity changes in brain areas distant from the site of stimulation.

The stimulation parameters used for hippocampus stimulation can induce long-term potentiation and kindling in animals. The increase in activity of the proenkephalinergic system, which has excitatory effects, and the decrease in the prodynorphin system, which may have mainly inhibitory effects on hippocampal pyramidal cells (Siggins and Gruol 1986), raise the intriguing possibility that the substantial alteration in opioid gene expression in granule cells may contribute to the maintainance of long-term potentiation and kindling.

A relatively long time period (more than 4 h) is required before changes in opioid peptide mRNA levels become manifest after stimulation. On the other hand, activation of voltage-dependent Ca^{2+} channels has been shown rapidly to induce (within minutes) the expression of the *fos* proto-oncogene (Morgan and Curran 1987). It is possible that c-*fos* or a similarly acting transcription factor plays a role in the early events of the gene expression of opioid peptides.

References

Auffray C, Rougeon F (1980) Purification of mouse immunoglobin heavy chain mRNAs from total myeloma tumor RNA. Eur J Biochem 303–312

Bancroft FC, Gick GG, Johnson ME, White BA (1985) Regulation of growth hormone and prolactin gene expression by hormones and calcium. In: Litwack G (ed) Biochemical actions of hormones, vol 12. Academic, New York, pp 173–183

Black IB, Adler JE, Dreyfus GM, Jonakait, Katz DM, LaGamma EF, Markey KM (1984) Neurotransmitter plasticity at the molecular level. Science 225:1266–1270

Chomzynski P, Sacchi N (1987) Single-step method of RNA isolation by acid guanidinium thiocyanate-phenol-chloroform extraction. Anal Biochem 162:156–159

Fischer-Colbrie R, Iacangelo A, Eiden LE (1988) Neural and humoral factors separately regulate neuropeptide Y, enkephalin and chromagranin A and B mRNA levels in rat adrenal medulla. Proc Natl Acad Sci USA 85:3240–3244

Kanamatsu T, Unsworth CD, Diliberto EJ, Viveros OH, Hong JS (1986) Reflex splanchnic nerve stimulation increases levels of proenkephalin A mRNA and proenkephalin A-related peptides in the rat adrenal medulla. Proc Natl Acad Sci USA 83:9245–9249

Kilpatrick DL, Howells RD, Fleminger G, Udenfriend S (1984) Denervation of rat adrenal glands markedly increases preproenkephalin mRNA. Proc Natl Acad Sci USA 81:7221–7223

Kley N, Loeffler JP, Pittius CW, Höllt V (1986) Proenkephalin A gene expression in bovine adrenal chromaffin cells is regulated by changes in electrical activity. EMBO J 5:967–970

LaGamma EF, White JD, Adler JE, Krause JE, McKelvy JF, Black IB (1985) Depolarization regulates adrenal preproenkephalin mRNA. Proc Natl Acad Sci USA 82:8252–8255

Morgan JI, Curran T (1986) Role of ion flux in the control of c-*fos* expression. Nature 322:552–555

Morris BJ, Haarmann I, Kempter B, Höllt V, Herz A (1986) Localization of prodynorphin messenger RNA in rat brain by in situ hybridization using a synthetic oligonucleotide probe. Neurosci Lett 69:104–108

Morris BJ, Moneta ME, ten Bruggencate G, Höllt V (1987) Levels of prodynorphin mRNA in rat dentate gyrus are decreased during hippocampal kindling. Neurosci Lett 80:298–302

Morris BJ, Feasey KJ, ten Bruggencate G, Herz A, Höllt V (1988) Electrical stimulation in vivo increases the expression of proenkephalin mRNA and decreases the expression of prodynorphin mRNA in rat hippocampal granule cell. Proc Natl Acad Sci USA 85:3226–3230

Naranjo JR, Mocchetti I, Schwartz JP, Costa E (1986) Permissive effect of dexamethasone on the increase of proenkephalin mRNA induced by depolarization of chromaffin cells. Proc Natl Acad Sci USA 83:1513–1517

Pittius CW, Kley N, Loeffler JP, Höllt V (1985) Quantitation of proenkephalin A messenger RNA in bovine brain, pituitary and adrenal medulla: correlation between mRNA and peptide levels. EMBO J 4:1257–1260

Siggins GR, Gruol DL (1987) Mechanisms of transmitter action in the vertebrate central nervous system. In: Bloom FE (ed) Handbook of physiology. The nervous system, vol 4. American Physiological Society, Bethesda, pp 1–114

von Dreden G, Loeffler JP, Grimm C, Höllt V (1988) Influence of calcium ions on proopiomelanocortin mRNA levels in clonal anterior pituitary cells. Neuroendocrinology 47:32–37

White BA, Bancroft FC (1982) Cytoplasmic dot hybridization. Simple analysis of relative mRNA levels in multiple small cells or tissue samples. J Biol Chem 257:8569–8573

Biosynthesis of Opioid Peptides

J. Rossier[1]

All endogenous opioid peptides have at their amino-terminal a characteristic amino acid sequence, Tyr-Gly-Gly-Phe-Met or Tyr-Gly-Gly-Phe-Leu. These sequences were initially discovered by Hughes et al. (1975) and named enkephalin. Later it was realized that the opioid peptides constitute three distinct families – endorphins, enkephalins, and dynorphins (Table 1) – organized in three different neuronal systems within the central nervous system (Patey and Rossier 1986). Molecular genetic techniques have shown that these three families of opioid peptides are synthesized by three distinct precursors:

Table 1. Amino acid sequences of the principal opioid peptides derived from the three different protein precursors

Peptides derived from proopiomelanocortin	
β-Endorphin (human):	*Tyr-Gly-Gly-Phe-Met*-Thr-Ser-Glu-Lys-Ser-Gln-Thr-Pro-Leu-Val-Thr-Leu-Phe-Lys-Asn-Ala-Ile-Ile-Lys-Asn-Ala-Tyr-Lys-Lys-Gly-Glu
β-Endorphin (1–27)	
β-Endorphin (1–26)	
α-Endorphin:	β-endorphin (1–16)
γ-Endorphin:	β-endorphin (1–17)
Peptides derived from proenkephalin (or proenkephalin A)	
[Met^{5}]enkephalin:	*Tyr-Gly-Gly-Phe-Met*
[Leu^{5}]enkephalin:	*Tyr-Gly-Gly-Phe-Leu*
Heptapeptide:	*Tyr-Gly-Gly-Phe-Met*-Arg-Phe
Octapeptide:	*Tyr-Gly-Gly-Phe-Met*-Arg-Gly-Leu
Peptides derived from prodynorphin (or proenkephalin B)	
Dynorphin A (1–17):	*Tyr-Gly-Gly-Phe-Leu*-Arg-Arg-Ile-Arg-Pro-Lys-Leu-Lys-Trp-Asp-Asn-Gln
Dynorphin A (1–8):	*Tyr-Gly-Gly-Phe-Leu*-Arg-Arg-Ile
Dynorphin B:	*Tyr-Gly-Gly-Phe-Leu*-Arg-Arg-Gln-Phe-Lys-Val-Val-Thr
α-Neoendorphin:	*Tyr-Gly-Gly-Phe-Leu*-Arg-Lys-Tyr-Pro-Lys
β-Neoendorphin:	*Tyr-Gly-Gly-Phe-Leu*-Arg-Lys-Tyr-Pro

[Met^{5}]enkephalin or [Leu^{5}]enkephalin sequences present in each peptide are in italics.

[1] Laboratoire de Physiologie Nerveuse du CNRS, 91198 Gif-sur-Yvette Cedex, France.

Neuropsychopharmacology
Edited by Bunney/Hippius/Laakmann/Schmauß

1. Proopiomelanocortin makes endorphins as well as adrenocorticotrophin hormone and melanotrophin hormones (Fig. 1).
2. Proenkephalin makes four copies of [Met^5]enkephalin, one copy of [Leu^5]enkephalin, and two other peptides derived from [Met^5]enkephalin, the heptapeptide [Met^5]enkephalin-Arg^6-Phe^7 and the octapeptide [Met^5]enkephalin-Arg^6-Gly^7-Leu^8 (Fig. 2). This molecule has been isolated in brain (Beaumont et al. 1985); fragments of it have been found in large amounts in the bovine adrenal medulla (Patey et al. 1984; Metters and Rossier 1987).
3. Prodynorphin leads to dynorphin A, dynorphin B (or rimorphin), and to α- and β-neoendorphins. All the prodynorphin-derived peptides have a sequence of [Leu^5]enkephalin at their amino-terminal (Fig. 3).

All the active opioid peptides are therefore synthesized in the form of preprohormones, usually having at their N-terminal extremity a hydrophobic sequence of about 20 amino acids known as the signal peptide. The biologically active peptide sequences are generally bracketed by pairs of basic amino acids which serve as signals to the enzymes involved in the maturation process of the precursor (Fig. 4).

The most common scheme for enzymatic maturation of precursors proposes the action of a trypsinlike endopeptidase followed by a carboxypeptidase B-like exopeptidase (Fig. 5). However, we have provided evidence that this combination of trypsinlike and carboxypeptidase B-like enzymes may not be the only mechanism for liberating enkephalin from low molecular weight enkephalin-containing peptides. Endo-oligopeptidase A, an enzyme known to hydrolyse the Phe^5-Ser^6 bond of bradykinin and the Arg^8-Arg^9 bond of neurotensin, has been shown to produce by a single cleavage [Leu^5]enkephalin or [Met^5]enkephalin from small enkephalin-containing peptides (Camargo et al. 1987; Toffoletto et al. 1988). The optimal substrate size was found to be 8–13 amino acids, with enkephalin the only product released from precursors in which this sequence is immediately followed by a pair of basic residues.

A great homology exists in the organization of precursors of the opioid peptides and their genes (Fig. 6). This is also true for several other families of neuropeptides. Like most of the proteins, precursors of opioid peptides have probably evolved from common gene ancestors. The organization of the three precursors of the opioid peptides is therefore very similar. The N-terminal parts, which represent at least one-third of the sequence, contain four to six cysteinyl residues. The multiple sequences of opioid peptides represent only 10%–15% of the whole sequence and are located toward the C-terminal sequence of precursors. Our recent studies on synenkephalin, the N-terminal part of proenkephalin, have shown that this sequence, which does not contain opioid peptides, is not destroyed during the processing of the precursor (Liston et al. 1983; Fig. 2). Synenkephalin is released in equimolar ratio along with the other peptides resulting from the maturation of the precursor (Liston and Rossier 1984). It must be stressed that when endorphinergic, enkephalinergic, or dynorphinergic neurons are activated, the opioid peptides released represent

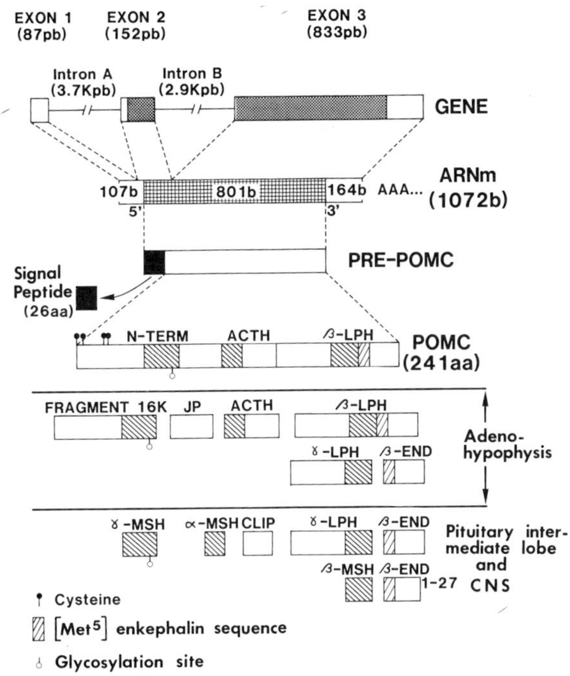

Fig. 1. Biosynthesis and maturation of proopiomelanocortin. The upper part of the figure illustrates the biosynthesis of human proopiomelanocortin from the corresponding gene. For practical reasons, the 5′ end of the gene upstream from the first exon and the 3′ end of the gene downstream from the third exon have not been represented in the figure. The gene is composed of three exons containing 87, 152, and 833 base pairs (*pb*), respectively, separated by two introns of 3.7 and 2.9 kilobasepairs (*kpb*). The three exons are transcribed into a messenger RNA (*ARNm*) 1072 bases long, to the 3′ end of which is added a polyadenylated tail (*AAA*...). This messenger RNA possesses a 5′ noncoding region 107 bases long and a 3′ noncoding region 164 bases long, which are not translated. Translation of the coding part of the messenger RNA (801 bases) gives rise to pre-proopiomelanocortin (*PRE-POMC*). Like other precursors of secreted peptides, its amino-terminal part is constituted by a short sequence of hydrophobic amino acids, the signal peptide. In the case of human pre-proopiomelanocortin, this peptide comprises the first 26 amino acids of the precursor. The signal peptide is cleaved by the signal peptidase during the transfer of the precursor across the membrane of the endoplasmic reticulum. Proopiomelanocortin (*POMC*), which results from this cleavage, undergoes proteolytic maturation and gives rise to biologically active peptides. Human proopiomelanocortin is a 241 amino acid long protein. Its amino-terminal part is glycosylated, rich in cysteine residues. Biologically active peptides are grouped in the carboxy-terminal part of the protein. In the lower part of the figure are represented the different peptides which result from the maturation of proopiomelanocortin in the anterior and intermediate lobes of the hypophysis and in the central nervous system. *MSH*, Melanophore-stimulating hormone; *ACTH*, adrenocorticotropin hormone; *END*, endorphin; *LPH*, lipotropin; *JP*, joining peptide; *CLIP*, corticotrophin-like intermediate lobe peptide

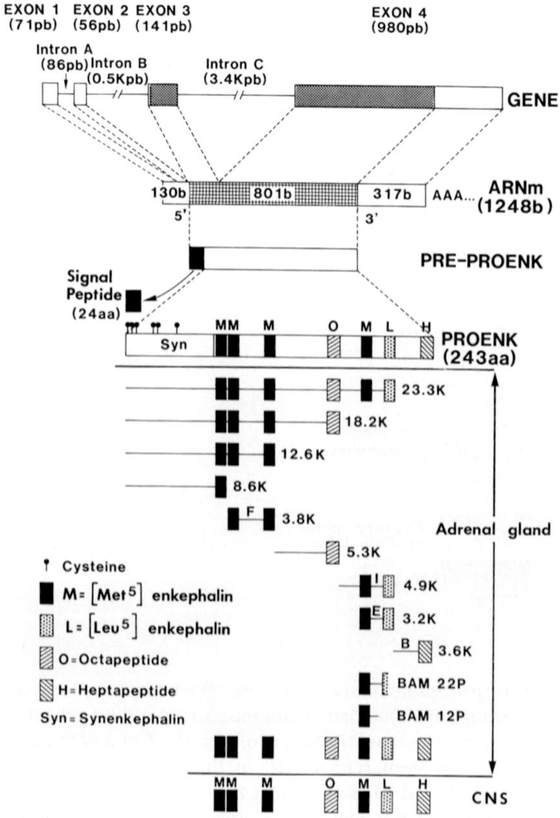

Fig. 2. Biosynthesis and maturation of proenkephalin. The upper part of the figure describes the biosynthesis of human proenkephalin from the corresponding gene. For practical reasons, the 5′ end of the gene upstream from the first exon and the 3′ end of the gene downstream from the fourth exon have not been represented in the figure. The gene is composed of four exons containing 71, 56, 141, and 980 basepairs (*pb*), respectively, separated by three introns of 86 base pairs, 0.5, and 3.4 kilobasepairs (*kpb*). The four exons are transcribed into a messenger RNA (*ARNm*) 1248 bases long, to the 3′ end of which is added a polyadenylated tail (*AAA*...). This messenger RNA possesses a 5′ noncoding region 130 bases long and a 3′ noncoding region 317 bases long, which are not translated. Translation of the coding part of the messenger RNA (801 bases) gives rise to pre-proenkephalin (*PRE-PROENK*). Like other precursors of secreted peptides, its amino-terminus is constituted by a short sequence of hydrophobic amino acids, the signal peptide. In the case of human pre-proenkephalin, this peptide comprises the first 24 amino acids of the precursor. The signal peptide is cleaved by the signal peptidase during the transfer of the precursor across the membrane of the endoplasmic reticulum. Proenkephalin (*PROENK*), which results from this cleavage, undergoes proteolytic maturation and gives rise to biologically active peptides. Human proenkephalin is a 243 amino acid long protein. Its amino-terminal part is rich in cystein residues and devoid of opioid activity and has been called synenkephalin (Liston et al. 1983). The sequences of opioid peptides are grouped in the carboxy-terminal part of the protein. In the lower part of the figure are schematically represented all the peptides derived from proenkephalin which have been purified or characterized from bovine adrenal medulla, as well as the opioid peptides [Met^5]enkephalin, [Leu^5]enkephalin, [Met^5]-enkephalin-Arg^6-Phe^7, and [Met^5]-enkephalin-Arg^6-Gly^7-Leu^8, which are also present in this tissue. These four opioid peptides have been found also in the central nervous system of several species

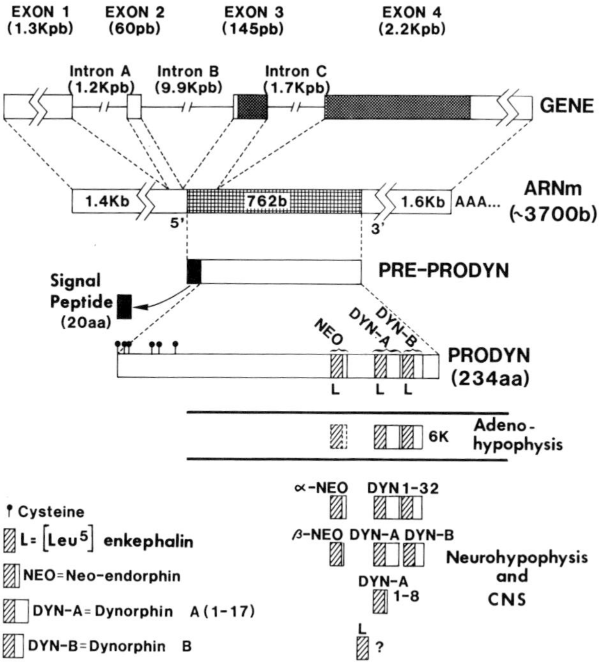

Fig. 3. Biosynthesis and maturation of prodynorphin. The upper part of the figure describes the biosynthesis of human prodynorphin from the corresponding gene. For practical reasons, the 5′ end of the gene upstream from the first exon and the 3′ end of the gene downstream from the fourth exon have not been represented in the figure. The gene is composed of four exons containing 1.3 kilobasepairs (*kpb*) 60 basepairs (*pb*) 145 basepairs, and 2.2 kilobasepairs, respectively, separated by three introns of 1.2, 9.9, and 1.7 kilobasepairs. The four exons of the gene are transcribed into a messenger RNA (*ARNm*) approximately 3700 bases long, to the 3′ end of which is added a polyadenylated tail (*AAA*...). This messenger RNA possesses a 5′ noncoding region 1.4 kilobases long and a 3′ noncoding region 1.6 kilobases long, which are not translated. Translation of the coding part of the messenger RNA (762 bases) gives rise to pre-prodynorphin (*PRE-PRODYN*). Like other precursors of secreted peptides, its amino-terminus is constituted by a short sequence of hydrophobic amino acids, the signal peptide. In the case of human pre-prodynorphin, this peptide comprises the first 20 amino acids of the precursor. The signal peptide is cleaved by the signal peptidase during the transfer of the precursor across the membrane of the endoplasmic reticulum. Prodynorphin (*PRODYN*), which results from this cleavage, undergoes maturation and gives rise to biologically active peptides. Human prodynorphin is a 234 amino acid long protein. Its amino-terminal part is rich in cysteine residues. The sequences of opioid peptides are grouped in the carboxy-terminal part of the protein. In the lower part of the figure are represented the peptides resulting from the maturation of prodynorphin in the anterior lobe of the hypophysis, in the neurohypophysis and the central nervous system

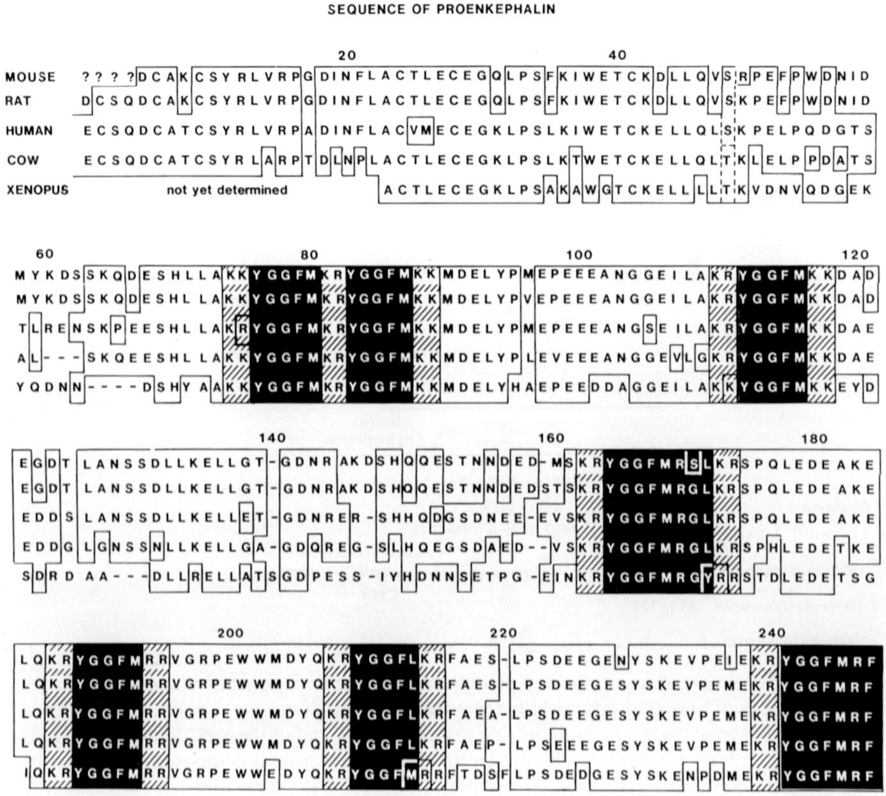

Fig. 4. Comparison of mouse, rat, human, bovine, and *Xenopus* proenkephalin sequences. This figure represents the amino acid sequences (expressed according to the one-letter code) of the five proenkephalin molecules known at the present time. The sequence of *Xenopus* and mouse proenkephalin is not yet completely known, as shown by the space in the first line. The sequences have been aligned as to obtain the maximum homologies. The sequences of the opioid peptides (Met-enkephalin, Leu-enkephalin, heptapeptide, and octapeptide) are represented on a *dark background*. Note that in the *Xenopus* proenkephalin the sequence of Leu-enkephalin is replaced by a sequence of Met-enkephalin, and that the last amino acid of the octapeptide is a tyrosine whereas the corresponding amino acid in the four other species is a leucine. Note also in the case of the mouse the presence of Ser[7] instead of Gly[7] in the octapeptide sequence. The most important homologies between the sequences are found in three regions. The first region is constituted by the amino-terminal half of synenkephalin. Synenkephalin is the amino-terminal part of proenkephalin, which extends to the first Met-enkephalin sequence. A marked homology between the proenkephalin sequences is found also in the region comprising the first three Met-enkephalin sequences. Finally, starting from the octapeptide sequence, the carboxy-terminal parts of the four proenkephalin sequences are almost identical. It is worth noting that certain regions in the sequences from species as far phylogenetically as human and *Xenopus* are identical, suggesting that these regions may play a major role in the structure and/or function of this protein

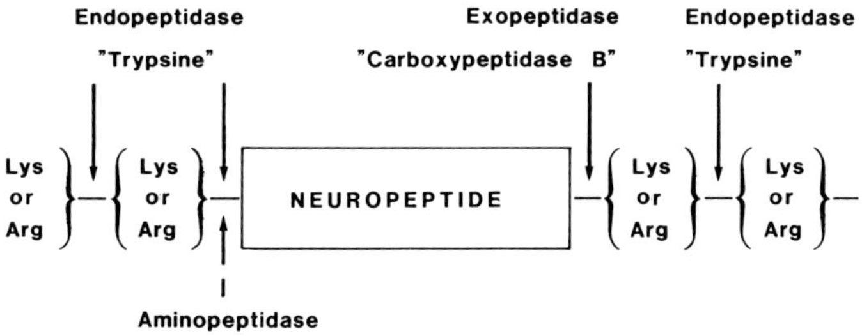

Fig. 5. Model of the maturation of neuropeptide precursors, involving two peptidases with substrate specificities close to those of trypsin and carboxypeptidase B, and possibly an aminopeptidase

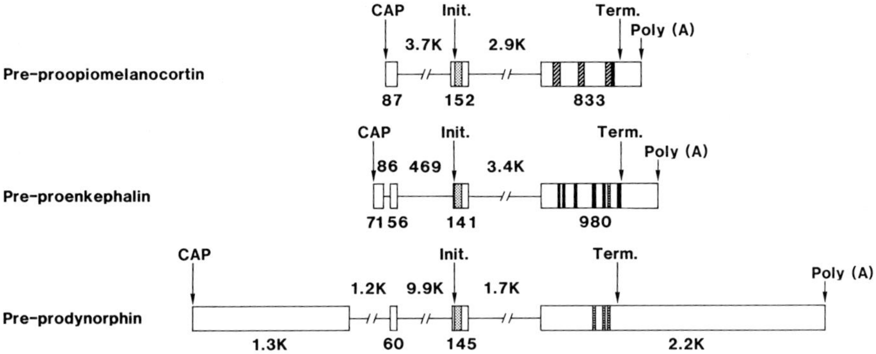

Fig. 6. Comparison of the structures of the human genes coding for the three precursors of opioid peptides. This figure represents the genes coding for human pre-proopiomelanocortin, pre-proenkephalin, and pre-prodynorphin. The 5′ end of the genes upstream from the first exons and the 3′ end of the genes downstream from the last exons are not represented on the figure. The exons are represented by *rectangles*. The length of each exon is indicated under the corresponding exon in basepairs or kilobasepairs (*k*). Introns are represented by the *lines between exons*; their lengths are indicated above each one. The sites of initiation (*Init.*) and termination (*Term.*) of translation into protein of the messenger RNA coded for by each gene are indicated above the corresponding gene. *Shaded area* in each gene represents the region of the gene coding for the signal peptide. *Cross-hatched areas* in the third exon of pre-proopiomelanocortin gene code for MSH sequences, and *thick black bar* after the last cross-hatched area represents the Met-enkephalin sequence of β-endorphin. *Thick black bars* in the fourth exon of the pre-proenkephalin gene code for the sequences of Met-enkephalin or related opioid peptides (heptapeptide and octapeptide), and *area containing horizontal bars* codes for the Leu-enkephalin sequence. In the fourth exon of the pre-prodynorphin gene, *areas containing horizontal bars* code for Leu-enkephalin sequences. *CAP*, Site of capping of messenger RNA; *Poly (A)*, site of polyadenylation of messenger RNA

only a small proportion of the material released by these neurons. What happens to the released nonopioid peptides? We may suppose that they are destroyed by the many membrane peptidases present in the CNS. The function of these peptidases would be not only to inactivate the active neuropeptides (Patey et al. 1985) but also to transform the inactive peptides into more diffusible amino acids.

What is the role of the synenkephalin and the other presumably inactive peptides that sometimes amount to more than 90% of the precursor sequence? We may presume that they are necessary to provide an adequate three-dimensional structure for the precursors. These three-dimensional structures should also allow the precursors to resist degradation by nonspecific peptidases. Recent experiments from our laboratory have also indicated that the three-dimensional structure is also important in targeting the appropriate cleavage by enzymes involved in the maturation process. The fragments of precursors, by-products of the maturation process, may also have physiological roles not yet defined. In the case of proopiomelanocortin, the N-terminal part would have a mitogenic effect on the adrenal cortex.

Several recent results show that the maturation process of precursors is not identical in all tissues. From the same precursor, different products can be obtained. This has been clearly shown for the three peptide opioid precursors (Liston et al. 1984). This heterogeneity among the final products might indicate the existence of several different enzymes implicated in the maturation of precursors.

Recently we have proposed that processing of proenkephalin could also take place in the blood by hydrolysis by the proleolytic enzyme known as plasma kallikrein (Metters et al. 1988). Plasma kallikrein is an enzyme involved in blood coagulation and also in the formation of the nonapeptide bradykinin from circulating kininogen of high molecular weight.

The ability of plasma kallikrein selectively to cleave *in vitro* several biologically active peptide precursors at sites shown to be cleaved *in vivo* has led to the proposal that this enzyme could play a widespread role in prohormone maturation (Metters et al. 1988). In a recent study it was shown that human plasma kallikrein also displays a strong preference for cleavage at pairs of basic amino acids within proenkephalin-derived peptides, suggesting that this enzyme may be involved in the processing of this precursor. The exact role that plasma kallikrein could play as a putative proenkephalin-converting enzyme remains to be established. An attractive model would postulate the involvement of plasma kallikrein in the extracellular maturation of precursors, either during or after their release into the circulation. This mechanism has already been proposed for the conversion of proatrial natriuretic factor into the major circulating form ANF_{99-126}. This type of model could also apply to the maturation of proenkephalin. The chromaffin granules of the adrenal medulla contain high concentrations of proenkephalin-derived peptides. Processing within this tissue is judged to be incomplete since the majority of enkephalin is present in the form of intermediates with higher molecular weights (Patey et al. 1984; Liston et al. 1984). Moreover, these biologically inactive, high molecular weight enkephalin precursors have been shown to be released both *in vitro* and *in vivo* in response to various stimuli (Chaminade et al. 1984; Rossier et al. 1988). Relatively little work has been done to characterize the circulating forms of proenkephalin-derived peptides. However, both enkephalin and enkephalin congeners have been detected in the plasma. Therefore, although several putative enkephalin-converting enzymes have been partially purified from bovine adrenal medulla chromaffin granules and may be responsible for the limited maturation within the gland, it is also possible that the released precursors are further processed extracellularly. Plasma kallikrein, displaying the strict selectivity of cleavage toward proenkephalin would be a good candidate enzyme for this style of maturation.

References

Beaumont A, Metters KM, Rossier J, Hughes J (1985) Identification of a proenkephalin precursor in striatal tissue. J Neurochem 44:934–939

Camargo ACM, Oliveira EB, Toffoletto O, Metters KM, Rossier J (1987) Brain endo-oligopeptidase A, a putative enkephalin converting enzyme. J Neurochem 48:1258–1263

Chaminade M, Foutz AS, Rossier J (1984) Co-release of enkephalins and precursors with catecholamines from the perfused cat adrenal gland in situ. J Physiol 353:157–169

Hughes J, Smith TW, Kosterlitz HW, Fothergill LA, Morgan BA, Morris HR (1975) Identification of two related pentapeptides from the brain with potent opiate agonist activity. Nature 258:577–579

Liston DR, Rossier J (1984) Synenkephalin is coreleased with Met-enkephalin from neuronal terminals *in vitro*. Neurosci Lett 48:211–216

Liston DR, Vanderhaeghen JJ, Rossier J (1983) Presence in brain of synenkephalin, a proenkephalin-immunoreactive protein which does not contain enkephalin. Nature 302:62–65

Liston DR, Patey G, Rossier J, Verbanck P, Vanderhaeghen JJ (1984) Processing of proenkephalin is tissue-specific. Science 225:734–737

Metters KM, Rossier J (1987) Affinity purification of synenkephalin-containing peptides, including a novel 23.3-kilodalton species. J Neurochem 49:721–728

Metters KM, Rossier J, Paquin J, Chrétien M, Seidah NG (1988) Selective cleavage of proenkephalin-derived peptides (<23,300 Daltons) by plasma kallikrein. J Biol Chem 263:12543–12553

Patey G, Rossier J (1986) Découverte, anatomie et biosynthèse des différentes familles de peptides opioïdes endogènes. Ann Endocrinol (Paris) 47:71–87

Patey G, Liston DR, Rossier J (1984) Characterization of new enkephalin-containing peptides in the adrenal medulla by immuno-blotting. FEBS Lett 172:303–307

Patey G, Cupo A, Mazarguil H, Morgat JL, Rossier J (1985) Release of proenkephalin-derived opioid peptides from rat striatum *in vitro* and their rapid degradation. Neurosci Lett 15:1035–1044

Rossier J, Barrès E, Cupo A, Edwards V (1988) The release of enkephalin-containing peptides from the adrenal gland in concious calves. In: Pickering BT, Wakerley JB, Summerlee AJS (eds) Neurosecretion: cellular aspects of the production and release of neuropeptides. Plenum, London, pp 53–59

Toffoletto O, Metters KM, Oliveira EB, Camargo ACM, Rossier J (1988) Enkephalin is liberated from metorphamide and dynorphin A_{1-8} by endooligopeptidase A, but not by metalloendopeptidase EC 3.4.24.15. Biochem J 252:35–38

Vanderhaeghen JJ, Lotstra F, Liston DR, Rossier J (1983) Proenkephalin, (Met)enkephalin, and oxytocin immunoreactivities are colocalized in bovine hypothalamic magnocellular neurons. Proc Natl Acad Sci USA 80:5139–5143

Modulation of Energy Metabolism by Vasoactive Intestinal Peptide, Adenosine, and K^+ in the Cerebral Cortex: Focus on the Cellular Level *

P. J. MAGISTRETTI [1,2], J.-L. MARTIN [1,2], and P. R. HOF [1,3]

Introduction

Energy substrates must be readily available to neurons for the maintenance of the multiple energy-consuming processes in which they are engaged. The major energy cost of neurons is represented by the activity of various ion-pumping systems in order to maintain proper ionic gradients across the cell membrane which represent the basis of neuronal excitability. The axonal transport of macromolecules from and to the perikaryon, the synthesis of neurotransmitters, and general cell metabolism are other neuronal energy-consuming processes (Siesjö 1978). These energy demands are generally thought to be met by the uptake of glucose and oxygen from the blood supply to a given brain region. It is, however, also well established that glycogen is the single largest energy reserve of the brain (Lajtha et al. 1981), and, although its concentration is much lower than that present in muscle or liver, its turnover rate is extremely rapid, thus indicating a constant utilization by the nervous tissue (Lajtha et al. 1981). It is therefore conceivable that at least part of the immediate increases in local energy demands may be met by the hydrolysis of glycogen.

In fact, careful consideration of the neuronal microenvironment indicates that for glucose to reach a group of neurons with increased energy demands, various cellular barriers have to be crossed from the vascular lumen, such as the capillary endothelium and the membranes of pericytes and of astrocytes. In contrast, glycogen, owing to the fact that it is stored predominantly in astrocytes, can release glucose or other metabolic intermediates from a source that is in close association with neurons. This mechanism would therefore provide a rapid increase in the availability of energy substrates to meet immediate energy demand increases with considerable efficiency as well as spatial and temporal precision. In support of this view is the fact that glycogen levels within the CNS are controlled by a number of intercellular messengers

* This research was supported by a grant from the Fonds National Suisse de la Recherche Scientifique (no. 3.357-0.86) to P.J.M.

[1] Department of Pharmacology, Centre Medical Universitaire, 9 av. de Champel, 1211 Geneva 4, Switzerland.

[2] *Present address:* Institut de Physiologie, 7, rue du Bugnon, 1005 Lausanne, Switzerland.

[3] *Present address:* Fishberg Research Center for Neurobiology, The Mount Sinai School of Medicine, New York, NY 10029-6574, USA.

Neuropsychopharmacology
Edited by Bunney/Hippius/Laakmann/Schmauß

such as the monoamines noradrenaline (NA), serotonin (5-HT), and histamine, by the neuropeptide vasoactive intestinal peptide (VIP), and by adenosine and K^+ (Quach et al. 1978, 1980, 1982; Magistretti et al. 1981, 1986; Hof et al. 1988). In this chapter we review our work on the regulation of glycogenolysis by VIP, adenosine, and K^+ in mouse cerebral cortical slices.

Glycogen in the Nervous System

Glycogen is the single largest energy reserve of the brain (Siesjö 1978; Lajtha et al. 1981). It is localized predominantly in astrocytes (Cataldo and Broadwell 1986a); however glycogen has also been identified in the choroid plexus and ependymal epithelia (Cataldo and Broadwell 1986b) and to a lesser extent in endothelium and pericytes (Cataldo and Broadwell 1986b). Glycogen can also be visualized in certain neurons (Sotelo and Palay 1968). At the ultrastructural level, glycogen appears predominantly as electron-dense isodiametric beta particles within the cytoplasm. The size of these particles ranges between 10 and 30 nm in diameter (Cataldo and Broadwell 1986a). Glycogen undergoes a very fast turnover (Gatfield et al. 1966; Lajtha et al. 1981); enzymes for its synthesis and degradation, e.g., synthase and phosphorylase, have been identified in the nervous system, and their kinetic properties have been characterized (Breckenridge and Crawford 1961; Breckenridge and Norman 1962). The activity of these enzymes is regulated by intracellular messengers such as cyclic-AMP and Ca^{2+} (Edwards et al. 1974; Ververken et al. 1982). Several reviews have appeared in recent years on glycogen in the nervous system (see for example Koizumi 1974; Ibrahim 1975).

Stimulation of Glycogenolysis by VIP

Mouse cerebral cortical slices maintained in Krebs-Ringer bicarbonate buffer containing [^{3}H]glucose synthesize [^{3}H]glycogen in a time-dependent manner, reaching a steady state within 30–40 min of incubation (see Quach et al. 1978; Magistretti et al. 1981 for methodological details). When VIP is added at this point in time, a concentration-dependent glycogen breakdown with an EC_{50} of 26 n*M* is observed (Fig. 1). This action of VIP is rapid ($t_{\frac{1}{2}}$, 1 min) and is reversible (Magistretti et al. 1981, 1984). This glycogenolytic action is shared by peptide histidine isoleucine (PHI) and secretin, with potencies that are in direct relationship with the degree of homology of their sequences with that of VIP (Magistretti et al. 1984). Thus PHI and secretin promote glycogenolysis with EC_{50} of 300 and 500 n*M*, respectively (Magistretti et al. 1984). In contrast, growth hormone releasing factor (GRF), which has a degree of homology with VIP similar to that of secretin, is inactive (Magistretti et al. 1986). However some of the amino acids that GRF and VIP have in common are different from

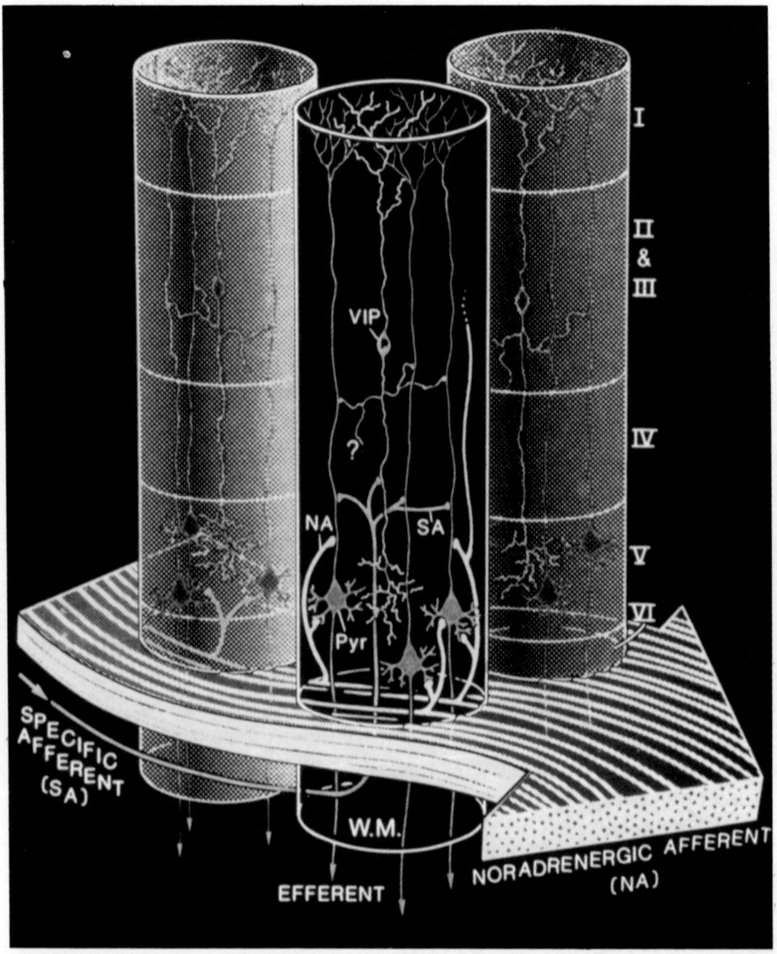

Fig. 1. Diagrammatic representation of the anatomic substrate for the metabolic actions of NA and VIP. *VIP*, VIP-containing bipolar cell; *NA*, noradrenergic afferent; *Pyr*, pyramidal cell furnishing major efferent projections: *SA*, specific afferent (i.e., from thalamus or from other cortical areas); *W.M.*, subcortical white matter; cortical layers denoted by *roman numerals*. Note tangential orientation of NA fibers and radially restricted domain of VIP-containing neuron. For graphic clarity, only the VIP-containing (*VIP*) and the pyramidal cells (*Pyr*) have been represented here. In particular, the principal target cells of the thalamocortical afferents, i.e., the small stellate cells in layer IV, have been omitted. However, any cell with the capacity for dendritic reception in layer IV may receive thalamic inputs (White 1981). Furthermore, also for graphic clarity, only one VIP neuron per cylinder has been drawn, in representation of a group of VIP neurons. (From Magistretti and Morrison 1988)

Table 1. Substances inactive in promoting [^{3}H]glycogenolysis in mouse cerebral cortical slices

γ-Aminobutyric acid	Met-enkephalin
Glutamate	Leu-enkephalin
Aspartate	Corticotropin-releasing factor
Carbamylcholine[a]	Vasopressin
Somatostatin-14	Oxytocin
Somatostatin-28	VIP fragments 6–28, 16–28, 21–28
Cholecystokinin-8	

[a] Stable analog of acetylcholine.

those that VIP shares with secretin. This observation may point to some key amino acids in the sequence of VIP that are necessary for the expression of its glycogenolytic activity. VIP fragments 6–28, 11–28, and 21–28 are also without effect on cortical glycogen levels (Magistretti et al. 1984).

As shown in Table 1, several neurotransmitters of the cerebral cortex do not stimulate glycogenolysis, thus stressing the specificity of the metabolic action of VIP. In particular, it is interesting to note that neurotransmitters with clear-cut primary actions on neuronal excitability such as the amino acids glutamate, aspartate, and γ-aminobutyric acid (GABA) do not promote glycogen breakdown (Magistretti et al. 1981). This observation would therefore appear to exclude the possibility that the metabolic action of VIP is secondary to alterations in neuronal excitability which, by increasing the metabolic demands of the target cells, could bring about the hydrolysis of glycogen. VIP is, however, not the only glycogenolytic neurotransmitter in the cerebral cortex; the monoamines NA, 5-HT, and histamine display a similar metabolic action (Quach et al. 1978, 1980, 1982). Thus NA promotes the hydrolysis of glycogen by acting at β-adrenergic receptors with an EC_{50} of 500 nM (Quach et al. 1978). The effect of 5-HT and histamine occurs with EC_{50} of 20 and 3 µm, respectively (Quach et al. 1980, 1982). The glycogenolysis elicited by histamine is mediated by H_1 receptors and shows rapid desensitization (Quach et al. 1980, 1981).

Morphological Correlates

VIP-containing neurons in the cerebral cortex, i.e., the CNS region where we have observed the glycogenolytic effect of VIP, have been identified and characterized by indirect immunohistochemistry (Lorén et al. 1979; Connor and Peters 1984; Morrison et al. 1984). These represent a rather homogeneous neuronal population with over 90% of the cells displaying the following characteristics. VIP neurons are bipolar cells oriented perpendicularly to the pial surface and arborizing only minimally (60–100 μm) in the horizontal plane, predominantly in layers I and IV–V (Fig. 1; Connor and Peters 1984; Morrison et al. 1984). The axonal arborization of a given VIP-containing neuron is also radially restricted. Thus, each VIP cortical neuron defines a column that spans from layers I to V with a diameter not exceeding 100 μm (Morrison et al. 1984; Magistretti and Morrison 1985). These morphological constraints indicate that VIP neurons are in a position to exert input-output functions locally, within narrow and radially oriented transcortical volumes. In particular, this geometric arrangement of VIP-containing neurons indicates that the glycogenolytic action of VIP in the cerebral cortex described earlier, operates within cortical columns (Fig. 1). Based on these considerations, we have proposed that VIP neurons may regulate the availability of energy substrates locally, within discrete cortical regions (Magistretti et al. 1981).

Functional Complementarity with the Noradrenergic System

As described above, the monoamines NA, 5-HT and histamine also stimulate cortical glycogenolysis. An examination of the morphological characteristics of the neuronal circuits that contain these neurotransmitters reveals striking differences with the domain of action of the VIP-containing neurons. In particular, in contrast to the VIP intracortical system, noradrenergic neurons originate in the nucleus locus coeruleus in the brainstem, from which they project to several CNS regions, including the cerebral cortex (Dahlstrom and Fuxe 1964; Morrison et al. 1978). Here the noradrenergic fibers enter from the rostral (i.e., anterior) aspect and proceed caudally (i.e., posteriorly) in a tangential plane (i.e., in a plane parallel to the pial surface). This trajectory, which is therefore orthogonal to the plane of orientation of the bipolar VIP-containing neurons, endows the noradrenergic fibers with the capacity to modulate neuronal activity synchronously and globally across a vast rostrocaudal expanse of cerebral cortex (Morrison et al. 1981). Such a cortical domain stands in striking contrast with the columnar arrays which the VIP-containing cells are positioned to regulate (Morrison and Magistretti 1983; Magistretti and Morrison 1988; see Fig. 1, 2).

The hydrolysis of glycogen induced by VIP and NA results, at the cellular level, in an increased availability of energy substrates. This action, when viewed in relation to the morphological characteristics of the VIP- and NA-containing neurons indicates the existence of two complementary systems which participate in the regulation of energy metabolism within the cerebral cortex: (a) the intracortical VIP-containing system, endowed with the capacity to regulate glycogenolysis locally, within individual cortical columns of 60–100 μm diameter, and (b) the tangentially organized noradrenergic fibers, exerting their action globally and synchronously across functionally distinct cortical regions (Magistretti et al. 1981; Morrison and Magistretti 1983; Magistretti and Morrison 1988).

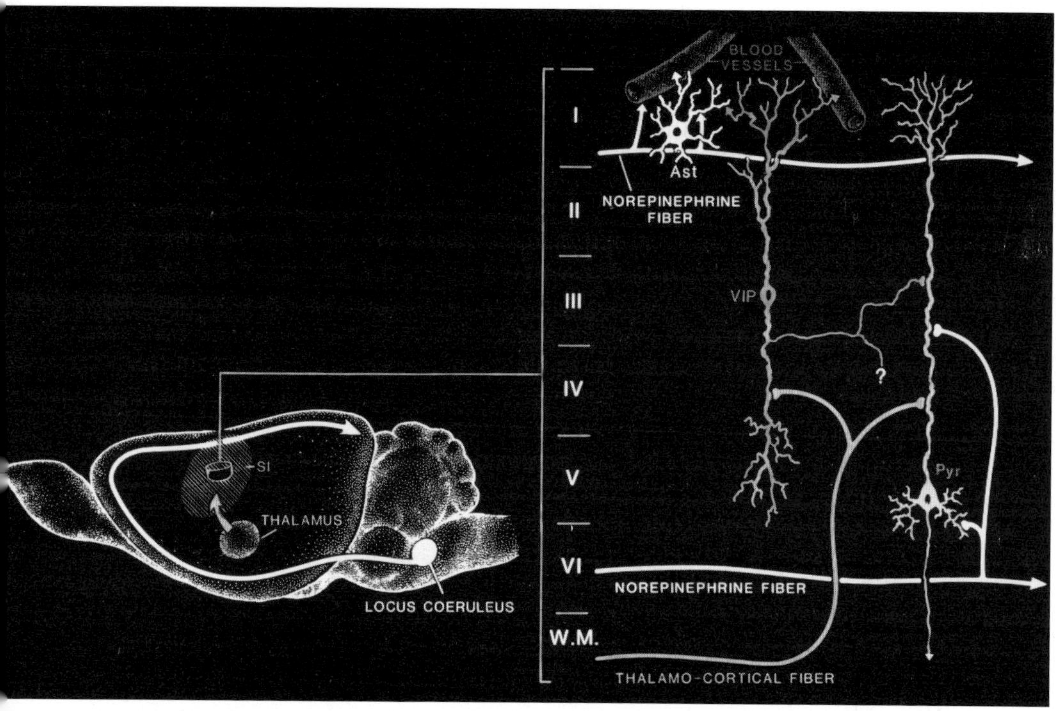

Fig. 2. Schematic drawing of the anatomic organization and putative targets of the intracortical NA and VIP systems (see text for details). Note contrast of local, radial VIP system (*right panel*) and global, tangential NA system (*left panel*). Both the VIP and NA systems can interact with two distinct cellular partners: (a) synaptic interaction with neuronal targets predominantly in the intervening layers and (b) nonsynaptic interaction with nonneuronal elements (astrocytes and blood vessels), primarily in layer I. Cortical layers are designated with *roman numerals*; *Ast*, astrocyte; *Pyr*, pyramidal cell; *SI*, primary somatosensory cortex; *W.M.*, subcortical white matter. (From Magistretti and Morrison 1988)

The function of the glycogenolysis promoted by VIP and NA may be to prepare discrete neuronal ensembles for incoming activity. The position in cortical circuitry of the VIP-containing intracortical system stresses the possibility for these neurons to translate an increase in activity of specific cortical afferents into a cellular metabolic message in their target cells. The spatial domain of such a metabolic regulation would then be determined by the resolution and pattern of activity of the specific corticocortical and thalamocortical afferents that drive the VIP-containing neurons (Figs. 1, 2).

Studies in Cultured Astrocytes

The nervous system is a cellularly heterogeneous tissue. Therefore, an effect observed following the application of a neurotransmitter onto a brain slice may occur in one of the following cell types: neurons, astrocytes, oligodendrocytes, the microglia, and cells of the vasculature such as pericytes and the vascular endothelium. As indicated earlier, ultrastructural analysis has revealed that most of the CNS glycogen is localized in astrocytes (Cataldo and Broadwell 1986a). We have therefore subjected to experimental test the hypothesis that VIP, NA, and the other monoamines exert the observed glycogenolytic action in astrocytes. To this end, primary cultures of astrocytes were prepared from rat and mouse neonatal cerebral cortex. In this preparation, which consists for over 90% of astrocytes (Manthorpe et al. 1979) as determined by their immunoreactivity to the selective marker glial fibrillary acidic protein (Bignami et al. 1972), VIP and NA promoted an approximately 60% hydrolysis of [^{3}H]glycogen newly synthesized from [^{3}H]glucose (Magistretti et al. 1983). The monoamines 5-HT and histamine were also active, although with a reduced potency. In contrast, GABA and cholecystokinin-8 were devoid of glycogenolytic properties, in keeping with their inactivity in cerebral cortical slices (Magistretti et al. 1981). These observations, if representative of interactions also occurring *in vivo*, indicate that neurotransmitters released from active neurons may vehiculate a message onto surrounding astrocytes that results in the mobilization of energy stores for the active neuronal environment. Thus a functional coupling between neurons and astrocytes geared at maintaining energy metabolism homeostasis may be operative within the cerebral cortex, and possibly within other CNS regions. In this context it is interesting to note that VIP is a potent relaxant of pial vessels (McCulloch and Edvinsson 1980; Wei et al. 1980) and stimulates cyclic-AMP formation in intracortical microvessel preparations (Huang and Rorstad 1983, 1984). Thus VIP neurons may act in a functionally coordinated fashion to increase the availability of energy substrates by stimulating glycogenolysis and by increasing local blood flow (Fig. 2).

Stimulation of Glycogenolysis by Adenosine and Potassium

In addition to the neurotransmitters discussed thus far, two other neuroactive agents have been recently shown to promote glycogenolysis (Magistretti et al. 1986; Hof et al. 1988); these are adenosine and K^+. When neurons are activated, they release adenosine in the extracellular space up to concentrations ranging between 150 and 400 μM (Pull and McIlwain 1972). Two adenosine receptor subtypes inversely coupled to adenylate cyclase have been described (van Calker et al. 1979; Daly 1985). Thus, the A_1 subtype, upon which adenosine acts at nanomolar concentrations, is negatively coupled to adenylate cyclase, whereas stimulation of the A_2 subtype by adenosine at micromolar concentrations leads to an increased cyclic-AMP formation. In view of this latter action we have examined the effect of adenosine on cortical glycogen. We have observed that in mouse cerebral cortical slices, adenosine stimulates a concentration-dependent glycogenolysis with an EC_{50} of 7 μM (Magistretti et al. 1986). This effect is inhibited by the adenosine receptor antagonist theophylline with an IC_{50} of 80 μM (Magistretti et al. 1986) and is mimicked by various adenosine analogs with a rank-order of potencies that is characteristic of A_2 receptor activation (Magistretti et al. 1986). These observations therefore support the notion that adenosine may play a modulatory role in the coupling between neuronal activity and energy metabolism in the CNS (Magistretti et al. 1986).

Potassium ions are also released in the extracellular space during neuronal activity (Nicholson 1981; Sykova 1983). The concentrations reached by the ion under these conditions range between 5 and 12 mM (Gardner-Medwin and Nicholson 1983). We have recently described in mouse cerebral cortex the existence of a K^+-evoked glycogenolysis which is dependent on the presence of extracellular Ca^{2+} (Hof et al. 1988). Ca^{2+} can act as second messenger, and in the case of glycogen level regulation, the mechanisms leading to Ca^{2+}-mediated glycogenolysis have been elucidated. The final step in the cascade of intracellular events that triggers glycogenolysis is the conversion of phosphorylase from "*b*" (less active) to "*a*" (active) forms. This conversion occurs by a phosphorylation via phosphorylase kinase. Phosphorylase kinase in turn can be activated either by a cyclic-AMP dependent protein kinase or directly by Ca^{2+} (Cohen 1982). Therefore an increase in intracellular free Ca^{2+} concentration can trigger the hydrolysis of glycogen. In fact, Ververken et al. (1982) have demonstrated a crucial role for Ca^{2+} in the activation of phosphorylase "*b*" in the cerebral cortex.

Three types of Ca^{2+} channels have recently been described, denominated T, N, and L, which present different electrical properties and pharmacological sensitivities (Fox et al. 1986; Nowycky et al. 1985; Tsien 1987). The pharmacological sensitivity of the various channel subtypes is the following: T channels are blocked by Ni^{2+} (80% block at 0.1 mM) but are weakly sensitive to Cd^{2+} and ω-conotoxin, and are insensitive to dihydropyridines; in contrast, N and L channels are weakly sensitive to Ni^{2+} but are blocked by Cd^{2+} and ω-conotoxin; in addition, L channels are blocked by dihydropyridines and activated by BAY K 8644 (Fox et al. 1986; Tsien 1987). The glycogenolytic effect of K^+ is inhibited by Ni^{2+} at 0.1 mM (Fig. 1) but not by Cd^{2+} at 20 μM (Table 2), a concentration of the ion that almost completely blocks voltage-sensitive Ca^{2+} channels of the L and N subtypes (Fox et al. 1986; Miller 1987). Furthermore, the action of K^+ is insensitive to nifedipine, diltiazem, verapamil, BAY K 8644 and ω-conotoxin. This pharmacological profile of blockade therefore strongly suggests that activation of T channels mediates the glycogenolytic effect of K^+.

The glycogenolysis elicited by K^+ is operative at concentrations reached by the ion in the extracellular space during neuronal activity (Hof et al. 1988). These results further delineate the role of K^+ in intercellular communication in the nervous system. They also suggest that K^+, released from active neurons, could mobilize energy substrates in regions of increased neuronal activity. Whether this mechanism is concurrent or sequentially related to the adenosine-stimulated glycogenolysis remains to be determined.

An important difference between the glycogenolysis elicited by VIP and the monoamines and that promoted by adenosine and K^+ should be stressed. The two latter agents are released by all neurons during cellular activation, whereas the neurotransmitters VIP and the monoamines are contained in discrete populations of neurons, with precise geometric arrangements. Thus, in contrast to adenosine- and K^+-stimulated glycogenolysis, the metabolic action of VIP and the monoamines becomes operative exclusively upon activation of specific neuronal circuits within spatially defined domains of action.

Table 2. [^{3}H]Glycogenolysis elicited by K^+ in homozygous (*qk/qk*), heterozygous (+/*qk*), and control (+/+) mice

[^{3}H]glycogen hydrolysis (%)		
	Younger than 7 weeks	Older than 7 weeks
qk/qk	26.7 ± 2.8	55.9 ± 1.7^a
+/*qk*	28.4 ± 1.1	30.7 ± 3.2
+/+	27.6 ± 4.5	29.5 ± 2.7

[a] Significantly different ($p < 0.05$) from +/*qk* and +/+.

Studies in Spontaneously Epileptic Mouse Mutants

Dramatic perturbations of energy metabolism are observed in epileptic brains, both in humans and in laboratory animals (Siesjö 1978). Various animal models of epilepsy have been described, and these fall into two main categories: drug-induced epilepsies in otherwise normal animals and spontaneously epileptic mutants. The latter models of inherited epilepsies provide the unique opportunity to examine the consequences of mutations occurring at specific gene loci on the regulation of neuronal excitability and energy metabolism. For these reasons we sought to examine the regulation of glycogenolysis in the neocortex of *quaking* and *tottering* mice, two spontaneously epileptic mutants.

The *quaking* (*qk*) mutant presents a recessive monogenic mutation located on chromosome 17 (Sidman et al. 1964). This mutant is characterized by a deficient myelination due to an impaired differentiation of oligodendrocytes (Wisniewski and Morell 1971). The epileptic symptomatology is characterized by the following features: a tremor of voluntary movement, spontaneous tonic-clonic convulsions occurring predominantly during paradoxical sleep, manipulation-induced tonic-clonic fits, and audiogenic seizures (Maurin et al. 1985). A cytological anomaly observed in *qk* mice is an increase (up to 50%) of noradrenergic neurons in the mid-portion of the locus coeruleus accompanied by a developmentally regulated enhancement in the density of α_1- and α_2-adrenergic receptors restricted to the brain stem (Maurin et al. 1985).

The glycogenolytic effect of K^+ on cerebral cortical slices prepared from *qk/qk*, +/*qk*, and +/+ mice was examined, and the results are shown in Table 2. In animals older than 7 weeks, K^+ 8 m*M* hydrolyzed 55.9 ± 1.7% of basal [^{3}H]-glycogen levels in *qk/qk* mutants, whereas this value reached only 30.7 ± 3.2% in the +/*qk* and 29.5 ± 2.7% in the +/+. In younger animals no difference was observed between the three groups (Table 2). These results indicate the existence of a marked supersensitivity in the cerebral cortex of the *qk/qk* mutant to the glycogenolytic action of K^+ at a concentration reached by the ion in the extracellular space during neuronal activity. This supersensitivity was only observed after 7 weeks, an age at which the epileptic symptomatology is fully expressed.

The *tottering* (*tg*) mouse presents a delayed-onset (3–4 weeks postnatally) stereotyped pattern of spontaneous spike-wave discharges in the neocortex and hippocampus accompanied by behavioral absence seizures that resemble petit mal (Noebels and Sidman 1979). The mutation affects a gene locus on chromosome 8, and its mode of transmission is autosomal recessive. The sole cytological anomaly observed thus far in homozygous mutants (*tg/tg*) is an increase in the number of noradrenergic axons in the terminal fields innervated by the nucleus locus coeruleus, including the hippocampus and neocortex (Levitt and Noebels 1981). This increase in axon number is accompanied by enhanced NA levels, up to 200%, in the corresponding CNS areas. Evidence for a causal link between noradrenergic hyperinnervation and the neurological disorder of *tg/tg* mice has been provided by experiments in which central noradrenergic axons were destroyed neonatally or later in development with the selective neurotoxin 6-hydroxydopamine; in such neurotoxin-lesioned mutants the epileptic symptomatology was prevented or reversed, respectively (Noebels 1984).

In view of the altered pattern of neocortical noradrenergic innervation we examined the postsynaptic sensitivity to the glycogenolytic action of NA in this spontaneously epileptic mouse mutant. Our observations indicate that the potency and efficacy of NA in promoting glycogenolysis were markedly decreased in homozygous *tg/tg* when compared to control mice (+/+). Thus, the EC_{50} for this action of NA, which is mediated by adrenergic receptors of the β subtype, were 1.7 μ*M* in *tg/tg* and 0.17 μ*M* in +/+ (Magistretti et al. 1987). A similar subsensitive response was observed with isoproterenol, a selective β-adrenergic agonist, which is not taken up by presynaptic noradrenergic terminals. This latter result stresses the postsynaptic nature of the subsensitive response.

It should be noted that this alteration in the regulation of glycogenolysis is specific to NA, since the response to VIP and K^+ is normally expressed in *tg/tg* mutants.

This set of observations indicates that cortical glycogen metabolism is markedly altered in certain murine models of epilepsy. Furthermore, by revealing the expression of single-locus mutations at the cellular level, they may represent a useful starting point for further investigations at the molecular level which could then provide a link between an allele and the altered synthesis or regulation of gene products in certain forms of epilepsy.

A Neuroendocrine System Within the Brain?

The fact that VIP and NA stimulate glycogenolysis in the cerebral cortex underscores the notion that neuronal systems may exist within the CNS that exert actions other than the classically described alterations in neuronal excitability. Thus neurotransmitters may also primarily trigger cellular processes that are an integral part of the mechanisms that maintain the stability of the neuronal microenvironment, and that regulate intracellular metabolism. The nature of these actions is therefore "hormonal" rather than "electrical." These actions are nevertheless exerted with great spatial and temporal precision, occurring in concert with changes in the activity of discrete neuronal circuits. Thus neuronal systems with a primarily hormonal function may exist within the CNS. It is proposed that these systems, which are subject to the constraints of synaptic transmission, may function spatially and temporally in parallel with those circuits that use as intercellular mediators neurotransmitters, such as glutamate or GABA, that affect neuronal excitability in a direct, rapid, and rapidly reversible fashion. VIP- and NA-containing neuronal circuits within the cerebral cortex may constitute an example of such neuronal systems with hormonal function. Similar systems may also exist in other CNS regions and use other chemical messengers.

Acknowledgement. The authors wish to thank Ms. Sylvianne Bonnet for expert secretarial help.

References

Bignami A, Eng LF, Dahl D, Uyeda CT (1972) Localization of the glial fibrillary acidic protein in astrocytes by immunofluorescence. Brain Res 43:429–435

Breckenridge BM, Crawford EJ (1961) The quantitative histochemistry of the brain. Enzymes of glycogen metabolism. J Neurochem 7:234–240

Breckenridge BM, Norman JH (1962) Glycogen phosphorylase in brain. J Neurochem 9:383–392

Cataldo AM, Broadwell RD (1986a) Cytochemical identification of cerebral glycogen and glucose-6-phosphatase activity under normal and experimental conditions. I. Neurons and glia. J Electron Microsc (Tokyo) 3:413–437

Cataldo AM, Broadwell RD (1986b) Cytochemical identification of cerebral glycogen and glucose-6-phosphatase activity under normal and experimental conditions. II. Choroid plexus and ependymal epithelia, endothelia and pericytes. J Neurocytol 15:511–524

Cohen P (1982) The role of protein phophorylation in neural and hormonal control of cellular activity. Nature 296:613–620

Connor JR, Peters A (1984) Vasoactive intestinal polypeptide-immunoreactive neurons in rat visual cortex. Neuroscience 12:1027–1044

Dahlstrom A, Fuxe K (1964) Evidence for the existence of monoamine-containing neurons in the central nervous system. I. Demonstration of monoamines in the cell bodies of brain stem neurons. Acta Physiol Scand 62 (Suppl 232):1–55

Daly JW (1985) Adenosine receptors. Adv Cyclic Nucleotide Protein Phosphorylation Res 19:29–46

Edwards C, Nahorski SR, Rogers KJ (1974) *In vivo* changes of cerebral cyclic adenosine 3′,5′-monophosphate induced by biogenic amines: association with phosphorylase activation. J Neurochem 22:565–572

Fox AP, McCleskey EW, Nowycky MC, Tsien RW (1986) Different types of neuronal calcium channels. In: Magistretti PJ, Morrison JH, Reisine TD (eds) Discussions in neurosciences, vol 3/3. FESN, Geneva, pp 87–93

Gardner-Medwin AR, Nicholson C (1983) Changes of extracellular potassium activity induced by electric current through brain tissue in the rat. J Physiol (Lond) 335:375–392

Gatfield PD, Lowry OH, Schulz DW, Passonneau JV (1966) Regional energy reserves in mouse brain and changes in ischemia and anaesthesia. J Neurochem 13:185–195

Hof PR, Pascale E, Magistretti PJ (1988) K^+ at concentrations reached in the extracellular space during neuronal activity promotes a Ca^{2+}-dependent glycogen hydrolysis in mouse cerebral cortex. J Neurosci 8:1922–1928

Huang M, Rorstad OP (1983) Effects of vasoactive intestinal polypeptide, monoamines, prostaglandins, and 2-chloroadenosine on adenylate cyclase in rat cerebral microvessels. J Neurochem 40:719–726

Huang M, Rorstad OP (1984) Cerebral vascular adenylate cyclase: evidence for coupling to receptors for vasoactive intestinal peptide and parathyroid hormone. J Neurochem 43:849–856

Ibrahim MZ (1975) Glycogen and its related enzymes of metabolism in the central nervous system. Adv Anat Embryol Cell Biol 52:3–89

Koizumi J (1974) Glycogen in the central nervous system. Prog Histochem Cytochem 6:1–37

Lajtha AL, Maker HS, Clarke DD (1981) Metabolism and transport of carbohydrates and amino acids. In: Siegel GJ, Albers RW, Agranoff RW, Katzman R (eds) Basic neurochemistry. Little, Brown, Boston, pp 329–353

Levitt P, Noebels JL (1981) Mutant mouse tottering: selective increase of locus coeruleus axons in a defined single-locus mutation. Proc Natl Acad Sci USA 78:4630–4634

Lorén I, Emson PC, Fahrenkrug J, Björklund A, Alumets J, Hakanson R, Sundler F (1979) Distribution of vasoactive intestinal polypeptide in the rat and mouse brain. Neuroscience 4:1953–1976

Magistretti PJ, Morrison JH (1985) VIP neurons in the neocortex. TINS 8:7–8

Magistretti PJ, Morrison JH (1988) Noradrenaline- and vasoactive intestinal peptide-containing neuronal systems in neocortex: functional convergence with contrasting morphology. Neuroscience 24:367–378

Magistretti PJ, Morrison JH, Shoemaker WJ, Sapin V, Bloom FE (1981) Vasoactive intestinal polypeptide induces glycogenolysis in mouse cortical slices: a possible regulatory mechanism for the local control of energy metabolism. Proc Natl Acad Sci USA 78:6535–6539

Magistretti PJ, Manthorpe M, Bloom FE, Varon S (1983) Functional receptors for vasoactive intestinal polypeptide in cultured astroglia from neonatal rat brain. Regul Pept 6:71–80

Magistretti PJ, Morrison JH, Shoemaker WJ, Bloom FE (1984) Morphological and functional correlates of VIP neurons in cerebral cortex. Peptides 5:213–218

Magistretti PJ, Hof PR, Martin JL (1986) Adenosine stimulates glycogenolysis in mouse cerebral cortex: a possible coupling mechanism between neuronal activity and energy metabolism. J Neurosci 6:2558–2562

Magistretti PJ, Hof PR, Celio MR (1987) Noradrenergic sub-sensitivity in the cerebral cortex of the tottering mouse, a spontaneously epileptic mutant. Brain Res 403:181–185
Manthorpe M, Adler R, Varon S (1979) Development, reactivity and GFA immunofluorescence of astroglia-containing monolayer cultures from rat cerebrum. J Neurocytol 8:605–621
Maurin Y, Le Saux F, Graillot C, Baumman N (1985) Altered postnatal ontogeny of α_1- and α_2-adrenoceptor binding sites in the brain of a convulsive mutant mouse (quaking). Dev Brain Res 22:229–235
McCulloch J, Edvinsson L (1980) Cerebral circulatory and metabolic effects of vasoactive intestinal polypeptide. Am J Physiol 238:H449–H456
Miller RJ (1987) Multiple calcium channels and neuronal function. Science 235:46–52
Morrison JH, Magistretti PJ (1983) Monoamines and peptides in cerebral cortex. TINS 6:146–151
Morrison JH, Grzanna R, Molliver M, Coyle JT (1978) The distribution and orientation of noradrenergic fibers in neocortex of the rat: an immunofluorescence study. J Comp Neurol 181:17–40
Morrison JH, Molliver ME, Grzanna R, Coyle JT (1981) The intra-cortical trajectory of the coeruleo-cortical projection in the rat: a tangentially organized cortical afferent. Neuroscience 6:139–158
Morrison JH, Magistretti PJ, Benoît R, Bloom FE (1984) The distribution and morphological characteristics of the intracortical VIP-positive cell: an immunohistochemical analysis. Brain Res 292:269–282
Nicholson C (1981) Brain-cell microenvironment as a communication channel. In: Schmitt FO, Worden FD (eds) The neurosciences, fourth study program. MIT Press, Cambridge, pp 457–476
Noebels JL (1984) A single gene error of noradrenergic axon growth synchronizes central neurones. Nature 310:409–411
Noebels JL, Sidman RL (1979) Inherited epilepsy: Spike-wave and focal motor seizures in the mutant mouse tottering. Science 204:1334–1336
Nowycky MC, Fox AP, Tsien RW (1985) Three types of neuronal calcium channel with different calcium agonist sensitivity. Nature 316:440–443
Pull I, McIlwain H (1972) Adenine derivatives as neurohumoral agents in the brain. The quantities liberated on excitation of superfused cerebral tissues. Biochem J 130:975–981
Quach TT, Rose C, Schwartz JC (1978) (^{3}H)-glycogen hydrolysis in brain slices: responses to neurotransmitters and modulation of noradrenaline receptors. J Neurochem 30:1335–1341
Quach TT, Duchemin AM, Rose C, Schwartz JC (1980) ^{3}H-glycogen hydrolysis elicited by histamine in mouse brain slices: selective involvement of H_1-receptors. Mol Pharmacol 17:301–308
Quach TT, Duchemin A-M, Rose C, Schwartz J-C (1981) Specific desensitization of histamine H_1 receptor-mediated [^{3}H]glycogen hydrolysis in brain slices. Mol Pharmacol 20:331–338
Quach TT, Rose C, Duchemin AM, Schwartz JC (1982) Glycogenolysis induced by serotonin in brain: identification of a new class of receptor. Nature 298:373–375
Sidman RL, Dickie MM, Appel SH (1964) Mutant mice (quaking and jimpy) with deficient myelination in the central nervous system. Science 144:309–311
Siesjö BK (1978) Brain energy metabolism. Wiley, New York
Sotelo C, Palay SL (1968) The fine structure of the lateral vestibular nucleus in the rat. I. Neurons and neuroglial cells. J Cell Biol 36:151–179
Sykova E (1983) Extracellular K^+ accumulation in the central nervous system. Prog Biophys Mol Biol 42:135–189
Tsien RW (1987) Calcium currents in heart cells and neurons. In: Kaczmarek LK, Levitan IB (eds) Neuromodulation. Oxford University Press, New York, pp 206–242
van Chalker D, Muller M, Hamprecht B (1979) Adenosine regulates via two different types of receptors, the accumulation of cyclic AMP in cultured brain cells. J Neurochem 33:999–1005

Ververken D, Van Veldhoven P, Proost C, Carton H, De Wulf H (1982) On the role of calcium ions in the regulation of glycogenolysis in mouse brain cortical slices. J Neurochem 38:1286–1295

Wei EP, Kontos HA, Said SI (1980) Mechanism of action of vasoactive intestinal polypeptide on cerebral arterioles. Am J Physiol 239:H765–H768

White EL (1981) Thalamocortical synaptic relations. In: Schmitt FO, Worden FG, Adelman G, Dennis SG (eds) The organization of the cerebral cortex. MIT Press, Cambridge, pp 153–161

Wisniewski H, Morell P (1971) Quaking mouse: ultrastructural evidence for arrest of myelinogenesis. Brain Res 29:63–73

How Neuropeptides Alter Neuronal Excitability *

G. R. SIGGINS [1] and W. ZIEGLGÄNSBERGER [2]

Introduction

The task of this chapter is to highlight something of our current understanding of neuropeptide electrophysiology. This task is both intimidating and exciting for the same reason: that there is an ever-increasing number of peptides – we count some 20–50 in total – that could eventually qualify as playing a role in central nervous function, even outside the hypothalamic-pituitary axis. Because of this large number we cannot possibly do justice to all of them and therefore must apologize for omitting some important peptides. Rather, we try to illustrate some basic principles of neuropeptide action using examples from only three peptide systems: (a) the opioid peptide family, (b) the somatostatin (SS) family, and (c) corticotropin-releasing factor (CRF).

It has become clear over the past decade that exogenously applied neuropeptides, like neurotransmitter candidates in general, can exert many kinds of actions on vertebrate neurons. Many of these actions are not typical of classic neurotransmitters, as recently reviewed (Siggins and Gruol 1986). Table 1 summarizes and describes several categories of actions reported for peptides acting on vertebrate neurons (see Pittman 1980; Siggins and Gruol

Table 1. Categories of exogenous neuropeptide action on central neurons

1.	Presynaptic modulation of the release of other transmitters
2.	Postsynaptic modulation of the action of other transmitters
3.	Classical transmitter action (opens ion channels)
4.	Closes ion channels
5.	Acts on voltage-dependent channels (opens or closes)
6.	Acts on ion-dependent (calcium-dependent) channels (opens or closes)

* The original research reported here was supported by United States Public Health Service grants MH-44346, DA-03665, AA-06420, and AA-07456 and by the Alexander von Humboldt Stiftung (to G.R.S.), Bundesministerium für Forschung und Technik and Sonderforschungsbereich 220 (to W.Z.). G.R.S. especially thanks Bissendorf Peptide for the Bissendorf Lecture Award supporting his participation at the meeting.

[1] Research Institute of Scripps Clinic, 10666 North Torrey Pines Road, La Jolla, CA 92037, USA.
[2] Max-Planck-Institut für Psychiatrie, Kraepelinstraße 2, 8000 München 40, FRG.

Neuropsychopharmacology
Edited by Bunney/Hippius/Laakmann/Schmauß

1986, for review). As the present review makes clear, the most excitement in this area seems to be centered on: (a) the modulatory action of peptides, (b) neuropeptide actions on voltage-dependent or ion-dependent conductances, and (c) the mediation of peptide effects by second messengers, especially GTP-binding proteins. The methods used to examine peptide actions on neurons have ranged from iontophoresis or pressure application with extracellular recording in vivo (via multibarrel pipettes), as in earlier studies, to intracellular voltage or current recordings combined with bath or local application of peptides to relatively isolated neurons.

Opioid Peptides

The opioid family of peptides provides an excellent example of the ability of one peptide family to exert many types of action, depending upon the neuron under study. In general, the opioids appear to exert predominantly inhibitory effects on cell firing, although via at least four major mechanisms. In extracellular recordings, the preponderant stereospecific action of opiate alkaloids or opioid peptides in most neurons is depression of spontaneous, synaptically, or chemically evoked neuronal single-unit discharge activity. The depresssions are generally blocked by naloxone, suggesting involvement of the empirically defined opiate receptors. Some major exceptions to the usual depressions exist, such as the naloxone-reversible excitatory responses seen in hippocampal pyramidal cells (Nicoll et al. 1977; Zieglgänsberger et al. 1979), in spinal cord cells (Davies 1976), in the brain stem (Satoh et al. 1979), and in the substantia nigra (Gysling and Wang 1983) (see Siggins and Gruol 1986; Zieglgänsberger 1986, for review).

In the hippocampus, both in vivo studies and in vitro intracellular recording revealed excitatory responses of hippocampal pyramidal neurons to opioid agonists. Blockade of GABA responses by bicuculline and transmitter release by Mg^{2+} indicate that excitation may actually be indirect, resulting from a primary inhibitory effect on neighboring inhibitory interneurons and leading to the excitation of pyramidal cells by disinhibition (Zieglgänsberger et al. 1979; see below). It is possible that the opiate-induced excitations seen in other areas may also derive from disinhibitory opiate actions. However, intracellular recording is usually required to test more strictly the disinhibition hypothesis and is obligatory for determining the possible ionic mechanisms involved in opiate function.

Recent intracellular studies have revealed four or more general types of opioid mechanisms. The first type, *presynaptic modulation*, may in fact derive from the operation at the presynaptic level of one or more of the other three mechanisms. Unfortunately, the difficulty of recording from presynaptic terminals in mammalian CNS generally precludes direct examination of the acute mechanisms involved. However, there have been several studies indicating that opioids can reduce release of synaptic transmitters (Jessel and Iversen

1977; Macdonald and Nelson 1978; Mudge et al. 1979), thus indicating a presynaptic site of action.

A second opioid mechanism, *postsynaptic modulation*, was one of the first described (Zieglgänsberger and Bayerl 1976; Zieglgänsberger and Tulloch 1979). In this case, we define modulation as an alteration in the action of the other transmitters by the opioids without direct action on the excitability of the postsynaptic neuronal membrane (Siggins and Gruol 1986). Early studies, involving the intracellular recording of cat spinal cord neurons with simultaneous extracellular microiontophoretic drug application, suggested that morphine and opioid peptides did not change the membrane potential or resting membrane resistance but did decrease the magnitude and rate of rise of evoked excitatory postsynaptic potentials (EPSPs) and depressed glutamate-induced depolarization (Zieglgänsberger and Bayerl 1976; Zieglgänsberger and Tulloch 1979). As microiontophoretically applied L-glutamate increases the postsynaptic membrane conductance to Na^+ and K^+, it was postulated that the opiates interfere with the chemically excitable cationic channels opened by synaptically released excitatory transmitters.

To some extent, the antiglutamate action of opioid peptides in vivo has been confirmed for mouse spinal neurons grown in culture, where a noncompetetive blocking action on the glutamate-activated conductances was observed (Barker et al. 1978). A similar antiglutamate effect of opioids has been shown as well as for hippocampal and cortical pyramidal neurons in slice preparations (Sutor and Zieglgänsbeger 1984, 1987; Deisz et al. 1988). In addition, opiates have been reported to reduce evoked EPSPs in hippocampal CA1 neurons (Siggins and Zieglgänsberger 1981), in dentate granule cells (Moore et al. 1988a), and in nucleus accumbens neurons (Deisz et al. 1988) without significant alteration of postsynaptic membrane properties.

In an extracellular study, antagonism of L-glutamate responses by an enkephalin analogue in substantia gelatinosa neurons recorded in a slice preparation of adult rat spinal cord has been shown (Zieglgänsberger and Sutor 1983). Nonetheless, several intracellular studies on acutely isolated or hemisected spinal cord preparations in vitro did not confirm an opioid antagonism of glutamate excitatory actions (Nicoll 1982) and/or have recorded opioid-induced hyperpolarizations (Nicoll 1982; Suzue et al. 1981; Yoshimura and North 1983). Two of these three studies involved sucrose gap recordings of hemisected frog spinal cord and measured only small (0.5–1.0 mV) membrane potential changes. However, the other study (Yoshimura and North 1983) used intracellular recording of substantia gelatinosa neurons in a rat spinal cord slice and revealed hyperpolarizations that averaged 8 mV in about 50% of the cells tested. Opioid activation of a K^+ conductance was suggested (see also below). In contrast, a more recent preliminary report showed that bath application of a μ-preferring agonist in concentrations that did not have a measurable effect on postsynaptic resting membrane properties produced a depression of the EPSP induced by activation of small primary afferents in dorsal horn neurons of the rat spinal cord (Jeftinija 1988). It is possible that some of the discrepancies in the literature with respect to the effects of the opioids on membrane potential and responses to glutamate in spinal cord could arise from species, methodological or cell-type differences.

A third general opiate mechanism, *reduced* Ca^{2+} influx, is illustrated by studies of cultured dorsal root ganglia neurons (Dunlop and Fischbach 1981; Werz and Macdonald 1982; Crain 1988). In these neurons (derived from either chick or rat neonates), none of the opioid peptides tested altered membrane potential, but they did reduce the duration of the Ca^{2+}-dependent action potential. It was initially thought that this reduction was due to interference with a voltage-dependent Ca^{2+} conductance (Dunlop and Fischbach 1981). However, this opioid effect might arise from the enhancement of some K^{+} conductance (e.g., Ca^{2+}-dependent K^{+} conductance or delayed rectifier), as suggested by the studies of μ- and δ-receptor activation in these neurons (Werz and Macdonald 1983, 1984). In these studies, the effect of enkephalin on the action potential duration, but not the response to dynorphin, was abolished by intracellular Cs^{+} injection, which eliminates most K^{+} conductances. Second messengers such as a GTP-binding protein and cyclic AMP may be involved in these opioid responses (Crain 1988). Regardless of the primary mechanism, the net effect of such an action would be a reduction in calcium entry into the cell. Such a reduction, if it also occurred in the terminals of these cells in the spinal cord (e.g., in substantia gelatinosa), could provide the mechanism for the reported opioid-induced inhibition of transmitter release (mechanism number 1, above). Notwithstanding, there are other data (e.g., that dorsal root ganglion cells acutely isolated from adult rats do not show this opiate effect; Williams and Zieglgänsberger 1981) that confound this hypothesis. Recent studies performed in neuroblastoma × glioma hybrid cells employing tight-seal whole-cell recording and Fura-II measurements revealed that μ and δ-preferring opioid agonists reduce a calcium-current. These results are in accord with previous investigations reporting the activation of a perfussis toxin (PTX) sensitive G-protein as an essential step in mediating the inhibition of this voltage-activated Ca^{2+} channel (Zieglgänsberger and Neher 1988).

The fourth major mechanism reported, *classic transmitter action*, derives originally from in vitro intracellular recordings of myenteric plexus and locus ceruleus (LC) neurons (e.g., Pepper and Henderson 1980) that show hyperpolarizing responses to the opioid peptides associated with an increased conductance. The group of North (Williams et al. 1982) has presented evidence that the opioid-induced hyperpolarization in LC is sensitive to naloxone, and that the increased conductance involves K^{+}. An almost identical series of findings have been reported from the same laboratory for substantia gelatinosa neurons of the rat spinal cord slice preparation (Yoshimura and North 1983), again suggesting a classic neurotransmitter-like action for the opioid peptides. However, more recent data from this laboratory suggests that the K^{+} channels involved in the opioid-induced hyperpolarization in LC (and in submucous ganglion) neurons are the same voltage-dependent (inwardly rectifying) channels activated by several other inhibitory transmitters (including SS; see below), and that such activation involves a PTX-sensitive GTP-binding protein but not cyclic AMP (Aghajanian and Wang 1987; North et al. 1987).

In contrast, the sum of our findings, derived from intracellular recordings of several diverse brain regions (Hippocampus CA1, cortex, dentate gyrus, nucleus accumbens) in vitro and carried out in two different laboratories, indicate that the most pronounced effect of low concentrations of the enkephalin peptides falls into the first or second category of mechanisms, pre- or postsynaptic modulation (Deisz et al. 1988; Moore et al. 1988a). However, preliminary studies of CA3 hippocampal pyramidal neurons in vitro (Moore et al. 1988b) have shown that dynorphin in low concentrations (50–100 nM), and the κ-preferring agonist U-50 488H, can augment another K^+ conductance, the so-called M-current (Brown and Adams 1980; Halliwell and Adams 1982). This is a voltage- and time-dependent conductance sustained and primarily activated at membrane potentials (-10 to about -65 mV) somewhat depolarized to resting levels (Fig. 1; see "Somatostatins" below). In sympathetic ganglia, muscarinic inactivation of this current cases the slow EPSP (Adams et al. 1982). Interestingly, higher dynorphin concentrations (1 μM), that can also activate μ- and δ-receptors as well as κ-receptors, and D-Ala^2, D-Leu^5 enkephalin, the μ/δ receptor activator, both reduce the size of the M-current (Moore et al. 1988b). These new data suggest that opioids can alter neuronal excitability by a fifth mechanism: *reciprocal alteration of the M-current*. As the M-current is a K^+ channel with a net hyperpolarizing effect, we would predict that the κ preferring agonists should hyperpolarize CA3 pyramidal neurons and inhibit their firing, whereas μ/δ-preferring agonists should depolarize and excite these neurons, provided that the cells are already

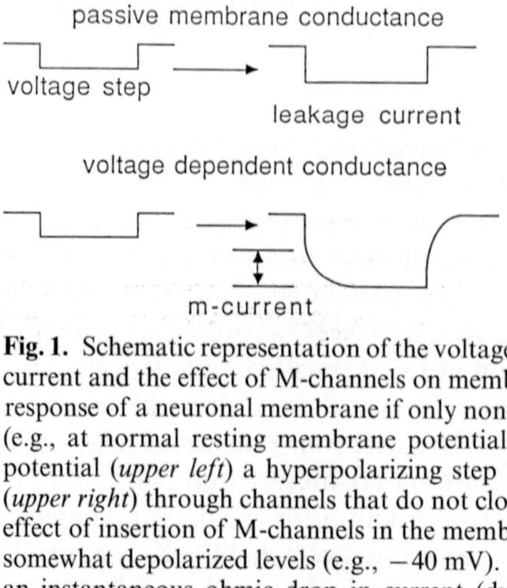

Fig. 1. Schematic representation of the voltage-clamp method of estimating the size of the M-current and the effect of M-channels on membrane current responses. *Top*, "ohmic" current response of a neuronal membrane if only non-voltage-dependent, leakage channels are open (e.g., at normal resting membrane potentials in some neurons). In a cell held at resting potential (*upper left*) a hyperpolarizing step "command" results in the passage of current (*upper right*) through channels that do not close at the new hyperpolarized potential. *Lower*, effect of insertion of M-channels in the membrane when holding the membrane potential at somewhat depolarized levels (e.g., -40 mV). An abrupt hyperpolarizing step now produces an instantaneous ohmic drop in current (due to ions passing through "leak" and other channels that have not had time to close), followed by a slowly settling current "relaxation" due to the time-dependent closing of M-channels at the new hyperpolarized potential. The difference between instantaneous current and steady-state current at the end of the hyperpolarizing command constitutes a measure of the M-current amplitude at a given holding potential. Inward currents are down by convention. (From Siggins et al. 1989)

somewhat depolarized to the point (about 60 mV) that M-channels are open. These opioid actions would thus constitute another example of voltage-dependent peptide effects.

Somatostatins

Both in vivo and in vitro studies (Pittman and Siggins 1981; Mancillas et al. 1986; Yamashita et al. 1987; Oomura and Mizuno 1986; North et al. 1987; Mihara et al. 1987; Moore et al. 1988c; Jacquin et al. 1988; see also Siggins and Gruol 1986, for review) indicate that the SSs (principally the tetradecapeptide, SS-14) also predominantly inhibit central and peripheral neurons (but see Olpe et al. 1980; Dodd and Kelly 1978; Delfs and Dichter 1983; Müller et al. 1986, for excitatory actions). However, Mancillas et al. (1986) noticed that SS-14 applied by iontophoresis had inhibitory effects on spontaneous firing in vivo unless acetylcholine (ACh) was included in the multibarrel iontophoresis assembly. Leakage of ACh was noted to favor excitatory responses to SS-14, both in the dorsal hippocampus and the parietal cortex, where fields of SS-containing and cholinergic nerve terminals overlap. SS-14, when applied alone, directly depressed spontaneous discharge rate in about 90% of these cells, with a slow onset and offset of its effects. However, when tested concurrently with either brief pulses or small amounts of ACh continuously leaked from an iontophoretic pipette, SS-14 caused a dose-dependent enhancement of the usual ACh-induced facilitations, while glutamate exitations were usually depressed (see also below). These data could explain the apparent contradictory or inconsistent effects of SS-14 reported by different groups (Siggins and Gruol 1986); the reported excitatory actions (see above) could have resulted from unrecognized influences of ACh, either allowed to leak (purposely or inadvertently) from an iontophoretic pipette or released spontaneously from endogenous sources. From the results of these extracellular studies, SS-14 could be conceived to have a bidirectionally *conditional* effect on hippocampal and cortical neurons.

The mechanism(s) of this SS-ACh interaction may derive from one or more of the several mechanisms utilized by ACh or SS individually. Electrophysiological studies indicate that activation of cholinergic muscarinic receptors mostly excites pyramidal neurons, via multiple mechanisms, including presynaptic actions and suppression of several different postsynaptic K^+ currents (Dodd et al. 1981; Benardo and Prince 1981; Madison et al. 1987), including the M-current (Halliwell and Adams 1982). The action of SS-14 in several brain regions has been partially clarified by intracellular in vitro studies. Thus, the SS-14 or SS-28 elicited inhibitions and hyperpolarizations of hippocampal CA1 pyramidal neurons are associated with a reduction in input resistance (Pittman and Siggins 1981; Watson and Pittman 1986) involving an increase in K^+ conductance (Watson and Pittman 1986).

Moore et al. (1988c) and Jacquin et al. (1988) have pursued the mechanisms of the interaction of SS and ACh using intracellular current and voltage-clamp recording techniques in the rat hippocampal and brain stem slice preparations. In current-clamp recordings, superfusion of SS-28 or SS-14 (0.2–1.0 μ*M*) elicited hyperpolarizations in most nucleus tractus solitarius and CA1 pyramidal cells, in association with reduced firing of spontaneous spikes and a small (15–30%) reduction in input resistance. No cells were depolarized by SS-28 or SS-14. In voltage clamp mode in the presence of 1 μ*M* tetrodotoxin, (TTX), when neurons were clamped either at resting or more positive membrane potentials, SS-14 and SS-28 superfusion usually (81% of cells) produced a steady outward current of up to 400 pA in association with a slight increase in conductance (Fig. 2).

The voltage- and time-dependent K^+ conductance, termed the M-current, is seen best with holding potentials around −40 mV and long hyperpolarizing command steps of 5–20 mV, when it appears as a slow inward current relaxation following the instantaneous (ohmic) inward current drop (Fig. 1; Brown and Adams 1980; Halliwell and Adams 1982). As the instantaneous current jump at command onset is larger than that at command offset, the relaxation represents the slow inactivation of an outward (K^+) current rather than the slow activation of an inward current. The difference between the instantaneous current at command onset and the steady-state current at the end of the command constitutes the magnitude of the M-current (Fig. 1), about 100–300 pA. Superfusion of SS-14 or SS-28 (0.5–1.0 μ*M*) increased the amplitude of the M-currents in hippocampal pyramidal cells (Fig. 2) by 15%–480% (mean ±SEM, 197 ± 27%, at −10 mV commands) in almost 85% of pyramidal neurons tested (Moore et al. 1988c). The relaxations were suppressed in all cells by superfusion or local pressure application of the muscarinic agonists carbachol or muscarine (25 or 50 μ*M*), even during their maximal augmentation by the SSs (Fig. 2).

Preliminary tests did not reveal effects of SS on other conductances altered by ACh, such as postburst afterhyperpolarizations (AHPs; generated by a Ca^{2+}-dependent K^+ current), Ca^{2+}-dependent spikes and the transient A-

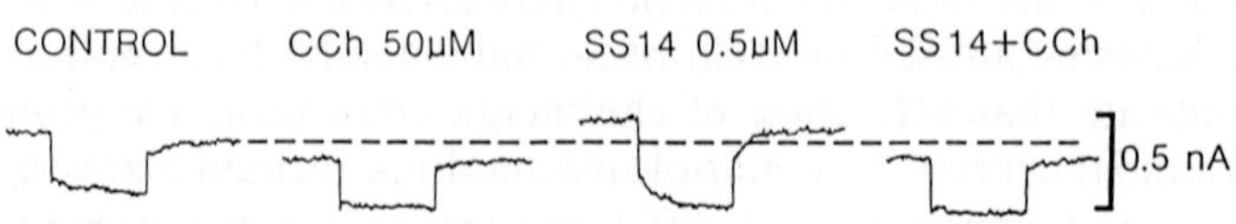

Fig. 2. Effect of carbachol (*CCh*), a muscarinic agonist, and somatostatin 14 (*SS-14*) on membrane currents recorded from a CA1 hippocampal pyramidal neuron in vitro in the presence of 1 μ*M* tetrodotoxin. The membrane potential was held at −40 mV (in the M-current range), and 1 s hyperpolarizing steps of −15 mV were applied. *Dashed line*, holding current in control conditions; note that CCh produces an overall inward steady current and SS-14 an overall outward current. During the command step, both the ohmic current drop and the M-current relaxation (see Fig. 1) are reduced by CCh, indicating an overall decrease in membrane currents recorded from a CA1 hippocampal pyramidal neuron in vitro in the presence of 1 μ*M* tetrodotoxin. The membrane potential was held at −40 mV (in the M-current range), and 1 s hyperpolarizing steps of −15 mV were applied. *Dashed line*, holding containing recording pipette. (Data of Moore et al. 1988c)

current (another K^+ conductance). The so-called Q-current, at least partially carried by K^+, was also not altered by the SSs (Moore et al. 1988c).

Thus, SS-14 and SS-28 specifically enhance a voltage-dependent K^+ current, the M-current. Voltage-clamp studies of neurons of the solitary tract complex have also shown SS-induced hyperpolarization and M-current augmentation (Jacquin et al. 1988). Although many agonists, including ACh and several neuropeptides such as luteinizing hormone releasing hormone (LH-RH) and bradykinin, have been shown to reduce the M-current (Brown 1988), this was first evidence in neurons for agonist-induced *enhancement* of the M-current. These data also show a reciprocal (opposing) regulation of a single type of voltage-dependent ionic channel by two different transmitters (ACh and SS). However, the SS-muscarinic interaction may be more complex than simple reciprocal regulation, since the in vivo studies indicate that SS alone has predominantly inhibitory actions on pyramidal neurons but is excitatory in the presence of ACh (Mancillas et al. 1986). This unusual interaction could result from the closing by ACh of the same M-channels opened by SS; in the presence of SS more M-channels are open for ACh to act upon (perhaps at lower ACh concentrations). ACh then predominates over the SS effect. However, more direct studies are needed to determine whether the other effects of ACh, for example, the voltage-independent depolarizations (Madison et al. 1987) and reduction of Ca^{2+} currents (Gähwiler and Brown 1987), are involved in the ACh-SS interaction. For example, SS has also been shown to decrease voltage-dependent Ca^{2+} conductances (Tsunoo et al. 1986; Luini et al. 1986).

In terms of function, it has been noted that the M-current acts to clamp the membrane potential at rest, thus braking regenerative phenomena such as spike bursts (Brown and Adams 1980; Adams et al. 1982). SS should accentuate this function. The recent finding by Vidal and Zieglgänsberger (1989) that SS blocks both glutamate and GABA evoked depolarizations and associated conductance increases in neocortical neurons in vitro could be explained by this clamping effect of the M-current augmentation by SS, although SS might also stimulate a slow uptake mechanism that decreases the extracellular amino acid concentration. By virtue of their overlapping terminal fields and physiological effects, selective SS-ACh, SS-glutamate, or SS-GABA interactions could be involved in disorders such as dementia or epilepsy or in the well-known role of the hippocampus and other cortical areas in normal behaviors such as memory and learning. The pronounced cortical loss of these transmitters and/or their receptors in dementia of the Alzheimer's type (Bartus et al. 1982; Rossor et al. 1980; Hyman et al. 1986; Greenamyre et al. 1985) further extends such implications. These findings also suggest that SS could be involved in prevention of epileptiform activity.

As shown by studies on several neuron types in other laboratories, SS and several other inhibitory agonists (opioid peptides, see above; α-adrenergic agonists, serotonin, baclofen, adenosine), may also activate another type of voltage-dependent K^+ channel (inward rectifying), probably through a common mechanism involving a PTX-sensitive GTP-binding protein (see North et al. 1987, for review). Studies in progress (S. Moore et al., in preparation) suggests that SS can also open inwardly rectifying K^+ channels in CA1 hippocampus. Thus, in many CA1 pyramidal neurons we also have seen SS elicit an outward current at membrane holding potentials (−65 to −75 mV) that should be outside the M-current activation range. As this SS current is blocked by PTX pretreatment (S. Moore et al., in preparation), which inactivates the GTP-binding proteins G_k, G_i, and G_o, we assume that SS activates the same GTP-binding protein mediated, inwardly rectifying K^+ channel as that reported for LC and certain peripheral neurons (North et al. 1987). However, the M-current and its activation by SS is PTX-insensitive (Moore et al., in preparation), suggesting that, if a G-protein is involved in the M-current, it must be something other than G_k, G_i, or G_o. A similar conclusion

Table 2. Actions of peptides on the M-current in vertebrate neurons

Neuropeptide	M-current amplitude
LH-RH, tLH-RH	Decrease
Angiotensin	Decrease
Substance P	Decrease
Bradykinin	Decrease
Enkephalins	Decrease (see text)
Somatostatin	Increase
Dynorphin	Increase (see text)

was reached by Dutar and Nicoll (1988), whose studies further suggest that the second messenger inositol triphosphate may mediate the muscarinic closure of M-channels in hippocampal pyramidal neurons. Combining these bits of data for the M-channel and inwardly rectifying K^+ channel leads us to postulate at least two possible voltage-dependent, receptor-channel sites of SS action in hippocampus, the M-channel and the inwardly rectifying K^+ channel. There are several other neuropeptides that act on the M-channel, as shown in Table 2 (see Brown 1988, for review). Most cause M-channel closure, and therefore are excitatory within the voltage range of M-channel activation.

In sum, data from several laboratories suggests that SSs can: (a) elicit presynaptic effects (Scharfman and Schwartzkroin 1988; Delfs and Dichter 1983); (b) postsynaptically modulate other transmitter effects; (c) activate at least two voltage-dependent K^+ channels; and (d) block voltage-dependent Ca^{2+} channels. GTP-binding proteins may be involved in some or all of these effects.

Corticotropin Releasing Factor

Considerable data from biochemical, physiological, and immunocytochemical studies indicate that central CRF immunoreactive neurons not only communicate through corticotropes to the rest of the organism but also with neurons of

CNS. These findings, combined with observation of potent effects of centrally injected CRF on autonomic (Brown et al. 1982) and behavioral (Sutton et al. 1982; Britton et al. 1982; Holsboer 1987) function in the rat, point to a role for CRF as an important neuromessenger in the CNS. The results of these studies and those reviewed below have led to suggestions that the neuronal effects of CRF may mediate the stresslike response seen in behaving animals with intracerebral CRF injections. Furthermore, the electrophysiological data provide a better understanding of the cellular and molecular mechanisms involved in the hypothalamic regulation of ACTH release from pituitary corticotropes.

In contrast to the peptides reviewed above, CRF appears to have predominantly excitatory actions. Thus, CRF administered intracerebroventricularly in low doses (10–100 ng) elicits EEG activation associated with increased (6–8 Hz) activity in the dorsal hippocampus and a desynchronization and decreased low frequency (less than 15 Hz) activity in cortex after a delay of 15–20 min (Ehlers et al. 1983). Higher doses (0.1–1.0 μg) produced a long-lasting EEG activation associated with increased locomotor and grooming behavior and in some rats after a delay of 2 h large interictal spikes spreading from amygdala to the dorsal hippocampus. At doses of 10–25 μg, CRF produced intense behavioral activation associated with interictal spikes and afterdischarges in amygdala. After a delay of 4–7 h motor seizures developed in some rats similar to amygdala "kindling."

One of several brain stem nuclei that appears to receive an innervation of CRF fibers is the LC. It is relevant that the LC has previously been implicated in behavioral activation and the mediation of stress responses (see Foote et al. 1980). In extracellular studies of single LC neurons recorded from anesthetized rats, CRF applied either intracerebroventricularly or by pressure from micropipettes increased spontaneous discharge rates in most LC cells (Valentino et al. 1983; Valentino and Foote 1987), while spike activity evoked by sensory stimulation was reduced (Valentino and Foote 1987). These and other data suggest that CRF has two distinct actions in the LC. Valentino et al. (1983) suggest that endogenous CRF, possibly released into the ventricular system or from fibers innervating the LC, may play a role in the activity of this nucleus. The effective intraventricular dose of CRF in this study is comparable to that reported to produce behavioral and autonomic activation (Brown et al. 1982; Sutton et al. 1982), providing evidence that CRF has actions on the autonomic and central nervous system akin to those of the stress syndrome. LC neurons are known to become more active during those behavioral states involved in heightened vigilance or orientation of the external environment (Foote et al. 1980).

In another extracellular in vivo study (Eberly et al. 1983), iontophoretically applied CRF increased spontaneous discharge in about half of the neurons of the cerebral cortex. In the thalamus, a larger percentage of the neurons tested were depressed than excited. In the preoptic, anterior, and ventromedial hypothalamic areas a majority of cells was activated whereas in lateral septum a majority was depressed. Thus, the results of this study (Eberly et al. 1983) show that, of those cells responding, the majority of hypothalamic and cortical neurons were excited by CRF, whereas thalamic and lateral septal neurons were more often depressed, suggesting region-specific effects of CRF on neuronal excitability. Unfortunately, it is not yet clear whether those cells tested would be likely targets for endogenous CRF-containing fibers.

The first intracellular studies of CRF were performed on the hippocampal slice preparation (Aldenhoff et al. 1983). Here, superfusion of CRF concentrations above 0.25 μ*M* usually depolarized both CA1 and CA3 pyramidal neurons, accompanied by elevations in spontaneous firing rate and a slight increase in input resistance (that is, a decrease in ionic conductance). At lower concentrations (10–200 n*M*), CRF also reduced the magnitude and duration of the AHPs following spontaneous or current-evoked trains of action potentials and increased discharge activity, with little apparent effect on membrane potential. More recently, similar effects of CRF have been seen in neurons of the nucleus tractus solitarious (G. Siggins, J. Champagnat, T. Jacquin, M. Saubie, in preparation).

These AHPs probably arise from Ca^{2+}-dependent K^+ conductance (Alger and Nicoll 1980; Hotson and Prince 1980; Schwartzkroin and Stafstrom 1980). As the size of the Ca^{2+}-dependent spikes recorded in the presence of TTX is not reduced by CRF, CRF probably diminishes the K^+ conductance directly rather than indirectly through alteration of Ca^{2+} conductances (Aldenhoff et al. 1983). Indeed, it is possible that a CRF-induced reduction of a Ca^{2+}-dependent K^+ conductance would lead to influx of greater amounts of Ca^{2+} during firing of spikes or bursts of spikes. Such an effect, if obtained also in corticotropes, could account for the enhanced release from these cells of ACTH via a calcium-dependent process (Vale et al. 1981).

It might be noted that the overall effect of CRF on hippocampal pyramidal neurons is similar to some of the actions of cholinergic muscarinic agonists on these cells (see Madison et al. 1987; Siggins and Gruol 1986, for review). Thus, muscarinic agonists depolarize these neurons with increased discharge, decreased ionic conductance, and a reduction of postburst AHPs. A portion of the muscarinic depolarization is attributable to inactivation of the M-current (see "Somatostatins" above). The effect of CRF on the M-current in hippocampal neurons has yet to be tested, but it could inactivate the M-current here like muscarinic agonists, and as CRF appears to do in human adenoma cells (see below). It is of interest, given the known antagonistic interaction of CRF and SS (Reisine and Axelrod 1983), that the M-current in pyramidal neurons is augmented by SS (see above). In the rat brain the hippocampus is a major target area for corticosterone. This structure displays the highest specific neuronal binding for corticosterone of any brain region (see Vidal et al. 1986 for references). Recent studies suggest that corticosterone hyperpolarizes hippocampal neurons by an increase in conductance to Cl^- and/or K^+ ions (Vidal et al. 1986; Zieglgänsberger et al., in preparation). It might be postulated that excitatory CRF actions are terminated by such a hyperpolarizing action of corticosterone (Holsboer 1987).

Hypothalamic neurons also seem to be likely targets for CRF-containing fibers (Bloom et al. 1982; Swanson et al. 1983). In preliminary extracellular studies of a hypothalamic slice preparation, most responsive cells of the arcuate area were depressed by 1 μM CRF (Siggins et al. 1985). In mostly extracellular recordings from neurons of the paraventricular nucleus, CRF superfusion (up to 1 μM) was more often effective than in the arcuate area. However, inhibition still predominated.

A recent intracellular electrophysiological study (Mollard et al. 1987) of the adrenocorticotropin-secreting adenoma, taken from patients with Cushing's disease and cultured in vitro, sheds considerable light on the mechanism(s) of CRF-evoked ACTH release. Dispersed cells from these tumors reveal calcium-dependent spikes whose duration of depolarization are markedly dependent upon K^+ conductances. In standard voltage recordings, CRF alone at low concentrations (10 nM) increased spike discharge and, at 10 times higher concentrations, caused slow depolarizations with: (a) increased firing, (b) increased input resistance, (c) increased duration and amplitude of the calcium-dependent spikes, and (d) decreased ionic conductance. CRF had no effect on the AHPs following single spikes; however, the effect of CRF on the long duration AHPs following bursts of spikes apparently was not examined.

These tumor cells possess a slow, voltage-dependent K^+ current that persists at the low resting potentials of these cells, and that is very similar to the M-current described for sympathetic ganglia (Brown and Adams 1980) and hippocampal neurons (Halliwell and Adams 1982). CRF, and the combination of angiotensin II and CRF, appears to reduce this persistent K^+ current, thus causing a net inward current at normal resting potentials in these adenoma cells (Mollard et al. 1987). These results suggest that the effect of reducing the K^+ conductance would be to depolarize the adenoma cells, thus causing increased action potential discharge and increasing the duration of each action potential. As the action potential currents appear to be carried mostly by calcium ions (the spikes are TTX resistant), the end result would be an increased calcium influx and enhanced ACTH release.

In sum, intracellular studies of hippocampal pyramidal neurons and human adenoma cells suggest inactivation of at least two K^+ conductance mechanisms (one ion-dependent and one voltage-dependent) for the excitatory action of CRF and may explain how CRF induces release of ACTH from corticotropes. Interestingly, the reduction of AHPs by block of a Ca^{2+}-dependent K^+ conductance has been described for the effects of other nonpeptide transmitters also in hippocampal pyramidal cells (see Siggins and Gruol 1986, for review). The end effect of such a process and the reduction of other K^+ currents (e.g., I_M) may lead not only to the increased firing of spikes (due to reduction of the inhibition afforded by the AHP) but also to a change in cellular Ca^{2+} physiology, including increased intracellular Ca^{2+}. Observations of excitatory actions of CRF in brain regions that may be involved in alerting behavior point to a role of CRF in the stress response of the extrahypothalamic brain as well as those areas concerned with ACTH and β-endorphin release.

Summary and Conclusion

It is evident from the foregoing review of only three peptide families that neuropeptides in general, and even a single neuropeptide alone, can exert a variety of actions (see Table 1) on central neurons. In many respects, peptides do not appear basically different from the nonpeptide neurotransmitter candidates (for review, see Siggins and Gruol 1986), although modulatory interactions with other transmitter effects may be more prevalent than for nonpeptides. As with the nonpeptide transmitters, it seems likely that the diversity of actions of an individual peptide may derive from the activation of multiple receptor subtypes for that peptide.

But now that we know that peptides can exert all the different general types of actions shown in Table 1, what do we really know? A major question remains: are all these multiple effects of even the same neuropeptide, at different concentrations in different cell types, meaningful with respect to the function of synaptic or endogenously released peptide? It seems possible, even likely, that only one of the various effects seen with exogenous peptide may be relevant to the "primary" action of the endogenous peptide.

It seems obvious by now that the only critical way to answer this most important question is to begin applying strictly, for each peptide in each brain region, the types of criteria already developed for identification of neurotransmitters and neuromodulators (see Siggins and Gruol 1986, for examples). The following brief criteria may thus be applied for identification of physiological roles for the neuropeptides:

1. The neuropeptide must be shown to be transported to, in some fashion, or contained within nerve elements projecting to, the target cell under study.
2. The peptide must be shown to be released onto the cell under study.
3. The effect of exogenously applied peptide must mimic the effect of the synaptically released or endogenous peptide, whether the effect is described as transmitterlike or modulatory.
4. Interacting drugs and ligands must alter the response to the exogenous peptide in the same direction as they alter the effect of the endogenously released peptide.

In reviewing these minimal, admittedly personal criteria, it should be noted that they have been satisfied for only very few peptides, principally LH-RH (Jan et al. 1980) and perhaps substance P (Tsunoo et al. 1982; Sejnowski 1982) in autonomic ganglia. In the CNS, satisfaction of the last two criteria have been the most difficult to realize, as with nonpeptide neurotransmitters (Siggins and Gruol 1986). Although some might consider current electrophysiological studies of exogenous peptides very inefficient, we submit that the present phase of "cataloguing" all the various actions of exogenous peptides is necessary for later comparison of the response to those resulting from synaptic release. Otherwise, how will we know what to look for among all the many possible expressions of endogenous ligand action? This will be especially critical in studies of the CNS, where selective activation of release of only one type of transmitter or peptide is very difficult and often nearly impossible.

Notwithstanding, we suggest that a concerted effort now be made to focus on the effects of synaptically released neuropeptide, under various conditions of stimulus rate, resting membrane potential, and the presence of other neurotransmitters. This task may require returning to the less isolated or less simplified model preparations that are more amenable to activation of peptide-containing afferents or networks. Then, interacting drugs or even antisera to the peptides might be used to parcel out the relevant peptide responses. Alternatively, other currently unimagined new methods will be needed.

Acknowledgement. We thank Nancy Callahan for typing the manuscript.

References

Adams PR, Brown DA, Constanti A (1982) M-currents and other potassium currents in bullfrog sympathetic neurones. J Physiol 330:537–572

Aldenhoff JB, Gruol DL, Rivier J, Vale W, Siggins GR (1983) Corticotropin releasing factor decreases post-burst hyperpolarizations and excites hippocampal pyramidal neurons in vitro. Science 221:875–877

Aghajanian GK, Wang YY (1987) Common α_2 and opiate effector mechanisms in the locus coeruleus: intracellular studies in brain slices. Neuropharmacology 26:793–799

Alger BE, Nicoll RA (1980) Epileptiform burst after-hyperpolarization: calcium-dependent potassium potential in hippocampal CA1 cells. Science 210:1122–1124

Barker JL, Neale JH, Smith TG, Macdonald RL (1978) Opiate peptide modulation of amino acid responses suggests novel form of neuronal communication. Science 199:1451–1453

Bartus RT, Dean RL, Beer B, Lippa AS (1982) The cholinergic hypothesis of geriatric memory dysfunction. Science 217:408–417

Benardo LS, Prince DA (1981) Acetylcholine induced modulation of hippocampal pyramidal neurons. Brain Res 211:227–234

Bloom FE, Battenberg ELF, Rivier J, Vale W (1982) Corticotropin releasing factor (CRF): immunoreactive neurons and fibers in rat hypothalamus. Regul Pept 4:43–48

Britton DR, Koob GF, Rivier J, Vale W (1982) Intraventricular corticotropin releasing factor enhances behavioral effects of novelty. Life Sci 31:363–367

Brown D (1988) M-currents: an update. Trends Neurosci 11:294–299

Brown DA, Adams PR (1980) Muscarinic suppression of a novel voltage-sensitive K^+ current in a vertebrate neurone. Nature 283:673–676

Brown MR, Fisher LA, Spiess J, Rivier C, Rivier J, Vale W (1982) Corticotropin-releasing factor (CRF): actions on the sympathetic nervous system and metabolism. Endocrinology 111:928–935

Crain SM (1988) Regulation of excitatory opioid responsivity of dorsal root ganglion neurons. In: Illes P, Farsang C (eds) Regulatory role of opioid peptides. VCH, Weinheim, pp 186–201

Davies J (1976) Effects of morphine and naloxone on Renshaw cells and spinal interneurons in morphine dependent and non-dependent rats. Brain Res 113:311–326

Deisz RA, Madamba S, Moore S, Siggins GR, Sutor B, Zieglgänsberger W (1988) Regulation of neuronal excitability by opioid peptides: intracellular analysis in several brain regions. In: Illes P, Farsang C (eds) Regulatory role of opioid peptides. VCH, Weinheim, pp 147–164

Delfs JR, Dichter MA (1983) Effects of somatostatin on mammalian cortical neurons in culture – physiological actions and unusual dose-response characteristics. J Neurosci 3 (6):1176–1188

Dodd J, Kelly JS (1978) Is somatostatin an excitatory transmitter in the hippocampus? Nature 273:674–675
Dodd J, Dingledine R, Kelly JS (1981) The excitatory action of acetylcholine on hippocampal neurones of the guinea pig and rat maintained in vitro. Brain Res 207:109–127
Dunlop K, Fischbach GD (1981) Neurotransmitters decrease the calcium conductance activated by depolarization of embryonic chick sensory neurones. J Physiol 317:519–535
Dutar P, Nicoll RA (1988) Classification of muscarinic responses in hippocampus in terms of receptor subtypes and second-messenger systems: electrophysiological studies in vitro. J Neurosci 8:4214–4224
Eberly LB, Dudley CA, Moss RL (1983) Iontophoretic mapping of corticotropin-releasing factor (CRF) sensitive neurons in the rat forebrain. Peptides 4:837–841
Ehlers CL, Henriksen SJ, Wang M, Rivier J, Vale W, Bloom FE (1983) Corticotropin releasing factor produces increases in brain excitability and convulsive seizures in rats. Brain Res 278:332–336
Foote S, Aston-Jones G, Bloom FE (1980) Impulse activity of locus coeruleus neurons in awake rats and squirrel monkeys is a function of sensory stimulation and arousal. Proc Natl Acad Sci USA 77:3033–3037
Gähwiler BH, Brown DA (1987) Muscarine affects calcium-currents in rat hippocampal pyramidal cells in vitro. Neurosci Lett 76:301–306
Greenamyre JT, Penney JB, Young AB (1985) Alterations in L-glutamate binding in Alzheimer's and Huntington's disease. Science 227:1496–1500
Gysling K, Wang RY (1983) Morphine-induced activation of A 10 dopamine neurons in the rat. Brain Res 277:119–127
Halliwell JV, Adams PR (1982) Voltage-clamp analysis of muscarinic excitation in hippocampal neurons. Brain Res 250:71–92
Holsboer F (1987) Psychoneuroendocrine strategies. Adv Psychosom Med 17:185–233
Hotson JR, Prince DA (1980) A calcium-activated hyperpolarization follows repetitive firing in hippocampal neurons. J Neurophysiol 43:409–419
Hyman BT, Van Hoesen GW, Damasio AR (1986) Glutamate depletion of the perforant pathway terminal zone in Alzheimer disease. Soc Neurosci Abstr 12:944
Jacquin T, Champagnat J, Madamba S, Denavit-Saubié M, Siggins GR (1988) Somatostatin depresses excitability in neurons of the solitary tract complex through hyperpolarization and augmentation of I_M, a noninactivating voltage-dependent outward current blocked by muscarinic agonists. Proc Natl Acad Sci USA 85:948–952
Jan YN, Jan LY, Kuffler SW (1980) Further evidence for peptidergic transmission in sympathetic ganglia. Proc Natl Acad Sci USA 77:5008–5012
Jeftinija S (1988) Opioid μ-receptor agonist inhibits synaptic transmission in the rat spinal dorsal horn. In: Illes P, Farsang C (eds) Regulatory role of opioids. VCH, Weinheim, pp 175–185
Jessel TM, Iversen LL (1977) Opiate analgesics inhibit substance P release from rat trigeminal nucleus. Nature 268:549–551
Luini A, Lewis D, Guild S, Schofield G, Weight F (1986) Somatostatin, an inhibitor of ACTH secretion, decreases cytostolic free calcium and voltage-dependent calcium current in a pituitary cell line. J Neurosci 6:3128–3132
Macdonald RL, Nelson PG (1978) Specific-opiate-induced depression of transmitter release from dorsal root ganglion cells in culture. Science 199:1449–1451
Madison DV, Lancaster B, Nicoll RA (1987) Voltage clamp analysis of cholinergic action in the hippocampus. J Neurosci 7:733–741
Mancillas JR, Siggins GR, Bloom FE (1986) Somatostatin selectively enhances acetylcholine-induced excitations in rat hippocampus and cortex. Proc Natl Acad Sci USA 83:7518–7521
Mihara S, North RA, Surprenant AM (1987) Somatostatin increases an inwardly rectifying potassium conductance in guinea-pig submucous plexus neurones. J Physiol 390:335–355
Mollard P, Vacher P, Guerin J, Rogawski MA, Dufy B (1987) Electrical properties of cultured adrenocorticotropin-secreting adenoma cells: effects of high K^+, corticotropin-releasing factor, and angiotensin II. Endocrinology 121:395–399

Moore SD, Madamba SG, Zieglgänsberger W, Siggins GR (1988a) Enkephalin analogues depress synaptic potentials in rat dentate granule cells recorded intracellularly in vitro. Neurosci Lett 91:71–76

Moore SD, Madamba SG, Siggins GR (1988b) Opioids reciprocally regulate the M-current in hippocampal CA3 pyramidal neurons in vitro. Soc Neurosci Abstr 14:464

Moore SD, Madamba SG, Joels M, Siggins GR (1988c) Somatostatin augments the M-current in hippocampal neurons. Science 239:278–280

Mudge AW, Leeman SE, Fischbach GD (1979) Enkephalin inhibits release of substance P from sensory neurons in culture and decreases action potential duration. Proc Natl Acad Sci USA 76:526–530

Müller AL, Kunkel DD, Schwartzkroin PA (1986) Electrophysiological actions of somatostatin (SRIF) in hippocampus: an in vitro study. Cell Mol Neurobiol 6:363–379

Nicoll RA (1982) Responses of central neurons to opiates and opioid peptides. In: Costa E, Trabucchi M (eds) Regulatory peptides: from molecular biology to function. Raven, New York, pp 337–346

Nicoll RA, Siggins GR, Ling N, Bloom FE, Guillemin R (1977) Neuronal actions of endorphins and enkephalins among brain regions: a comparative microiontophoretic study. Proc Natl Acad Sci USA 74:2584–2588

North RA, Williams JT, Surprenant AM, Christie MJ (1987) μ- And δ-receptors belong to a family of receptors that are coupled to potassium channels. Proc Natl Acad Sci USA 84:5487–5491

Olpe H-J, Balcar VJ, Bittiger H, Rink H, Sieber P (1980) Central actions of somatostatin. Eur J Pharmacol 63:127–133

Oomura Y, Mizuno Y (1986) Effect of somatostatin on the vagal motor neuron in the rat. Brain Res Bull 17:397–401

Pepper CM, Henderson G (1980) Opiates and opioid peptides hyperpolarize locus coeruleus neurons in vitro. Science 209:394–396

Pittman QJ (1980) Peptide modulation of neuronal electrical responses. In: Stark E, Makara GB, Halasz B, Rappay GY (eds) Endocrinology, neuroendocrinology, neuropeptides. Part 2. Advances in physiological sciences, vol 14. Pergamon, Oxford, pp 231–241

Pittman QJ, Siggins GR (1981) Somatostatin hyperpolarizes hippocampal pyramidal cells in vitro. Brain Res 221:402–408

Reisine T, Axelrod J (1983) Prolonged somatostatin pretreatment desensitizes somatostatin's inhibition of receptor-mediated release of adrenocorticotropin hormone and sensitizes adenylate cyclase. Endocrinology 113:811–813

Rossor MN, Emson PC, Mountjoy CQ, Roth M, Iversen LL (1980) Neurosci Lett 20:373–377

Satoh M, Akaike A, Takagi H (1979) Excitation by morphine and enkephalin of single neurons of nucleus reticularis paragigantocellularis in the rat: a probable mechanism of analgesic action of opioids. Brain Res 169:406–410

Scharfman HE, Schwartzkroin PA (1988) Selective depression of GABA-mediated IPSPs by somatostatin in area CA1 of rabbit hippocampal slices. Soc Neurosci Abstr 14:115

Schwartzkroin PA, Stafstrom CE (1980) Effects of EGTA on the calcium-activated after hyperpolarization in hippocampal CA3 pyramidal cells. Science 210:1125–1126

Sejnowski TJ (1982) Peptidergic synaptic transmission in sympathetic ganglia. Fed Proc 41:2923–2928

Siggins GR, Gruol DL (1986) Synaptic mechanisms in the vertebrate central nervous system. In: Bloom FE (ed) Handbook of physiology, Intrinsic regulatory systems of the brain. The American Physiological Society, Bethesda, pp 1–114

Siggins GR, Zieglgänsberger W (1981) Morphine and opioid peptides reduce inhibitory synaptic potentials in hippocampal pyramidal cells in vitro without alteration of membrane potential. Proc Natl Acad Sci USA 78:5235–5239

Siggins GR, Gruol D, Aldenhoff J, Pittman Q (1985) Electrophysiological actions of corticotropin-releasing factor in the central nervous system. Fed Proc 44:237–242

Siggins GR, Madamba SG, Moore SD (1989) Electrophysiological evaluation of acute ethanol effects on transmitter responses in central neurons. In: Deitrich R (ed) Initial Sensitivity to Ethanol. NIAA Research Monograph, Washington, D.C. (in press)

Sutor B, Zieglgänsberger W (1984) Actions of D-ala^2-D-leu^5-enkephalin and dynorphin A (1–17) on neocortical neurons in vitro. Neuropeptides 5:241–244

Sutor B, Zieglgänsberger W (1987) A low voltage activated, transient calcium current is responsible for the time-dependent depolarizing inward rectification of rat neocortical neurons in vitro. Pflügers Arch 410:102–111

Sutton RE, Koob GF, Le Moal M, Rivier J, Vale WW (1982) Corticotropin releasing factor produces behavioral activation in rats. Nature 297:331–333

Suzue T, Yanaihara N, Otsuka M (1981) Actions of vasopressin, gastrin releasing peptide and other peptides on neurons of newborn rat spinal cord in vitro. Neurosci Lett 26:137–142

Swanson LW, Sawchenko PE, Rivier J, Vale WW (1983) The organization of ovine corticotropin-releasing factor (CRF)-immunoreactive cells and fibers in the rat brain: an immunohistochemical study. Neuroendocrinology 36:165–186

Tsunoo A, Konishi S, Otsuka M (1982) Substance P as an excitatory transmitter of primary afferent neurons in guinea-pig sympathetic ganglia. Neuroscience 7:2025–2037

Tsunoo A, Yoshii M, Narahashi T (1986) Block of calcium channels by enkephalin and somatostatin in neuroblastoma-glioma hybrid NG 108-15 cells. Proc Natl Acad Sci USA 983:9832–9836

Vale WW, Spiess J, Rivier C, Rivier J (1981) Characterization of a 41-residue ovine hypothalamic peptide that stimulates secretion of corticotropin and β-endorphin. Science 213:1394–1397

Valentino RJ, Foote SL (1987) Corticotropin-releasing factor disrupts sensory responses of brain noradrenergic neurons. Neuroendocrinology 45:28–36

Valentino RJ, Foote SL, Aston-Jones G (1983) Corticotropin-releasing factor activates noradrenergic neurons of the locus coeruleus. Brain Res 270:363–367

Vidal C, Zieglgänsberger W (1989) Actions of somatostatin on rat neocortical neurons in vitro. Eur J Neurosci (in press)

Vidal C, Jordan W, Zieglgänsberger W (1986) Corticosterone reduces the excitability of hippocampal pyryamidal cells in vitro. Brain Res 383:54–59

Watson TWJ, Pittman QJ (1986) Somatostatin action in hippocampus. Soc Neurosci Abstr 12:150

Werz MA, Macdonald RL (1982) Heterogenous sensitivity of cultured dorsal root ganglion neurones to opioid peptides selective for μ- and δ-opiate receptors. Nature 299:730–733

Werz MA, Macdonald RL (1983) Opioid peptides selective for μ- and δ-opiate receptors reduce calcium-dependent action potential duration by increasing potassium conductance. Neurosci Lett 42:173–178

Werz MA, Macdonald RL (1984) Dynorphin decreases a voltage-dependent Ca conductance in mouse dorsal root ganglion neurons in cell culture. Neurosci Lett 46:185–190

Williams J, Zieglgänsberger W (1981) Mature spinal ganglion cells are not sensitive to opiate receptor mediated actions. Neurosci Lett 21:211–216

Williams JT, Egan TM, North RA (1982) Enkephalin opens potassium channels on mammalian central neurons. Nature 299:74–77

Yamashita N, Shibuya N, Ogata E (1986) Hyperpolarization of the membrane potential caused by somatostatin in dissociated human pituitary adenoma cells that secrete growth hormone. Proc Natl Acad Sci USA 83:6198–6202

Yamashita N, Kojima I, Shibuya N, Ogata E (1987) Pertussis toxin inhibits somatostatin-induced K^+ conductance in human pituitary tumor cells. Am J Physiol 253:E28–E32

Yoshimura M, North RA (1983) Substantia gelatinosa neurones in vitro hyperpolarized by enkephalin. Nature 305:529–530

Zieglgänsberger W (1986) Central control of nociception. In: Mountcastle VB, Bloom FE, Geiger SR (eds) Handbook of physiology, vol 4. The nervous system. IV. American Physiological Society, Bethesda, pp 581–645

Zieglgänsberger W, Bayerl J (1976) The activity of opiates in the spinal cord of cat. Brain Res 115:111–128

Zieglgänsberger W, Neher E (1988) μ- And δ-selective opioid agonists reduce a calcium-current in neuroblastoma × glioma hybrid cells analysed with tight-seal whole-cell recording. Proceedings, INRC conference, Albi, France
Zieglgänsberger W, Sutor B (1983) Responses of substantia gelatinosa neurones to putative neurotransmitters in an in vitro preparation of the adult rat spinal cord. Brain Res 279:316–320
Zieglgänsberger W, Tulloch IF (1979) The effects of methionine- and leucine-enkephalin on spinal neurons of the cat. Brain Res 167:53–64
Zieglgänsberger W, French ED, Siggins GR, Bloom FE (1979) Opioid peptides may excite hippocampal pyramidal neurons by inhibiting adjacent inhibitory interneurons. Science 205:415–417

13 Clinical Aspects of Neuropeptide Research

Corticotropin Releasing Factor, the Amygdaloid Complex, and Depression: A Hypothetical Interrelationship *

C. D. KILTS [1,2], P. D. BUTLER [1], and C. B. NEMEROFF [1,2]

Introduction

The neurochemical basis of the pathogenesis and pharmacotherapy of affective disorders has been the subject of much speculation and theorization. The early biogenic amine theories postulated a critical role for norepinephrine and serotonin in the etiology of depression (Schildkraut 1965; Jesberger and Richardson 1985) and the mechanism of action of antidepressant (Sulser et al. 1978; de Montigny and Aghajanian 1978). More recently, the concept of a peptidergic basis of depression has received considerable investigative attention (Nemeroff and Bissette 1986) with the majority of interest focused on the 41 amino acid neuropeptide corticotropin releasing factor (CRF; Nemeroff 1990). This discussion attempts to expand the involvement of CRF in depressive disorders to include specific actions in the amygdaloid complex, an integral component of the limbic system. To this end, a brief discussion of the evidence implicating CRF in depression is presented, followed by a review of evidence linking the amygdaloid complex and depressive disorders, and, finally, the case for a role of CRF as a neurotransmitter or neuromodulator in the amygdaloid complex is presented. The causal relationships proposed result from our contention that the amygdaloid nuclear complex represents a common anatomical substrate for a seemingly diverse group of psychiatric disorders (e.g., schizophrenia, depression, anxiety) which utilize distinct amygdaloid neurotransmitter systems as elements of neural circuits mediating affected behaviors.

Involvement of CRF in the Pathogenesis of Depressive Disorders

Support for the role of CRF in depression is largely derived from clinical and preclinical findings and from evidence supporting a stress diathesis for depressive disorders. An extensive review of these data and the relevant role of CRF as an integral component in the hypothalamic-pituitary-adrenal (HPA) axis and

* This research was supported by NIMH grants 39967 and 42088.
Departments of [1] Psychiatry and [2] Pharmacology, Duke University Medical Center, Durham, NC 27710, USA.

Neuropsychopharmacology
Edited by Bunney/Hippius/Laakmann/Schmauß

in HPA axis abnormalities in depression is beyond the intent of this discussion. The interested reader is referred to several recent reviews (Gold and Chrousos 1985; Amsterdam et al. 1988; Nemeroff 1990; Butler and Nemeroff 1990) for more detailed discussion. The presence of supranormal concentrations of CRF in cerebrospinal fluid (CSF) of patients with depression has been well documented (Nemeroff et al. 1984; Banki et al. 1987). The concomitant decrease in depressive symptoms and pretreatment CSF CRF concentrations following a mean of 8.5 treatments with electroconvulsive therapy suggest that elevated CSF concentrations of CRF represent a state-dependent, rather than trait-dependent, marker of depression (Butler and Nemeroff 1990). The apparent hypersecretion of CRF in depressed patients may underlie, at least in part, the hypercortisolemia characteristic of a large subgroup of patients (Sachar et al. 1973; Carroll et al. 1976). It is not known whether CRF is hypersecreted at extrahypothalamic sites in depressed patients; no examinations of synaptic markers of CRF neurons (e.g., CRF concentration, CRF mRNA, CRF receptors, efficiency of CRF signal transduction) in postmortem brain regions from depressed patients have been conducted. However, frontal cortical CRF receptors are decreased in suicide victims, many of whom fulfill criteria for major depression (Nemeroff et al. 1988). By and large, however, the CNS sites of origin of the elevated CSF concentration of CRF in depression are unknown.

Preclinical studies indicate that the consequences of the central administration of CRF are strikingly similar to many of the cardinal signs and symptoms of depression. The intracerebroventricular administration of CRF to rats results in decreased food intake and subsequent weight loss (Britton et al. 1982; Morley and Levine 1982; Levine et al. 1983), diminished sexual behavior (Sirinathsinghji et al. 1983; Sirinathsinghji 1987), psychomotor activation (Sutton et al. 1982; Ehlers et al. 1983; Britton et al. 1986), and disrupted sleep (Ehlers et al. 1983). The central administration of CRF also induces an anxiogenic-like state in laboratory animals (Britton et al. 1982, 1985; Dunn and File 1987), an effect consistent with a role for CRF in anxiety disorders and of relevance to the present discussion due to the recognized parallels in the symptoms, treatment, and biology of anxiety and depressive disorders (Butler and Nemeroff 1990). Many of these effects of CRF have been demonstrated to be independent of its actions in regulating the activity of the HPA axis (Britton et al. 1986; Eaves et al. 1985). These findings support the contention that extrahypothalamic CRF influences similar brain functions to those disordered in depression, with psychopathology perhaps reflecting a hyperactivity of CRF neurons.

Additional indirect support for the involvement of CRF in the pathogenesis of depression is derived from the compelling data indicating a critical role for CRF in the organization of responses to stress and the increasingly supported contention that stress represents an exacerbant of the depressive process. The effects of the intracerebroventricular or intracerebral administration of CRF mimics many of the responses commonly observed following stress. Paralleling responses include activation of the autonomic nervous system (Brown et al.

1982; Lenz et al. 1987), activation of common neurotransmitter systems (Valentino et al. 1983; Dunn and Berridge 1987), alterations in neuroendocrine function (Donald et al. 1983; Rock et al. 1984; Rivier et al. 1986), and the elicitation of specific behavioral patterns (Koob and Bloom 1985). Moreover, studies utilizing the CRF antagonist α-helical CRF_{9-41} further support the contention that the enhanced release of CRF at extrahypothalamic sites in the CNS mediates many of the sequelae of exposure to stress. The central administration of α-helical CRF_{9-41} attenuates stress-induced effects including increases in autonomic nervous system activity (Brown et al. 1986), decreases in food consumption (Krahn et al. 1986), fighting (Tazi et al. 1987), inhibition of luteinizing hormone secretion (Rivier et al. 1986), and decreases in exploratory behavior (Berridge and Dunn 1987). Finally, we have demonstrated that exposure of rats to acute and chronic regimens of stress produces profound alterations in the concentration of CRF-like immunoreactivity in selectively responsive brain nuclei or areas, most notably the locus ceruleus and arcuate/median eminence area (Chappell et al. 1986). Collectively, these findings indicate that CRF neurons are recruited in organizing a diverse array of brain output systems in forming an integrated response to stress.

Involvement of the Amygdaloid Complex in the Pathogenesis and Pharmacotherapy of Depression

The amygdaloid nuclear complex is an aggregate of functionally, biochemically, and anatomically heterogeneous nuclei located in the temporal lobes and is central to every definition of the organization of the limbic system. While the component nuclear groups of the amygdaloid complex are phylogenetically preserved, their relative orientation and further subdivision differs across species (Price 1981). Initial support for a role of the amygdaloid complex in the pathogenesis of depressive disorders is derived by arraying the putative functions subserved by the amygdaloid complex and the major symptoms of depression as extremes on a physiological-pathological continuum of brain function. The amygdala has a long-recognized role as the primary substrate of affective expression (Kluver and Bucy 1939; Gloor 1986). Additional evidence supports the involvement of the amygdaloid complex in regulation of the HPA axis (Beaulieu et al. 1987), sleep (Kluver and Bucy 1939), feeding behavior (Fonberg 1981), sexual behavior (Kling and Dunne 1976) and social behavior (Rosvold et al. 1954) – brain functions which are preferentially disordered in depressive disorders. However, it should be noted that the constellation of brain functions affected by stimulation or ablation of the amygdaloid complex is not identical to the constellation of affected functions which form the major signs and symptoms of depression. This does not necessarily weaken the case for the amygdaloid complex as an anatomical substrate of depression but rather reflects the limitations inherent in this inferential approach to defining cause-effect relationships. Species differences, differences in the neurochemical and anatomical specificity of functional alterations produced by experimental manipulations versus pathology, and perhaps most importantly the probability that the amygdaloid complex is not exclusively involved in the pathogenesis of depression undoubtedly contribute to the expected mismatch between experimental and clinical observations.

A more convincing argument for the involvement of the amygdaloid complex in depressive disorders is derived from preclinical studies of the effects of the intra-amygdaloid microinjection of antidepressants in animal behavioral models of depression. A diverse collection of animal behavioral paradigms varying in predictive, face, and construct validity have been proposed to represent models of clinical depression (Willner 1984; Jesberger and Richardson 1985). The intra-amygdaloid microinjection of antidepressants mimics the effects of their systemic administration in a striking number of diverse animal models of depression. When microinjected into the amygdaloid complex, tricyclic antidepressants inhibit muricidal behavior in rats (Horowitz 1966) and reverse the performance deficits occurring in olfactory bulbectomized rats (Broekkamp et al. 1982). Furthermore, the systemic administration of tricyclic antidepressants suppresses seizure activity kindled from amygdaloid sites of stimulation (Penaloza-Rojas et al. 1961; Minabe et al. 1987).

Mice or rats reexposed to an inescapable water swim task rapidly assume an immobile posture. The onset of immobility in response to retesting in this behavioral despair model of depression (Porsolt et al. 1978) is delayed by pretreatment with an impressively wide variety of antidepressant treatments including tricyclic antidepressants, monoamine oxidase inhibitors, atypical antidepressants, electroconvulsive therapy, and rapid eye movement sleep deprivation (Browne 1979; Gorka and Wojtasik 1980; Porsolt et al. 1977, 1978; Porsolt 1981; Schecter and Chance 1979). A unique, significant positive correlation between clinical potency and the potency of antidepressants in behavioral despair paradigms has been reported (Willner 1984); the use of chronic rather than acute drug administration regimens enhanced the effects of antidepressants (Kitada et al. 1981) and reduced the incidence of false positives (Kitada et al. 1981; Kawashima et al. 1986). Thus, behavioral despair paradigms exhibit important elements of predictive and face validity supporting their utility as animal behavioral models of depression. It is therefore of interest that the intra-amygdaloid microinjection of tricyclic antidepressants or a monoamine oxidase inhibitor significantly reduced the duration of immobility in the retesting component of a forced swim behavioral despair paradigm (Araki et al. 1984; Duncan et al. 1986). Drug injections into the nucleus accumbens, caudate nucleus, and anterior amygdaloid area were ineffective.

Consistent with the organization of the amygdaloid complex into functionally distinct nuclear groups, the effects of the intra-amygdaloid administration of antidepressants in forced swim tasks appear to be localized to specific component nuclei of the amygdaloid complex, notably the central, lateral, or basal nuclei (Duncan et al. 1986) or medial nucleus (Araki et al. 1984). Furthermore, electrolytic lesions of the amygdaloid complex largely confined to the basolateral (Gorka et al. 1979) or medial (Shimazoe et al. 1988) nucleus blocked the effects of systemically administered imipramine on performance in a forced swim paradigm. The effects of the systemic administration of imipramine or desipramine on duration of immobility were attenuated by neurotoxin-induced lesions of catecholaminergic, but not serotonergic, neurons innervating the amygdaloid complex (Araki et al. 1985). These findings indicate that the amygdaloid complex is an important site of action for antidepressants in mediating their effects on performance in animal behavioral models of depression. The strength and significance of this contention are dependent on the value of behavioral despair paradigms in testing theorization concerning the sites and mechanisms of action of the therapeutic effects of antidepressants.

The plausible interrelationship between the critical role of the amygdaloid complex in the ability to organize a response to stress (see below) and a stress diathesis for depression provides additional support for the involvement of the amygdaloid complex in depressive disorders. An extensive literature implicates the amygdaloid complex in neuroendocrine (Beaulieu et al. 1987), autonomic and cardiovascular (Galeno et al. 1984), gastric (Henke 1981), and behavioral (Blanchard and Blanchard 1972) responses to stress. Moreover, the unit activity in the central amygdaloid nucleus is significantly altered by stress (Henke 1988), and electrical stimulation of this nucleus produces somatic (Henke 1988) and autonomic (Iwata et al. 1987) responses highly reminiscent of responses to stressful situations. The effects of stress and tricyclic antidepressants on amygdaloid function suggests that these distinct influences may use amygdaloid neurons as a common means of exacerbating and attenuating, respectively, the depressive process.

CRF as a Neurotransmitter or Neuromodulator in the Amygdaloid Nuclear Complex

A hallmark of the limbic system is the richness of content and diversity of neuropeptides in brain structures which comprise its anatomical organization (Palkovits 1984). The amygdaloid complex is exemplary in this regard as many neuropeptides are well represented and unevenly distributed among its component nuclei (Roberts et al. 1982; Shiosaka et al. 1983). Immunohistochemical mapping techniques demonstrate a high density of CRF immunopositive cells and fibers in the amygdaloid complex, the densest localization of CRF neurons being found in the central amygdaloid nucleus (Merchenthaler 1984; Olschowka et al. 1982; Sakanaka et al. 1987). These CRF cells project to the parabrachial nucleus, mesencephalic nucleus of the trigeminal nerve, and bed nucleus of the stria terminalis; the cells of the corticomedial amygdaloid nucleus provide a distinct CRF innervation of the ventromedial nucleus of the hypothalamus (Sakanaka et al. 1986). The combination of micropunch dissection and radioimmunoassay techniques indicate a nuclei-variable distribution of CRF in the amygdaloid complex with the greatest concentration in the central amygdaloid nucleus (Palkovits et al. 1985; Skofitsch and Jacobowitz 1985; Kilts et al. 1987).

In addition to CRF immunoreactivity, a number of additional markers of CRF synapses are well represented in the amygdaloid complex. The mapping of ^{125}I-labeled CRF binding sites using in vitro quantitative autoradiography indicates an intermediate to high density of CRF receptors in the amygdaloid complex (De Souza et al. 1985). The highest density of CRF receptors was noted in the basolateral amygdaloid nucleus, a component nucleus containing only low to intermediate densities of CRF immunoreactive fibers and CRF content. In the central amygdaloid nucleus, the content of mRNA encoding the amino acid sequence of CRF is similar to that of the CRF mRNA-rich paraventricular nucleus (PVN) of the hypothalamus (Thompson et al. 1987; Beyer et al. 1988). However, in contrast to the PVN, the CRF mRNA of the central amygdaloid nucleus is not under the regulatory influence of adrenal corticosteroids (Beyer et al. 1988). This differential regulation indicates that CRF neurons in the central amygdaloid nucleus are involved in brain functions other than the regulation of the synthesis and release of pituitary ACTH, the principal role of PVN CRF neurons (Lundblad and Roberts 1988). Independent of intrinsic CRF neurons, the amygdaloid complex is, however, involved in regulation of the HPA axis, as indicated by the presence of high concentrations of glucocorticoid receptors in the central amygdaloid nucleus (Reul and DeKloet 1985) and the observation that the amygdaloid nuclei exert profound influences on corticosterone secretion (Dunn and Whitener 1986). The apparently unique functions of amygdaloid CRF neurons reinforce the concept of distinct functional roles for different populations of CRF neurons in the CNS and the fact that CRF subserves brain functions other than as a corticotropin releasing factor. Thus, dysregulation of amygdaloid CRF-containing neurons may be involved in the signs and symptoms of depression other than hypercortisolemia.

Before CRF neurons in the amygdaloid complex can be implicated in the pathogenesis of depressive disorders, the question of the neuroactivity of CRF in the amygdaloid complex and its involvement in specific amygdaloid functions needs to be addressed. While much more work is clearly necessary, several recent reports support the contention that CRF is a neuroregulator in the amygdaloid complex. First, the intracerebroventricular administration of CRF to rats results in the delayed expression of electrographic and behavioral signs of seizure activity which originate in the amygdaloid complex (Ehlers et al. 1983). These signs were indistinguishable from those produced by electrical kindling of the amygdala. Secondly, the bilateral intra-amygdaloid administration of CRF produces a facilitated retention of a passive avoidance response and decreased activity and frequency of specific behaviors in an open field apparatus (Liang and Lee 1988). These results suggest that CRF neurons modulate the output of the amygdaloid complex, although the results of more focused electrophysiological, molecular, behavioral, and biochemical studies are needed to establish the physiological significance of amygdaloid CRF neurons.

Amygdaloid CRF Neurons and Depression: An Integration of Findings

Based upon the preceding discussion we propose the following role for amygdaloid CRF neurons in the pathogenesis of depressive disorders. Depressed patients and perhaps individuals predisposed to depression would be characterized by a hyperfunctioning of amygdaloid CRF neurons. The sustained enhanced synaptic release of CRF would result in a "kindling" of CRF-receptive cells in the amygdaloid complex; these cells represent elements of neural circuits which are critical determinants of the affective state of the individual. The amygdaloid complex is well recognized as a particularly sensitive substrate for the induction of kindled phenomena (Goddard et al. 1969), and kindling processes have been previously suggested to be involved in the development of psychopathology (Post et al. 1981). Indeed, amygdaloid-kindled seizures have been proposed as models of depression and a means of assessing potential antidepressant properties of pharmacological and somatic treatments (Babington 1981; Post et al. 1986; Adamec and Stark-Adamec 1983). The kindled state would be distinct from the seizure state induced by repeated electrical stimulation of the amygdaloid complex or high intracerebroventricular doses of CRF, perhaps due to the differential (graded?) effects of physiological versus pharmacological doses of CRF and/or the neurochemically selective influence of CRF versus electrical stimulation. Progressive and long-lasting alterations in brain function and behavior unrelated to seizure activity can be reliably evoked by mild kindling conditions applied to the amygdaloid complex (Adamec 1978). Presumably, the therapeutic effects of antidepressants would reflect a direct or indirect action on amygdaloid CRF neurons to rebalance their influence or counteracting CRF-independent actions on CRF-modulated neural circuits originating in the amygdaloid complex.

Stress represents, perhaps, an important unifying feature in this hypothetical interrelationship between CRF, the amygdaloid complex, and depression. It has been often suggested that stressful life events may predispose an individual to or precipitate major depression (Lesse 1982; Blazer et al. 1987). The role of the amygdaloid complex in emotional behavior and as a determinant of the impact of stressful stimuli on the organism has been increasingly emphasized (Henke 1988). Alterations in the functional activity of the amygdaloid complex, particularly the central nucleus, contribute critically to some forms of stress-related somatic disorders (Henke 1981, 1988). The enhanced neuronal excitability associated with partial, subconvulsant electrical kindling of the centromedial area of the amygdaloid complex resulted in an increased susceptibility to stress-induced gastric pathology (Henke and Sullivan 1985). It is plausible that the amygdaloid complex also is highly involved in the psychological manifestations of stress (Hitchcock and Davis 1986; Rosen and Davis 1988). Thus, in this model the affective symptoms associated with a CRF-induced kindling of amygdaloid neuronal circuits, perhaps in particular those involving the CRF-rich central amygdaloid nucleus, would be exacerbated by stressful life events. Such a CRF-kindled state would also render the individual more susceptible to the deleterious effects of stress. Therefore, the postulated hypersecretion of amygdaloid CRF neurons may predispose the individual to a decreased resistance to the negative effects of stress on affective states, and/or earlier life stress may facilitate the kindling process by enhancing the release or actions of CRF in the amygdaloid complex.

The proposed causal relationship between amygdaloid CRF neurons and depressive disorders represents a heuristic model for studying the role of CRF in the pathogenesis of affective disorders. This model results from evidence supporting (a) a role for CRF in depression, (b) a role for the amygdaloid complex in depression, and (c) a role for CRF as a neuroregulator in the amygdaloid complex. This model provides a framework or guide for the design of preclinical and clinical experiments intended to determine the anatomical and neurochemical substrates of the pathogenesis and pharmacotherapy of depression.

Acknowledgement. The authors are grateful to Mary Kolodny for valuable assistance in literature review and the preparation of this manuscript.

References

Adamec R (1978) Normal and abnormal limbic system mechanisms of emotive biasing. In: Livingston KE, Hornykiewicz O (eds) Limbic mechanisms. Plenum, New York

Adamec RE, Stark-Adamek C (1983) Limbic kindling and animal behavior – implications for human psychopathology associated with complex partial seizures. Biol Psychiatry 18:269–293

Amsterdam JD, Maeslin G, Winokur A, Berwisly N, Kling M, Gold PW (1988) The oCRH stimulation test before and after clinical recovery from depression. J Affective Disord 14:213–222

Araki H, Kawashima K, Aihara H (1984) The difference in the site of actions of tricyclic antidepressants and methamphetamine on the duration of the immobility in the behavioral despair test. Jpn J Pharmacol 35:67–72

Araki H, Kawashima K, Uchiyama Y, Aihara H (1985) Involvement of amygdaloid catecholaminergic mechanism in suppressive effects of desipramine and imipramine on duration of immobility in rats forced to swim. Eur J Pharmacol 113:313–318

Babington RG (1981) Neurophysiological techniques and antidepressant activity. In: Enna SJ, Malick JB, Richelson E (eds) Antidepressants: neurochemical, behavioral and clinical perspectives. Raven, New York, pp 157–173

Banki CM, Bissette G, Arato M, O'Connor L, Nemeroff CB (1987) CSF corticotropin-releasing factor-like immunoreactivity in depression and schizophrenia. Am J Psychiatry 144:873–877

Beaulieu S, Di Paolo T, Cote J, Barden N (1987) Participation of the central amygdaloid nucleus in the response of adrenocorticotropin secretion to immobilization stress: opposing roles of the noradrenergic and dopaminergic systems. Neuroendocrinology 45:37–46

Berridge CW, Dunn AJ (1987) A corticotropin-releasing factor antagonist reverses the stress-induced changes of exploratory behavior in mice. Horm Behav 21:393–401

Beyer HS, Matta SG, Sharp BM (1988) Regulation of the messenger ribonucleic acid for corticotropin-releasing factor in the paraventricular nucleus and other brain sites of the rat. Endocrinology 123:2117–2123

Blazer D, Hughes D, George LK (1987) Stressful life events and the onset of a generalized anxiety syndrome. Am J Psychiatry 144:1178–1183

Britton DR, Koob GF, Rivier J, Vale W (1982) Intraventricular corticotropin-releasing factor enhances behavioral effects of novelty. Life Sci 31:363–367

Britton KT, Morgan J, Rivier J, Vale W, Koob GF (1985) Chlordiazepoxide attenuates response suppression induced by corticotropin-releasing factor in the conflict test. Psychopharmacology 86:170–174

Britton KT, Lee G, Dana R, Risch SC, Koob GF (1986) Activating and anxiogenic' effects of corticotropin releasing factor are not inhibited by blockade of the pituitary-adrenal system with dexamethasone. Life Sci 39:1281–1286

Broekkamp CL, Garrigou D, Lloyd KG (1982) The importance of the amygdala in the effect of antidepressants on olfactory bulbectomised rats. In: Costa E, Racagni G (eds) Advances in biochemical psychopharmacology, vol 31. Raven, New York, pp 371–377

Brown MR, Fisher LA, Spiess J, Rivier C, Rivier J, Vale W (1982) Corticotropin releasing factor: actions on the sympathetic nervous system and metabolism. Endocrinology 111:928–931

Browne RG (1979) Effects of antidepressants and anticholinergics in a mouse "behavioural despair" test. Eur J Pharmacol 58:331–334

Butler PD, Nemeroff CB (1990) Corticotropin-releasing factor as a possible cause of comorbidity in anxiety and depressive disorders. In: Maser JD, Cloninger CR (eds) Comorbidity of mood and anxiety disorders. Amer Psychiat Assn Press, Washington, DC, pp 413–438

Carroll BJ, Curtis GC, Davies BM, Mendels J, Sugerman AA (1976) Urinary free cortisol excretion in depression. Psychol Med 6:43–50

Chappell PB, Smith MA, Kilts CD, Bissette G, Ritchie J, Anderson C, Nemeroff CB (1986) Alterations in corticotropin-releasing factor-like immunoreactivity in discrete rat brain regions after acute and chronic stress. J Neurosci 6(10):2908–2914

de Montigny C, Aghajanian GK (1978) Tricyclic antidepressants: long-term treatment increases responsivity of rat forebrain neurons to serotonin. Science 202:1303–1306

De Souza EB, Insel TR, Perrin MH, Rivier J, Vale WE, Kuhar MJ (1985) Corticotropin-releasing factor receptors are widely distributed within the rat central nervous system: an autoradiographic study. J Neurosci 5:3189–3203

Donald RA, Redekopp C, Cameron V, Nicholls MG, Bolton J, Livesey J, Espiner EA, Rivier J, Vale W (1983) The hormonal actions of corticotropin-releasing factor in sheep: effect of intravenous and intracerebroventricular injection. Endocrinology 113:866–870

Duncan GE, Breese GR, Criswell H, Stumpf WE, Mueller RA, Covey JB (1986) Effects of antidepressant drugs injected into the amygdala on behavioral responses of rats in the forced swim test. J Pharmacol Exp Ther 238:758–762

Dunn AJ, Berridge CW (1987) Corticotropin-releasing factor administration elicits a stress-like activation of cerebral catecholaminergic systems. Pharmacol Biochem Behav 27:685–691

Dunn AJ, File SE (1987) Corticotropin-releasing factor has an anxiogenic action in the social interaction test. Horm Behav 21:193–202

Dunn JD, Whitener J (1986) Plasma corticosterone responses to electrical stimulation of the amygdaloid complex: cytoarchitectural specificity. Neuroendocrinology 42:211–217

Eaves M, Thatcher-Britton K, Rivier J, Vale W, Koob GF (1985) Effects of corticotropin-releasing factor on locomotor activity in hypophysectomized rats. Peptides 6:923–926

Ehlers CL, Hendriksen SJ, Wang M, Rivier J, Vale W, Bloom FE (1983) Corticotropin releasing factor produces increases in brain excitability and convulsive seizures in rats. Brain Res 278:332–336

Fonberg E (1981) Specific versus unspecific functions of the amygdala. In: Ben-Ari Y (ed) INSERM symposium 20. Elsevier/North-Holland Biomedical, New York

Galeno TM, Van Hoesen GW, Brody MJ (1984) Central amygdaloid nucleus lesion attenuates exaggerated hemodynamic responses to noise stress in the spontaneously hypertensive rat. Brain Res 291:249–259

Gloor P (1986) Role of the human limbic system in perception, memory, and affect: lessons from temporal lobe epilepsy. In: Doane BK, Livingston KE (eds) The limbic system: functional organization and clinical disorders. Raven, New York, pp 159–169

Goddard GV, McIntyre DC, Leech CK (1969) A permanent change in brain function resulting from daily electrical stimulation. Exp Neurol 25:295–330

Gold PW, Chrousos GP (1985) Clinical studies with corticotropin releasing factor: implications for the diagnosis and pathophysiology of depression, Cushing's disease, and adrenal insufficiency. Psychoneuroendocrinology 10:401–419

Gorka Z, Wojtasik A (1980) The effect of antidepressants on behavioral despair in rats. Pol J Pharmacol 32:463

Gorka Z, Ossowska K, Stach R (1979) The effect of unilateral amygdala lesion on the imipramine action in behavioural despair in rats. J Pharm Pharmacol 31:647–648

Henke PG (1981) Attenuation of shock-induced ulcers after lesions in the medial amygdala. Physiol Behav 27:143–146

Henke PG (1988) Electrophysiological activity in the central nucleus of the amygdala: emotionality and stress ulcers in rats. Behav Neurosci 102:77–83

Henke PG, Sullivan RM (1985) Kindling in the amygdala and susceptibility to stress ulcers. Brain Res Bull 14:5–18

Hitchcock J, Davis M (1986) Lesions of the amygdala, but not of the cerebellum or red nucleus, block conditioned fear as measured with the potentiated startle paradigm. Behav Neurosci 100:11–22

Horovitz ZP (1966) The amygdala and depression. In: Garattini S, Dukes M (eds) Antidepressant drugs. Excerpta Medica, Amsterdam, pp 121–129

Iwata J, Chida K, LeDoux JE (1987) Cardiovascular responses elicited by stimulation of neurons in the central amygdaloid nucleus in awake but not anesthetized rats resemble conditioned emotional responses. Brain Res 418:183–188

Jesberger JA, Richardson JS (1985) Animal models of depression: parallels and correlates to severe depression in humans. Biol Psychiatry 20:764–784

Kawashima K, Araki H, Aihara H (1986) Effect of chronic administration of antidepressants on duration of immobility in rats forced to swim. Jpn J Pharmacol 40:199–204

Kilts CD, Bissette G, Krishnan KRR, Smith MA, Chappel P, Nemeroff CB (1987) In: Halbreich U (ed) Hormones and depression. Raven, New York, pp 297–311

Kitada Y, Miyauchi T, Satoh A, Satoh S (1981) Effects of antidepressants in the rat forced swimming test. Eur J Pharmacol 72:145–152

Kling A, Dunne K (1976) Social-environmental factors affecting behavior and plasma testosterone in normal and amygdala lesioned *Macaca speciosa*. Primates 17:23–42

Kluver H, Bucy PC (1939) Preliminary analysis of functions of the temporal lobes in monkeys. Arch Neurol Psychiatry 42:979–1000

Koob GF, Bloom FE (1985) Corticotropin-releasing factor and behavior. Fed Am Soc Exp Biol 44:259–263

Krahn DD, Gosnell BA, Grace M, Levine AS (1986) CRF antagonist partially reverses CRF- and stress-induced effects on feeding. Brain Res Bull 17:285–289

Lenz HJ, Raedler A, Greten H, Brown MR (1987) CRF initiates biological actions within the brain that are observed in response to stress. Am J Physiol 252:34–39

Lesse S (1982) The relationship of anxiety to depression. Am J Psychother 36:332–348

Levine AS, Rogers B, Kneip J, Grace M, Morley JE (1983) Effect of centrally administered corticotropin releasing factor (CRF) on multiple feeding paradigms. Neuropharmacology 22:337–339

Liang KC, Lee EHY (1988) Intra-amygdala injections of corticotropin releasing factor facilitate inhibitory avoidance learning and reduce exploratory behavior in rats. Psychopharmacology (Berlin) 96:232–236

Lundblad JR, Roberts JL (1988) Regulation of proopiomelanocortin gene expression in pituitary. Endocr Rev 9:135

Merchenthaler I (1984) Corticotropin releasing factor (CRF)-like immunoreactivity in the rat central nervous system: extrahypothalamic distribution. Peptides 5 (Suppl 1):53–69

Minabe Y, Tanii Y, Kurachi M (1987) Acute effect of some psychotropic drugs on low-frequency amygdaloid kindled seizures. Biol Psychiatry 22:1444–1450

Morley JE, Levine AS (1982) Corticotropin releasing factor, grooming and ingestive behavior. Life Sci 31:1459–1464

Nemeroff CB (1990) Corticotropin-releasing factor. In: Nemeroff CB (ed) Neuropeptides and psychiatric disorders. American Psychiatric Association, Washington

Nemeroff CB, Bissette G (1986) Neuropeptides in psychiatric disorders. In: Berger PA, Brodie HKH (eds) American handbook of psychiatry, vol 7. Basic Books, New York, pp 64–110

Nemeroff CB, Owens MJ, Bissette G, Andorn AC, Stanley M (1988) Reduced corticotropin-releasing factor (CRF) binding sites in the frontal cortex of suicides. Arch Gen Psychiatry 45:577–579

Olschowka JA, O'Donohue TL, Mueller GP, Jacobowitz DM (1982) The distribution of corticotropin releasing factor-like immunoreactive neurons in rat brain. Peptides 3:995–1015

Palkovits M (1984) Distribution of neuropeptides in the central nervous system: a review of biochemical mapping studies. Prog Neurobiol 23:151–189

Palkovits M, Brownstein MJ, Vale W (1985) Distribution of corticotropin-releasing factor in rat brain. Fed Proc 44:215–219

Penaloza-Rojas JH, Bach-Y-Rita G, Rubio-Chevannier HF, Hernandez-Peon R (1961) Effects of imipramine upon hypothalamic and amygdaloid excitability. Exp Neurol 4:205–213

Porsolt RD (1981) Behavioural despair. In: Enna SJ, Malick JB, Richelson E (eds) Antidepressants: neurochemical, behavioural and clinical perspectives. Raven, New York, pp 121–139

Porsolt RD, LePichon M, Jalfre M (1977) Depression: a new animal model sensitive to antidepressant treatment. Nature 266:730–732

Porsolt RD, Anton G, Blavet N, Jalfre M (1978) Behavioural despair in rats, a new model sensitive to antidepressant treatments. Eur J Pharmacol 47:379–391

Post RM, Ballenger JC, Uhde TW, Putnam FW, Bunney WE Jr (1982) Kindling and drug sensitization: implications for the progressive development of psychopathology and treatment with carbamazepine. In: Sandler M (ed) The psychopharmacology of anti-convulsants. Oxford University Press, Oxford, pp 27–53

Post RM, Putnam F, Uhde TW, Weiss SRB (1986) Electroconvulsive therapy as an anticonvulsant. Implications for its mechanism of action in affective illness. Ann NY Acad Sci 462:376–388

Price JL (1981) Toward a consistent terminology for the amygdaloid complex. In: Ben-Ari Y (ed) INSERM symposium 20. Elsevier/North-Holland Biomedical, New York

Reul JMHM, de Kloet ER (1985) Two receptor systems for corticosterone in rat brain: microdistribution and differential occupation. Endocrinology 117:2505–2511

Rivier C, Rivier J, Vale W (1986) Stress-induced inhibition of reproductive functions: role of endogenous corticotropin-releasing factor. Science 20:607–609

Roberts GW, Woodhams PL, Polak JM, Crow TJ (1982) Distribution of neuropeptides in the limbic system of the rat: the amygdaloid complex. Neuroscience 7:99–131

Rock JP, Oldfield EH, Schulte HM, Gold PW, Kornblith PL, Loriaux L, Chrousos GP (1984) Corticotropin releasing factor administered into the ventricular CSF stimulates the pituitary-adrenal axis. Brain Res 323:365–368

Rosen JB, Davis M (1988) Enhancement of acoustic startle by electrical stimulation of the amygdala. Behav Neurosci 102:195–202

Rosvold HE, Mirsky AF, Pribram KH (1954) Influence of amygdalectomy on social behavior in monkeys. J Comp Physiol Psychol 47:173–178

Sachar EJ, Hellman L, Roffwarg H (1973) Disrupted 24 hour patterns of cortisol secretion in psychotic depression. Arch Gen Psychiatry 28:19–24

Sakanaka M, Shibasaki T, Lederis K (1986) Distribution and efferent projections of corticotropin-releasing factor-like immunoreactivity in the rat amygdaloid complex. Brain Res 382:213–238

Sakanaka M, Shibasaki T, Lederis K (1987) Corticotropin releasing factor-like immunoreactivity in the rat brain as revealed by a modified cobalt-glucose oxidase-diaminobenzidine method. J Comp Neurol 260:256–298

Schecter MD, Chance WT (1979) Non-specificity of "behavioural despair" as an animal model of depression. Eur J Pharmacol 60:139–142

Schildkraut JJ (1965) The catecholamine hypothesis of depression: a review of supporting evidence. Am J Psychiatry 122:509–522

Shimazoe T, Shibata S, Yatsugi S, Ueki S (1988) Involvement of the medial amygdaloid nucleus in the action of imipramine in rats subjected to the forced swimming test. J Pharmacobiodyn 11:137–139

Shiosaka S, Sakanaka M, Inagaki S, Senba E, Hara Y, Takatsuki K, Takagi H, Kawai Y, Tohyama M (1983) Putative neurotransmitters in the amygdaloid complex with special reference to peptidergic pathways. In: Emson PC (ed) Chemical neuroanatomy. Raven, New York, pp 359–389

Sirinathsinghji DJS (1987) Inhibitory influence of corticotropin releasing factor on components of sexual behaviour in the male rat. Brain Res 407:185–190

Sirinathsinghji DJS, Rees LH, Rivier J, Vale W (1983) Corticotropin-releasing factor is a potent inhibitor of sexual receptivity in the female rat. Nature 305:230–235

Skofitsch G, Jacobowitz DM (1985) Distribution of corticotropin releasing factor-like immunoreactivity in the rat brain by immunohistochemistry and radioimmunoassay: comparison and characterization of ovine and rat/human CRF antisera. Peptides 6:319–336

Sulser F, Vetulani J, Mobley PL (1978) Mode of action of antidepressant drugs. Biochem Pharmacol 27:257–261

Sutton RE, Koob GF, Le Moal M, Rivier J, Vale W (1982) Corticotropin releasing factor produces behavioural activation in rats. Nature 297:331–333

Tazi A, Dantzer R, LeMoal M, Rivier J, Vale W, Koob GF (1987) Corticotropin-releasing factor antagonist blocks stress-induced fighting in rats. Regul Pept 18:37–42

Thompson RC, Seasholtz AF, Herbert E (1987) Rat corticotropin-releasing hormone gene: sequence and tissue-specific expression. Mol Endocrinol 1:363

Valentino RJ, Foote SL, Aston-Jones G (1983) Corticotropin-releasing factor activates noradrenergic neurons of the locus coeruleus. Brain Res 270:363–367

Willner P (1984) The validity of animal models of depression. Psychopharmacology 83:1–16

Clinical Aspects of Neuropeptide Research *

D. L. Evans [1], R. N. Golden [2], C. B. Nemeroff [3], C. A. Pedersen [2], C. F. McCartney [4], J. J. Haggerty, Jr. [2], J. S. Simon [5], and D. Raft [1†]

Introduction

Increasing evidence suggests that depression is found in a high percentage of patients with cancer (Petty and Noyes 1981; Buckberg et al. 1984), but depression appears to be both underdiagnosed and inadequately treated in cancer patients. There is also a growing body of evidence suggesting that experimentally induced stress in animals as well as psychiatric illness and stressful life experience in humans are associated with alterations in both neuroendocrine and immune function. Alterations in immune function have been found in patients with major depression (Kronfol et al. 1983; Schliefer et al. 1984, 1985), and there is one report suggesting an epidemiologic relationship between depression and cancer (Shekelle et al. 1981). However, it is not known whether the alterations in immune function found in depression are of clinical significance, and there have been no comprehensive studies of both neuroendocrine and immune function in depressed cancer patients.

We have been investigating both clinical and neuroendocrine aspects of depression in cancer patients as well as clinical, neuroendocrine, and immune characteristics of depressed psychiatric patients. We review here our findings of depression in the cancer patient and integrate these findings with our neuroendocrine and immune assessments of depressed psychiatric patients. This review sets the stage for future studies that will be necessary to assess the relationship between depression, immune function, and cancer.

* Supported in part by Public Health Service Grant R 2517973 awarded by the National Cancer Institute to D.L.S., C.F.M., and D.R. by a University of North Carolina United Way research grant and North Carolina mental health research funds to D.L.E.; by NIMH grant MH-33127 to D.L.E.; and by NIMH Grant MH-40159 and MH-42088 to C.B.N.

† Dr. Raft died October 15, 1985.

[1] Departments of Psychiatry and Medicine, University of North Carolina School of Medicine, Chapel Hill, NC 27514, USA.

[2] Department of Psychiatry, University of North Carolina School of Medicine, Chapel Hill, NC 27514, USA.

[3] Departments of Psychiatry and Pharmacology and the Center for Aging and Human Development, Duke University Medical Center, Durham, NC 27710, USA.

[4] Departments of Psychiatry and of Obstetrics and Gynecology, University of North Carolina School of Medicine, Chapel Hill, NC 27514, USA.

[5] Department of Psychiatry, University of Wisconsin, Mt. Sinai Medical Center, Milwaukee, WI 53201, USA.

Neuropsychopharmacology
Edited by Bunney/Hippius/Laakmann/Schmauß

Depression and Cancer Patients

Clinical Findings

The assessment of depression in the cancer patient is rendered difficult because the descriptive diagnostic criteria for major depression include signs and symptoms that may result from the cancer itself. Major depressive criteria such as appetite loss, weight loss, insomnia, loss of interest in usual activities, and loss of energy may be secondary to the underlying cancer per se or be due to side effects of the cancer treatment. Although recent studies have found a high prevalence rate of depression in cancer patients, physicians may underestimate the severity of depression in cancer patients (Derogatis et al. 1976). In fact, relatively few cancer patients are referred for psychiatric consultation (Levine et al. 1978), and there is evidence that cancer patients do not receive adequate antidepressant treatment (Derogatis et al. 1979; Haggerty et al. 1986). Clearly, both the assessment and treatment of depression in cancer patients is less than optimal (Evans et al. 1986).

In addition to the difficulty in assessing depression in the cancer patient, it has been suggested that depression in cancer patients may differ qualitatively from primary depression (Plumb and Holland 1977; Buckberg et al. 1984). We have studied a uniform population of patients with gynecologic cancer and have found a high prevalence rate (47%) of depression (Evans et al. 1986). Nineteen (23%) of the 83 patients studied met DSM-III criteria for major depression and 20 (24%) of the patients met criteria for minor depression (adjustment disorder, $n=15$; dysthymic disorder, $n=4$; uncomplicated bereavement, $n=1$). Six (7%) of the patients met criteria for other, nondepressive diagnoses, and 38 (46%) received no DSM-III diagnosis.

The clinical presentation of major depression in these cancer patients was similar to the clinical features seen in a subgroup of major depressed psychiatric inpatients (Evans and Nemeroff 1987). None of the major depressed cancer patients exhibited melancholic or psychotic symptoms; unlike major depression in many psychiatric patients these depressed cancer patients did not show anhedonia, marked psychomotor retardation, or excessive guilt. In fact, thoughts of suicide were rare, and none of the cancer patients were judged to be an acute suicide risk. In addition, the severity of depression as measured by the Hamilton Rating Scale for Depression (HRS) and the Carroll Rating Scale for Depression (CRS) were indicative of significant depression; however, the scores are not as high as are generally seen in unipolar and bipolar depressed psychiatric patients. The mean scores $\pm$SD on the HRS and the CRS, respectively, of patients in the depression groups were: major depression, 19.8 ± 4.4 and 19.9 ± 11.1; minor depression 13.0 ± 4.0 and 11.4 ± 8.7. These clinical findings lend support to the view that depression in the hospitalized cancer patient usually does not include the full range of depressive symptoms seen in psychiatric inpatients (Plumb and Holland 1977; Buckberg et al. 1984; Lansky et al. 1987); the clinical characteristics of depression in the cancer patient resemble the characteristics of nonmelancholic major depression (Evans et al. 1986).

Neuroendocrine Findings

In addition to qualitative descriptive phenomena, we have further evidence from neuroendocrine challenge studies to suggest that depression in the cancer patient is similar to depression in nonmelancholic, depressed psychiatric patients. We used two neuroendocrine challenge studies, the dexamethasone suppression test (DST) and the thyrotropin-releasing hormone (TRH) stimulation test to assess the depressed cancer patients. We have DST ($n = 47$) and TRH test ($n = 27$) results from the initial group of 83 patients with gynecologic cancer (Evans et al. 1986). Using a standard (1 mg) overnight DST with serum cortisol concentrations measured in blood samples obtained at 4 P.M. and 11 P.M. the following day, we found that six of the 15 major depressed cancer patients (40%) exhibited hypercortisolism as measured by nonsuppression of serum cortisol following dexamethasone. This rate of nonsuppression is very similar to the 48% nonsuppression rate that we found in psychiatric inpatients with DSM-III major depression without melancholia (Evans and Nemeroff 1987). Not only is the rate of nonsuppression similar between the cancer patients with major depression without melancholia and the depressed psychiatric patients with this DSM-III diagnosis, but the postdexamethasone serum cortisol concentrations at 4 P.M. and 11 P.M. were similar in these two patient groups.

We found a blunted thyroid-stimulating hormone response to TRH in 29% of the cancer patients with major depression and in 8% of cancer patients with no psychiatric diagnosis. This is consistent with previous findings in depressed psychiatric patients (Loosen and Prange 1982; Extein et al. 1981). These neuroendocrine findings suggest a similar endocrine alteration in both depressed psychiatric patients and depressed cancer patients.

Summary

The clinical and neuroendocrine findings taken together suggest similarity between nonmelancholic major depression in psychiatric patients and nonmelancholic major depression in cancer patients. These observations argue that cancer patients should be evaluated carefully for depression. Furthermore, the clinical and neuroendocrine similarities between depression in psychiatric patients and depression in cancer patients suggest that the depressed cancer patient would in fact benefit from somatic antidepressant treatment. However, there has been little systematic study of the effects of antidepressant treatment in depressed cancer patients.

Treatment of Depression in Cancer Patients

It has been our clinical practice to treat depressed cancer patients with antidepressants. Preliminary findings from a naturalistic, pilot study suggest that cancer patients with major depression (and perhaps minor depression as well) benefit from antidepressants and may also have a better psychosocial adjustment to cancer following antidepressant medication treatment (Evans et al. 1988 a).

We have preliminary findings in 22 cancer patients who were chosen by one of us (D.R.) to receive antidepressant treatment. This investigation is a follow-up of a subset of depressed patients in our previous study of gynecologic oncology patients (Evans et al. 1986) who were referred for antidepressant treatment. We assessed the response to antidepressant treatment by evaluating the severity of depression and the quality of life of these patients. We assessed depressed patients who received adequate antidepressant treatment versus depressed patients who received inadequate or no antidepressant treatment. Of the 22 patients (major depression, $n = 12$; minor depression, $n = 10$), ten did not fulfill criteria for satisfactory antidepressant treatment (imipramine dose ≥ 150 mg per day for at least 4 weeks of treatment). Thus, two comparison groups emerged: the treated group ($n = 12$) and the inadequately treated ("untreated") group ($n = 10$). All 22 patients were reevaluated after discharge (mean $\pm$SD, 8.6 ± 4.8 months). Each patient received both a HRS and a Psychosocial Adjustment to Illness Scale (PAIS). The PAIS is a semistructured interview that samples seven areas in a patient's life. This instrument has been validated and used extensively to assess life adaptation in cancer patients (Derogatis 1986) and in other medically and surgically ill populations (Gundle et al. 1980; Raft et al. 1985).

Mean scores on the HRS obtained at follow-up were significantly lower than baseline HRS for the treated group but not for the untreated group. In addition, the mean posttreatment HRS scores were lower than baseline HRS for both treatment groups but were significantly lower only in the treated major depressed group. The PAIS score was also significantly lower for the group receiving treatment.

These preliminary results suggest that depressed cancer patients who receive adequate antidepressant treatment demonstrate significant improvement in depression. Although major depressed cancer patients who were not adequately treated also showed some improvement in depression, they showed considerably less improvement in depression and continued to have elevated depression ratings. The treated major depression patients also exhibited better life adaptation (PAIS) when compared to depressed cancer patients who remained untreated. Patients with minor depression who received somatic treatment had similar levels of adaptation as did treated patients with major depression. In addition, the untreated minor depressed patients exhibited a poorer adjustment to cancer, as measured by the PAIS, and had similar PAIS scores as the untreated major depressed patients. These preliminary findings suggest that major depressed cancer patients (and perhaps cancer patients with minor depression) will benefit from antidepressant treatment and experience a better quality of life than depressed cancer patients who do not receive antidepressant treatment, or who receive inadequate antidepressant treatment.

Depression, Endocrine, and Immune Relationships

Is there any reason to believe that depression or the treatment of depression might be related to the cancer process or the progression of cancer? Recent studies have suggested alterations in immune function in patients with major depression (Kronfol et al. 1983; Schliefer et al. 1984, 1985). The clinical significance of these findings remains unknown, but there is epidemiologic evidence linking depression (as measured by the MMPI) and increased risk for cancer morbidity and mortality at 17-year follow-up (Shekelle et al. 1981). Furthermore, the considerable evidence of hypercortisolism as measured by nonsuppression of serum cortisol following dexamethasone in depressed psychiatric patients (Stokes et al. 1975; Carroll and Mendels 1976; Schlesser et al. 1980; Carroll et al. 1981; Evans 1988; Evans and Nemeroff 1983, 1984, 1987; Evans et al. 1983, 1987; Schatzberg et al. 1983; Holsboer 1983; Arana et al. 1985; Rubin et al. 1987; Evans and Golden 1987) and in a significant number of cancer patients with depression (Evans et al. 1986), coupled with the immunosuppressive characteristics of cortisol, suggest a potential relationship between depression, endocrine state, immune alterations, and physical illness such as cancer.

The relationship between immune function and hypothalamic-pituitary-adrenal (HPA) activity in patients with major depression has not been well studied (see Evans and Nemeroff 1988, for review). Preclinical studies have suggested that corticosteroids are immunosuppressive and are associated with lymphocytopenia, thymus involution, and a decrease in spleen and lymph node tissue mass (Riley 1981; Stein et al. 1981). Although there is evidence that stress induces immunosuppression and earlier cancer appearance in animals, there is also evidence that stress induces enhancement of immunocompetence and a delay in cancer appearance (see Riley et al. 1981 and Fox 1981 for review). It should be noted that while most preclinical work has been conducted in species which are relatively sensitive to the effects of steroids, man is relatively steroid insensitive by comparison (Claman 1972). Thus, one-to-one comparisons between endocrine and immune interrelationships in animals and in man are rendered difficult (Fox 1981).

No consistent relationship between immune function and cortisol state has been found in psychiatric patients with major depression or in individuals undergoing stressful life experiences (Bartrop et al. 1977; Dorian et al. 1982; Schliefer et al., 1984; Keicolt-Glaser et al. 1984a, b; Kronfol et al. 1985). We have studied the relationship between major depression and the endocrine and immune state by measuring the total lymphocyte count and T-cell subpopulations in patients with major depression and in psychiatric control subjects shortly after admission to an acute inpatient psychiatric unit. Lymphocyte subpopulations were identified by monoclonal antibodies directed against various T-lymphocyte cell surface proteins, and cell populations were enumerated by flow cytometry.

We studied 21 patients (DSM-III major depression, $n = 14$; psychiatric controls with depressive symptoms, $n = 7$) and found that recently admitted major depressed patients showed a significant decrease in natural killer cell number and a trend for lower leukocyte count when compared to recently admitted psychiatric control subjects with depressive symptoms who did not fulfill criteria for major depression. We also studied the relationship between the immune and the endocrine states as assessed by a standard DST and found that, irrespective of diagnosis, patients who exhibited DST nonsuppression showed a trend for lower numbers of natural killer cells, helper cells, and suppressor cells on admission compared to DST suppressors (Evans et al. 1988 b).

We also investigated the relationship between the endocrine and the immune system by studying the effects of dexamethasone on the T-cell and discrete T-cell subpopulations. We found that major depressed patients showed different lymphocyte responses to dexamethasone on admission compared to psychiatric control subjects; major depressed patients were resistent to the glucocorticoid lowering effect on T-cell and T-cell subpopulations compared to the psychiatric controls. However, DST nonsuppressors did not differ from DST suppressors in this T-cell and T-cell subpopulation sensitivity (Pedersen et al., in press). Thus, these preliminary findings suggest that major depressed patients may have altered cellular immunity as demonstrated by lower numbers of natural killer cells and may exhibit T-cell resistance to the glucocorticoid lowering effect on T-cell population number. The relationship between these measures of immunity and the endocrine state as measured by postdexamethasone serum cortisol will require further study. We are now extending these preliminary studies and are assessing the immune state through a more sophisticated analysis of both lymphocyte phenotyping and lymphocyte activity as measured by mitogen stimulation, lymphokine (interleukin 2, interferon) release and natural killer cell activity.

Alteration of immune function, as mediated by endocrine function, could conceivably alter the development and course of malignancy. However, it should be stressed that the relationship between depression and immune function in the cancer patient is not known. There is evidence that the natural opioids, endorphins (Morley et al. 1985), and enkephalins (Plotnikoff et al. 1985), as well as the corticosteroids (Riley 1981) exert a modulatory effect on the immune system; the endorphins and the enkephalins have been shown to be immunoenhancing, and cortisol has been shown to be immunosuppressive. Plotnikoff et al. (1985) have suggested that enkephalins and endorphins modulate the corticosteroid effects on immune function during times of stress when the activity of the HPA axis includes concomitant release of ACTH and endorphin from the anterior pituitary along with release of adrenocorticosteroids and enkephalins from the adrenal. Further study of these endocrine systems in major depression is necessary to determine their role as mediating factors in immune alterations in major depression.

Conclusion

Converging lines of evidence from both preclinical and clinical studies suggest a potential relationship between depression and cancer. The high prevalence rate of depression in the cancer patient coupled with the independent observation of alterations in the endocrine state and in the immune state in depression argue for a simultaneous assessment of psychological state, endocrine state, and immune state in patients with cancer. Because alterations in the immune state could effect the course of cancer, future studies should assess the relationship between psychological state, neuroendocrine-neuroimmune state, and the course of cancer in patients with malignancies. Both cross-sectional and longitudinal studies will be necessary to assess not only the benefits of antidepressant medication treatment in cancer patients with major and minor depression, as well as the relationship between depression and psychosocial adjustment to cancer, but also the relationship between depression and the cancer process as well as the progression of cancer. Further study of the immune alterations in major depression and the relationship with the endocrine state should help determine any clinical relevance for the depressed cancer patient.

References

Arana GW, Baldessarini RJ, Ornsteen M (1985) The dexamethasone suppression test for diagnosis and prognosis in psychiatry. Arch Gen Psychiatry 42:1193–1204

Bartrop RW, Luckhurst E, Lazarus L, Kiloh LG, Penny R (1977) Depressed lymphocyte function after bereavement. Lancet 2:834–836

Bukberg J, Penman D, Holland JC (1984) Depression in hospitalized cancer patients. Psychosom Med 46:199–212

Carroll BJ, Mendels J (1976) Neuroendocrine regulation in affective disorders. In: Sachar EJ (ed) Hormones, behavior, and psychophathology. Raven, New York

Carroll BJ, Feinberg M, Smouse PE, Rawson SG, Greden JF (1981) The Carroll Rating Scale for Depression. Br J Psychiatry 138:194–200

Claman HN (1972) Corticosteroids and lymphoid cells. N Engl J Med 287:388–389

Derogatis LR (1986) The psychosocial adjustment to illness scale (PAIS). J Psychosom Res 30(1):77–91

Derogatis LR, Abeloff MD, McBeth CD (1976) Cancer patients and their physicians in the perception of psychological symptoms. Psychosomatics 17:197–201

Derogatis LR, Feldstein M, Morrow G, Schmal A, Schmitt M, Gates C, Murawski B, Holland J, Penman D, Melisaratos N (1979) A survey of psychotropic drug prescriptions in an oncology population. Cancer 44:1919–1929

Dorian B, Garfinkel P, Brown G, Shore A, Gladman D, Keystone E (1982) Aberrations in lymphocyte subpopulations and function during psychological stress. Clin Exp Immunol 50:132–138

Evans DL (1988) Use of the dexamethasone suppression test in clinical psychiatry. In: Nemeroff CB, Schatzburg AS (eds) Recent advances in the hypothalamic-pituitary-adrenal axis: physiology and pathophysiology. Raven, New York

Evans DL, Golden RN (1987) The dexamethasone suppression test – a review. In: Nemeroff CB, Loosen PT (eds) Handbook of clinical psychoneuroendocrinology. Guilford, New York

Evans DL, Nemeroff CB (1983) Use of the dexamethasone suppression test using DSM-III criteria on an inpatient psychiatric unit. Biol Psychiatry 18:505–511

Evans DL, Nemeroff CB (1984) The dexamethasone suppression test in organic affective syndrome. Am J Psychiatry 141:1465–1467

Evans DL, Nemeroff CB (1987) The clinical use of the DST in DSM-III affective disorders: correlation with the severe depression subtypes of melancholia and psychosis. J Psychiatr Res 21:185–194

Evans DL, Nemeroff CB (1988) Depression and aging: psychoneuroendocrinology and psychoneuroimmunology. Prog Neuroendocrinol 1 (4):21–27

Evans DL, Burnett GB, Nemeroff CB (1983) The dexamethasone suppression test in the clinical setting. Am J Psychiatry 140:586–589

Evans DL, McCartney CF, Nemeroff CB, Raft D, Quade D, Golden RN, Haggerty JJ, Holmes V, Simon JS, Droba M, Mason GA, Fowler WC (1986) Depression in women treated for gynecological cancer: clinical and neuroendocrine assessment. Am J Psychiatry 143:4:447–452

Evans DL, Nemeroff CB, Haggerty JJ, Pedersen CA (1987) Use of the dexamethasone suppression test with DSM-III criteria in psychiatrically hospitalized adolescents. Psychoneuroendocrinology. 12:203–209

Evans DL, McCartney CF, Haggerty JJ, Nemeroff CB, Golden RN, Simon JS, Quade D, Holmes V, Droba M, Mason GA, Fowler WC, Raft D (1988a) Treatment of depression in cancer patients is associated with better life adaptation: a pilot study. Psychosom Med 50:72–76

Evans DL, Pedersen CA, Folds JD (1988b) Depression and immunity: evidence of decreased natural killer cell populations. Prog Neuropsychopharmacol Biol Psychiatry 12:739–748

Extein I, Potash ALC, Gold MS (1981) The thyrotropin-releasing hormone test in the diagnosis of unipolar depression. Psychiatry Res 5:311–316

Fox B (1981) Psychosocial factors and the immune system in human cancer. In: Adler R (ed) Psychoneuroimmunology. Academic, New York

Gundle MJ, Reeves BR, Tate S, Raft D, McLaurin LP (1980) Psychosocial outcome after coronary artery surgery. Am J Psychiatry 137:159

Haggerty JJ, Evans DL, McCartney CF, Raft D (1986) Psychotropic prescribing patterns of non-psychiatric residents in a general hospital in 1973 and 1982. Hosp Community Psychiatry 37:357–361

Holsboer F (1983) The dexamethasone suppression test in depression: clinical and biochemical aspects. J Steroid Biochem 19:251–257

Keicolt-Glaser JK, Ricker D, George J, Messick G, Speicher CE, Garner W, Glaser R (1984a) Urinary cortisol levels, cellular immunocompetancy, and loneliness in psychiatric inpatients. Psychosom Med 46:14–23

Keicolt-Glaser JK, Garner W, Speicher C, Penn GM, Holliday J, Glaser R (1984b) Psychosocial modifiers of immunocompetence in medical students. Psychosom Med 46:7–14

Kronfol Z, Silva J, Greden J, Dembinski S, Gardner R, Carroll B (1983) Impaired lymphocyte function in depressive illness. Life Sci 33:241–247

Kronfol Z, Nasrallah HA, Chapman S, House JD (1985) Depression, cortisol metabolism and lymphocytopenia. J Affective Disord 9:169–173

Lansky SB, List MA, Ritter-Sterr C (1987) Recognizing depression in oncology patients. American Psychiatric Association 140th annual meeting. Abstract no 108, p 242

Levine PM, Silverfarb PM, Lipowski ZJ (1978) Mental disorders in cancer patients. Cancer 42:1385–1391

Loosen PT, Prange AJ (1982) Serum thyrotropin response to thyrotropin-releasing hormone in psychiatric patients: a review. Am J Psychiatry 139:405–416

Morley JE, Kay N, Allen J, Moon T, Billington CJ (1985) Endorphins, immune function, and cancer. Psychopharmacol Bull 21:485–488

Pedersen CA, Folds J, Evans DL (in press) Dexamethasone effects on lymphocyte number in major depression. Prog Neuropsychopharmacol Biol Psychiatry

Petty F, Noyes R, (1981) Depression in cancer. Biol Psychiatry 16:1203–1221

Plotnikoff NP, Murgo AJ, Miller GC, Corder CN, Faith RE (1985) Enkephalins: immunomodulators. Fed Proc 44:118–122

Plumb MM, Holland J (1977) Comparative studies of psychological function in patients with advanced cancer. I. Self-reported depressive symptoms. Psychosom Med 39:264–276

Raft D, McKee DC, Popio KA, Haggerty JJ (1985) Life adaptation after percutaneous transluminal coronary angioplasty and coronary artery bypass grafting. Am J Cardiol 56:395–398

Riley V (1981) Psychoneuroendocrine influences on immunocompetence and neoplasia. Science 212:1100–1109

Rubin RT, Poland RE, Lesser IM, Winston RA, Blodgett ALN (1987) Neuroendocrine aspects of primary endogenous depression: cortisol secretory dynamics in patients and matched controls. Arch Gen Psychiatry 44:328–336

Schatzberg AF, Rothschild JJ, Stahl JB, Bond TC, Rosenbaum AH, Lofgren SB, McLaughlin RA, Sullivan MA, Cole JO (1983) The dexamethasone suppression test: identification of subtypes of depression. Am J Psychiatry 140:88–91

Schlesser MA, Winokur G, Sherman BM (1980) Hypothalamic-pituitary-adrenal axis activity in depressive illness. Arch Gen Psychiatry 37:737–743

Schliefer SJ, Keller SE, Meyerson AT, Raskin MJ, Davis KL, Stein M (1984) Lymphocyte function in major depressive disorder. Arch Gen Psychiatry 41:484–486

Schliefer SJ, Keller SE, Siris SG, Davis KL, Stein M (1985) Depression and immunity. Arch Gen Psychiatry 42:129–133

Shekelle RB, Raynor WJ, Ostfeld AM, Garron DC, Bieliauskas LA, Liu SC, Maliza C, Paul O (1981) Psychological depression and 17-year risk of death from cancer. Psychosom Med 43:117–125

Stein M, Keller SE, Schleifer SJ (1981) The hypothalamus and the immune response. In: Weiner H, Hofer MA, Stunkard AJ (eds) Brain, behavior and bodily disease. Raven, New York, pp 45–65

Stokes PE, Pick GR, Stoll PM, Nunn WD (1975) Pituitary-adrenal function in depressed patients: resistance to dexamethasone suppression. J Psychiatr Res 12:271–281

Thyroid Axis Stimulation Tests in Psychiatry

C. M. Banki[1], M. Arato[2], G. Bissette[3], and C. B. Nemeroff[3]

Introduction

The unprecedented popularity of the dexamethasone suppression test has greatly facilitated the penetration of neuroendocrinology into psychiatric research; various psychoneuroendocrine tests, most of them applicable in clinical settings, have been developed and widely investigated. Among these, the hypothalamic-pituitary-thyroid axis has received particular attention since the late 1960s, and following the availability of the synthetic thyrotropin-releasing hormone (TRH) the TRH stimulation test became one of the first neuroendocrine procedures used in psychiatric patients (Loosen and Prange 1982; Kastin et al. 1972; Prange et al. 1972). Subsequently, data with the TRH test have been published in more than 55 papers covering at least 1200 patients (Loosen and Banki 1988).

Apart from being an empirically established procedure, the rationale to use the TRH stimulation test – i.e., the evaluation of the serum thyrotropin (TSH) response to an intravenous test dose of 0.2–0.6 mg synthetic TRH – in psychiatry is based on the following observations:

- Both hypo- and hyperthyroidism have long been known to cause psychiatric disorders; these may be quite severe and sometimes the first manifestations of the thyroid disease (Whybrow et al. 1969; Prange et al. 1969).
- Thyroid hormones, particularly triiodothyronine, can potentiate the effect of tricyclic antidepressants; this observation has been confirmed under strictly controlled double-blind circumstances (Prange et al. 1969, 1984; Goodwin et al. 1982).
- TRH itself is widely distributed extrahypothalamically in the brain, localized at the synaptic level, released at synaptic terminals, attached to specific receptors which alter the neuronal activity, etc. – i.e., it is probably a neurotransmitter in the brain (Griffiths 1985).
- TRH has several behavioral or "psychotropic" properties (Nemeroff et al. 1984; Griffiths 1985) although its clinical use as a potential antidepressant

[1] Regional Neuropsychiatric Institute, 4321 Nagykallo, Hungary.
[2] National Institute for Nervous and Mental Diseases, 1281 Budapest, Hungary.
[3] Department of Psychiatry, Duke University Medical Center, Durham, NC 27710, USA.

Neuropsychopharmacology
Edited by Bunney/Hippius/Laakmann/Schmauß

has yielded controversial results (Prange et al. 1984; Garbutt and Loosen 1984).

- The release of TRH is under monoaminergic control (Reichlin 1975; Vagenakis 1979); monoamine disturbances are thought to play a role in the pathogenesis of the major psychoses.
- Psychotropic drugs may affect thyroid function; in this respect lithium is the best known example, but others include neuroleptics (Extein et al. 1984) and carbamazepine (Joffe et al. 1984).

Previous reviews (Loosen and Prange 1982; Loosen 1985; Extein et al. 1984; Loosen and Banki 1988) have summarized the practical value of the TRH test in psychiatry, with the following main results:

- The TSH response to TRH is blunted in 25%–55% of patients with major depression (and mania) while in less than 5% of healthy controls.
- The specificity of the test against other psychiatric conditions is variable; alcohol abuse, stress, chronic pain, borderline personality disorder, etc. are also often associated with blunted TSH responses to TRH.
- Under certain conditions the continuing blunted response in depressed patients may predict early relapse or poor antidepressant effect (Kirkegaard 1981; Targum 1983) while normalization of the test is correlated with better clinical improvement.
- TSH blunting in depression may be related to (violent) suicidal behavior (Linkowski et al. 1983).
- Other hormonal responses to TRH, in particular prolactin (PRL) or growth hormone (GH) elevation, may yield additional information about the functional state of the hypothalamic-pituitary-thyroid axis (Brambilla et al. 1978; Winokur et al. 1983).

In our investigations using a low-dose (0.2 mg) TRH stimulation (Banki et al. 1984a) we focused attention on the specific association of the TSH blunting to depression and/or suicide and to test specificity against other psychiatric disorders.

The TRH Test in Depression and Suicide

In an early study (Banki et al. 1984b) made in a mixed psychiatric patient population including only a small number of major depressives we found an inverse relationship between TSH blunting and suicidal behavior; patients with a recent violent suicide attempt had less blunting than nonsuicidal subjects. This observation was most probably due to the effect of diagnostic heterogeneity in a relatively small sample, because in a much larger population containing both suicidal and nonsuicidal patients separately in the depressed and the nondepressed group (including schizophrenia, alcohol dependence, or adjustment disorder) there was no such effect demonstrable (Fig. 1). The TSH responses to TRH were clearly and markedly smaller in the patients with major

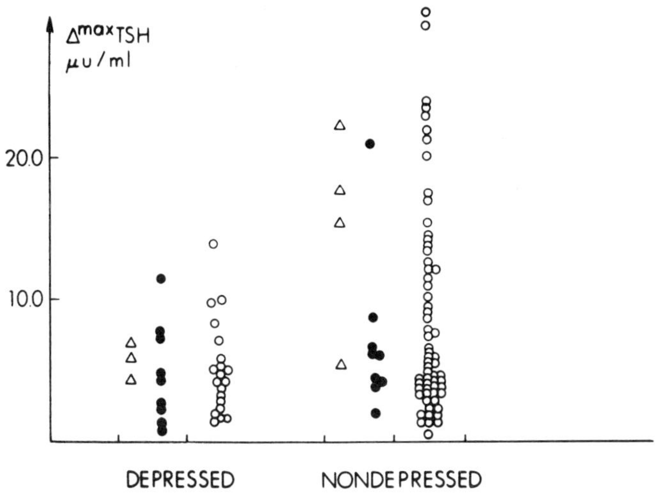

Fig. 1. TRH-induced TSH responses in depressed ($n = 33$) and nondepressed ($n = 75$) psychiatric patients. *Triangles*, violent suicide attempters; *filled circles*, nonviolent (sedative overdose) attempters; *open circles*, nonattempters

depression (with no difference between unipolar and bipolar subjects), but there was no tendency at all for a specific blunting related to either violent or nonviolent suicidal behavior in either group. This conclusion is based on a multiple regression analysis of the TSH data using the dichotomous variables depression and suicide as independent variables (Table 1). Although our results are at variance with that of Linkowski et al. (1983), the patient populations were different. In the depressed group only, both studies contained very few patients with recent violent attempts so that chance findings were likely; the pattern of the nonviolent attempters in depression was in fact quite similar; and the result in our nondepressed suicidal patients might be related to sociocultural factors probably underlying a large proportion of the very high incidence figures of suicidal behavior in Hungary. The latter may have different biological correlates, if any, than that observed in depressed suicides and which is thought to be identifiable by the TRH stimulation test.

It is difficult to interpret the association of TSH blunting with depression (and possibly suicidal behavior). The TSH response is dependent on several factors, such as the pituitary TSH reserve, the sensitivity of the pituitary

Table 1. Multiple regression analysis of TSH responses to TRH ($n = 108$)

Independent variable	R^2	F	p	ΔR^2	F	p
Depression	0.108	12.83	<0.001	–	–	–
Suicide	0.155	6.17	<0.001	0.043	2.03	ns
(Violent suicide)	–	–	–	0.011	1.35	ns
(Nonviolent suicide)	–	–	–	0.037	3.44	ns

thyrotrope cell receptors to TRH, the endogenous TRH level, and the feedback effect of the thyroid hormone levels. The regulation of TRH secretion itself is complex, involving a multiplicity of factors (Fig. 2). One such factor, brain serotonin, has been repeatedly shown to be possibly involved in the facilitation of suicidal behavior. Most psychiatric patients who had attempted suicide shortly before admission (with the exception of some bipolar subgroups) had low levels of the serotonin metabolite 5-hydroxyindoleacetic acid (5-HIAA) in

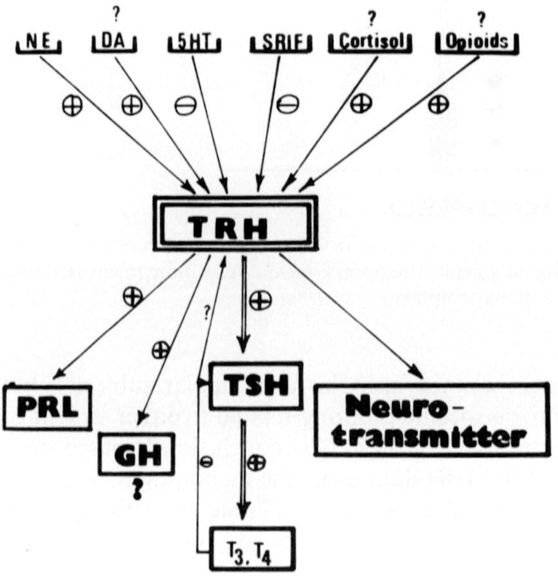

Fig. 2. Multiple regulating factors and effects of TRH. *NE*, Norepinephrine; *DA*, dopamine; *5HT*, serotonin; *SRIF*, somatostatin; *PRL*, prolactin; *GH*, growth hormone; T_3, triiodothyronine, T_4, thyroxine

the cerebrospinal fluid (CSF) as compared to the nonsuicidal patients (Åsberg et al. 1976; Banki et al. 1984b). Serotonin deficiency – which may be present in melancholia per se (Åsberg et al. 1984) – may lead to increased TRH release in the hypothalamus and, if persisting for a prolonged period of time, to a down-regulation in pituitary TRH receptors. If this hypothesis were true, than depressed patients (those with the most severe illness being most likely to attempt suicide) would be characterized by low CSF 5-HIAA and high endogenous TRH in the CSF together with a blunted TSH response to exogenous TRH.

The first attempt to measure endogenous TRH in the CSF was made by Kirkegaard et al. (1979) who reported a very marked elevation in endogenous depression. No particular attention to suicide was made. Because of technical difficulties to raise sufficiently specific antibodies against the TRH the replication of this study could be made only most recently by ourselves (Banki et al. 1988). A strong, almost threefold elevation of CSF TRH was found in 14 patients with major depression (mean, 12.8 pg/ml ± 5.7 pg/ml), highly significant when compared to the control group (4.4 ± 1.8 pg/ml, $n = 16$). In

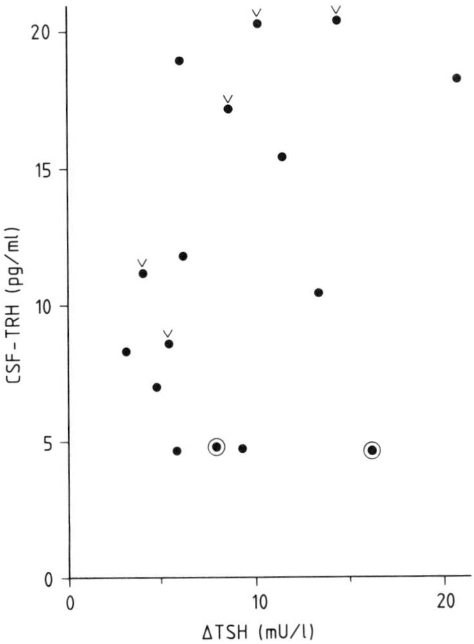

Fig. 3. Relationship between CSF TRH and TSH response to TRH in depressed patients. *V*, Violent attempters; *circles*, manic patients. $r = 0.32$ (NS)

addition, there was a tendency for the five violent suicide attempters to have even higher (15.65 ± 5.37 pg/ml) CSF TRH levels than the nonsuicidal depressed patients (11.17 ± 5.53), although this difference fell short of any statistical significance.

There was, however, no significant correlation between the CSF TRH immunoreactivity level and the TSH response to TRH in 14 depressed and 2 manic patients (Fig. 3). This is not surprising because it is known that a large proportion of the TRH in the CNS is extrahypothalamic, and the lumbar CSF probably contains only about 30% TRH originating from the hypothalamus (Griffiths 1985; Nemeroff et al. 1984). Here again, the TSH responses of the violent suicide attempters occupied a middle position within the depressed group; no particular tendency to further blunting was seen. The two manic patients had normal CSF TRH levels and also normal TSH responses to TRH. Basal TSH, triiodothyronine, and thyroxine levels – all within normal ranges – were also correlated to CSF TRH in these 16 affective patients: none of the coefficients were significant.

Until more data are available, we believe it is fairly plausible to assume that the increased central TRH release – with or without a consequent blunting of the TSH response – plays a role in the biological pathogenesis of major depression. Whether this is related to a more central serotonin deficit and is thus also associated to the development of a suicide risk in certain populations remains to be clarified.

Multiple Hormonal Responses to TRH

Exogenous TRH stimulates, in addition to the TSH, also PRL and GH secretion. PRL responses in depression have been found to be either blunted (Linnoila et al. 1979) or normal (Loosen et al. 1983) concomitantly with blunted TSH responses. Positive GH responses are generally considered as abnormal because they do not occur in healthy controls but are often observed in medical and psychiatric disorders (Maeda et al. 1975).

In a considerable sample of 63 psychiatric patients and 15 healthy controls we simultaneously measured the TSH, PRL, and GH responses to 0.2 mg TRH (Banki et al. 1985). The purpose of this study was to derive, if possible, specific hormonal patterns to major depression, schizophrenia, alcohol dependence, and adjustment disorder to separate these from controls and perhaps from each other. The results basically confirmed those of Brambilla et al. (1978) and Winokur et al. (1983). Although all three responses were more often abnormal in depression than in controls (where in fact only one PRL response was considered blunted), many patients with other psychiatric diagnosis shared the same endocrine pattern. To further analyze the results we derived, in multiple steps, the best canonical discrimination (Dillon and Goldstein 1984); starting from six variables (three baseline and three response variates) only one significant function emerged retaining only three variables (TSH and PRL responses and basal TSH). This function classified the patients and controls as shown in Table 2.

Table 2. Number of patients classified as "control" and "depressive" by a canonical discriminant function

Clinical diagnosis	"Depressed"	"Control"
Healthy volunteers	1	14
Major depression	15	4
Schizophrenia	13	7
Alcohol withdrawal	6	3
Adjustment disorder	9	5

From the above results we concluded the following:

- The TRH stimulation test has some value in separating major depression from the psychiatrically healthy state; this separation can be increased to a remarkable level by adding further hormonal variables (such as the PRL response) to the test. It is, however, evident that this separation needs no biological test at all in any clinical situation.
- The test is not specific for depression and is unable to separate depression from schizophrenia, alcohol withdrawal state, or adjustment disorder with emotional features. Adding further variables to the test fails to increase its specificity.

- There may be some subgroups of depressed patients in which violent suicide attempts are associated with particularly strong TSH blunting; but this is not generally the case, and suicidal behavior per se does not imply abnormal TRH test results.

Opiate Stimulation of TSH Secretion

Some authors have found morphine and other opiate agonists to increase serum TSH in man (Grossman et al. 1981; Devilla et al. 1985) while other authors have found no change (Tolis et al. 1975; Rolandi et al. 1984). In a previous study we measured several hormonal responses, including that of TSH, to 0.1 mg/kg morphine administered intravenously in 22 female psychiatric patients and 5 healthy controls (Banki and Arato 1987). Only a weak, nonsignificant tendency to increase serum TSH was seen after morphine administration, without any difference in baseline levels and response pattern between patients and controls.

Recently a potent and relatively μ-receptor specific opiate agonist, fentanyl, was used by our group to investigate opiate-sensitive hormonal changes; in addition, the hormonal responses to fentanyl were determined twice in each subject (at 9:00 A.M. and 9:00 P.M.) to detect diurnal changes in the opiate-induced hormonal responses (Frecska et al. 1987). This study revealed that there was a marked, significant circadian rhythm in the serum TSH level both in healthy controls (ten women) and in the ten female depressed patients. With a few exceptions, all individual TSH levels were higher in the evening than in the morning (Fig. 4). In the morning, 0.1 mg intravenous fentanyl elicited practically no TSH response at all either in controls or in depressed patients; on

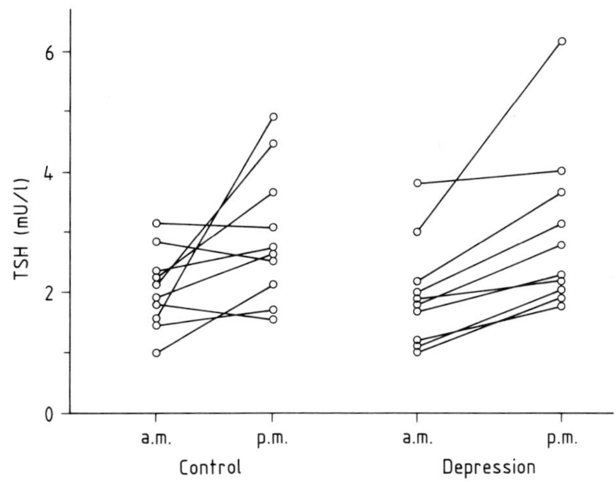

Fig. 4. Serum TSH level in the morning (*am*) and in the evening (*pm*)

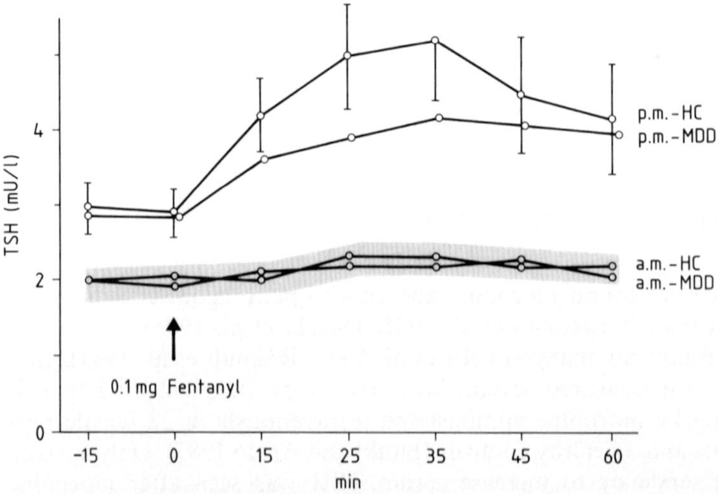

Fig. 5. TSH response to fentanyl. *HC*, healthy controls; *MDD*, major depressive disorder; *dotted area* mean ± SEM of the control range for morning values

the other hand, the same dose in the evening (tested in a randomized order, 36 h apart) induced a clear, marked TSH response in both groups. Using profile analysis (Morrison 1967) there was a significant interaction effect between the 20 morning and 20 evening samples ($F_{6,33} = 2.57$, $p < 0.04$) showing different profiles, i.e., a significantly different response pattern in the evening as compared to no response in the morning. Furthermore, there was no significant group effect but again a significant interaction when comparing control and depressive response curves in the evening only ($F_{5,13} = 3.22$, $p < 0.045$). This is interpreted as a significantly smaller, blunted TSH response curve to fentanyl in depression compared to the controls. No such difference was detectable in the morning samples. The overall situation is illustrated in Fig. 5.

The fact that the opiate agonist fentanyl caused a marked TSH response in the evening (with a significant difference between controls and depressed patients) while no response and no difference was seen in the morning raises the possibility that the regular TRH stimulation test would also be worth investigating in the evening since it may behave differently at the two times. To our knowledge, only one such study has been made to date, confirming the above expectation in eight healthy controls (Caroff and Winokur 1984).

Discussion

There is solid empirical evidence for the involvement of the hypothalamic-pituitary-thyroid axis in psychiatric disorders, particularly of the affective type.

Although therapeutic trials to date have not provided conclusive evidence, the development of clinically applicable, long-acting TRH analogs that reach the central TRH receptors in effective concentrations will probably help to evaluate the role of this peptide in affective disorders (Griffiths 1985; Prange et al. 1984). Repeated TRH administration diminishes the TSH response even if given at weekly intervals (Winokur et al. 1984), which raises the possibility that a primary hypersecretion of endogenous TRH is capable of inducing a prolonged alteration in pituitary responsiveness as detected by the usual TRH stimulation test. There is now strong suggestive evidence that during depression TRH *is* hypersecreted in the CNS (Kirkegaard et al. 1979; Banki et al. 1988) although it remains to be elucidated which brain regions are responsible for this phenomenon, which appears to be fairly specific to major depression. Both we and Kirkegaard et al. failed to find a correlation between the CSF TRH immunoreactivity level and the TSH response; this argues against the direct interpretation that the TRH stimulation test simply measures central TRH release (provided that the pituitary and the thyroid glands are healthy). It would be highly interesting to investigate CSF TRH concentrations in recovered and in chronic nonrecovering depressed patients, for this would enable us to determine whether the TRH overactivity is a state or a trait feature, and whether it covaries with changes in the TRH stimulation test results.

From a practical point of view, the TRH stimulation test remains a research tool to evaluate one aspect of the thyroid axis in selected patients. The accumulated clinical data do not support its use as a clinical diagnostic aid because of its low specificity, low sensitivity, and the numerous confounding factors to be considered (Loosen and Banki 1988). The measurement of TRH-induced PRL and GH responses have, similarly, no established clinical value in psychiatry; although the presence of two or more endocrine abnormalities increases the probability of diagnosing major depression with melancholia (Winokur et al. 1983; Banki et al. 1985), this is more evident when other endocrine tests (e.g., DST, insuline tolerance test) are combined. Further research is required to determine whether there is a clinically applicable new form of the thyroid axis stimulation test which would more closely reflect central TRH changes and thus eventually provide diagnostic, therapeutic, or prognostic information. Such a new test may involve either a different stimulus than the TRH or a different response to be measured. Opiate stimulation is a tentative way to explore alternative testing mechanisms (Frecska et al. 1987).

References

Åsberg M, Träskman L, Thorén P (1976) 5HIAA in the cerebrospinal fluid: a biochemical suicide predictor? Arch Gen Psychiatry 33:1193–1197

Åsberg M, Bertilsson L, Mårtensson B, Scalia-Tomba GP, Thorén P, Träskman-Bendz L (1984) CSF monoamine metabolites in melancholia. Acta Psychiatry Scand 69:201–219

Banki CM, Arató M (1987) Multiple hormonal responses to morphine, relationship to diagnosis and dexamethasone suppression. Psychoneuroendocrinology 12:3–11

Banki CM, Arató M, Papp Z (1984a) Thyroid stimulation test in healthy subjects and psychiatric patients. Acta Psychiatr Scand 70:295–303

Banki CM, Arató M, Papp Z, Kurcz M (1984b) Biochemical markers in suicidal patients. J Affective Disord 6:341–350

Banki CM, Vojnik M, Arató M, Papp Z, Kovacs Z (1985) Dexamethasone suppression and multiple hormonal responses to TRH in some psychiatric disorders. Eur Arch Psychiatr Neurol Sci 235:32–37

Banki CM, Bissette G, Arató M, Nemeroff CB (1988) Elevation of immunoreactive thyrotropin-releasing hormone (TRH) in cerebrospinal fluid of depressed patients. Am J Psychiatry 145:1526–1531

Brambilla F, Smeraldi E, Sacchetti E, Negri F, Cocci E, Muller EE (1978) Deranged anterior pituitary responsiveness to hypothalamic hormones in depressed patients. Arch Gen Psychiatry 35:1231–1238

Caroff SN, Winokur A (1984) Hormonal response to thyrotropin-releasing hormone following rest-activity reversal in normal men. Biol Psychiatry 19:1015–1025

Devilla L, Pende A, Morgano A, Giusti M, Lotti G (1985) Morphine-induced TSH release in normal and hypothyroid subjects. Neuroendocrinology 40:303–308

Dillon WR, Goldstein M (1984) Multivariate analysis, methods and application. Wiley, New York

Extein I, Pottash ALC, Gold MS, Cowdry RW (1984) Changes in TSH response to TRH in affective Illness. In: Post RM, Ballenger JC (eds) Neurobiology of mood disorders. Wilkins and Williams, Baltimore, pp 297–310

Frecska E, Arató M, Banki CM, Bagdy G, Perenyi A, Fekete MIK (1987) Diurnal variation in fentanyl-induced hormonal responses and side effects. Presented at the 140th annual meeting of the American Psychiatric Association, May 9–14, Chicago

Garbutt JC, Loosen PT (1984) A dramatic behavioral response to thyrotropin-releasing hormone following low-dose neuroleptics. Psychoneuroendocrinology 9:311–314

Goodwin FK, Prange AJ, Post RM, Muscettola G, Lipton MA (1982) Potentiation of antidepressant effects by triiodothyronine in tricyclic nonresponders. Am J Psychiatry 139:34–38

Griffiths EC (1985) Thyrotropin releasing hormone: endocrine and central effects. Psychoneuroendocrinology 10:225–235

Grossman A, Stubbs WA, Gaillard RC, Delitala G, Besser GM (1981) Studies on the opiate control of prolactin, GH, and TSH. Clin Endocrinol (Oxf) 14:381–386

Joffe RT, Gold PW, Uhde TW, Post RM (1984) The effects of carbamazepine on the thyrotropin response to TRH. Psychiatry Res 12:161–166

Kastin AJ, Ehrenring RH, Schalch DS, Anderson MS (1972) Improvement in mental depression with decreased thyrotropin response after adminsitration of TRH. Lancet 2:740–742

Kirkegaard C (1981) The thyrotropin response to thyrotropin-releasing hormone in endogeneous depression. Psychoneuroendocrinology 6:189–212

Kirkegaard C, Faber J, Hummer L, Rogowski P (1979) Increased levels of TRH in cerebrospinal fluid from patients with endogenous depression. Psychoneuroendocrinology 4:227–235

Linkowski P, Van Wettere JP, Kerkhofs M, Brauman H, Mendlewicz J (1983) Thyrotrophin response to thyrostimulin in affectively ill women, relationship to suicidal behaviour. Br J Psychiatry 143:401–405

Linnoila M, Lamberg BA, Rosberg G, Karonen SL, Welin MG (1979) Thyroid hormones and TSH, prolactin, and GH responses to repeated TRH and LRH injections in depressed patients. Acta Psychiatr Scand 59:536–544

Loosen PT (1985) The TRH-induced TSH response in psychiatric patients: a possible neuroendocrine marker. Psychoneuroendocrinology 10:237–260

Loosen PT, Banki CM (1988) The use of nonopiate neuropeptides as diagnostic tools in psychiatric and neurological disorders. In: Nemeroff CB (ed) Neuropeptides in psychiatric and neurological disorders. John Hipkins University Press, Baltimore, pp 18–48

Loosen PT, Prange AJ (1982) Serum thyrotropin response to thyrotropin-releasing hormone in psychiatric patients: a review. Am J Psychiatry 139:405–416

Loosen PT, Kistler K, Prange AJ (1983) Use of the TSH response to TRH as an independent variable. Am J Psychiatry 140:700–706

Maeda K, Kato Y, Yamaguchi N, Chihara K, Iwasaki Y, Moridera K, Imura H (1975) GH and prolactin release after injection of TRH in patients with depression. J Clin Endocrinol Metab 40:501–505

Morrison DF (1967) Multivariate statistical methods. McGraw-Hill, New York

Nemeroff CB, Kalivas PW, Golden RN, Prange AJ (1984) Behavioral effects of hypothalamic hypophysiotropic hormones, neurotensin, substance P, and other neuropeptides. Pharmacol Ther 24:1–56

Prange AJ, Wilson IC, Rabon AM (1969) Enhancement of imipramine antidepressant action by hormones. Am J Psychiatry 126:457–469

Prange AJ, Wilson IC, Lara PP, Alltop LB, Breese GR (1972) Effects of TRH in depression. Lancet 2:999–1002

Prange AJ, Loosen PT, Wilson IC, Lipton MA (1984) The therapeutic use of hormones of the thyroid axis in depression. In: Post RM, Ballenger JC (eds) Neurobiology of mood disorders. Wilkins and Williams, Baltimore, pp 311–322

Reichlin S (1975) Regulation of the hypophysiotropic secretions of the brain. Arch Intern Med 135:1350–1361

Rolandi E, Franceschini R, Marabini A, Messina V, Barreca T (1984) Serum concentrations of PRL, GH, LH, FSH, TSH, and cortisol after single administration of a new synthetic narcotic analgesic butorphanol. Eur J Clin Pharmacol 26:563–565

Targum SD (1983) The application of serial neuroendocrine challenge studies in the management of depressive disorder. Biol Psychiatry 18:3–19

Tolis G, Hickey J, Guyda H (1975) Effects of morphine on serum growth hormone, cortisol, prolactin, and thyroid stimulating hormone in man. J Clin Endocrinol Metab 41:797–800

Vagenakis AG (1979) Regulation of TSH secretion. In: Tolis G, Labrie F, Martin JB, Naftolin F (eds) Clinical neuroendocrinology. Raven, New York, pp 329–343

Whybrow PC, Prange AJ, Treadway CR (1969) Mental changes accompanying thyroid gland dysfunction. Arch Gen Psychiatry 20:48–62

Winokur A, Amsterdam JD, Oler J, Mendels J, Snyder PJ, Brunswick DJ (1983) Multiple hormonal responses to protirelin (TRH) in depressed patients. Arch Gen Psychiatry 40:525–531

Winokur A, Caroff SN, Amsterdam JD, Maislin G (1984) Administration of thyrotropin-releasing hormone at weekly intervals results in a diminished thyrotropin response. Biol Psychiatry 19:695–701

Corticotropin-Releasing Hormone and the Proopiomelanocortin-Derived Peptides in Depression

B. G. Charlton [1] and I. N. Ferrier [2]

A wide range of abnormalities of the hypothalamo-pituitary-adrenal (HPA) axis have been described in depressed subjects. This chapter reviews these abnormalities and attempts to synthesise them into a testable hypothesis.

Substantial research attention has been devoted to the abnormalities of the dexamethasone suppression test (DST) in depression (Arana et al. 1985; Braddock 1986). While it has not proved to be specific to the condition, hypercortisolaemia remains the best validated biochemical abnormality in depression. However, this emphasis has tended to focus the attention of researchers on measuring cortisol in plasma samples, and it is often neglected that cortisol is only the last element in a whole system of hormones: the HPA axis.

The HPA axis consists of a chain of stimulatory hormones and feedback loops and is under control from higher cerebral centres which determine its overall level of activity (Hall et al. 1981). Corticotropin-releasing hormone (CRH) is a 41 amino acid peptide which is secreted into the hypophysial portal venous system (linking the hypothalamus with the anterior pituitary). Secretion of CRH is influenced by a variety of neurotransmitters including acetylcholine (stimulatory), γ-aminobutyric acid, catecholamines (both inhibitory) and perhaps serotonin and a variety of peptides (Gillies and Grossman 1985). CRH is generally considered to be the principal factor responsible for stimulating adrenocorticotropic hormone (ACTH) release from the anterior pituitary, but there is evidence that vasopressin has a synergistic role to play (Gillies and Grossman 1985) and may be of equal physiological importance (Plotsky et al. 1985).

ACTH is cleaved from a precursor glycoprotein termed proopiomelanocortin (POMC). Cleavage of POMC produces a whole family of peptides along with ACTH; indeed it is possible that ACTH is itself subject to further processing to form α-melanocyte stimulating hormone (MSH; ACTH 1–13; Charlton et al. 1987a). Other products include β-lipotropic hormone, of no known physiological function, which is further processed to produce the endogenous opiate β-endorpin from its carboxy-terminal. Another peptide, derived from the amino-terminal of POMC, is *N*-proopiomelanocortin (*N*-

[1] Anatomy Department, Glasgow University, Glasgow G12 8QQ, United Kingdom.
[2] MRC Neurochemical Pathology Unit, Newcastle General Hospital, Newcastle-upon-Tyne NE4 6BE, United Kingdom.

Neuropsychopharmacology
Edited by Bunney/Hippius/Laakmann/Schmauß

POMC, also known as pro-γ-MSH; Lowry 1984). Its possible functions are discussed below. ACTH is released into the systemic circulation where it acts on the adrenal to stimulate the release of cortisol. The other POMC-derived peptides are co-secreted in equimolar quantities along with ACTH (Nakao et al. 1980).

The HPA system is kept in check by negative feedback from cortisol on both CRH and ACTH secretion, and there is an overall circadian rhythm, probably controlled from the suprachiasmatic nucleus of the hypothalamus (Krieger 1979a). The most powerful influences on acutely increasing the activity of the HPA axis encompass a wide variety of aversive environmental factors including pain, exercise, surgery, physical illness and emotions such as fear or anger (commonly, and unhelpfully, grouped together under the term of "stress").

As can be seen, the system is complex and offers a wide range of possible sites for abnormality underlying the reported changes in cortisol secretion in depression. Applying the model of HPA axis function quoted above, it would seem to be inevitable that disorders in cortisol secretion would be accompanied by parallel changes in ACTH. In fact, establishing this link has proved far from straightforward. Part of the difficulty is associated with problems of measuring ACTH concentrations in plasma using the usual radioimmunoassay (RIA) techniques (Krieger 1979b). Mainly due to the relatively low affinity of the antibodies available, these RIAs are prone to inerference from cross-reacting molecules and tend to be insensitive and unreliable. Our group has employed a two-site recognition immunoradiometric assay developed by Lowry's team (Hodgkinson et al. 1984). This assay performs better due to having affinity-purified antibodies (added in excess) directed at both ends of the ACTH molecule; this makes it highly specific as well as sensitive.

In addition to difficulties with the RIAs, a further problem with some published research on ACTH secretion in depression has been that a normal control group was not used, comparisons being made only among depressed patients (Kalin et al. 1982; Reus et al. 1983; Yerevanian and Woolf 1983). Bearing in mind these drawbacks, other studies are broadly in support of the two main findings of our group (Charlton et al. 1987b; Ferrier et al. 1988): that basal concentrations of ACTH are normal in depression (Linkowski et al. 1985; a multiple timepoint sampling study over 24 h), but that ACTH is relatively resistant to suppression by dexamethasone (Kalin et al. 1982; Reus et al. 1983; Roy et al. 1986 – although the latter group also reported elevated basal levels). This pattern of abnormality is anomalous according to the standard model of HPA axis function (Hall et al. 1981), because in depression basal cortisol is raised without significant change in ACTH while both cortisol and ACTH are resistant to dexamethasone supression. Interestingly, this pattern of dissociation between ACTH and cortisol has also been reported in a variety of other situations (after haemorrhage in dogs, Gann 1979; following pain in cats, Berieter et al. 1982; with increased intracranial pressure in humans, Feibel et al. 1983). It would seem that the relationship between ACTH and cortisol is much less straightforward than is sometimes assumed.

These observation suggest that in depression (a) the adrenal has an increased sensitivity to basal ACTH, and (b) there is a down-regulation of glucocorticoid receptors at either or both hypothalamic and pituitary levels, with the result that dexamethasone has only a blunted effect in suppressing ACTH and/or CRH secretion.

There is evidence from several studies to support the hypothesis of adrenal hyperresponsivity or hypertrophy in depression. For example, there is an increased cortisol secretory response to a given dose of intravenous ACTH 1–24 (Amsterdam et al. 1983; Jaekle et al. 1987). Also when CRH is given as an intravenous bolus, depressed subjects have a smaller ACTH response than controls, but this reduced ACTH stimulus nevertheless produces a normal-sized cortisol response (Gold et al. 1984; Holsboer et al. 1986). These findings point to enhanced adrenal responsivity to ACTH, which may be speculated to be associated with enlargement of the adrenal cortex and therefore of the whole gland. This is supported by preliminary reports of enlarged adrenals in depressed patients who were DST non-suppressors when the whole glands were examined using computer tomographic (CT) scanning in living subjects (there was no significant difference, however, between the mean volumes of the groups of depressed and control subjects; Amsterdam et al. 1987). Also, increased adrenal weight at post mortem was noted in victims of violent suicide compared with controls dying of natural causes (Dorovini-Zis and Zis 1987). However the proportion of depressed subjects in the suicide group was not known.

But there is a further implication. Although basal ACTH is not increased, neither is it decreased, despite the greater negative feedback from prevailing high cortisol levels. This seems to point to an increased drive to ACTH secretion which balances the feedback effect of increased suppression from cortisol. The most likely cause of enhanced ACTH secretion is increased hypothalamic CRH production. While there is no evidence for increased CRH levels in the hypophysial portal system in depression, there are reports of elevated CRH concentrations in the cerebrospinal fluid of depressed patients (Nemeroff et al. 1984; Banki et al. 1987). This may reflect CRH changes in the hypothalamus, although the link is not established. CRH has been measured in the plasma of depressed subjects (Charlton et al. 1986), but concentrations do not seem to relate to HPA axis activity, and it seems likely that plasma CRH derives from a peripheral source. CRH has also been located in the human cortex (Bissette et al. 1985; Charlton et al. 1987c), where it probably functions as a neurotransmitter or neuromodulator.

Gold and co-workers (1984) have suggested that depression may be associated with an underlying hyperactivity of cerebral CRH systems, both in the hypothalamus and generally throughout the brain (Gold et al. 1984). In support of this idea Nemeroff et al. (1988) have found reduced numbers of CRH binding sites in the frontal cortex of suicide victims compared with controls. This finding could represent down-regulation of receptors in response to CRH hypersecretion (although other explanations are possible), but it must be emphasized that there was no clinical evidence as to whether or not these suicide victims were depressed. In contrast, post-mortem comparisons of cortical CRH concentrations between groups of clinicaly depressed suicide subjects and controls have shown no significant difference (Charlton et al. 1988). This negative result is confirmed by a recent study of both CRH concentrations and CRH binding sites in depressed subjects who died in mental hospitals of coincident illness (I. N. Ferrier and A. Leake, unpubished observations). On balance, there is at present no compelling evidence of generalised cerebral CRH overactivity, and no *direct* evidence concerning the status of hypophysial portal CRH secretion.

The other question concerns the mechanism of production of increased adrenal sensitivity to ACTH. As basal ACTH concentrations are normal, it seems unlikely that hypertrophy could be caused by ACTH alone: in fact there is considerable evidence that ACTH does not produce adrenal growth (Lowry 1984). For example, ACTH inhibits cell proliferation in vitro; physiological doses "in vivo" fail to stimulate compensatory hyperplasia of the remaining adrenal following unilateral adrenalectomy; and chronic treatment of the living animal with anti-ACTH antiserum does not affect adrenal size. It has been proposed that adrenal growth is produced by interaction with *N*-POMC (Lowry 1984). Intact *N*-POMC (1–76) and also the carboxy-terminal (γ-3-MSH) have been found to potentiate the steroidogenic effect of ACTH on adrenal cells in vitro (Pedersen et al. 1980) and in animal studies (Al Dujaili et al. 1981). The amino-terminal portion of the peptide promotes adrenal cell proliferation in the rat (Lowry et al. 1983). Lowry (1984) has proposed that the circulating form of *N*-POMC (which acts synergistically with ACTH on cortisol secretion) can be enzymically cleaved within the adrenal under the control of autonomic nerves which link the ventromedial nucleus of hypothalamus with the adrenal cortex (Dallman et al. 1977). Adrenal nerves are considered to be responsible for compensatory adrenal hypertrophy following unilateral adrenalectomy and also for hypertrophy of the contralateral gland following manipulation under anaesthetic – responses which can be blocked by spinal cord section. These responses can also be blocked by anti-*N*-POMC antiserum, which implies a humoral component to the response. Lowry et al. (1983) have proposed that following neural activation proteolytic enzymic cleavage liberates the active amino-terminal of *N*-POMC to promote adrenal cell proliferation.

It must be emphasised that the evidence for an adrenal growth-promoting role of *N*-POMC is derived from in vitro and animal studies, and there is at present no direct evidence concerning the role of *N*-POMC in humans. *N*-POMC is found to be present in depressed subjects with a similar pattern of abnormality to that of ACTH (Charlton et al. 1988), that is, normal basal levels but with a relative resistance to dexamethasone suppression. A similar degree of dexamethasone resistance has been reported for the other POMC family members β-endorpin and β-lipotropic hormone (Brambilla et al. 1981; Matthews et al. 1982), although there is some disagreement in the literature (Cohen et al. 1984; Ball et al. 1987). On balance, however, there is good evidence for a dysregulation of POMC-derived peptides characterised by a blunted suppressive effect of dexamethasone. This evidence reinforces the conclusion that the glucocorticoid receptors for dexamethasone (and by implication of cortisol) are down-regulated in depression: reduced in number and/or affinity.

It is now possible to pool the above information to produce a model for HPA axis dysfunction in depression. This model incorporates certain features proposed by Gold et al. (1984). Gold's group suggested that all the HPA axis changes in depression are the result of increased CRH drive, which caused raised ACTH and in turn adrenal hypertrophy with raised cortisol. The raised cortisol acts to suppress the ACTH back to normal levels. However the normal concentration of ACTH causes the secretion of higher than normal cortisol concentrations due to adrenal hypertrophy. The theory of Gold et al. has several flaws, such as the probability that ACTH cannot alone produce adrenal hypertrophy (Lowry 1984), the lack of evidence for a raised basal ACTH level early in the illness that is required to cause adrenal hypertrophy (Charlton et al. 1987b), and the lack of any means of maintainig adrenal hypertrophy when ACTH levels have been suppressed back to normal by the raised cortisol.

To account for the full range of reported abnormalities in depression it is necessary to postulate two primary mechanisms, one being an increased secretion of CRH into the hypophysial portal system and the other being increased adrenal responsivity to ACTH. Both abnormalities may be caused by changes in the hypothalamus. We propose that there is a simultaneous increase in activity in the paraventricular nucleus (where the cell bodies responsible for secreting both CRH and vasopressin are situated) and the ventromedial nucleus (site of the cell bodies which activate the adrenal autonomic neurones). Increased CRH secretion cases increased drive to ACTH secretion which is balanced by increased negative feedback from elevated plasma cortisol, leading to normal basal ACTH levels. The adrenal cortex is hyperresponsive due to increased proteolytic enzyme activation (potentiated by the autonomic nerves), increasing cleavage of *N*-POMC to liberate the growth promoting amino-terminal peptide. DST non-suppression of both cortisol and the POMC-derived peptides (including ACTH) is explained in terms of reduced glucocorticoid receptor numbers and/or affinity (down-regulation) in response to the high prevailing cortisol concentrations. High basal cortisol also acts to blunt the ACTH response to intravenous CRH.

The idea that the hypothalamus is important in depression is not a new one. The possibility is suggested by the striking similarity between the biological features of depression and behaviours which the hypothalamus regulates: e.g. appetite, sleep, sexual drive and circadian rhythms. However, previous authors who proposed a hypothalamic dysfunction in depression (Sachar et al. 1973) tended to emphasise that this was secondary to limbic system (and therefore neurotransmitter) changes – the idea of the "neuroendocrine window" on the brain (Rubin 1985). The recent expansion of knowledge concerning the neurotransmitter regulation of hormone secretion has led to an increased awareness of the complexity of these neuroendocrine interactions, involving numerous factors of varying importance (as described above for CRH). This has resulted in a greater degree of caution in interpreting peripheral endocrine changes in terms of specific neurotransmitter changes. We believe that such speculations are not useful at present, given our current level of understanding of the cerebral regulation of the HPA axis; however it is hoped that future advances will allow such links between blood and brain to be made.

This hypothesis has several immediate implications for research. It predicts that the glucocorticoid receptors at hypothalamic and/or pituitary levels are down-regulated, and these could be examined using post-mortem tissue. Another focus for post-mortem studies could be to measure indices of CRH and vasopressin activity (peptide concentrations, receptors and metabolites, mRNA content) in the paraventricular nucleus of the hypothalamus, the median eminence and the anterior pituitary, where changes would be expected. Adrenal changes would also be predicted. Post-mortem studies (and imaging techniques, if definition is adequate) could concentrate on the adrenal cortex (rather than the whole gland including medulla) to measure volume and weight, histology may provide clues to altered function. Adrenal enzymes involved in *N*-POMC cleavage are a further possible area for future study. Clearly, more research is required to establish the role of adrenal cortex innervation in the human, although there is good evidence of its importance in the rat (Holzwarth et al. 1987).

It is becoming apparent that the HPA axis abnormalities described above may not occur in a single subgroup of depressed patients but instead form a variety of overlapping groups (Meller et al. 1988). If this is the case, it implies that the endocrine profile of individual subjects may be more variable than has been believed. Following on from this the model also points towards an increased emphasis on longitudinal studies of individual depressed patients rather than the cross-sectional method of taking a "snapshot" of endocrine status in a group of patients with illnesses of varied duration and severity. Another factor is that the hormones of the HPA axis have a dynamic inter-relationship, characterised by pulsatile secretion and complex feedback modulations. It would be valuable, in this context, to follow patients through the sequence of hormone changes as a depressive illness develops and resolves.

We would also stress the limitations of this model. In particular, it has been necessary to choose between conflicting experimental results in establishing the basic "ingredients", and this has inevitably introduced a measure of subjective judgement. We have combined a range of different studies from many centres which have used a variety of clinical criteria and hormone measurement systems. It must not be forgotten that HPA axis abnormalities occur in only about half of depressed subjects. Furthermore, depression is a heterogeneous disorder, and it is unlikely that a single aetiology underlies the multiplicity of clinical forms. Despite these limitations we feel that a clear and comprehensive hypothesis such as this can act fruitfully to stimulate debate and focus experiment.

Acknowledgements. Thanks are due to Mr. Alan Leake and Prof. Jim Edwardson of the MRC Neurochemical Pathology Unit and to Prof. Phil Lowry of Reading University for discussions which were important to the formulation of ideas proposed in this paper.

References

Al-Dujaili EAS, Hope J, Estivariz FE, Lowry PJ, Edwards CRW (1981) Circulating human pituitary pro-gamma-melanotropin enhances the adrenal response to ACTH. Nature 291:156–158

Amsterdam JD, Winokur A, Abelman E, Lucki I, Rickel K (1983) Cosynotropin (ACTH 1–24) stimulation test in depressed patients and healthy subjects. Am J Psychiatry 140:907–909

Amsterdam JD, Marinelli DL, Arger P, Winokur A (1987) Assessment of adrenal gland volume by computed tomography in depressed patients and healthy volunteers: a pilot study. Psychiatry Res 21:189–197

Arana GW, Baldessarini RJ, Ornsteen M (1985) The dexamethasone suppression test for diagnosis and prognosis in psychiatry. Arch Gen Psychiatry 42:1193–1204

Ball R, Howlett T, Silverstone T, Rees L (1987) The inter-relationship of beta-endorphin, ACTH and cortisol in depressive illness: a controlled study. Psychol Med 17:31–37.

Banki CM, Bissette G, Arato M, O'Connor L, Nemeroff CB (1987) CSF corticotropin-releasing factor-like immunoreactivity in depression and schizophrenia. Am J Psychiatry 144:873–877

Berieter DA, Plotsky PM, Gann DS (1982) Tooth pulp stimulation stimulates the adrenocorticotropin response to haemorrhage in cats. Endocrinology 111:907–909

Bissette G, Reynolds GP, Kilts CD, Widerlov E, Nemeroff CB (1985) Corticotropin-releasing factor-like immunoreactivity in senile dementia of the Alzheimer type. JAMA 254:3067–3069

Braddock L, (1986) The dexamethasone suppression test: fact and artefact. Br J Psychiatry 148:363–374

Brambilla F, Genazzani AR, Facchinetti F, Parrini D, Petraglia F, Sacchetti E, Scarone S, Gnastalla A, D'Antona N (1981) Beta-endorphin and beta-lipotrophin plasma levels in chronic schizophrenia, primary affective disorders and secondary affective disorders. Psychoneuroendocrinology 6:321–330

Charlton BG, Leake A, Ferrier IN, Linton EA, Lowry PJ (1986) Corticotropin-releasing factor in plasma of depressed patients and controls. Lancet i:161–162

Charlton BG, Ferrier IN, Gibson AM, Biggins JA, Leake A, Wright C, Edwardson JA (1987a) A preliminary study of alpha-MSH concentrations in depressed patients and controls. Biol Psychiatry 22:1276–1279

Charlton BG, Leake A, Wright C, Griffiths HW, Ferrier IN (1987b) A combined study of cortisol, ACTH and dexamethasone concentrations in major depression: multiple timepoint sampling. Br J Psychiatry 150:791–796

Charlton BG, Ferrier IN, Perry RH (1987c) Distribution of corticotropin-releasing factor-like immunoreactivity in human brain. Neuropeptides 10:329–334

Charlton BG, Ferrier IN, Leake A, Edwardson JA, Eccleston D, Crowcombe K, Jackson S, Mclean C, Lowry PJ (1988) A multiple timepoint study of N-terminal pro-opiomelanocortin in depression using a two-site recognition immunoradiometric assay. Clin Endocrinol 28:165–172

Charlton BG, Cheetham SC, Horton RW, Katona CLE, Crompton MR, Ferrier IN (1988) Corticotropin-releasing factor immunoreactivity in post-mortem brain from depressed suicides. J Psychopharmacol 2:13–18

Cohen MR, Pickar D, Extein I, Gold MS, Sweeney DR (1984) Plasma cortisol and beta-endorphin immunoreactivity in nonmajor and major depression. Am J Psychiatry 141:628–632

Dallman MF, Engeland WC, McBride MH (1977) The neural regulation of compensatory adrenal growth. In: Krieger DT, Ganong WF (ed) ACTH and related peptides: structure, regulation and action. New York Academy of Sciences, New York, pp 373–392

Dorovini-Zis K, Zis AP (1987) Increased adrenal weight in victims of violent suicide. Am J Psychiatry 144:1214–1215

Feibel J, Kelly M, Lee L, Woolf P (1983) Loss of adrenocortical suppression after acute brain injury. J Clin Endocrinol Metab 57:1245–1250

Ferrier IN, Pascual J, Charlton BG, Wright C, Leake A, Griffiths HW, Fairbairn AF, Edwardson JA (1988) Cortisol, ACTH and dexamethasone concentrations in a psychogeriatric population. Biol Psychiatry 23:252–260

Gann DS (1979) Cortisol secretion after haemorrhage. Nephron 23:119–124

Gillies G, Grossman A (1985) The CRFs and their control: chemistry, physiology and clinical implications. Clin Endocrinol Metab 14:821–843

Gold PW, Crousos GP, Kellner C, Post R, Roy A, Augerinos P, Schulte H, Oldfield E, Lynn Loriaux D (1984) Psychiatric implications of basic and clinical studies with corticotropin-releasing factor. Am J Psychiatry 141:619–627

Hall R, Anderson J, Smart GA, Besser M (1981) Fundamentals of clinical endocrinology. Pitman, Glasgow

Hodgkinson SC, Allolio B, Landon J, Lowry PJ (1984) Development of a non-extracted two-site immunoradiometric assay for corticotropin utilising extreme amino and carboxy terminally directed antibodies. Biochem J 218:703–711

Holsboer F, Gerken A, Von Bardelbeau U, Grimm W, Beyer H, Muller OA, Stalla GK (1986) Human corticotropin-releasing hormone in depression: correlation with thyrotropin secretion following thyrotropin-releasing hormone. Biol Psychiatry 21:601–611

Holzwarth MA, Cunningham LA, Kleitman N (1987) The role of adrenal nerves in the regulation of adrenocortical functions. Ann NY Acad Sci 512:449–464

Jaeckle RS, Kathol RG, Lopez JF, Meller WH, Krummel SJ (1987) Enhanced adrenal sensitivity to exogenous cosynotropin (ACTH 1–24) stimulation in major depression. Arch Gen Psychiatry 44:233–240

Kalin NH, Weiler SJ, Sheldon SE (1982) Plasma ACTH and cortisol concentration before and after dexamethasone. Psychiatry Res 7:87–92

Krieger DT (1979a) Rhythms in CRF, ACTH and corticosteroids. In: Krieger DT (ed) Comprehensive endocrinology: endocrine rhythms. Raven, New York

Krieger DT (1979b) Plasma ACTH and corticosteroids. In: Degroot LJ (ed) Endocrinology. Grune and Stratton, New York

Linkowski P, Mendlewicz J, Leclerq R, Brasseur M, Mubain P, Golstein J, Copinschi G, Cauter EV (1985) The 24 hour profile of adrenocorticotropin and cortisol on major depressive illness. J Clin Endocrinol Metab 61:429–438

Lowry PJ (1984) Pro-opiocortin: the multiple adrenal hormone precursor. Biosci Rep 4:467–482

Lowry PJ, Silas L, Maclean C, Linton EA, Estivariz FE (1983) Pro-gamma-melanocyte stimulating hormone cleavage in adrenal gland undergoing compensatory growth. Nature 306:70–73

Matthews J, Akil H, Greden J, Watson S (1982) Plasma measures of beta-endorphin-like immunoreactivity in depressives and other psychiatric subjects. Life Sci 31:1897–1870

Meller W, Kathol RG, Jaeckle RS, Grambsch P, Lopez JF (1988) HPA axis abnormalities in depressed patients with normal response to the DST. Am J Psychiatry 145:318–324

Nakao K, Oki S, Tanaka I, Nakai Y, Imura H (1980) Concomitant secretion of gamma-MSH with ACTH and beta-endorphin in humans. J Clin Endocrinol Metab 51:1205–1207

Nemeroff CB, Widerlov E, Bissette G, Wallens H, Karlsson I, Eklund K, Kilts CD, Lossen PT, Vale WW (1984) Elevated concentrations of CSF corticotropin-releasing factor-like immunoreactivity in depressed patients. Science 226:1342–1344

Nemeroff CB, Owens MJ, Bissette G, Andorn AC, Stanley M (1988) Reduced corticotropin releasing factor binding sites in the frontal cortex of suicide victims. Arch Gen Psychiatry 45:577–579

Pedersen RC, Brownie AC, Ling N (1980) Pro-adrenocorticotropin/endorpin-derived peptides. Science 208:1044–1045

Plotsky PM, Bruhn TO, Vale W (1985) Hypophysiotropic regulation of adrenocorticotropin secretion in response to insulin-induced hypoglycemia. Endocrinology 117:323–329

Reus VI, Marshall J, Dallman M (1983) Regulation of ACTH and cortisol in depression. Peptides 4:786–788

Roy A, Gold PW, Pickard D, Wolkouritz OM, Chrousos G, Paul SM (1986) Pre- and post-dexamethasone ACTH levels in depressed patients and normal controls. J Affective Disord 10:95–99

Rubin RT (1985) The prospects for clinical psychoneuroendocrinology: has the curtain been drawn across the neuroendocrine window? Psychol Med 15:451–454

Sachar EJ, Hellman MD, Roffwarg HP, Halpern FS, Fukushima DH, Gallagher TF (1973) Disrupted 24-hour patterns of cortisol secretion in psychotic depression. Arch Gen Psychiatry 28:19–24

Yerevanian BG, Woolf PD (1983) Plasma ACTH levels in primary depression. Psychiatry Res 9:45–51

Alterations in Neuropeptide Systems in Alzheimer's Disease *

L. L. Cook, G. Bissette, and C. B. Nemeroff [1]

Introduction

The high concentration of neuropeptides in cortical interneurons, their neurotransmitter or neuromodulator roles, and their colocalization with conventional neurotransmitters have served as an impetus for studies of neuropeptide systems in Alzheimer's disease (AD). Substantial progress in biochemical characterization of AD has been obtained from studies of neurotransmitter systems in postmortem tissue. Alterations in cholinergic neurons have been demonstrated consistently in patients with histologically verified AD. The most reproducible finding has been that of marked reductions in the activity of choline acetyltransferase (ChAT), a marker of intact cholinergic neurons, in the neocortex and hippocampus as well as in the nucleus basalis of Meynert (substantia innominata) in AD (see Davies and Wolozin 1987 for review). Similarly, alterations in noradrenergic and serotonergic neurons (Adolfsson et al. 1979; Tomlinson et al. 1981; Perry et al. 1981a; Gottfries et al. 1983; Yates et al. 1983a; Arai et al. 1984a; Iversen et al. 1984) in AD have been demonstrated, although a recent study suggested that these deficits may be apparent only in severely demented patients exhibiting widespread neuronal loss, while cholinergic deficits may occur in more moderate cases of AD (Palmer et al. 1987). Widespread reductions in the concentration of γ-aminobutyric acid (GABA), a major inhibitory neurotransmitter of intrinsic cortical neurons, as well as of the excitatory neurotransmitter glutamic acid, have also been reported (Ellison et al. 1986). These studies have clearly demonstrated that both cortical interneurons and cortical afferent projection terminals are pathologically involved in AD. Reviews of neuropeptide abnormalities in dementia and AD have been published previously (Kragh-Sorensen et al. 1986; Rossor et al. 1986; Cain and Nemeroff 1987; Bouras et al. 1986; Beal et al. 1987a; Nemeroff and Bissette 1986).

* This research was supported by the following grants: NIMH MH-40524, NIA AG-05128, and NRSA ES-07031.

[1] Departments of Psychiatry and Pharmacology, Duke University Medical Center, Durham, NC 27710, USA.

Neuropsychopharmacology
Edited by Bunney/Hippius/Laakmann/Schmauß

Somatostatin (SRIF)

SRIF Concentration in Brain Tissue

The study of neuropeptide alterations in AD was pioneered by Davies and his colleagues who reported marked decreases in somatostatin (somatotropin releasing inhibitory factor, SRIF) concentration in the hippocampus, frontal and parietal cortices, and the superior temporal gyrus (Davies et al. 1980; Davies and Terry 1981). SRIF reductions have been reported to be more marked in the frontal and temporal cortex than in other cortical or subcortical regions (Francis et al. 1987; Rossor et al. 1980 a; Nemeroff et al. 1983), to occur in brain regions with the highest plaque counts (Rossor et al. 1980 a), and to be present in patients with early-onset AD (Davis and Terry 1981; Rossor et al. 1984 b). Reductions in SRIF concentration have not generally been observed in subcortical regions (Beal et al. 1986 a, b). Ferrier et al. (1983) reported reduced SRIF concentrations in the frontal, temporal, and parietal cortices and septum, while the SRIF concentration of the nucleus accumbens and amygdala were not altered in AD. Arai et al. (1984 b) reported SRIF reductions in the orbital cortex, hippocampus, and putamen but not in the substantia innominata. Our group found SRIF reductions in the frontal and temporal cortices and the hypothalamus but not in the parietal cortex, amygdala, caudate nucleus, nucleus accumbens, or posterior hippocampus (Nemeroff et al. 1983). In contrast, Candy et al. (1985) reported reduced concentrations of multiple molecular weight species of SRIF in the amygdala.

Reductions in SRIF concentration in AD have been correlated with alterations in morphology and neurochemistry as well as deficits in cognition. SRIF reductions have been correlated with the number of neuritic plaques and neurofibrillary tangles in the temporal cortex (Dawbarn et al. 1986) and with reduced ChAT activity in the parietal cortex (Tamminga et al. 1985). In addition, Reinikainen et al. (1987) recently reported reductions in both SRIF and ChAT in all cortical areas studied (frontal, temporal, and parietal) but not in the thalamus or putamen in AD.

Using immunohistochemical methods, SRIF-containing neurons have been shown to be either lost or reduced in size in frontal (layers III and V) and temporal cortex and in the hippocampus in AD (Joynt and McNeil 1984; Chan-Palay 1987). SRIF immunoreactivity has also been observed in 30%–50% of cortical plaques in postmortem brain tissue of AD (Armstrong et al. 1985; Morrison et al. 1985).

Measurement of SRIF in Cerebrospinal Fluid

Studies in which the concentration of SRIF in CSF of AD patients was measured have been reviewed recently (Beal and Growdon 1986). The SRIF concentration in CSF has been reported to be reduced in patients with both senile dementia (Oram et al. 1982) and AD (Wood et al. 1982; Serby et al. 1984;

Beal et al. 1986c), and these CSF SRIF reductions are correlated with cognitive deficits (Reinikanen et al. 1987; Soininen et al. 1984). In collaboration with Widerlov and colleagues, we reported a marked decrease in CSF SRIF concentrations in senile dementia, but reductions in patients with major depression and schizophrenia were also observed (Bissette et al. 1986). In another study, Tamminga et al. (1987) reported a correlation between a reduction in CSF SRIF in AD patients with deficits in cognitive performance and a decline in cortical glucose utilization.

Consistent with the tissue studies described above, almost all studies of CSF in AD have found reductions in SRIF. However, this finding is relatively nonspecific in view of the reduction of CSF SRIF in patients with other psychiatric and neurological disorders (Bissette et al. 1986).

SRIF Receptors

High-affinity binding sites, putative SRIF receptors, have been identified in the brain, pituitary and peripheral tissue (Beal et al. 1985). Beal and colleagues (1985) recently reported a 50% reduction in SRIF receptor density in the frontal (Brodmann's areas, BA, 6, 9, and 10) and temporal cortex (BA 21), with no change in receptor affinity; no changes in the cingulate cortex, postcentral gyrus, temporal pole, or superior temporal gyrus were observed. In confirmation, we have recently reported a 40% reduction in B_{max} of SRIF binding in the frontal cortex (BA 10) and temporal cortex (BA 38; Knight et al. 1988).

The widespread reduction in cortical SRIF concentrations in AD has been interpreted as either degeneration of intrinsic SRIF cortical neurons or markedly reduced biosynthesis (Beal et al. 1987a). Interpretation of the observed reduction in SRIF receptor density is problematic because postsynaptic receptor density up-regulation is usually observed following diminished availability of the presynaptically released neurotransmitter as, for example, in the CRF system (see below). Thus, these findings suggest that SRIF receptors may be reduced in density due to their location either on presynaptic SRIF terminals or on postsynaptic neurons that are vulnerable to degeneration in AD, or to a reduction in receptor synthesis.

Corticotropin-Releasing Factor

Corticotropin-releasing factor (CRF) is a 41 amino acid containing peptide that is the major physiological regulator of the pituitary-adrenal axis. In addition to its neuroendocrine role, CRF has been shown to fulfill many of the requisite neurotransmitter criteria, including enrichment in synaptosomal fractions, heterogeneous distribution in the brain, release from brain slices following depolarization, and electrophysiological effects after microiontophoretic application (Merchenthaler 1984; Vale et al. 1983; DeSouza 1985).

CRF has been identified in intrinsic cerebrocortical neurons as well as in neurons of the hypothalamus, brain stem, amygdala, and basal forebrain in rat (Olschowka et al. 1982; Swanson et al. 1983; Crawley et al. 1985) and human (Bissette et al. 1985; Charlton et al. 1987). Cortical CRF-containing neurons in rodents have cell bodies predominantly in cortical layers II and III and terminal fields in laminae I and IV, where CRF receptor density is high (Desouza 1985; Olschowka et al. 1982; Swanson et al. 1983).

We have previously reported that CRF concentrations in AD are reduced by 50% in the frontal cortex (BA 10) and temporal cortex (BA 38), and reduced by 70% in the caudate nucleus (Bissette et al. 1985). The concentration of CRF in the hypothalamus, nucleus accumbens, hippocampus, amygdala, cingulate gyrus, and substantia innominata was not reduced compared to normal controls. These findings have been confirmed and extended by DeSouza et al. (1986) who reported a decrease in CRF concentration in the frontal, temporal, and occipital cortices along with an inversely related increase in CRF receptor density. These changes were also correlated with decrements in ChAT activity. Reductions in the CSF concentration of CRF has been reported in some chronically hospitalized patients with AD (Mouradian et al. 1986; May et al. 1987). A recent study by Whitehouse et al. (1987) has demonstrated reductions in cortical CRF immunoreactivity in patients with AD, Parkinson's disease (PD), and progressive supranuclear palsy; reductions were greatest in AD and in PD with AD neuropathology. They demonstrated decreased concentrations of CRF in the frontal, temporal, and occipital cortices in AD and in PD with AD neuropathology and interpreted these findings as abnormalities in intrinsic cortical neurons. We have recently reviewed the role of CRF in neurodegenerative disorders (DeSouza et al. 1990).

Neuropeptide Y

Neuropeptide Y (NPY) is a 36 amino acidcontaining peptide which is widely distributed in both the rat and human brain (Adrian et al. 1983; Allen et al. 1983; Dawbarn et al. 1984; Chronwall et al. 1985; Lundberg et al. 1984; Chan-Palay et al. 1985a). Although NPY has been shown to be colocalized with SRIF in both cortical and striatal neurons (Hendry et al. 1984; Vincent et al. 1982, 1983; Kowall et al. 1986), NPY concentrations have been reported to be unaltered in four cortical regions and to be increased in the substantia innominata in AD (Allen et al. 1984). Recent studies in AD have shown that NPY is not altered in the frontal (BA 10) or parietal (BA 21, 39, and 40) cortices, regions exhibiting reductions in ChAT activity and SRIF concentration (Foster et al. 1986; Dawbarn et al. 1986). In contrast, Beal et al. (1986d) have recently reported a widespread reduction in NPY concentration in AD which significantly correlated with reduced SRIF concentration. Maximal (60%–70%) reductions were observed in the temporal lobe, and alterations were also seen in the locus ceruleus and central nucleus of the amygdala. These authors reported no alterations in SRIF and NPY concentrations in subdivisions of the striatum in normal and AD patients (Beal et al. 1987b). Differences in patient age and disease severity, as well as differences in antisera characteristics, may account for the discordant results between these and earlier studies. In addition, a recent study by Chan-Palay et al. (1985b) demonstrated structural changes in cortical NPY neurons in AD. Neuronal alterations including enlarged cell somata and reduced, thickened, and gnarled dendrites were found in the temporal, parietal, and frontal cortices. Dawbarn and Emson (1985) reported that 10%–20% of neuritic plaques in the cortex and hippocampus of AD patients contained NPY.

Thyrotropin-Releasing Hormone

In agreement with studies by Biggins and colleagues (1983) and Yates et al. (1983b), we reported that the concentration of thyrotropin-releasing hormone (TRH) was unaltered in AD (Nemeroff et al. 1983). Using the antiserum available to us at that time, cortical TRH was undetectable. However, the concentration of TRH in CSF, as well as that of gonadotropin-releasing hormone, was reduced in AD patients (Oram et al. 1982). The availability of more sensitive TRH antisera clearly will permit more definitive studies of TRH in AD.

Vasopressin

Vasopressin (AVP), also known as antidiuretic hormone, is best known as the neurohypophyseal hormone that is released from the posterior pituitary in response to alterations in plasma osmolarity. AVP has been shown to have a wide extrahypothalamic distribution in rodents (Dogterom and Buijs 1980) and humans (Rossor et al. 1981a). AVP is of particular interest in AD because of its purported involvement in learning and memory in experimental animals (DeWeid et al. 1984; Kovacs et al.1979) and man (Weingartner et al. 1981; Beckwith et al. 1984). In an early study, the concentration of AVP in different areas of the brain showed little or no differences in AD patients (Rossor et al. 1980b). Recent studies by Mazurek and colleagues (Beal et al. 1987a; Mazurek et al. 1985, 1986a) have shown reductions of AVP in the globus pallidus, nucleus accumbens, and hippocampus in AD patients but no changes in other subcortical and cortical regions. However, in another recent study, the mean AVP concentration was shown to be significantly reduced in BA 4, 7, and 10 in nine patients with AD (Fujiyoshi et al. 1987). In addition, the CSF concentration of AVP has been shown to be reduced in patients with dementia of the Alzheimer's type (Sorensen et al. 1983; Mazurek et al. 1986b; Raskind et al. 1986).

It is of interest that AVP reductions do not parallel other pathological and neurochemical changes in AD. Unlike the SRIF deficits which presumably occur in intrinsic cortical neurons, the spared AVP content in the cortex and elsewhere may reflect the preservation of AVP cell bodies extrinsic to the cortex (Mazurek et al. 1986a).

Neurotensin

Neurotensin (NT), a tridecapeptide, fulfills many criteria for neurotransmitter status in the mammalian CNS (Nemeroff et al. 1980). We have shown that the concentration of NT in histologically verified cases of AD was reduced by 30% in the amygdala, but not in five other brain regions, compared to age- and sex-matched controls (Nemeroff et al. 1983). Ferrier et al. (1983) reported a decrease in NT concentration in the septum but not in 13 other brain regions in AD. However, other investigators have reported that NT was not changed significantly in AD in the cortex, hippocampus, or amygdala (Biggins et al. 1983; Rossor et al. 1984a). Yates et al. (1985) also reported that NT levels were not altered in the temporal cortex or in several subcortical regions in AD, although it was increased in the caudate and cortex in younger Down's syndrome patients.

Substance P

The concentration of substance P (SP), an undecapeptide, was reported to be reduced in the frontal, parietal, temporal, and occipital cortices of patients with AD in an early study (Crystal and Davies 1982). In contrast, Yates et al. (1983b) reported no changes in SP concentration in postmortem AD brain, and Ferrier et al. (1983) reported a reduction in SP in the putamen only in a study of 14 brain areas including cortical areas with documented SRIF reductions. However, in a recent study, Beal and Mazurek (1987) observed 20%–40% reductions of SP in the hippocampus and several cortical regions of AD brains; the most pronounced reduction was in the inferior temporal gyrus. Whether this reduction is a result of alterations in intrinsic cortical neurons or afferent terminals has not been established. There is some evidence of colocalization of SP with either SRIF, GABA, or NPY in the monkey cortex (Jones and Hendry 1986).

Vasoactive Intestinal Peptide

Vasoactive intestinal peptide (VIP) is a 28 amino acid neuropeptide with a widespread distribution in the human (Emson et al. 1979) and rat (Fuxe et al. 1977; Loren et al. 1979) brain; the limbic cortex, amygdala, hippocampus and hypothalamus, and human CSF (Fahrenkrug et al. 1977) contain relatively high concentrations. Current evidence suggests that the concentration of VIP is not reduced in either cortical or subcortical sites in AD (Perry et al. 1981 b; Ferrier et al. 1983; Rossor et al. 1980c). Wikkelso et al. (1985) reported that CSF VIP concentrations are not altered in patients with AD but were reduced in multi-infarct dementia and normal pressure hydrocephalus.

Oxytocin

Oxytocin is best known as a neurohypophyseal hormone released from the posterior pituitary in response to suckling. It is found in hypothalamic neurons which project not only to the posterior pituitary but to other brain regions as well (Poulain et al. 1980). Like AVP, oxytocin may have particular relevance in the study of AD because of its putative involvement in learning and memory. In contrast to the purported enhancement of memory by AVP, oxytocin inhibits memory storage and retrieval in animal models (Bohus et al. 1978). Raskind et al. (1986) reported that the concentration of oxytocin was not altered in the CSF of AD patients compared to normal elderly and normal young subjects. Mazurek et al. (1987) have recently reported that the concentration of oxytocin is increased by 33% in the hippocampus and temporal cortex of 12 cases of histologically confirmed AD compared to controls but normal in other cortical and subcortical regions.

Other Neuropeptides

β-Endorphin, a product of proopiomelanocortin, is an opioid peptide contained in neurons originating in the arcuate nucleus of the hypothalamus. Because certain animal studies suggest that β-endorphin, like AVP, enhances memory (DeWeid et al. 1978), recent reports of its reduction in CSF in AD patients are of interest (Ueki and Namba 1983; Jolkkonen et al. 1985). These findings were not replicated, however, in a later study (Raskind et al. 1986). Jolkkonen et al. (1987) recently reported a marginal reduction in CSF β-endorphin in severely demented, but not marginally demented, AD patients. Rossor et al. (1982) reported that Met-enkaphalinlike immunoreactivity in the neocortex and hippocampus was not altered in AD compared to a control group.

α-Melanocyte stimulating hormone (α-MSH), the NH_2-terminal fragment (1–13) of adrenocorticotrophic hormone (ACTH), is widely distributed in extrahypothalamic regions as well as in the hypothalamus of the rat (Swaab et al. 1981) and human brain (Arai et al. 1986). α-MSH is of particular relevance in AD because of its purported role in learning and memory (Bohus and deWied 1981) and influence on the septo-hippocampal cholinergic neurons (Wood et al. 1978; Botticelli and Wurtman 1981). In a recent study of 21 regions in postmortem brains of five AD patients and eight normal subjects, α-MSH was found to be reduced in the cingulate cortex, caudate, and substantia nigra (Arai et al. 1986).

Cholecystokinin (CCK), a 33 amino acid containing peptide, appears to be a CNS neurotransmitter. It is of particular interest to study CCK in AD because this peptide is found in extraordinarily high concentrations in interneurons of the cerebral cortex. However, the concentration of CCK in the cortex has been found to be unchanged in AD (Perry et al. 1981 a, b; Rossor et al. 1981 b; Ferrier et al. 1983).

Conclusion

Two neuropeptides are consistently reduced in the hippocampus and cortex in AD: SRIF and CRF. The absence of confirmed alterations of neurons containing NT, VIP, and CCK, as well as the increase in oxytocin concentration in hippocampus and cortex, demonstrate a specific vulnerability of SRIF and CRF neurons in AD. Future studies are needed to resolve the discordant findings concerning VIP, NPY, and SP in AD.

Studies focusing on alterations in the concentration and function of neuropeptides in AD may provide new insights regarding the selective neuronal vulnerability observed in this disease. Studies designed to evaluate a possible modulatory relationship between SRIF and CRF neurons with cholinergic and GABAergic systems in AD also are suggested. In addition, the reduction in the concentration of SRIF, but not in those of NPY and GABA with which SRIF is colocalized, suggests studies which evaluate specific impairments in intracellular mechanisms responsible for the synthesis and storage of SRIF. Whether SRIF or CRF receptor agonists would modify any of the cognitive deficits observed in AD remains unknown.

Acknowledgement. The authors are grateful to Shelia Walker for preparation of this manuscript.

References

Adolfsson R, Gottfries CG, Roos BE, Winblad B (1979) Changes in brain catecholamines in patients with dementia of Alzheimer type. Br J Psychiatry 135:216–223

Adrian TE, Allen JM, Bloom SR, Ghatei MA, Rossor MN, Roberts GW, Crow TJ, Tatemoto K, Polak JM (1983) Neuropeptide Y distribution in human brain. Nature 306:584–586

Allen JM, Ferrier IN, Roberts GW, Cross AJ, Adrian TE, Crow TJ, Bloom SR (1984) Elevation of neuropeptide Y (NPY) in substantia innominata in Alzheimer's type dementia. J Neurol Sci 64:325–331

Allen YS, Adrian TE, Allen JM, Tatemoto K, Crow TJ, Bloom SR, Polak JM (1983) Neuropeptide Y distribution in the rat brain. Science 221:877–879

Arai H, Kosaka K, Iizuka T (1984a) Changes in biogenic amines and their metabolites in postmortem brains from patients with Alzheimer's type dementia. J Neurochem 43:388–393

Arai H, Moroji T, Kosaka K (1984b) Somatostatin and vasoactive intestinal polypeptide in postmortem brains from patients with Alzheimer-type dementia. Neurosci Lett 52:73–78

Arai H, Moroji T, Kosaka K, Iizuka R (1986) Extrahypophyseal distribution of alpha-melocyte stimulating hormone (alpha-MSH)-like immunoreactivity in postmortem brains from normal subjects and Alzheimer-type dementia patients. Brain Res 377:305–310

Armstrong DM, LeRoy S, Shields D, Terry RD (1985) Somatostatin-like immunoreactivity within neuritic plaques. Brain Res 338:71–79

Beal MF, Growdon JH (1986) CSF neurotransmitter markes in Alzheimer's disease. Prog Neuropsychopharmacol Biol Psychiatry 10:259–270

Beal MF, Mazurek MF (1987) Substance P-like immunoreactivity is reduced in Alzheimer's disease cerebral cortex. Neurology 37:1205–1209

Beal MF, Mazurek MF, Tran VT, Chatta G, Bird ED, Martin JB (1985) Reduced numbers of somatostatin receptors in the cerebral cortex in Alzheimer's disease. Science 229:289–291

Beal MF, Mazurek MF, Svendsen CN, Bird ED, Martin JB (1986a) Widespread reductions of somatostatin-like immunoreactivity in the cerebral cortex in Alzheimer's disease. Ann Neurol 20:489–495

Beal MF, Benoit R, Mazurek MF, Bird ED, Martin JB (1986b) Somatostatin-28 (1–12)-like immunoreactivity is reduced in Alzheimer's disease cerebral cortex. Brain Res 368:380–383

Beal MF, Growdon JH, Mazurek MF, Martin JB (1986c) CSF somatostatin-like immunoreactivity in dementia. Neurol 36:294–297

Beal MF, Mazurek MF, Chattha GK, Svendsen CN, Bird ED, Martin JB (1986d) Neuropeptide Y immunoreactivity is reduced in cerebral cortex in Alzheimer's disease. Ann Neurol 20:282–288

Beal MF, Kowall NW, Mazurek MF (1987a) Neuropeptides in Alzheimer's disease. J Neural Transm [Supp] 24:163–174

Beal MF, Mazurek MF, McKee MA (1987b) The regional distribution of somatostatin and neuropeptide Y in control and Alzheimer's disease striatum. Neurosci Lett 79:201–206

Beckwith BE, Till RE, Schneider V (1984) Vasopressin analog (DDAVP) improves memory in human males. Peptides 5:819–822

Biggins JA, Perry EK, McDermott JR, Smith AI, Perry RH, Edwardson JA (1983) Postmortem levels of thyrotropin-releasing hormone and neurotensin in the amygdala in Alzheimer's disease, schizophrenia and depression. J Neurol Sci 58:117–122

Bissette G, Reynolds GP, Kilts CD, Widerlov E, Nemeroff CB (1985) Corticotropin-releasing factor-like immunoreactivity in senile dementia of the Alzheimer type. JAMA 254:3067–3069

Bissette G, Widerlov E, Walleus H, Karlsson I, Eklund K, Forsman A, Nemeroff CB (1986) Alterations in cerebrospinal fluid concentrations of somatostatinlike immunoreactivity in neuropsychiatric disorders. Arch Gen Psychiatry 43:1148–1151

Bohus B, deWied D (1981) Actions of ACTH- and MSH-like peptides on learning preformance, and retention. In: Martinez JL, Jensen RA, Messing RB et al. (eds) Endogenous peptides and learning and memory processes. Academic, New York, p 59

Bohus B, Kovacs GL, deWied D (1978) Oxytocin, vasopressin and memory: opposite effects on consolidation and retrieval processes. Brain Res 157:414–417

Botticelli LJ, Wurtman RJ (1981) Corticotropin regulates trans-synaptically the activity of septohippocampal cholinergic neurons. Nature 289:309–327

Bouras C, de St Hilaire-Kafi S, Constantinidis J (1986) Neuropeptides in Alzheimer's disease: a review and morphological results. Prog Neuropsychopharmacol Biol Psychiatry 10:271–286

Cain ST, Nemeroff CB (1987) Neuropeptides and neurotransmitters in Alzheimer's disease. In: Maddox GL, Busse EW (eds) Aging, the universal human experience. Springer, New York, p 63

Candy JM, Gascoigne AD, Biggins JA, Smith IA, Perry RH, Perry EK, McDermott JR, Edwardson JA (1985) Somatostatin immunoreactivity in cortical and some subcortical regions in Alzheimer's disease. J Neurol Sci 71:315–323

Chan-Palay V (1987) Somatostatin immunoreactive neurons in the human hippocampus and cortex shown by immunogold/silver intensification on vibratome sections: coexistence with neuropeptide Y neurons, and effects in Alzheimer-type dementia. J Comp Neurol 260:201–223

Chan-Palay V, Allen YS, Lang W, Haesler U, Polak JM (1985a) I. Cytology and distribution in normal human cortex of neurons immunoreactive with antisera against neuropeptide Y. J Comp Neurol 238:382–389

Chan-Palay V, Lang W, Allen YS, Haesler U, Polak JM (1985b) II. Cortical neurons immunoreactive with antisera against neuropeptide Y are altered in Alzheimer's-type dementia. J Comp Neurol 238:390–400

Charlton BG, Ferrier IN, Perry RH (1987) Distribution of corticotropin-releasing factor-like immunoreactivity in human brain. Neuropeptides 10:329–334

Chronwall BM, Chase TS, O'Donohue TL (1985) Coexistence of neuropeptide Y and somatostatin in rat and human cortical and rat hypothalamic neurons. Neurosci Lett 52:213–217

Crawley JN, Olschowka JA, Diz DI, Jacobowitz DM (1985) Behavioral investigation of the coexistence of substance P, corticotropin-releasing factor, and acetylcholinesterase in lateral dorsal tegmental neurons projecting to the medial frontal cortex of the rat. Peptides 6:891–901

Crystal HA, Davies P (1982) Cortical substance P-like immunoreactivity in cases of Alzheimer's disease and senile dementia of the Alzheimer type. J Neurochem 38:1781–1784

Davies P, Terry RD (1981) Cortical somatostatin-like immunoreactivity in cases of Alzheimer's disease and senile dementia of the Alzheimer type. Neurobiol Aging 2:9–14

Davies P, Wolozin BL (1987) Recent advances in the neurochemistry of Alzheimer's disease. J Clin Psychiatry 48:(Suppl) 5 23–30

Davies P, Katzman R, Terry RD (1980) Reduced somatostatin-like immunoreactivity in cerebral cortex from cases of Alzheimer's disease and Alzheimer's senile dementia. Nature 288:279–280

Dawbarn D, Emson PC (1985) Neuropeptide Y-like immunoreactivity in neuritic plaques of Alzheimer's disease. Biochem Biophys Res Commun 126:289–294

Dawbarn D, Hunt SP, Emson PC (1984) Neuropeptide Y: regional distribution, chromatographic characterization and immunohistochemical demonstration in post-mortem human brain. Brain Res 296:168–173

Dawbarn D, Rossor MN, Mountjoy CQ, Roth N, Emson PC (1986) Decreased somatostatin immunoreactivity but not neuropeptide Y immunoreactivity in cerebral cortex in senile dementia of Alzheimer type. Neurosci Lett 70:154–159

DeSouza EB (1985) Corticotropin-releasing factor. Compr Ther 11:3–5

DeSouza EB, Whitehouse PJ, Kuhar MJ, Price D, Vale WW (1986) Reciprocal changes in corticotropin-releasing factor (CRF)-like immunoreactivity and CRF receptors in cerebral cortex of Alzheimer's disease. Nature 319:593–595

DeSouza EB, Bissette G, Whitehouse PJ, Powers RE, Price D, Vale WW, Nemeroff CB (1990) Abnormalities in corticotropin-releasing factor (CRF) in neurodegenerative diseases. In: DeSouza EB, Nemeroff CB (eds) Corticotropin-releasing factor: basic and clinical studies of a neuropeptide. CRC, Boca Raton, p 335

DeWied D, Bohus B, Van Ree JM, Urban I (1978) Behavioral and electrophysiological effects of peptides related to lipotropin (β-LPH). J Pharmacol Exp Ther 204:570–580

DeWied D, Gaffori O, van Ree JM, de Jong W (1984) Central target for the behavioral effects of vasopressin neuropeptides. Nature 308:276–278

DiMaggio DA, Chronwall BM, Buchanan K, O'Donohue TL (1985) Pancreatic polypeptide immunoreactivity in rat brain is actually neuropeptide Y. Neuroscience 15:1149–1157

Dogterom J, Buijs RM (1980) Vasopressin and oxytocin distribution in rat brain; radioimmunoassay and immunocytochemical studies. In: Marson CA, Traczyk WZ (eds) Neuropeptides and neural transmission. Raven, New York, p 307

Ellison DW, Beal MF, Mazurek MF, Bird ED, Martin JB (1986) A postmortem study of amino acid neurotransmitters in Alzheimer's disease. Ann Neurol 20:616–621

Emson PC, Fahrenkrug J, Spokes EGS (1979) Vasoactive intestinal polypeptide (VIP): distribution in normal human brain and in Huntington's disease. Brain Res 173:174–178
Fahrenkrug J, Schaffalitzky de Muckadell OB, Fahrenkrug A (1977) Vasoactive intestinal polypeptide (VIP) in human cerebrospinal fluid. Brain Res 124:581–584
Ferrier IN, Cross AJ, Johnson JA, Roberts GW, Crow TJ, Corsellis JAN, Lee YC, O'Shaughnessey D, Adrian TE, McGregor GP, Baracese-Hamilton AJ, Bloom SR (1983) Neuropeptides in Alzheimer type dementia. J Neurol Sci 62:159–170
Foster NL, Tamminga CA, O'Donohue TL, Tanimoto K, Bird ED, Martin JB (1986) Brain choline acetyltransferase activity and neuropeptide Y concentrations in Alzheimer's disease. Neurosci Lett 63:71–75
Francis PT, Bowen DM, Lowe SL, Neary D, Mann DMA, Snowden JS (1987) Somatostatin content and release measured in cerebral biopsies from demented patients. J Neurol Sci 78:1–16
Fujiyoshi K, Suga H, Okamoto K, Nakamura S, Kameyame M (1987) Reduction of arginine-vasopressin in the cerebral cortex in Alzheimer type senile dementia. J Neurol Neurosurg Psychiatry 50:929–932
Fuxe K, Hokfelt T, Said SI, Mutt V (1977) Vasoactive intestinal polypeptide and the nervous system: immunohistochemical evidence for localization in central and peripheral neurons, particularly intracortical neurons of the cerebral cortex. Neurosci Lett 5:241–246
Gottfries CG, Adolfsson R, Aquilonius SM, Carlson A, Eckernas S-A, Norberg A, Oreland L, Svennerholm L, Wiberg A, Winblat B (1983) Biochemical changes in dementia disorders of Alzheimer type (AD/SDAT). Neurobiol Aging 4:261–271
Hendry SHC, Jones EG, Emson PC (1984) Morphology, distribution, and synaptic relations of somatostatin- and neuropeptide Y-immunoreactive neurons in rat and monkey neocortex. J Neurosci 4:2497–2517
Iversen LL, Rosser MN, Reynolds GP, Hills R, Roth M, Mountjoy CQ, Foote SL, Morrison JH, Bloom FE (1984) Loss of pigmented dopamine-β-hydroxylase positive cells from locus coeruleus in senile dementia of Alzheimer's type. Neurosci Lett 39:95–100
Jolkkonen JT, Soininen HS, Riekkinen PJ (1985) Reduced beta-endorphin-like immunoreactivity in CSF of patients with Alzheimer's disease. Neurology 35 (Suppl 1):218
Jolkkonen JT, Soininen HS, Riekkinen PJ (1987) β-Endorphin-like immunoreactivity in cerebrospinal fluid of patients with Alzheimer's disease and Parkinson's disease. J Neurol Sci 77:153–159
Jones EG, Hendry SHC (1986) Co-localization of GABA and neuropeptides in neocortical neurons. Trends Neurosci 9:71–76
Joynt RJ, McNeil TH (1984) Neuropeptides in aging and dementia. Peptides 5 (Suppl):269–274
Kovacs G, Bohus B, Versteg DHG, De Kloet R, DeWied D (1979) Effect of oxytocin and vasopressin on memory consolidation: sites of action and catecholaminergic correlates after local microinjection into limbic-midbrain structures. Brain Res 175:303–314
Knight DL, Bissette G, Kilts CD, Reynolds GP, Nemeroff CB (1988) Selective reductions in cerebrocortical somatostatin receptor binding density in Alzheimer's disease. Soc Neurosci Abstr 14:667
Kowall NW, Beal MF, Martin JB (1986) Neuropeptide Y, somatostatin and NADPH-diaphorase neurons do not contain neurofibrillary tangles in Alzheimer's disease. Neurol 36 (Suppl 1):224
Kragh-Sorensen P, Olsen RB, Lund S, van Riezen H, Steffensen K (1986) Neuropeptides: ACTH-peptides in dementia. Prog Neurospychopharmacol Biol Psychiatry 10:479–492
Loren I, Emson PC, Fahrenkrug A, Bjorklund A, Alumets J, Hakanson R, Sundler F (1979) Distribution of vasoactive intestinal polypeptide in the rat and mouse brain. Neuroscience 4:1953–1976
Lundberg JM, Terenius L, Hokfelt T, Tatemoto K (1984) Comparative immunohistochemical and biochemical analysis of pancreatic polypeptide-like peptides with special reference to presence of neuropeptide Y in central and peripheral neurons. J Neurosci 4:2376–2386

May C, Rapoport SI, Tomai TP, Chrousos GP, Gold PW (1987) Cerebrospinal fluid concentrations of corticotropin-releasing hormone (CRF) and corticotropin (ACTH) are reduced in patients with Alzheimer's disease. Neurology 37:535–538

Mazurek MF, Beal MF, Martin JB (1985) Vasopressin in Alzheimer's disease: a study of postmortem brain concentrations. Ann Neurol 20:665–670

Mazurek MF, Beal MF, Bird ED, Martin JB (1986a) Vasopressin in postmortem Alzheimer brain. Ann Neurol 18:143–144

Mazurek MF, Growdon JH, Beal MF, Martin JB (1986b) CSF vasopressin concentration is reduced in Alzheimer's disease. Neurology 36:1133–1137

Mazurek MF, Beal MF, Bird ED, Martin JB (1987) Oxytocin in Alzheimer's disease: postmortem brain levels. Neurology 37:1001–1003

Merchenthaler I (1984) Corticotropin releasing factor (CRF)-like immunoreactivity in the rat central nervous system. Extrahypothalamic distribution. Peptides 5 (Suppl 1):153–169

Morrison JH, Rogers J, Scherr S, Benoit R, Bloom F (1985) Somatostatin immunoreactivity in neuritic plaques of Alzheimer's patients. Nature 314:90–92

Mouradian MM, Farah JH, Mohr E, Fabbrini G, O'Donohue TL, Chase TN (1986) Spinal fluid CRF reduction in Alzheimer's disease. Neuropeptides 8:393–400

Nemeroff CB, Bissette G (1986) Neuropeptides in psychiatric disorders. In: Berger PA, Brodie HKH (eds) American handbook of psychiatry, 2nd edn. Basic Books, New York, p 64

Nemeroff CB, Luttinger D, Prange AJ (1980) Neurotensin-central nervous system effects of a neuropeptide. Trends Neurosci 3:212–215

Nemeroff CB, Bissette G, Busby WH, Youngblood WW, Rossor M, Roth M, Kizer JS (1983) Regional brain concentrations of neurotensin, thyrotropin-releasing hormone and somatostatin in Alzheimer's disease. Soc Neurosci Abstr 9:1052

Olschowka JA, O'Donohue TL, Mueller GP, Jacobowitz DM (1982) The distribution of corticotropin-releasing factor-like immunoreactive neurons in rat brain. Peptides 3:995–1015

Oram JJ, Edwardson J, Millard PH (1982) Investigation of cerebrospinal fluid neuropeptides in idiopathic senile dementia. Gerontology 27:216–223

Palmer AM, Wilcock GK, Esiri MM, Francis PT, Bowen DM (1987) Monoaminergic innervation of the frontal and temporal lobes in Alzheimer's disease. Brain Res 401:231–238

Perry EK, Blessed G, Tomlinson BE, Perry RH, Crow TJ, Cross AJ, Dockray GJ, Dimeline R, Arregui A (1981a) Neurochemical activity in human temporal lobe related to aging and Alzheimer-type changes. Neurobiol Aging 4:251–256

Perry RH, Dockray GJ, Dimeline R, Perry EK, Blessed G, Tomlinson BE (1981b) Neuropeptides in Alzheimer's disease and schizophrenia. J Neurol Sci 51:465–472

Poulain DA, Ellendorf F, Vincent JD (1980) Septal connections with identified oxytocin and vasopressin neurones in the supraoptic nucleus of the rat. An electrophysiological investigation. Neuroscience 5:379–387

Raskind MA, Peskind ER, Lampe TH, Risse SC, Taborsky GJ, Dorse D (1986) Cerebrospinal fluid vasopressin, oxytocin, somatostatin and β-endorphin in Alzheimer's disease. Arch Gen Psychiatry 43:382–388

Reinikanen KJ, Riekkinen PJ, Jolkkinen J, Kosma V-M, Soininen H (1987) Decreased somatostatin-like immunoreactivity in cerebral cortex and cerebrospinal fluid in Alzheimer's disease. Brain Res 402:103–108

Rossor MN, Emson PC, Mountjoy M, Roth M, Iversen LL (1980a) Reduced amounts of immunoreactive somatostatin in the temporal cortex in senile dementia of Alzheimer type. Neurosci Lett 20:373–377

Rossor MN, Iversen LL, Mountjoy CQ, Roth M, Hawthorne J, Ang YY, Jenkins JS (1980b) Arginine vasopressin and choline acetyltransferase in brains of patients with Alzheimer type senile dementia. Lancet 2:1367–1368

Rossor M, Fahrenkrug J, Emson P, Mountjoy C, Iversen L, Roth M (1980c) Reduced cortical choline acetyltransferase activity in senile dementia of Alzheimer type is not accompanied by changes in vasoactive intestinal polypeptide. Brain Res 201:249–253

Rossor MN, Iversen LL, Hawthorn J, Ang VTY, Jenkins JS (1981a) Extrahypothalamic vasopressin in human brain. Brain Res 214:349–355

Rossor MN, Rehfeld JF, Emson PC, Mountjoy CQ, Roth M, Iversen LL (1981b) Normal cortical concentration of cholecystokinin-like immunoreactivity with reduced choline acetyltransferase activity in senile dementia of Alzheimer type. Life Sci 29:405–410

Rossor MN, Emson PC, Mountjoy M, Roth M, Iversen LL (1982) Neurotransmitters of the cerebral cortex in senile dementia of Alzheimer type. Exp Brain Res (Suppl 5):153–157

Rossor MN, Emson PC, Iversen LL, Mountjoy CQ, Roth M (1984a) Patterns of neuropeptide deficits in Alzheimer's disease. In: Wurtman RJ, Corkin SH, Growden J (eds) Alzheimer's disease: advances in basic research and therapies. Proceedings of the Third Meeting of the International Study Group on the Treatment of Memory Disorders Associated with Aging. Zurich, pp 29–37

Rossor MN, Iversen LL, Reynolds GP, Mountjoy CQ, Roth M (1984b) Neurochemical characteristics of early and late onset types of Alzheimer's disease. Br Med J 288:961–964

Rossor MN, Emson PC, Dawbarn D, Mountjoy CQ, Roth M (1986) Neuropeptides and dementia. In: Emson PC, Rossor MN, Tohayama M (eds) Prog Brain Res 66:143

Serby M, Richardson SB, Twente, S, Siekierski J, Corwin J, Rotrosen J (1984) CSF somatostatin in Alzheimer's disease. Neurobiol Aging 5:187–189

Soininen HS, Jolkkonen JT, Reinikainen KH, Halonen TO, Riekkinen PJ (1984) Reduced cholinesterase activity and somatostatin-like immunoreactivity in the cerebrospinal fluid of patients with dementia of the Alzheimer's type. J Neurol Sci 63:167–172

Sorensen PS, Hammer M, Vorstrup S, Gjerros F (1983) CSF and plasma vasopressin concentrations in dementia. J Neurol Neurosurg Psychiatry 46:911–916

Swaab DF, Achterberg PW, Boer GJ, Dogterom J, van Leeman FW (1981) The distribution of MSH and ACTH in the rat and human brain and its relation to pituitary stores. In: Martinez JL, Jensen RA, Messing RB et al. (eds) Endogenous peptides and learning and memory processes. Academic, New York, p 7

Swanson LW, Sawchenko PE, Rivier J, Vale WW (1983) Organization of ovine corticotropin-releasing factor immunoreactive cells and fibers in the rat brain: an immunohistochemical study. Neuroendocrinology 36:166–186

Tamminga CA, Foster NL, Chase TN (1985) Reduced brain somatostatin levels in Alzheimer's disease. N Engl J Med 14:1294–1295

Tamminga CA, Foster NL, Fedio P, Bird ED, Chase TN (1987) Alzheimer's disease: low cerebral somatostatin levels correlate with impaired cognitive function and cortical metabolism. Neurology 37:161–165

Tomlinson BE, Irving D, Blessed G (1981) Cell loss in the locus coeruleus in senile dementia of Alzheimer type. J Neurol Sci 49:419–428

Ueki H, Namba M (1983) Decreased level of β-endorphin-like immunoreactivity in cerebrospinal fluid of patients with senile dementia of Alzheimer type. Life Sci 33:1039–1043

Vale WW, Rivier C, Brown MR, Spiess J, Koob G, Swanson L, Bilezikjian L, Bloom R, Rivier J (1983) Chemical and biological characterization of corticotropin-releasing factor. Recent Prog Horm Res 39:245–270

Vincent SR, Johansson O, Hokfelt T, Mayerson B, Sachs C, Elde RP, Terenius L, Kimmel J (1982) Neuropeptide coexistence in human cortical neurons. Nature 298:65–67

Vincent SR, Johansson O, Hokfelt T, Skirboll L, Elde RP, Terenius L, Kimmel J, Goldstein M (1983) NADPH-diaphorase: a selective histochemical marker for striatal neurons containing both somatostatin- and avian pancreatic polypeptide (APP)-like immunoreactivities. J Comp Neurol 217:252–263

Weingartner H, Gold P, Ballenger JC, Smallberg SA, Summers R, Rubinow DR, Post RM, Goodwin FK (1981) Effects of vasopressin on human memory functions. Science 211:601–603

Whitehouse PJ, Vale WW, Zweig RM, Singer HS, Mayeux R, Kuhar MJ, Price D, DeSouza EB (1987) Reductions in corticotropin-releasing factor-like immunoreactivity in cerebral cortex in Alzheimer's disease, Parkinson's disease, and progressive supranuclear palsy. Neurology 37(6):905–909

Wikkelso C, Fahrenkrug J, Blomstrand C, Johansson BB (1985) Dementia of different etiologies: vasoactive intestinal polypeptide in CSF. Neurology 35:592–595

Wood PL, Cheney DL, Costa E (1978) Modulation of the turnover rate of hippocampal acetylcholine by neuropeptides: possible site of action of α-melanocyte-stimulating hormone, adrenocorticotrophic hormone and somatostatin. J Pharmacol Exp Ther 209:97–103

Wood PL, Etienne P, Lal S, Gauthier S, Cajal S, Nair NPV (1982) Reduced lumbar CSF somatostatin levels in Alzheimer's disease. Life Sci 31:2073–2079

Yates CM, Simpson J, Gordon A, Maloney AFJ, Allison Y, Ritchie IM, Urquhart A (1983a) Catecholamines and cholinergic enzymes in pre-senile and senile Alzheimer-type dementia and Down's syndrome. Brain Res 280:119–126

Yates CM, Harmar AJ, Rosie R, Sheward J, Sanchez De Levy G, Simpson J, Maloney AFJ (1983b) Thyrotropin-releasing hormone, luteinizing-hormone-releasing hormone and substance P immunoreactivity in post-mortem brain from cases of Alzheimer-type dementia and Down's syndrome. Brain Res 258:45–52

Yates CM, Fink G, Bennie JG, Gordon A, Simpson J, Eskay RL (1985) Neurotensin immunoreactivity in post-mortem brain is increased in Down's syndrome but not in Alzheimer-type dementia. J Neurol Sci 67:327–335

Endocrine Response to Tricyclic Antidepressants and Peptides in Depression with Special Regard to Growth Hormone Secretion *

G. Laakmann [1], A. Hinz [1], U. Voderholzer [1], H. Neuhauser [1], C. Daffner [1], M. Winkelmann [1], and O. A. Müller [2]

Introduction

Within the last 20 years neuroendocrinological investigations have become increasingly relevant in the context of depression research. The secretion of growth hormone (GH), ACTH/cortisol, and thyroid-stimulating hormone (TSH) have been studied extensively. The present paper primarily refers to the stimulation of GH secretion following the administration of tricyclic antidepressants and releasing hormones in depressive patients.

Since Mueller et al. (1969) reported that psychotic depressed patients responded to insulin-related hypoglycemia with significantly lower GH secretion than nonpsychotic depressed patients and healthy subjects, GH stimulation has been studied in depressive patients using various stimulating agents. By means of testing with insulin-induced hypoglycemia, Sachar et al. (1971), Gruen et al. (1975), Garver et al. (1975), Casper et al. (1977), and Czernik et al. (1980) demonstrated that the GH stimulation was lower in the majority of endogenous depressive patients than in healthy subjects or nonendogenous depressive patients. These results, however, were not confirmed by Berger et al. (1982) or by Koslow et al. (1982).

GH stimulation in endogenous depressive patients was not found to be different from that of neurotic depressed patients in most studies using the L-dopa test (Mendels et al. 1974; Sachar et al. 1975; Gold et al. 1976; Mendlewicz 1979; Maany et al. 1979), the apomorphine test (Mendels et al. 1974; Casper et al. 1977; Maany et al. 1979), or the amphetamine test (Checkley and Crammer 1977; Checkley 1979).

Following the administration of the α_2-adrenergic agonist clonidine, endogenous depressive patients showed a significantly lower stimulation of GH secretion than neurotic depressed patients or healthy subjects, as reported first by Matussek et al. (1980). This result has been essentially confirmed by a great number of studies (Checkley et al. 1981; Charney et al. 1982; Siever et al. 1982; Glass et al. 1982; Ansseau et al. 1984; Moeller et al. 1984; Boyer et al.

* All studies were supported by the Deutsche Forschungsgemeinschaft, Schwerpunktprogramme Neuroendokrinologie und Neuropeptide (La 418/3,4-1, 4-3, 5-1, 5-2).

[1] Psychiatrische Klinik der Universität München, Nußbaumstr. 7, 8000 München 2, FRG.

[2] Medizinische Klinik Innenstadt, Universität München, Ziemssenstr. 1, 8000 München 2, FRG.

Neuropsychopharmacology
Edited by Bunney/Hippius/Laakmann/Schmauß

1985; Lechin et al. 1985; Uhde et al. 1986; Checkley and Corn 1986; Amsterdam et al. 1989). By contrast, Dolan and Calloway (1986) did not find a difference between the GH stimulation in endogenous depressive patients and that in healthy controls.

Because the acute administration of desipramine (DMI), an antidepressant which primarily inhibits the reuptake of norepinephrine (NE) and secondarily of serotonin (5-HT), was shown to stimulate GH secretion in healthy subjects (Laakmann et al. 1977), the effects of DMI and other tricyclic antidepressants on GH, prolactin, and cortisol secretion were investigated in healthy male and female subjects. GH stimulation occurred after p.o. and i.v. administration of DMI (Laakmann et al. 1977) and was shown to be reproducible (Laakmann 1980b), dose dependent (Laakmann et al. 1981, 1985), and age and sex dependent (Laakmann 1980a; Laakmann et al. 1978; Matussek and Laakmann 1981; Laakmann et al. 1986a).

First studies on a relatively small group of endogenous depressive patients demonstrated a significantly lower GH stimulation following DMI in these patients than in neurotic depressed patients and healthy subjects (Laakmann and Benkert 1978; Laakmann et al. 1978, Laakmann 1980a, 1980b, 1981, 1982). This result was confirmed in studies by Potter et al. (1981), Sawa et al. (1982), Calil et al. (1984), and Meesters et al. (1985). Asnis et al. (1986), however, found similar DMI-induced GH stimulation in endogenous depressive patients, diagnosed according to the Research Diagnostic Criteria (RDC), and healthy subjects. Similarly, Gilles and Mendlewicz (1986) did not report any difference in GH secretion between endogenous depressive patients, nonendogenous depressive patients, and healthy subjects. In this study, premenopausal endogenous and nonendogenous depressive women showed a comparable GH stimulation following DMI; this was significantly lower than that of healthy controls. There was also a trend toward a lower GH stimulation in the group of postmenopausal depressive women. Ryan et al. (1988) reported a significantly lower GH response to DMI in 20 adolescents with major depressive disorder, diagnosed according to RDC, than in 23 healthy adolescents. In 1989 Wilkins et al. tested 15 (9 females, 6 males) patients between the ages of 62 and 95 suffering from major depressive disorder, as defined by the Diagnostic and Statistical Manual (DSM-III), and also demonstrated a blunted DMI-induced GH stimulation. They did not, however, examine a control group corresponding in age and sex.

Based on these findings the question arises whether the stimulation of GH secretion could have any diagnostic value in psychiatric disorders. This examination strategy should at least be reviewed critically. Regarding the different studies on GH stimulation, it must be mentioned that the patients were diagnosed according to different diagnostic classifications such as the International Classification of Diseases (ICD9), RDC, or DSM-III, which can only be compared to a certain extent. Other factors such as the age and sex of patients and pharmacological pretreatments which influence the GH stimulation must also be considered. Premedication with adrenergic receptor blockers or agonists, for example, was shown to influence the GH stimulation

(Laakmann et al. 1983; Laakmann 1985; Laakmann et al. 1986b, 1986c, 1986d). The influence of antidepressants on the GH stimulation, which has been shown after long-term administration of DMI, also has to be considered. In this case, the GH stimulation is lower but not lacking (Laakmann and Benkert 1978).

We compared the GH stimulation in patients who had never been treated with psychotropic drugs with that in patients who had received antidepressants up to 3 days prior to the test. The GH stimulation was not significantly different in the two groups (Laakmann 1987). A pretreatment with neuroleptic drugs, which not only inhibit dopamine receptors but also bind to other central aminergic receptors to a various extent, could also influence the GH stimulation. In this context only a few systematically gathered results have been published (Sherman et al. 1971; Frantz et al. 1972; Beumont et al. 1974a, b; Laakmann and Benkert 1978; Koulu et al. 1980; Martin and Reichlin 1987). With regard to neuroleptic pretreatment, a sufficiently long wash-out phase prior to a stimulation test seems necessary.

Stimulation of GH Secretion Following Administration of Desipramine in Depressive Patients and Healthy Subjects

Continuing the examinations on the DMI-induced stimulation of GH secretion in endogenous depressive patients which we had started in 1978, an overall evaluation of all DMI tests, which had been performed in our hospital, was carried out (Laakmann 1987). Some of the data obtained are presented in the following. A total of 93 male and female patients, 48 of whom could be included in the analysis sample, were tested with DMI 75 mg i.m. All of them were suffering from a depressive disorder, which was diagnosed according to ICD as either mono- or bipolar endogenous depression (ICD 296.1/3) or neurotic depression (ICD 300.4). Forty-five patients had to be excluded because they were suffering from somatic diseases or other psychiatric disorders such as schizophrenia or addiction. Pretreatment with electroconvulsive therapy (ECT), gestation, or puerperium were also exclusion criteria. The wash-out period prior to each test was 3 days for benzodiazepines and antidepressants, 7 days for neuroleptics and 14 days for depot neuroleptics.

Since our investigations with healthy subjects had shown that the stimulation of GH secretion induced by DMI is dependent on age and sex, a group of healthy subjects were tested with DMI 75 mg i.m. in order to provide a comparison with the patients. The 48 depressive patients from the analysis sample were matched with 44 healthy subjects corresponding in age and sex and divided into different groups according to diagnosis (ICD) and sex.

The mean stimulation of GH secretion in endogenous depressive male patients (ICD 296.1/3; $n = 16$; mean age 42.1) was 7.0 ± 2.2 ng/ml 60 min after administration of DMI 75 mg i.m., the healthy subjects (mean age 41.1) showed a mean DMI-induced stimulation of GH secretion of 14.5 ± 2.0 ng/ml.

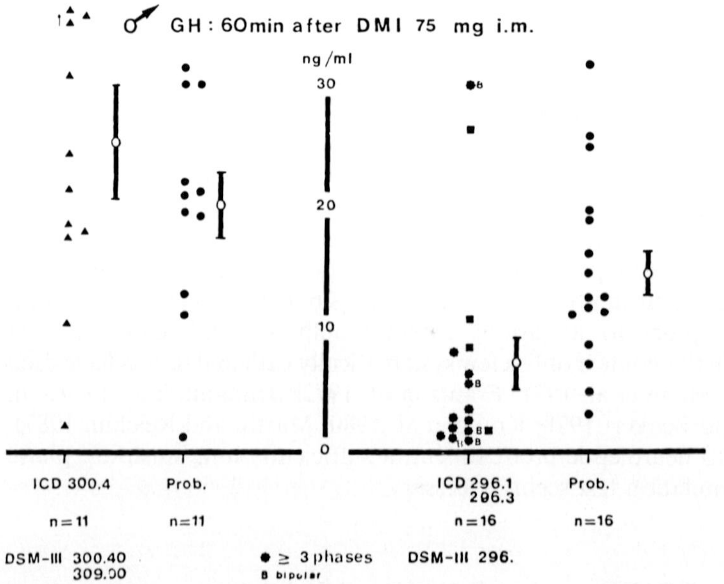

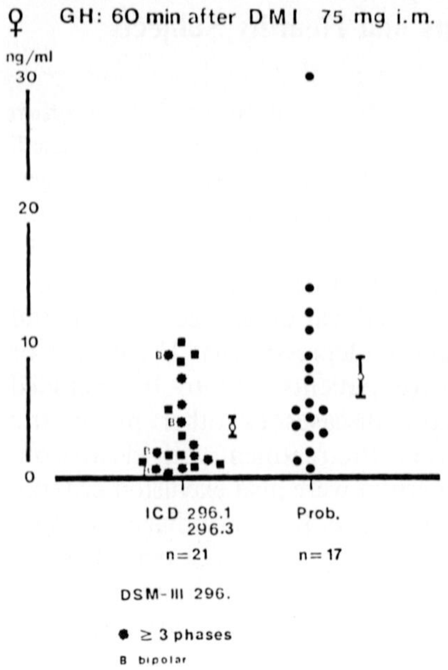

Fig. 1. GH (ng/ml) 60 min after administration of DMI 75 mg i.m. in neurotic depressive male patients (ICD 300.4; $n = 11$) and healthy male subjects ($n = 11$), in endogenous depressive male patients (ICD 296.1/3; $n = 16$) and healthy male subjects ($n = 16$), in endogenous depressive female patients (ICD 296.1/3; $n = 21$) and healthy female subjects ($n = 17$)

The comparison of the areas under the curve (AUC) using Student's t-test showed the GH stimulation to be significantly lower in endogenous depressive patients than in controls ($p < 0.05$; Fig. 1).

By contrast, the mean DMI-induced stimulation of GH secretion in neurotic depressed male patients (ICD 300.4; $n = 11$; mean age 27.6) was

25.2 ± 4.8 ng/ml, which was slightly but not significantly higher than the mean stimulation of GH secretion of 20.0 ± 2.7 ng/ml measured in healthy subjects ($n = 11$; mean age 27.4; Fig. 1).

In endogenous depressive female patients (ICD 296.1/3; $n = 21$; mean age 45.9) the mean stimulation of GH secretion was 3.6 ± 0.7 ng/ml 60 min after the administration of DMI, whereas in healthy female subjects ($n = 17$; mean age 40.2) the mean stimulation was 7.3 ± 1.7 ng/ml and thus significantly higher ($p < 0.05$; Fig. 1).

These investigations demonstrate that the DMI-induced stimulation of GH secretion in both male and female endogenous depressive patients (ICD 296.1/3) is significantly lower than that of age and sex matched healthy subjects. By contrast, neurotic depressed patients (ICD 300.4) do not significantly differ from a corresponding group of healthy subjects.

This result agrees with the previous studies mentioned above in which insulin-related hypoglycemia and clonidine were used and which also demonstrated that some endogenous depressive patients show a blunted response to GH stimulation. The question arises which underlying pathomechanism is-responsible for this disturbed GH stimulation. Studies with DMI in combination with various receptor blockers and antagonists in healthy subjects demonstrated that the stimulatory effect on GH secretion which the tricyclic antidepressant DMI induces can be explained by the drug's inhibiting effect on the reuptake of NE, i.e., by a central noradrenergic stimulation which is transmitted by α_2-adrenergic receptors and inhibited by β-adrenergic receptors (Laakmann et al. 1986b). This suggests that the disturbed GH secretion in endogenous depressive patients could be caused by a diminished responsiveness of central α_2-adrenergic receptors. Matussek et al. (1980), who found a blunted GH response to the α_2-adrenergic agonist clonidine in endogenous depression, explained their results in a similar way. These interpretations, however, were based on the hypothesis that there is no disturbance at the pituitary level such as a diminished GH production or a secretion of somatotrophs in endogenous depressive patients. In this case an undisturbed GH response to growth hormone releasing hormone (GHRH) must be expected.

Growth Hormone Stimulation Following the Administration of Desipramine and Growth Hormone Releasing Hormone in Endogenous Depressive Patients and Healthy Subjects

After GHRH became available for clinical trials (Guillemain et al. 1982; Rivier et al. 1982), it was possible to test the hypothesis that there is no disturbance at the pituitary level in endogenous depressive patients. First we compared the GH secretion following the administration of GHRH 100 µg i.v. with that following DMI 75 mg i.m. in ten healthy male subjects (mean age 25.9).

Following the administration of GHRH or DMI, the healthy male subjects showed a distinct GH stimulation with comparable mean maximal values of

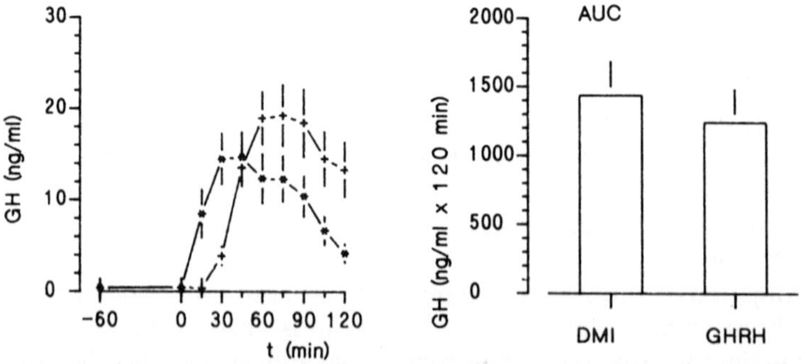

Fig. 2. GH mean value graphs ($\bar{x} \pm$ SE; ng/ml) and AUCs ($\bar{x} \pm$ SE; ng/ml × 120 min) after administration of DMI 75 mg i.m. (*plus sign*) and GHRH 100 µg i.v. (*asterisk*) in healthy male subjects ($n = 10$)

14.7 ± 2.5 ng/ml at $t = 45$ min after GHRH and 19.2 ± 3.1 ng/ml at $t = 75$ min after DMI (Hinz et al. 1988; Fig. 2).

In first tests on four endogenous depressive patients, the GH stimulation following DMI and GHRH was comparable, too. However, it was markedly lower in the patients than in the healthy subjects (Laakmann et al. 1986e).

Further examinations of nine endogenous depressive patients (mean age 37.9) confirmed these preliminary results. The mean maximum values of GH secretion in endogenous depressive patients were 8.1 ± 2.5 ng/ml after DMI and 7.1 ± 1.4 ng/ml after GHRH (Fig. 3). A group of age matched healthy subjects showed a mean maximum stimulation of GH secretion of 18.0 ± 3.0 ng/ml following DMI. The difference between the endogenous depressive patients and the healthy subjects was statistically significant ($p < 0.01$; Neuhauser und Laakmann 1988).

These results demonstrate that the antidepressant DMI, which acts on the central nervous system, and GHRH, which directly affects pituitary cells, have

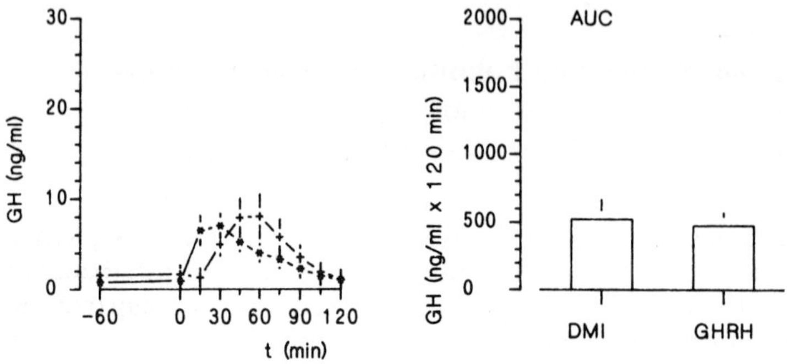

Fig. 3. GH mean value graphs ($\bar{x} \pm$ SE; ng/ml) and AUCs ($\bar{x} \pm$ SE; ng/ml × 120 min) after administration of DMI 75 mg i.m. (*plus sign*) and GHRH 100 µg i.v. (*asterisk*) in endogenous depressive male patients (ICD 296.1/3; $n = 9$)

a similar stimulatory capacity. Therefore, a disturbance at the pituitary level has to be considered as an explanation for the diminished GH stimulation in endogenous depressive patients. This could be caused by a diminished responsiveness of the pituitary cells to GHRH or by a lower production of GH.

The diminished GH stimulation following GHRH in endogenous depression was also found by Lesch et al. (1987, 1988a, b), Risch et al. (1986), Chiarini et al. (1987), and Müller et al. (1989). Lesch et al. (1988a) compared the GH stimulation following GHRH with that after clonidine in endogenous depressive patients. They found that in both tests the GH stimulation was comparable in the patients, but significantly lower than in healthy subjects. The patients also showed significantly increased somatomedin C concentrations.

GH, Cortisol, and TSH Stimulation Following Simultaneous Administration of Growth Hormone Releasing Hormone (GHRH), Corticotropin Releasing Hormone (CRH), Gonadotropin Releasing Hormone (GnRH), and Thyrotropin Releasing Hormone (TRH) in Healthy Subjects and Psychiatric Patients

To further clarify the cause of disturbed GH stimulation in endogenous depressive patients, we performed a combined pituitary stimulation test using the simultaneous administration of GHRH, CRH, GnRH, and TRH in order to investigate different hypothalamus-pituitary-axes to get information on whether abnormalities in GH secretion are associated with disturbances of other hormones.

A comparison of the combined i.v. administration of four releasing hormones (GHRH 100 μg, CRH 100 μg, GnRH 100 μg, and TRH 200 μg) with the individual administration of each of these releasing hormones in six healthy male subjects (mean age 26.8) shows a comparable GH stimulation. The mean maximal values were 28.1 ± 3.2 μg/ml after GHRH alone and 29.2 ± 5.8 μg/ml after the combined administration of GHRH, CRH, GnRH, and TRH. Similar findings were obtained by Sheldon et al. (1985), Schopohl et al. (1986), and Holl et al. (1988), who also found a comparable GH stimulation following the combined administration of GHRH, CRH, GnRH, and TRH, whereas Cohen et al. (1986) reported a slightly but significantly higher GH response to GHRH alone compared with the combined administration.

ACTH and cortisol stimulation were shown to be comparable when using the combination of four releasing hormones or CRH alone as stimuli, whereas a tendency toward higher TSH stimulation was observed following combined administration than after TRH alone (see "The Simultaneous Use of Four Releasing Factors" in this volume).

Since the stimulation of GH secretion was shown to be comparable in healthy subjects using either the combined or single releasing hormone test, we used the combined test to study the pituitary hormone secretion of depressive patients. In these investigations, special interest focused on whether GH and cortisol abnormalities are connected.

Fifteen endogenous depressive female patients (ICD 296.1/3) were investigated using the simultaneous i.v. administration of GHRH 100 μg, CRH 100 μg, GnRH 100 μg, and TRH 200 μg. Eight of them had to be excluded because of increased basal GH values > 5.0 ng/ml at $t = -60$ and $t = 0$ min. The remaining seven patients (mean age 42.4 years) had a mean maximum stimulation of GH secretion of 12.3 ± 4.0 ng/ml, which was significantly lower than that of seven healthy female subjects (mean age 40.4 years) whose mean GH peak was 26.8 ± 6.1 ng/ml (Fig. 4). The mean maximum stimulation of cortisol secretion following GHRH, CRH, GnRH, and TRH was 18.4 ± 1.3 μg/100 ml in the endogenous depressive female patients compared with 22.0 ± 1.2 μg/100 ml in age-matched healthy female subjects. This difference was not statistically significant (Fig. 4). The TSH stimulation following the combined administration of releasing hormones showed a mean peak of 12.6 ± 3.1 μU/ml in endogenous depressive female patients which was lower than the mean maximum TSH increase of 19.4 ± 4.5 μU/ml in healthy female subjects. The statistical evaluation, however, did not show a significant difference (Fig. 4).

We are not presently aware of other studies which have tested depressive patients using the combined releasing hormone test. However, since, as described above, the combined administration of the releasing hormones and the administration of GHRH alone have a comparable effect on GH stimulation it seems possible to compare our results of the combined test with those of other authors who investigated the GH response to GHRH alone in depressive patients.

In our studies, the GH response to the administration of releasing hormones in endogenous depressive patients agrees with similar results of the GHRH test in endogenous depressive patients (Laakmann et al. 1986a; Risch et al. 1986; Lesch et al. 1987; Chiarini et al. 1987; Neuhauser and Laakmann 1988; Lesch et al. 1988a, b, 1989; Müller et al. 1989).

In our investigations using the simultaneous administration of four releasing hormones, the stimulation of cortisol secretion in endogenous depressive female patients was not significantly different from that in age matched healthy female subjects. Holsboer et al. (1986) and Amsterdam et al. (1989), who used CRH alone as a stimulus, also reported a comparable stimulation of cortisol secretion in endogenous depressive patients and healthy subjects.

Regarding the stimulation of TSH secretion, there was a trend toward lower values in endogenous depressive women than in age matched female controls in our investigations. This difference was, however, not significant. Prange et al. (1972), Loosen and Prange (1982), and Loosen et al. (1987) reported a blunted TSH response after the administration of TRH in the majority of endogenous depressive patients compared with the response in healthy subjects. Lesch et al. (1989) investigated 15 endogenous depressive patients using GHRH, CRH, and TRH on consecutive days. They also found

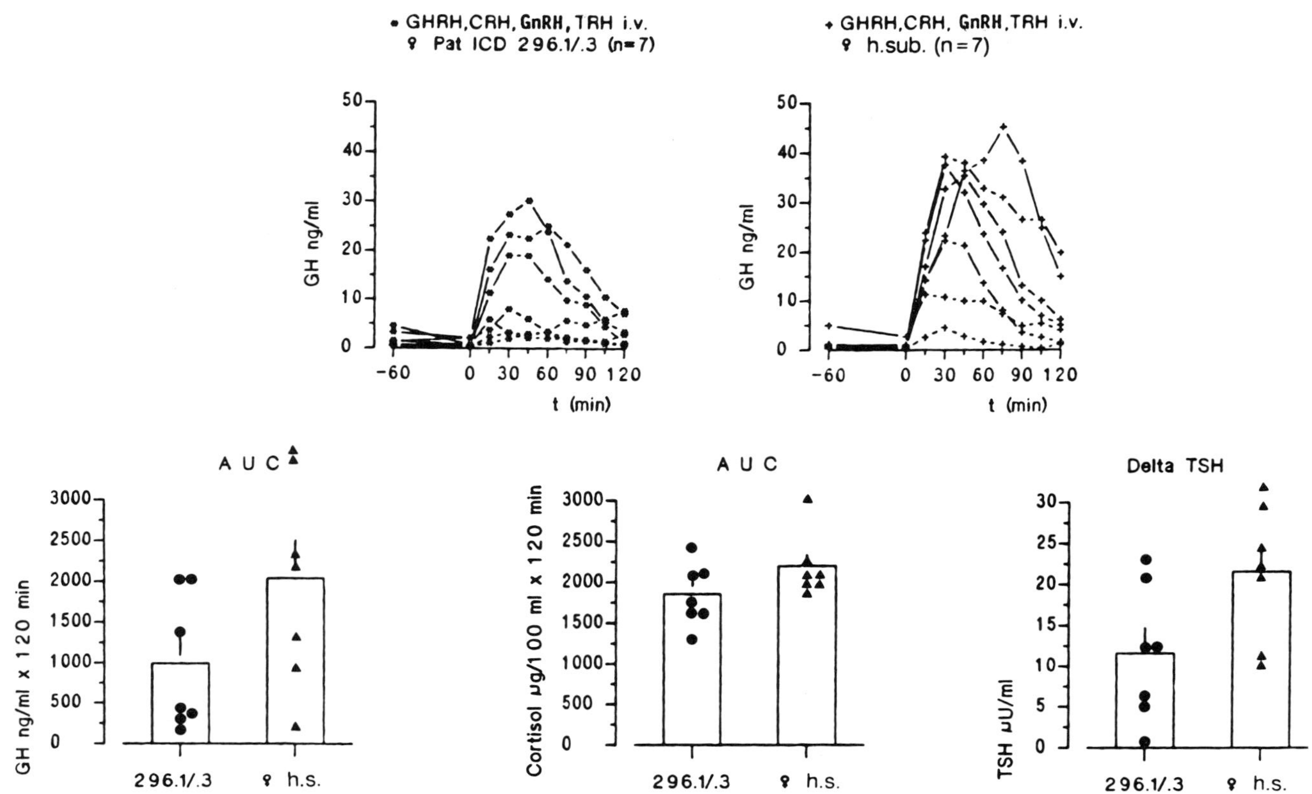

Fig. 4. GH graphs: (ng/ml) and AUC (ng/ml × 120 min), cortisol AUC (µg/100 ml × 120 min) and Delta TSH (µU/ml 0–30 min) after combined i.v. administration of GHRH 100 µg, CRH 100 µg, GnRH 100 µg, and TRH 200 µg in endogenous depressive female patients (ICD 296.1/3; $n = 7$) and healthy female subjects ($n = 7$)

the TSH response to TRH in the endogenous depressive patients to be lower than in healthy subjects.

The significantly diminished GH stimulation in endogenous depressive female patients in our studies using the simultaneous administration of GHRH, CRH, GnRH, and TRH was not associated with a disturbed cortisol secretion. This indicates that the lower GH stimulation was not caused by a modified cortisol secretion. The question whether there was a disturbance of the hypothalamus-pituitary-adrenal axis in our patients, can be answered only after the assessment of the ACTH values.

Concluding Remarks

There is at present no commonly accepted explanation for the diminished GH stimulation in endogenous depressive patients. There are, however, various possible ways to interpret this finding which are discussed in the following:

1. There is a tonic inhibition of the GH stimulation caused by a hyperactivity of central β-adrenergic receptors in endogenous depressive patients.
2. Endogenous depressive patients have a dysfunction of their pituitary somatotrophs.
3. Endogenous depressive patients have a pathological increase of the somatomedin C concentration which exerts negative feedback effects on the stimulation of GH secretion.

The interpretation described in the first point is based on pharmacological investigations by Sulser (1981) who found desensitization of β-adrenergic receptors following treatment with antidepressants. This led to the conclusion that endogenous depressive patients could have a hyperactivity of central β-adrenergic receptors resulting in a tonic inhibition of GH secretion. Imura et al. (1974) reported that pretreatment with the β-adrenergic blocker propranolol increased the GH response to insulin-related hypoglycemia in healthy subjects. Our investigations using the antidepressant DMI as GH-stimulating agent also demonstrated, that stimulated GH secretion increased after additional administration of the β-blocker propranolol, whereas the β-adrenergic agonist clenbuterol and the α_2-adrenergic antagonist yohimbine inhibited DMI-induced GH stimulation (Laakmann et al. 1986b; Laakmann 1987). It therefore seems possible that a hyperactivity of central β-adrenergic receptors in endogenous depression is responsible for the patients' diminished response to GH stimulation.

The interpretation in point two indicates that a disturbance at the pituitary level, such as a diminished GH production or a diminished responsiveness of the somatotrophs, could explain the diminished response to stimulated GH secretion in endogenous depressive patients in all tests. This explanation is mainly supported by the studies using GHRH or a combination of four releasing hormones as stimuli.

With regard to point three, increased concentrations of somatomedin C in endogenous depressive patients were reported by Lesch et al. (1988 b). Our own preliminary studies of somatomedin C concentrations in endogenous depressive patients confirmed these results (unpublished data). Somatomedin C is peripherally produced in positive dependency on GH concentration and exerts negative feedback effects on the pituitary GH secretion. An increased concentration of somatomedin C in endogenous depression would indicate a disturbed feedback regulation of pituitary GH release. This interpretation is also supported by the results of Mendlewicz et al. (1985), who reported a diurnal hypersecretion of GH in endogenous depressive patients. It remains, however, unclear why in this case the hypersecretion of GH is not inhibited by the increased somatomedin C concentrations.

It is not only of interest to ascertain what the underlying pathomechanism is, but also to investigate whether the diminished GH stimulation in endogenous depression could serve as a predictor of therapeutic response to antidepressant treatment.

References

Amsterdam JD, Maislin G, Skolnik B, Berwisch N, Winokur A (1989) Multiple hormone responses to clonidine administration in depressed patients and healthy volunteers. Biol Psychiatry 26:265–278

Ansseau M, Scheyvaerts M, Doumont A, Poirrier R, Legros JJ, Franck G (1984) Concurrent use of REM latency, dexamethasone suppression, clonidine, and apomorphine tests as biological markers of endogenous depression: a pilot study. Psychiatry Res 12:261–272

Asnis GM, Halbreich U, Rabinovich H, Puig-Antich J, Ryan ND (1986) The human growth hormone response to 75 mg i.m. desipramine in endogenous and normal controls. In: Shagass C et al. (eds) Biological psychiatry 1985: Proceedings of the VIth world congress of biological psychiatry. Elsevier, New York, pp 782–784

Berger M, Dörr P, Lund R, Bronisch T, von Zerssen D (1982) Neuroendocrinological and neurophysiological studies in major depressive disorders: are there biological markers for the endogenous subtype? Biol Psychiatry 17:1217–1242

Beumont P, Gelder M, Friesen H, Harris G, MacKinnon P, Mandelbrote B, Wiles D (1974 a) The effect of phenothiazines on endocrine function: I Patients with inappropriate lactation and amenorrhea. Br J Psychiatry 124:413–419

Beumont P, Corker C, Friesen H, Kolakowska T, Mandelbrote B, Marshall J, Murray M, Wiles D (1974 b) The effect of phenothiazines on endocrine function: II Effects in men and post-menopausal women. Br J Psychiatry 124:420–430

Boyer P, Davila M, Schaub C, Nassiet J (1985) Growth hormone response to clonidine stimulation in depressive states. Part I. Psychiatry and Psychobiol 1:189–195

Calil HM, Lesieur P, Gold PW, Brown GM, Zavadil AP III, Potter WZ (1984) Hormonal responses to zimelidine and desipramine in depressed patients. Psychiatry Res 13:231–242

Casper RC, Davis JM, Pandey GN, Garver DL, Dekirmenjian H (1977) Neuroendocrine and amine studies in affective illness. Psychoneuroendocrinology 2:105–113

Charney DS, Heninger GR, Sternberg DE (1982) Failure of chronic antidepressant treatment to alter growth hormone response to clonidine. Psychiatry Res 7:135–138

Checkley SA (1979) Corticosteroid and growth hormone responses to methylamphetamine in depressive illness. Psychol Med 9:107–115

Checkley SA, Crammer J (1977) Hormone responses to methylamphetamine in depression: A new approach to the noradrenaline depletion hypothesis. Br J Psychiatry 131:582–586

Checkley SA, Corn TH (1986) Factors responsible for reduced growth hormone (GH) responses to clonidine in patients with endogenous depression. In: Shagass C et al. (eds) Biological Psychiatry 1985: Proceedings of the VIth world congress of biological psychiatry. Elsevier, New York, pp 799–801

Checkley SA, Slade AP, Shur E (1981) Growth hormone and other responses to clonidine in patients with endogenous depression. Br J Psychiatry 138:51–55

Chiarini V, Graziano E, Cremonini N, Sforza A, Pezzoli A, Zampa G (1987) HGH response to hp-GHRH 1–44 in depression. J Endocrinol Invest 10 (Suppl 3):56

Cohen R, Bouquier D, Biot-Laporte S, Vermeulen E, Claustrat B, Cherpin MH, Cabrera P, Guidetti P, Ferry S, Bizollon CA, Sassolas G (1986) Pituitary stimulation by combined administration of four hypothalamic releasing hormones in normal men and patients. J Clin Endocrinol Metab 62:892–898

Czernik A, Kleesiek K, Steinmeyer EM (1980) Änderungen neuroendokrinologischer Parameter im Verlauf von Depressionen. Nervenarzt 51:662–667

Dolan RJ, Calloway SP (1986) The human growth hormone response to clonidine: relationship to clinical and neuroendocrine profile in depression. Am J Psychiatry 143:772–774

Frantz AG, Kleinberg DL, Noel GL, Suh K (1972) Effects of neuroleptics on the secretion of prolactin and growth hormone. In: Ebling ETG, Henderson TW (eds) Endocrinology. Elsevier, New York, pp 144–149

Garver DL, Pandey GN, Dekirmenjian H, DeLeon-Jones F (1975) Growth hormone and catecholamines in affective disease. Am J Psychiatry 132:1149–1153

Gilles C, Mendlewicz J (1986) Growth hormone stimulation tests in affective disorders and senile dementia of the Alzheimer's type. In: Shagass C et al. (eds) Biological psychiatry 1985: Proceedings of the VIth world congress of biological psychiatry. Elsevier, New York, pp 773–775

Glass IB, Checkley SA, Shur E, Dawling S (1982) The effect of desipramine upon central adrenergic function in depressed patients. Br J Psychiatry 141:372–376

Gold PW, Goodwin FK, Wehr T, Rebar R, Sack R (1976) Growth hormone and prolactin response to levodopa in affective illness. Lancet II:1308–1309

Gruen PH, Sachar EJ, Altman N, Sassin J (1975) Growth hormone responses to hypoglycemia in postmenopausal depressed women. Arch Gen Psychiatry 32:31–33

Guillemain R, Brazeau P, Böhlen P, Esch F, Ling N, Wehrenberg W (1982) Growth hormone-releasing factor from a human pancreatic tumor that caused acromegaly. Science 218:585–587

Hinz A, Laakmann G, Kropp G, Dick F (1988) Influence of growth hormone (GHRH) on the growth hormone (GH) secretion in healthy female and male subjects. Pharmacopsychiatry 21:445–446

Holl RW, Loos IJ, Hetzel WD, Heinze E, Fehm HL (1988) Combined pituitary stimulation test: interactions of hypothalamic releasing hormones on man. J Endocrinol Invest 111:219–223

Holsboer F (1986) Corticotropin-releasing hormone – a new tool to investigate hypothalamic-pituitary-adrenocortical physiology in psychiatric patients. Psychopharmacol Bull 22:907–912

Imura H, Nakai Y, Kato Y, Yoshimoto Y, Moridera K (1974) Propranolol-insulin stimulation test in the diagnosis of growth hormone deficiency. Horm Metab Res 6:343–346

Koslow S, Stokes P, Mendels J, Ramsey A, Casper R (1982) Insulin tolerance test: human growth hormone response and insulin resistance in primary unipolar depressed, bipolar Depressed and control Subjects. Psychol Med 12:45–55

Koulu M, Lammintausta R, Dahlström S (1980) Effects of some γ-aminobutyric acid (GABA)-ergic drugs on the dopaminergic control of human growth hormone secretion. J Clin Endocrinol Metab 51:124–129

Laakmann G (1980a) Beeinflussung der Hypophysenvorderlappen-Hormonsekretion durch Antidepressiva bei gesunden Probanden, neurotisch und endogen depressiven Patienten. Nervenarzt 51:725–732

Laakmann G (1980b) Neuroendocrinological findings in affective disorders after administration of antidepressants. Adv Biol Psychiatry 5:67–84

Laakmann G (1981) Diagnostic application of provocative stimuli for growth hormone release, with particular reference to the desimipramine test. In: Perris C, Struwe G, Jansson B (eds) Biological psychiatry 1981: Proceedings of the IIIrd world congress of biological psychiatry, Stockholm. Elsevier, Amsterdam, pp 321–324

Laakmann G (1982) Depression und Wachstumshormonstimulation. In: Beckmann H, Biologische Psychiatrie. Fortschritte psychiatrischer Forschung, Thieme, Stuttgart, pp 155–161

Laakmann G (1985) Pharmacoendocrinology and its clinical relevance. In: Pichot P, Berner P, Wolf R, Thau K (eds) Psychiatry – the state of the art, 2nd proceedings of the VIIth world congress of psychiatry, Wien, 1983. Plenum, New York, pp 257–262

Laakmann G (1987) Psychopharmakoendokrinologie und Depressionsforschung. Springer, Berlin Heidelberg New York Tokyo (Monographien aus dem Gesamtgebiete der Psychiatrie, Bd. 46.)

Laakmann G, Benkert O (1978) Effects of antidepressants on pituitary hormones. In: Garattine S (ed) Depressive disorders. Schattauer, Stuttgart New York, pp 255–266

Laakmann G, Schumacher G, Benkert O, von Werder K (1977) Stimulation of growth hormone secretion by desimipramin and chlorimipramin in man. J Clin Endocrinol Metab 44:1010–1013

Laakmann G, Benkert O, Neulinger E, von Werder K, Erhardt F (1978) Beeinflussung der Hypophysen-Vorderlappen-Hormon-Sekretion nach akuter und chronischer Gabe von Desipramin. Arzneimittelforschung/Drug Res. 28:1292–1294

Laakmann G, Schön HW, Wittmann M (1981) Desipramine and growth hormone secretion. Lancet II:996

Laakmann G, Schön HW, Wittman M, Zygan C (1983) Effect of receptor blockers on the desimipramine-induced stimulation of growth hormone and prolactin in man. In: Endröczi E et al. (eds) Integrative neurohumoral mechanisms. Elsevier, Amsterdam, pp 479–486

Laakmann G, Schön H, Blaschke D, Wittmann M (1985) Dosedependent growth hormone, prolactin and cortisol stimulation after i.v. administration of desimipramine in human subjects. Psychoneuroendocrinology 10:83–93

Laakmann G, Hinz A, Neulinger E, Strauß A, Wittmann M (1986a) DMI-induced growth hormone stimulation in healthy subjects and depressed patients. Pharmacopsychiatry 19:264–265

Laakmann G, Zygan K, Schön HW, Weiss A, Wittmann M, Meissner R, Blaschke D (1986b) Effect of receptor blockers (methysergide, propranolol, phentolamine, yohimbine and prazosin) on desimipramine-induced pituitary hormone stimulation in humans. I: Growth Hormone. Psychoneuroendocrinology 11:447–461

Laakmann G, Schön HW, Zygan K, Weiss A, Wittman M, Meissner R (1986c) Effects of receptor blockers (methysergide, propranolol, phentolamine, yohimbine and prazosin) on desimipramine-induced pituitary hormone stimulation in humans. II: Prolactin. Psychoneuroendocrinology 11:465–474

Laakmann G, Wittmann M, Schön HW, Zygan K, Weiss A, Meissner R, Müller OA, Stalla GK (1986d) Effects of receptor blockers (methysergide, propranolol, phentolamine, yohimbine and prazosin) on Desimipramine-induced pituitary hormone stimulation in humans. III: Hypothalamo-Pituitary-Adrenocortical Axis. Psychoneuroendocrinology 11:475–489

Laakmann G, Neuhauser H, Hinz A, Neulinger E, Wittman M (1986e) Stimulation of growth hormone, prolactin and cortisol by GHRH and DMI in depressed patients. Pharmacopsychiatry 19, 4:235–236

Lechin F, Van Der Dijs B, Jakubowicz D, Camero R, Villa S, Arocha L, Lechin A (1985) Effects of clonidine on blood pressure, noradrenaline, cortisol, growth hormone, and prolactin plasma levels in high and low intestinal tone. Neuroendocrinology 41:156–162

Lesch K, Laux G, Pfüller H, Erb A, Beckmann H (1987) Growth hormone (GH) response to GH-releasing hormone in depression. J Clin Endocrinol Metab 65:1278–1281

Lesch K, Laux G, Erb A, Pfüller H, Beckmann H (1988a) Growth hormone (GH) and prolactin responses to GH-releasing hormone in depression: correlation with GH release following clonidine. Psychiatry Res 25:301–310

Lesch K, Laux G, Erb A, Pfüller H, Beckmann H (1988b) Growth homone (GH) and prolactin responses after GH-releasing hormone in major depressive disorder: relationship to somatomedin C levels and dexamethasone suppressibility of cortisol. Psychoneuroendocrinology 13:255–263

Lesch K, Rupprecht R, Müller U, Pfüller H (1989) Comparison of GH responses after human GHRH-44 amide administration and TRH-induced TSH release in depressed patients. Biol Psychiatry 25:235–238

Loosen PT, Prange AJ, jr. (1982) Serum thyrotropin response to thyrotropin-releasing hormone in psychiatric patients: a review. Am J Psychiatry 4:405–416

Loosen PT, Garbutt JC, Prange AJ (1987) Evaluation of the diagnostic utility of the TRH-induced TSH response in psychiatric disorders. Pharmacopsychiatry 20:90–95

Maany I, Mendels J, Frazer A, Brunswick D (1979) A study of growth hormone release in depression. Neuropsychobiology 5:282–289

Martin JB, Reichlin S (1987) Clinical neuroendocrinology, 2nd edn. F. A. Davis Company, Philadelphia

Matussek N, Laakmann G (1981) Growth hormone response in patients with depression. In: Carlsson A et al. (eds) Recent Advances in the Treatment of Depression. Acta Psychiatr Scand 63 (Suppl 290):122–126

Matussek N, Ackenheil M, Hippius H, Müller F, Schröder HT, Schultes H, Wasilewski B (1980) Effect of clonidine on growth hormone release in psychiatric patients and controls. Psychiatry Res 2:25–36

Meesters P, Kerkhofs M, Charles G, Decoster C, Vanderelst M, Mendlewicz J (1985) Growth hormone release after desimipramine in depressive illness. Eur Arch Psychiatry Neurol Sci 235:140–142

Mendels J, Frazer A, Carroll BJ (1974) Growth hormone response in depression. Am J psychiatry 131:1154–1155

Mendlewicz J, Linkowski P, Van Cauter E (1979) Some neuroendocrine parameters in bipolar and unipolar depression. J Affective Disord 1:25–32

Mendlewicz J, Linkowski P, Kerkhofs M, Desmedt D, Golstein J, Copinschi G, Van Cauter E (1985) Diurnal hypersecretion of growth hormone in depression. J Clin Endocrinol Metab 60:505–512

Moeller HJ, Kissling W, Bottermann P (1984) Serial application of clonidine tests during antidepressiva treatment with clomipramine. Pharmacopsychiatry 17:184–187

Mueller PS, Heninger GR, McDonald RK (1969) Insulin tolerance test in depression. Arch Gen Psychiatry 21:587–594

Müller U, Lesch K, Rupprecht R, Kruse K, Schulte H (1989) Neuroendocrine dysfunction in depression: comparison of hormonal responses to GHRH, TRH and CRH. Acta Endocrinol (Copenh) 120, Suppl 1:220–221

Neuhauser H, Laakmann G (1988) Stimulation of growth hormone by GHRH as compared to DMI in depressed patients. Pharmacopsychiatry 21:443–444

Potter WZ, Calil HM, Extein I, Gold PW, Wehr TA, Goodwin FK (1981) Specific norepinephrine and serotonin uptake inhibitors in man: A crossover study with pharmacokinetic, biochemical, neuroendocrine and behavioral parameters. Acta Psychiatr Scand 63, Suppl 290:152–165

Prange AJ jr., Wilson IC, Lara PP, Alltop LB, Breese GR (1972) Effects of thyrotropin-releasing hormone in depression. Lancet II:999–1002

Risch S, Janowsky D, Judd L, Gillin J, Ehlers C (1986) Attenuated growth hormone response to human growth hormone releasing factor in depressed subjects vs. matched controls. In: 5th Collegium Internationale Neuro-Psychopharmacologicum Congress 14–17 December 1986, San Juan, Puerto Rico, p 197

Rivier J, Spiess J, Thorner M, Vale W (1982) Characterization of a growth hormone-releasing factor from a human pancreatic islet tumor. Nature 300:276

Ryan N, Puig-Antich J, Rabinovich H, Ambrosini P, Robinson D, Nelson B, Novacenko H (1988) Growth hormone response to desmethyliminpramine in depressed and suicidal adolescents. J Affective Disord 15:323–337

Sachar EJ, Finkelstein J, Hellman L (1971) Growth hormone responses in depressive illness. I. Response to insulin tolerance test. Arch Gen Psychiatry 25:263–269

Sachar EJ, Altman N, Gruen PH, Glassman A, Halpern FS, Sassin J (1975) Human growth hormone response to levodopa: Relation to menopause, depression and plasma dopa concentration. Arch Gen Psychiatry 32:502–503

Sawa Y, Odo SV, Nakazawa T (1982) Growth hormone secretion by tricyclic antidepressants in healthy volunteers and depressives. In: Langer SZ, Takahashi R, Segawa T, Briley M (eds) New vistas in depression. Pergamon, Oxford (Adv Biosci, vol 40) pp 309–315

Sheldon WR, deBold RC, Evans WS, DeCherney GS, Jackson RV, Island DP, Thorner MO, Orth DN (1985) Rapid sequential intraveneous administration of four hypothalamic releasing hormones as a combined anterior pituitary function test in normal subjects. J Clin Endocrinol Metab 60:623–630

Sherman L, Kim S, Benjamin F, Kolodny HCD (1971) Effects of chlorpromazine on serum growth hormone concentrations in man. New Engl J Med 284:72–74

Schopohl J, Losa M, König A, Müller OA, Stalla GK, von Werder K (1986) Combined pituitary function-test with four hypothalamic releasing hormones. Klin Wochenschr 64:314–318

Siever LJ, Uhde TW, Silberman EK, Jimerson DC, Aloi JA, Post RM, Murphy DL (1982) Growth hormone response to clonidine as a probe of noradrenergic receptor responsiveness in affective disorder patients and controls. Psychiatry Res 6:171–183

Sulser F (1981) New perspectives on the action of antidepressant drugs: regulation of central adrenergic function. Adv Biol Psychiatry 7:90–99

Uhde T, Roy-Byrne P, Post R (1986) Panic disorder and major depressive disorder: biological relationship. In: Shagass C et al. (eds) Biological psychiatry 1985: Proceedings of the VIth world congress of biological psychiatry. Elsevier, New York, pp 472–474

Wilkins JN, Spar JE, Carlson HE (1989) Desipramine increases circulating growth hormone in elderly depressed patients: a pilot study. Psychoneuroendocrinology 14, 3:195–202

14 Postmarketing Surveillance of Psychotropic Drugs

Relative Toxicity of Antidepressants Using Reports Independent of Observer Bias

S. A. Montgomery, D. Baldwin, and N. Fineberg [1]

The spontaneous confidential reporting of adverse drug reactions (ADRs) used in several countries has the advantage of being cheap and effective in drawing attention to unusual and unexpected reactions with new drugs. No system is perfect, and open reporting systems have their limitations. It is recognised that one of their important problems is the likelihood that for a number of reasons serious ADRs may be underreported.

The self-reporting system is concerned with measuring a pattern of ADRs seen with a particular drug. Many of these associations would be random and not necessarily caused by the drug. It is only when the pattern begins to appear consistently that a direct association with the drug becomes likely. There have been attempts by legal groups to take the individual reports of associations seen by clinicians to be an admission that the drug has caused an ADR. Such attempts at breaking the confidentiality of a reporting system may well result in clinicians becoming more wary of reporting possible associations.

Another problem with open reporting systems is that they appear to minimise the incidence of those ADRs which we have become accustomed to seeing, particularly with older drugs. The familiarity of the older drugs may lull clinicians into a false sense of security. Certain ADRs are well-known with older drugs, and clinicians may feel that it is no longer necessary to report them. A similar bias applies to published reports, in which editors are interested in publishing new findings with new drugs but not in repeating findings with old drugs. As a result estimates of the incidence of ADRs with older drugs which are based on data derived from spontaneous reporting systems are not reliable.

Most clinicians are alert to and have a high index of suspicion for ADRs when treating patients with new drugs, and they consequently tend to be more energetic in their reporting. A problem therefore arises when an assessment of the relative incidences of ADRs on new compounds compared with older ones is based on data derived from open reporting systems. It may well appear that a new compound is associated with a higher risk of ADRs than an older one simply because of the underreporting of ADRs with familiar drugs.

It would be unfortunate if a new and useful compound were rejected as a result of calculations based on the faulty premise that the reporting of ADRs

[1] Department of Psychiatry, St. Mary's Hospital, Praed Street, London W2 1NY, United Kingdom

Neuropsychopharmacology
Edited by Bunney/Hippius/Laakmann/Schmauß

remains constant between older and newer drugs. In order to establish the relative safety of a new drug compared with those already available, a system of assessment of ADRs is required which is less prone to bias than open reporting systems. This paper suggests two sources of comparative safety data which can be used to avoid this bias.

In the development of a potential antidepressant, a programme of double-blind clinical trials should be undertaken to assess the possible efficacy of a new compound in comparison with placebo and also to establish its efficacy relative to reference antidepressants. During these clinical trials all side effects and especially serious ADRs are monitored very closely and are usually reported by the investigator without knowledge of which compound, be it a new drug, reference antidepressant or placebo, is associated with the side effect. This provides a relatively unbiassed database from which estimates of ADRs with reference antidepressants might be derived.

A clear example of the value of this approach is provided by the different estimates of the incidence of convulsions associated with tricyclic antidepressants (TCAs): these appear substantially lower if open reporting systems are considered than if the data from clinical trials are examined. The incidence of convulsions associated with a drug is a useful model because the risk of convulsions is not dependent on a particular length of exposure. Some ADRs which are more likely to occur after some weeks of treatment, such as dyscrasias or hepatotoxicity, might be missed because of the short duration of treatment in trials, but this is less likely with convulsions.

The incidence of convulsions on imipramine reported in the clinical trials was 1%–2% (Geltzer 1986). The reports of convulsions associated with maprotiline during early clinical trials found a similar level of 0.46%–1.6% (28 of 1750 patients, Dillier 1982). In later trials conducted in the USA, the incidence with maprotiline was 0.41%. A higher level of convulsions was found in the dose-ranging trials in Europe. One explanation for this difference is that the doses used in the early studies in Europe were sometimes rather significantly higher than those used in trials in the USA (Geltzer 1986). There have been similar reports of an increased incidence of convulsions being associated with higher doses of dothiepin. A summary of the data with TCAs, based largely on imipramine data, suggests that a maximum acceptable benchmark figure for convulsions with the reference antidepressants is in the region of 0.5% during clinical trials. Anything higher than this is a cause for concern. High-dosage treatment with TCAs appears to be associated with an incidence of convulsions above this figure, which is worrying in view of the widespread belief that some TCAs are not effective at lower doses.

The model of examining the incidence of convulsions in clinical trials identified the association of an excessive number of convulsions with buproprion. The incidence in studies with patients suffering from depression was around 0.5%, but in studies with eating disordered patients it was sharply increased. The question now is whether the dose may be lowered to achieve a more acceptable level of convulsions and still retain efficacy. By comparison, two recently released antidepressants in Europe, fluoxetine and fluvoxamine, have an incidence of convulsions in the range of 0.2% in clinical trials, which is more acceptable compared with TCAs.

Another source of safety data which is independent of reporting bias is provided by the examination of deaths from overdose. In England and Wales fatal poisonings are reported at coroners' inquests, and the mortality statistics are published by the Office of Population and Censuses. The most direct measure of toxicity of an antidepressant in overdose is provided where the cause of death is attributed to a single drug rather than to many different drugs. An index of toxicity can be derived by relating the use of an antidepressant to the number of fatal overdoses reported. Several recent studies have based an assessment of relative toxicity of antidepressants on these statistics (Montgomery and Pinder 1987; Cassidy and Henry 1987). This index can be calculated as the ratio of total fatalities to prescriptions or as the ratio of fatalities to patients treated.

The Montgomery and Pinder study (1987) analysed data of widely used antidepressants by calculating the number of patients treated from the amount of drugs sold using defined daily doses and durations of treatment. The figures were based on Office of Population and Censuses and Surveys data and International Medical Statistics (IMS) market statistics for England and Wales for the period 1977–1984. They reported a wide variation in fatal poisonings with different antidepressants and showed that certain ones had notably greater toxicity than others. Amitriptyline and dothiepin appear to be the most toxic and dangerous in overdose.

A very similar rank order of the toxicity of antidepressants in overdosage was reported by Cassidy and Henry (1987). Their analysis was based on National Health Service prescription data from England, Wales and Scotland for the period 1975–1984. The older TCAs as a group were shown to be associated with significantly more deaths from overdose per million prescriptions than the average ratio for all antidepressants. The newer antidepressants mianserin, lofepramine and trazodone had a significantly lower ratio of fatalities per million prescriptions than the average.

The agreement between these separate analyses, which have used different approaches, is encouraging. Both point to the toxicity in overdose of the older TCAs and in particular to the danger of amitriptyline and dothiepin in comparison with other antidepressants. Maprotiline, which has a tricyclic structure but which is sometimes misleadingly referred to as a tetracyclic, does not seem to have escaped the toxicity associated with the earlier TCAs. The newer nontricyclic antidepressants appear to be significantly safer than the older TCAs. Of the newer TCAs, only lofepramine appears to be clearly safer in overdose.

These calculations of relative toxicity are based on the assumption that overdoses in a given population receiving antidepressants are randomly distributed. This may or may not be true. For example, there is evidence that the assumption does not hold for patients taking benzodiazepines, which are reported to produce disinhibition and to cause an increase in both aggression and suicide attempts (Gardner and Cowdry 1985). Recent warnings caution

doctors to be particularly careful in precribing benzodiazepines to patients who are potentially suicidal (Committee on Safety of Medicines 1988). Alcohol is reported likewise to increase the suicide rate by a rather similar mechanism, and the number of deaths associated with the ingestion of alcohol is high.

The idea that all antidepressants are neutral in relation to suicidal thoughts and suicidal acts is an assumption which needs to be examined. The suicide rate may possibly be affected in different ways. The question arises whether some antidepressants provoke suicide attempts: alternatively, some antidepressants may reduce suicidal thoughts or impulses.

A rather clear exception to the danger in overdose of the older TCAs is provided by clomipramine, of which the death from overdose index is low in both the Montgomery and Pinder and the Cassidy and Henry analyses. This is confusing in view of the high number of deaths from ADRs (5 per million prescriptions; Committee on Safety of Medicines 1985) and the substantial levels of anticholinergic effects reported in clinical practice. Clomipramine is known to be rather toxic and appears to be more dangerous than other TCAs in combination with MAOIs. In particular, deaths have been attributed to the combination of clomipramine and tranylcypramine. The relatively low apparent toxicity of clomipramine in overdose is therefore surprising and suggests that the low suicide rate may be a direct pharmacological effect.

Is there something specific to clomipramine which lowers the suicide rate? It is unlikely that clomipramine protects against the toxicity of other drugs since it has a high adverse drug interreaction profile. It is more likely that clomipramine reduces suicidal thoughts or impulses, thus protecting the individual from overdosing.

One test of this intriguing notion would be to see whether the suicidal thoughts or rates are selectively improved by clomipramine compared with other drugs in controlled studies. Unfortunately, the number of patients included in controlled studies has been too small to provide adequate data on this issue. There is interesting indirect evidence from the studies of the 5-HT reuptake inhibitors which appear to reduce selectively suicidal thoughts compared with standard antidepressants (Montgomery et al. 1981; de Wilde et al. 1985; Muijen et al. 1989). This finding fits nicely with the hypothesis that there is a link between serotonin and suicide attempts (Asberg et al. 1976) and impulse control (Linnoila et al. 1984). It may well be that 5-HT uptake inhibitors, including clomipramine, have a role in reducing impulsivity and may consequently reduce the suicidal attempt rate.

Conclusion

The relative incidence of serious ADRs with drugs is difficult to obtain. Differences in the way data are collected, particularly between old established drugs and newer drugs, makes the use of data from open reporting systems unreliable. The two techniques of avoiding bias suggested in this paper allow the relative safety of drugs to be compared. From this perspective, it appears that the older TCAs are associated with rather more ADRs and danger than is generally appreciated.

References

Asberg M, Traskman L, Thoren P (1976) 5-HIAA in the cerebrospinal fluid: a biochemical suicide predictor? Arch Gen Psychiatr 33:1193–1197

Cassidy S, Henry J (1987) Fatal toxicity of antidepressant drugs in overdose. Br Med J 295:1021–1024

Committee on Safety of Medicines (1985) Adverse reactions to antidepressants. Br Med J 291:1638

Committee on Safety of Medicines (1988) Benzodiazepines, dependence and withdrawal symptoms. Current Problems 21

de Wilde J, Mertens C, Fredricson Overo K, Hepfner Petersen HE (1985) Citalopram versus mianserin, a controlled double-blind trial in depressed patients. Acta Psychiatr Scand 72:89–96

Dillier N (1982) Worldwide clinical experience with Ludiomil. Act Nerv Super (Praha) 24:40–52

Gardner DL, Cowdry RW (1985) Alprazolam-induced dyscontrol in borderline personality disorder. Am J Psychiatry 142:98–100

Geltzer J (1986) Limits to chemotherapy of depression. Psychopathology 19:108–117

Linnoila M, Virkkunen M, Scheinin M, Muutila A, Rimon R, Goodwin FK (1984) Low cerebrospinal fluid 5-hydroxyindoleacetic acid concentration differentiates impulsive from nonimpulsive violent behaviour. Life Sci 33:2609–2414

Montgomery SA, Pinder RM (1987) Do some antidepressants promote suicide? Psychopharmacology 92:265–266

Montgomery SA, McAuley R, Rani SJ, Roy D, Montgomery D (1981) A double blind comparison of zimelidine and amitriptyline in endogenous depression. Acta Psychiatr Scand 63 [Suppl 290]:314–327

Muijen M, Roy D, Silverstone T, Mehmet A, Christie M (1988) A comparative clinical trial of fluoxetine, mianserin, and placebo with depressed outpatients. Acta Psychiatr Scand 78:384–390

Assessment of Drug Utilization and Adverse Drug Reactions in the Federal Republic of Germany

B. MÜLLER-OERLINGHAUSEN [1]

Phase IV studies are often seen only in terms of regulatory or safety aspects. This, however, is a rather narrow view of their actual value. The results of phase IV drug testing and drug surveillance can play a major role in improving the level of medical practice and performance – issues which have been much discussed by the public and by the medical profession in recent years. Furthermore, as emphasized in a recent draft of the proposed World Health Organization (WHO) guidelines on the clinical evaluation of psychotropic drugs, data on the actual use of a drug under routine conditions may generate new ideas about particular treatment strategies and can provide a soundbasis for therapeutic recommendations, for continuous education in psychopharmacology, and for appropriate measures to be taken by the regulatory authorities.

In the Federal Republic of Germany (FRG) it has taken a long time, much longer than for instance in some Nordic European countries, for it to be accepted that the manufacturers, medical profession, insurance companies, and public health authorities all gain valuable information from phase IV studies and should therefore encourage and support continuous evaluation of therapeutic compounds.

Postmarketing studies are directed mainly to objectives: (a) assessment of the drug efficacy in a routine use, (b) drug surveillance or assessment of adverse drug reactions (ADRs), and (c) drug utilization studies, which are an important factor in interpreting ADR figures from voluntary reporting systems (VRS). The present study examines what has been achieved in the FRG (including West Berlin) in recent years concerning the latter two aspects.

According to the WHO (1977) definition, drug utilization refers to "the marketing, distribution, prescribing and use of drugs in a society, with special emphasis on the resulting medical, social, and economic consequences." Rather than a drug-oriented issue, drug utilization can thus be seen as a problem-oriented, comprehensive, and continuous medical, social, and health-economic audit.

In the FRG, general and special health care is provided mainly by physicians in private practice, the costs for prescription being covered mainly by a national social security scheme. Thus, the patient usually does not himself pay directly for a prescribed drug. A regular, centralized evaluation of a 1‰

[1] Institut für Klinische Psychopharmakologie, Abteilung für Psychiatrie, Freie Universität Berlin, Eschenallee 3, 1000 Berlin 19 (West), FRG.

Neuropsychopharmacology
Edited by Bunney/Hippius/Laakmann/Schmauß

sample of these prescriptions was initiated in 1980 by the National Health Insurance System (Gesetzliche Krankenversicherung, GKV), and the findings of this so-called GKVindex are published annually. In addition, detailed sales and prescription statistics are collected by the drug manufacturers; their results, however, are not – at least not legally – available for other interested parties.

There are two prerequisites to performing sound drug utilization studies: first, the use of an internationally accepted drug classification system, and, second, an internationally accepted system for the calculation of prescribed or consumed amounts of drugs. Both have been developed mainly in the Scandinavian countries in cooperation with WHO, and it is most important that they be adopted by other nations in order to make the data from drug utilization studies more beneficial to the medical community.

A number of difficulties prevent a reliable comparison of FRG data with those of other countries. First the figures of the GKVindex are based on defined daily doses, however these are not yet fully comparable with the figures from Scandinavia. Second, drugs are not classified according to the anatomical/therapeutic/chemical (ATC) system but to the national drug compendium of the West German manufacturers' association. Third, figures refer only to patients of the 67000 physicians in private practice. And fourth, due to rigid data protection laws in this country, the figures cannot be related to morbidity data, which is, however, possible in some Scandinavian countries.

Figure 1 presents an overview of the total number of defined daily doses prescribed for various classes of psychotropic drugs in 1986 and 1987.

To obtain a more detailed insight into the prescribing behavior of general practitioners, internists, and psychiatrists in private practice, a comprehensive survey was carried out, supported by the Ministry of Labor and based on a quarterly self-audit system. This study took place between 1984 and 1986 in

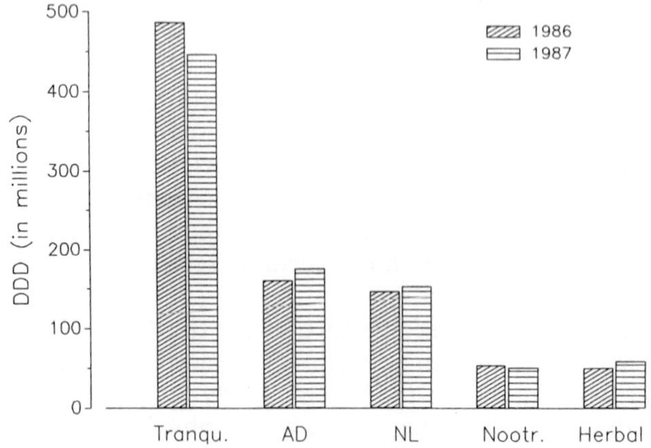

Fig. 1. Prescriptions of psychotropic drugs in the FRG in 1986 and 1987. *DDD*, Defined daily dose; *Tranqu.*, tranquilizers; *AD*, antidepressants; *NL*, neuroleptics; *Nootr.*, nootropics; *Herbal*, herbal drugs. (From Schwabe and Paffrath 1988)

Dortmund, a representative industrial area with 600000 inhibitants and 485 physicians, including 15 psychiatrists (Friebel et al. 1987, 1988). This survey showed that psychotropic drugs constitute about 10% of the total number of prescriptions by internists and general practitioners. It was also observed that, whereas the ranking of the most frequently prescribed antidepressants in psychiatric practice was very similar to the corresponding profile among internists, marked differences occurred in the rankings of the prescribed tranquilizers. Some 18%–50% of the individual compounds which a given physician prescribes to his patients per year are substituted by other drugs.

Several studies have also provided information on the prescripton of psychotropic drugs. As regards drug utilization in hospitalized psychiatric patients, accurate data are available for the University Hospital of the Free University in Berlin (Schmidt et al. 1988), which were collected in connection with an ongoing project (see Grohmann et al., this volume). In addition, a cross-section study on drug prescription by 44 psychiatrists in private practice was performed in West Berlin, in which particular attention was given to the level of polypharmacy in psychiatric practice (Schüssler and Müller-Oerlinghausen 1984). Data on the long-term use of benzodiazepines in a representative sample of the West German population can be derived from the Munich Blood Pressure Study (Koenig et al. 1987).

Utilization or prescription of a drug should be preceded by a risk/benefit appraisal by the doctor or the patient. However, the necessary quantitative information on either the benefit or the risk of even the widely used compounds is often lacking. There is as yet no law compelling manufacturers to provide quantitative data on the occurrence and severity of ADRs or to identify populations especially at risk after a sufficient number of patients have been treated with an individual drug.

The most important system for assessing ADRs in this country, as in many others, is the VRS, which is directed principally by the Drug Commission of the German Medical Profession in Cologne, established in 1958. Physicians or

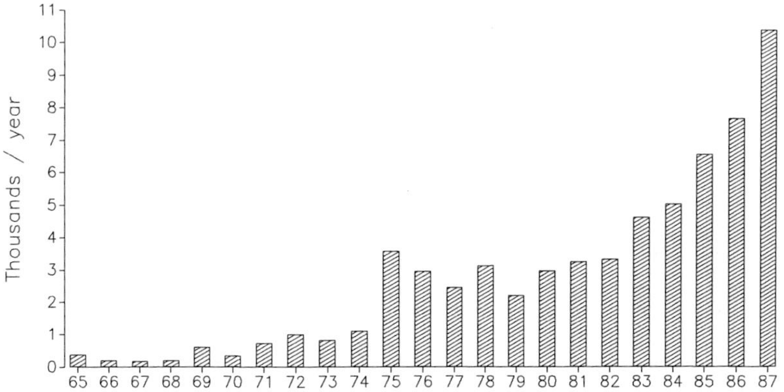

Fig. 2. Frequency of ADR reports received at the Drug Commission in Cologne, FRG, between 1965 and 1987

manufacturers can also report to the Federal Health Office in West Berlin, and a joint data bank of these two institutions is now being implemented (Kimbel and Müller-Oerlinghausen 1986). Figure 2 presents the annual frequency of reports received at our secretariate in Cologne. A total of some 1900 reports with approximately 2900 ADRs of antidepressants were on file in 1987. On the average, one report refers to 1.4 ADRs. Incoming reports are screened immediately by an experienced group of physicians who select special problem cases to be discussed in regular advisory committee meetings. ADRs are subdivided into 24 organ classes. All reporting physicians receive a personal letter commenting on their individual observation. Potential warnings generated by the VRS are discussed in routine sessions of the Federal Health Office. In addition, a special committee with selected experts from the Drug Commission and the Federal Health Office was established in 1987 that will have regular meetings in the future. As in the other 23 European countries with VRS, this national center also reports to WHO. The WHO data (approximately 400000 reports) are available to the national centers for confidential use.

Since incidence figures cannot be calculated from VRS data the most important source of information for comparing risks of individual drugs are therefore the so-called ADR profiles (Inman 1980), which examine the proportion of various ADR groups among all reported ADRs of a single drug. An example is shown in Fig. 3.

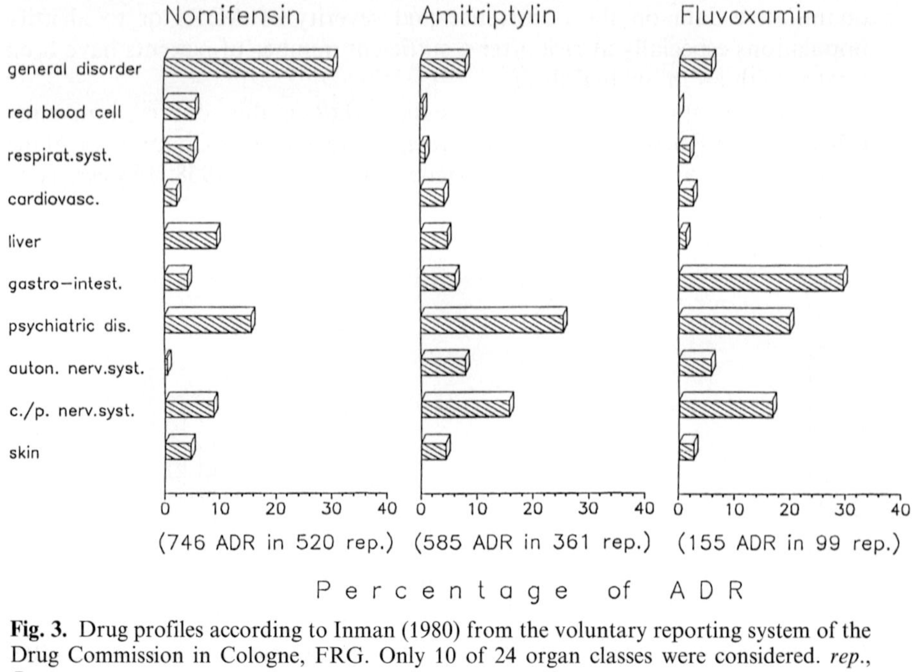

Fig. 3. Drug profiles according to Inman (1980) from the voluntary reporting system of the Drug Commission in Cologne, FRG. Only 10 of 24 organ classes were considered. *rep.*, *Reports*

VRS serves mainly as an early warning system, but it cannot provide information on the frequency, severity, or final outcome of ADRs. VRS must therefore be complemented by retrospective or prospective comprehensive drug surveillance systems, such as case control studies or intensive hospital-based monitoring. The project described by Grohmann et al. (this volume) presents such a comprehensive system regarding the medication of psychiatric patients. Another comprehensive approach is that of Medical Record Linkage, which is, however, often not feasible in the FRG due to data protection laws. Unfortunately, prescription event monitoring, a rather cheap but effective comprehensive drug-oriented system designed by Inman (1980) in the United Kingdom, has not yet been used on a large scale in this country. Another important instrument in the FRG is the "early warning system," which evaluates interviews with known drug addicts and provides a regular updating of the most frequently abused legal and illegal drugs.

In summary, a number of promising steps toward improved drug surveillance have been taken in the FRG. Drug safety, however, depends on safe physicians, and drug safety can only be as good as the average clinical-pharmacological education of medical students. In this respect the FRG still has much to learn and to adopt from other countries in the West and in the East.

References

Friebel H, Schäfer T, Balthasar R, Dinnendahl V, Hoffmans-Hohn M, Müller-Oerlinghausen B, Overhoff H (1987) Arzneimitteltransparenz und -beratung in Dortmund. Zum Verordnungsverhalten niedergelassener Ärzte (2. Mitteilung). Pharmazeutische Zeitung 33:1981–1990

Friebel H, Schäfer T, Balthasar R, Dinnendahl V, Feyerabend H, Hoffmans-Hohn M, Müller-Oerlinghausen B, Overhoff H (1988) Arzneimitteltransparenz und -beratung in Dortmund (3. Mitteilung, Teil 2). Pharmazeutische Zeitung 13:932–940

Inman WHW (ed) (1980) Monitoring for drug safety. MTP Press, Lancaster

Kimbel KH, Müller-Oerlinghausen B (1986) Spontanerfassung unerwünschter Arzneimittelwirkungen. In: Dölle W, Müller-Oerlinghausen B, Schwabe U (eds) Grundlagen der Arzneimitteltherapie. Bibliographisches Institut, Wissenschaftsverlag, pp 292–300

Koenig W, Rüther E, Remmers A, Keil U (1987) Comparison of psychotropic drug intake in two populations in West Germany. Results from the Munich Blood Pressure Study 1980/81 and the Luebeck Blood Pressure Study 1984. Pharmacopsychiatry 20:111–115

Schmidt LG, Lammers V, Stöckel M, Müller-Oerlinghausen B (1988) Recent trends of prescribing psychotropic drugs in a university hospital (1981–84). Pharmacopsychiatry 21:126–130

Schüssler G, Müller-Oerlinghausen B (1984) Polypharmacy in psychiatric practice. Compr Psychiatry 25:566–574

Schwabe U, Paffrath D (eds) (1988) Arzneiverordnungsreport '88. Aktuelle Daten, Kosten, Trends und Kommentare. Fischer, Stuttgart

World Health Organization (1977) The selection of essential drugs: report of a WHO expert committee. World Health Organization Report Series, no 615

Drug Surveillance in Psychiatric Patients in the Federal Republic of Germany

R. GROHMANN[1], L. G. SCHMIDT[2], and E. RÜTHER[3]

Introduction

In 1979 a study for drug surveillance in psychiatric patients (Arzneimittelüberwachung in der Psychiatrie, AMÜP) was initiated by the Arbeitsgemeinschaft für Neuropsychopharmakologie und Pharmakopsychiatrie, financed by the Federal Health Agency (Bundesgesundheitsamt) of the Federal Republic of Germany. The main aim of the study was to assess data on adverse drug reactions (ADRs) under conditions of everyday clinical practice. Data on type and frequency of ADRs for various psychotropic drugs are available from clinical trials, however in everyday clinical practice patients of all age groups, including the elderly, are treated; some patients have concomitant physical diseases, and frequently drug combinations are used, as polypharmacy is a common practice in psychiatry worldwide (Clark and Holden 1987; Grohmann et al. 1986; Schmidt et al. 1987; Swett 1979). As the need for additional information on the occurence of ADR under these treatment conditions had not previously been met by any large-scale drug surveillance study, the AMÜP study was undertaken.

This chapter describes in- and outpatient surveillance in the AMÜP study and presents some of its overall results.

Methods and Materials

Definitions. ADR is defined as any drug-related manifestation in a patient that is unintended and undesired by the prescribing physician (Seidl et al. 1965). Symptoms due to intoxication and inefficacy are not rated as ADRs.

The *probability of a causal relationship* between unwanted manifestation and drug treatment is assessed following the criteria given by Seidl et al. (1965) and Hurwitz and Wade (1969). The categories used are the following:

[1] Psychiatrische Klinik der Ludwig-Maximilian-Universität München, Nußbaumstr. 7, 8000 München 2, FRG.
[2] Psychiatrische Klinik der Freien Universität Berlin, Eschenallee 3, 1000 Berlin 19, FRG.
[3] Psychiatrische Klinik der Universität Göttingen, von-Sieboldstr. 5, 3400 Göttingen, FRG.

Neuropsychopharmacology
Edited by Bunney/Hippius/Laakmann/Schmauß

- *Possible:* Adverse reaction not characteristic for the drug in question, and/or time sequence not in accordance with previous experience, or, a probability of alternative cause for unwanted effect over 50%.
- *Probable:* Adverse reaction to drug in question generally accepted; time sequence in accordance with previous experience; probability of alternative cause under 50%.
- *Definite:* In addition to the criteria necessary for a "probable" rank, reappearance of ADR following rechallenge with drug(s) in question is necessary.

The reliability of these criteria was demonstrated in an interrater reliability study which resulted in a high agreement rate; the percent age of agreement exceeded that obtained with the algorithm proposed by Kramer et al. (1979) which has been used comparitively (Dirschedl et al. 1986).

Severity of the ADR was determined by rating the impact on therapy of the ADR as follows:

- *Grade I:* ADR leads to no change in medication.
- *Grade II:* ADR leads to a change in medication consisting of dose reduction and/or additional treatment to counteract the ADR.
- *Grade III:* ADR leads to discontinuation of the medication suspected of causing the ADR (including cases in which the drug would be discontinued if it were not vital).

In addition, a judgement was made on clinical grounds as to whether an ADR was severe or even life threatening. A specially trained psychiatrist acted as drug monitor, obtaining all necessary information from the treating physicians and recording it suitably for computer evaluation. The patients themselves were not examined by the drug monitor.

Inpatient Surveillance. Two different methods of inpatient surveillance were used. One was intensive drug monitoring (IDM). With IDM a randomly selected sample of patients (approximately 150 per year) were monitored for all ADRs throughout their stay in hospital. All signs and symptoms not rated as ADR were also recorded so that IDM was essentially an event-monitoring method (Finney 1965). The other form of surveillance was organized spontaneous reporting (OSR). With OSR only ADRs of grade III were assessed in all the other inpatients of participating hospitals. Drug use per year was assessed continually for the calculation of relative risk rates. More detailed descriptions of the methodological approach have been published earlier along with initial results (Rüther et al. 1980; Grohmann et al. 1984; Schmidt et al. 1984). In addition, inpatient surveillance included assessment of patients with drug abuse or dependence at the time of admission (Wolf et al. 1989), drug-related admissions (Schmidt and Langscheid-Schmidt 1987), and suicide attempts with psychotropic drugs before admission.

The Psychiatric Departments of the Universities of Berlin and Munich participated from the beginning, contributing to all aspects of inpatient surveillance. The Psychiatric Department of the University of Göttingen participated in IDM in the 1st year; thereafter only drug abuse data were contributed. In 1984–1985 the Psychiatric Department of the University of Mainz participated in IDM and OSR. In addition, state hospitals participated in the study. IDM was conducted for 1 year in a chronic ward in the regional hospital of Haar; (von Oefele and Rüther 1985). In addition, prevalence of tardive dyskinesia was assessed in two Bavarian state hospitals, those in Haar and Mainkofen (Haag 1983).

Outpatient Surveillance. In outpatients only grade III ADRs were assessed. In West Berlin 32 psychiatrists in private practice participated for 6 months in 1982, reporting grade III ADRs for all psychotropic drugs; drug use was not assessed. In 1986–1987, 12 psychiatrists reported grade III ADRs and prescriptions for some newly marketed antidepressants and low-dose fluspirilene. In Munich, five psychiatrists in private practice contributed data on grade III ADRs and prescriptions for all psychotropic drugs in the period 1982–1984. In 1986 this surveillance scheme was extended to 15 psychiatrists. More details as to methodology and initial results have been reported by Bürke et al. (1986) and Schmidt et al. (1985).

Results

The results reported here relate to data obtained in the two main participating centers, those in Berlin and Munich. If not otherwise noted, data pertain only to ADRs rated as probable or definite.

Overall ADR Rates. For inpatients ADRs of all grades were observed in 59% of 1100 patients monitored with IDM from May 1979 to December 1986. ADRs with some impact on therapy (grades II and III) were observed in 40%. Grade III ADRs were observed in 10% of about 15000 inpatients monitored with OSR in 1979–1986. In outpatients a similar rate of grade III ADRs was observed in Munich (where drug use and ADR data were assessed); in 11% of psychotropic drug treated patients ADRs led to drug discontinuation.

ADR Rates for Drug Groups. In relating ADRs to single drugs or drug groups the problem of polypharmacy must be considered. As an example, Table 1 presents data on drug combinations for the two most frequently used neuroleptics, haloperidol and perazine, which demonstrate the considerable frequency of this mode of treatment. The frequency of polypharmacy suggests that ADRs must often be attributed not to a single drug but to a combination of drugs. Therefore, ADR rates for the different drug groups, as obtained with IDM, are presented in two ways in Table 2, showing rates for all ADRs and for those ADRs in which drugs from only one group were suspected. Neuroleptics were most frequently associated with ADR, followed by antidepressants and

Table 1. Drug combinations with neuroleptics

	Haloperidol ($n=323$)	Perazine ($n=292$)
No other psychotropic drugs	1%	5%
Other psychotropic drugs simultaneously ≧7 days	78%	61%
Other neuroleptic	43%	31%
Antiparkinsonian drug	42%	15%
Antidepressant	17%	21%
Benzodiazepine	12%	11%
Lithium	9%	9%

Table 2. Rates of ADRs for drug groups

	n	Percentage with ADR	
		All[a]	Alone
Neuroleptics	576	64	59
Antidepressants	341	46	36
Lithium salts	81	30	17
Antiparkinsonian drugs	247	9	2
Tranquillizers	259	8	4
Hypnotics	388	2	1

[a] Includes cases of polypharmacy.

lithium salts. Antiparkinsonian drugs, tranquilizers, and hypnotics were only rarely associated with ADR and in most cases in combination with other drug groups.

ADR Profiles. Figures 1–3 show the types of grade III ADRs (OSR data) for haloperidol, perazine, and for amitriptyline, the most frequently used antidepressant. Although a direct, statistically valid comparison between the drugs is impossible due to the frequent combinations among them, differences in ADR profiles between the two neuroleptic drugs are obvious. With haloperidol (Fig. 1) extrapyramidal motor disturbances formed the bulk of grade III ADRs, mostly attributed to haloperidol alone (6.9% for haloperidol alone, 7.7% for all extrapyramidal motor symptoms involving haloperidol). Psychic disturbances (excluding toxic delirium, a separate category not observed with haloperidol) were next in frequency for haloperidol (2.9% for all cases), mostly sedation, agitation, and depression. For perazine (Fig. 2) EPMS were observed in only 1.2% of grade III ADRs and mostly (0.6%) in combination with other drugs. Similar frequencies were observed for increase of liver enzymes (1.2% for all cases), psychic disturbances, mostly sedation, and toxic delirium (1%

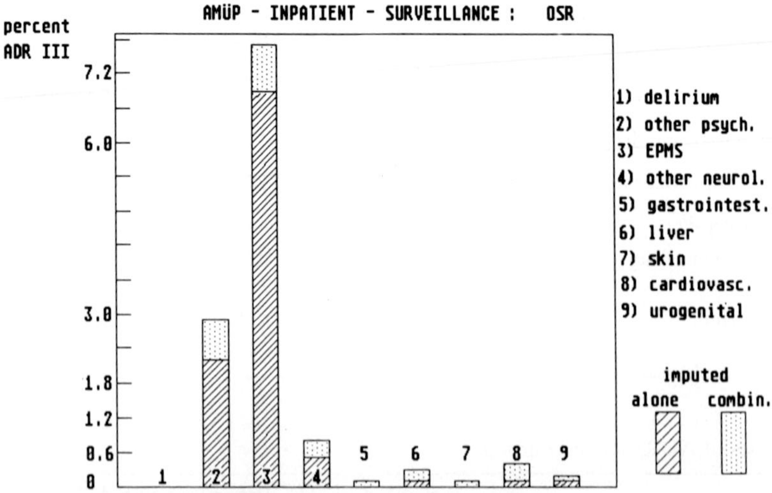

Fig. 1. Frequency of grade III ADRs observed with haloperidol. Organized spontaneous reporting among inpatients ($n = 3810$) in the period 1979–1984

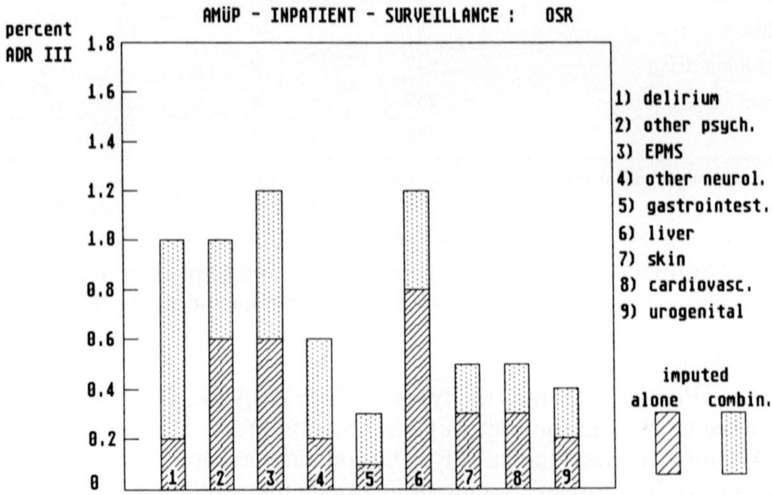

Fig. 2. Frequency of grade III ADRs observed with perazine. Organized spontaneous reporting among inpatients ($n = 3291$) in the period 1979–1984

each), the latter mostly in combination with other anticholinergic drugs. For amitriptyline (Fig. 3) toxic delirium was the most frequent type of grade III ADR (1.6% of cases), again frequently in combination with other drugs. Among the other psychic disturbances (1.3% of cases) sedation prevailed; other neurological disturbances (1.2% of cases) included tremor, ataxia, and dysarthria.

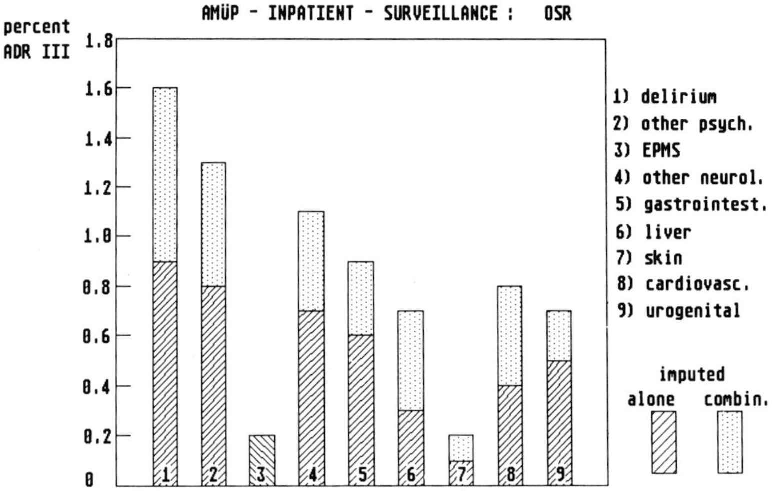

Fig. 3. Frequency of grade III ADRs observed with amitriptyline. Organized spontaneous reporting among inpatients ($n = 1843$) in the period 1979–1984

Severe ADRs. ADRs rated as severe (Table 3), were observed in 1.5% of inpatients. Among CNS reactions, toxic delirium (114 cases, 105 probable definite) were the most frequent form of ADR by far; seizures were observed in 19 cases (13 cases probable/definite) and neuroleptic syndrome (severe EPMS plus stupor) in 16 cases (11 cases probable/definite), all due to high-potency neuroleptics. In another two cases the full picture of malignant neuroleptic syndrome was observed. Depression was observed as an instance of severe ADR in 14 cases, but only five of these were rated as probable, which reflects the difficulty of causality assessment in this controversial type of ADR. In six cases a severe CNS crisis with coarse tremor, hyperthermia, and blood pressure instability (leading to death in one case) was observed with the combination of the monoamine oxidase inhibitor tranylcypromine with clomipramine (von Oefele et al. 1986). Cardiovascular reactions included conduction disturbances, arrhythmias, signs of beginning heart failure, and some cases of sudden death (but not among the only six probable ADRs). Gastrointestinal reactions were

Table 3. Severe ADRs in 11 225 patients

	All cases ($n = 210$)	Probable/definite ($n = 165$)
CNS	171	142
Cardiovascular	21	6
Gastrointestinal tract	9	9
Hematological	3	3
Other	6	5

principally ileus or subileus. In all three cases of agranulocytosis the tricyclic neuroleptic perazine was involved; in two cases almost complete disappearance of granulocytes occurred when leukocytes were still above 3000/mm.

Conclusions

The 9-year experience from the AMÜP study shows that its methodological approach was appropriate for a study designed to continue over several years. Continuous data assessment over a protracted period is required in any drug surveillance study in order to obtain the necessary number of patients. Even then frequent polypharmacy severely restricts the possibilities of statistical evaluation. Still, data on the frequency of ADRs show the extent to which ADRs influence treatment under conditions of everyday practice. Distinct ADR profiles for different types of drugs emerge. The rarer, severe adverse events can be observed and allow comparative risk assessments (e.g., excess risk of severe CNS ADRs with the combination of clomipramine and tranylcypromine; risk of agranulocytosis for medium-potency perazine versus neuroleptic syndrome and malignant neuroleptic syndrome for haloperidol).

Thus, among the various methodological approaches developed in the field of ADR research (Venulet 1977), drug surveillance schemes such as the AMÜP study form an important part of the work necessary for improvement of drug safety.

References

Bürke H, Grohmann R, Rüther E (1986) Psychiatric outpatients treatment: developing methods of drug surveillance. Pharmacopsychiatry 19:298–299

Clark AF, Holden L (1987) The persistence of prescribing habits: a survey and follow-up of prescribing to chronic hospital in-patients. Br J Psychiatry 150:88–91

Dirschedl P, Grohmann R, Schmidt LG (1986) Reliability of adverse drug reaction assessment. Pharmacopsychiatry 19:292–293

Finney DJ (1965) The design and logic of a monitor of drug use. J Chron Dis 18:77–98

Grohmann R, Hippius H, Müller-Oerlinghausen B, Rüther E, Scherer J, Schmidt LG, Strauß A, Wolf B (1984) Assessment of adverse drug reactions in psychiatric hospitals. Eur J Clin Pharmacol. 26:727–734

Grohmann R, Dirschedl P, Rennig E, Scherer J, Schmidt LG (1986) Methodological problems in assessment of adverse drug reactions with drug combinations. Pharmacopsychiatry 19:300–301

Haag H (1983) Spätdyskinesie. Eine epidemiologische Untersuchung. Thesis, Ludwig Maximilians University, München

Hurwitz N, Wade OL (1969) Intensive hospital monitoring of adverse reactions to drugs. Br Med J 1:531–536

Kramer MS, Leventhal JM, Hutchinson TA, Feinstein AR (1979) An algorithm for the operational assessment of adverse drug reactions. I: Background, description, and instruction for use. JAMA 242:623–632

Rüther E, Benkert O, Eckmann F, Eckmann I, Grohmann R, Helmchen H, Hippius H, Müller-Oerlinghausen B, Poser W, Schmidt LG, Stille G, Strauß A, Überla K (1980)

Drug Monitoring in psychiatrischen Kliniken. Bericht der Arbeitsgruppe für Medikamenten-Überwachung in der Psychiatrie. Arzneimittelforschung/Drug Res 30:1181–1183
Schmidt LG, Langscheid-Schmidt K (1987) Neuroleptika-bedingte Aufnahmen in einer psychiatrischen Universitätsklinik (Aus dem AMÜP-Projekt). Nervenarzt 58:379–382
Schmidt LG, Grohmann R, Helmchen H, Langscheid-Schmidt K, Müller-Oerlinghausen B, Poser W, Rüther E, Scherer J, Strauß A, Wolf B (1984) Adverse drug reactions. Acta Psychiatr Scand 70:77–89
Schmidt LG, Schüssler G, Linden M, Müller-Oerlinghausen B (1985) Impact of adverse drug reactions on treatment of psychiatric outpatients. Pharmacopsychiatry 17:40–41
Schmidt LG, Czerlinsky H, Stöckel M (1987) Longitudinal assessment of psychotropic drug use in acutely-ill psychiatric inpatients. Int J Clin Pharmacol Ther Toxicol 25:244–250
Seidl LG, Thornton GF, Cluff LE G (1965) Epidemiological studies of adverse drug reactions. Am J Publ Health 55:1170–1175
Swett C (1979) Patterns of drug use in psychiatric inpatient wards. J Clin Psychiatry 16:464–468
Venulet J (1977) Methods of monitoring adverse reactions to drugs. Proc Drug Res 21:231–292
von Oefele K, Rüther E (1985) Adverse drug reaction monitoring in long-term psychiatric inpatients. Pharmacopsychiatry 18:33–34
von Oefele K, Grohmann R, Rüther E (1986) Adverse drug reactions in combined tricyclic and MAO I-therapy. Pharmacopsychiatry 19:243–244
Wolf B, Grohmann R, Biber D, Brenner P, Rüther E (1989) Benzodiazepine abuse and dependence in psychiatric in patients. Pharmacopsychiatry 22:54–60

Surveillance of Toxicity of Antidepressants

B. E. LEONARD [1]

Introduction

To market a drug in the 1980s, it is essential in most countries for the pharmaceutical company concerned to provide evidence of the drug's safety and efficacy. Such evidence must, by its very nature, be limited as it depends on the pre-marketing phase of development which is usually restricted to studying the drug on a relatively small number of selected patients for a short period. This situation contrasts to the large numbers of unselected patients who eventually receive the drug following its release onto the market. Thus additional epidemiological information on the clinical effects of a new drug is essential once the drug has been marketed, and this has led to the establishment of post-marketing surveillance programmes in most industrialized countries of the world.

Post-marketing surveillance may be viewed as a process that systematically and comprehensively monitors the patterns of use and the beneficial and harmful effects of drugs as used in clinical practice. It is self-evident that, irrespective of the legislative requirements for pre-marketing studies, only following the introduction of a drug to the marketplace can full potential (both therapeutic and adverse) be determined under conditions of clinical use. A primer on post-marketing surveillance has recently been published under the auspices of the Committee on Clinical Safety Surveillance of the Medical Section of the Pharmaceutical Manufacturers Association (Hagler et al. 1987), which summarizes the methods used to undertake such surveillance in the United States and United Kingdom.

Post-Marketing Surveillance in the United States

In the United States, the Food and Drug Administration (FDA) has established several programmes that provide post-marketing surveillance information about drugs. Such programmes include: (a) spontaneous voluntary reporting of adverse effects to the FDA; (b) literature reports of the drug

[1] Pharmacology Department, University College, Galway, Republic of Ireland.

Neuropsychopharmacology
Edited by Bunney/Hippius/Laakmann/Schmauß

effects to the professional community (essentially a voluntary system); (c) post-marketing surveillance studies requested of the pharmaceutical company by the FDA (such studies are referred to as phase IV studies, and while the FDA does not have a statutory right to have such studies implemented, most companies comply with the request to prevent undue delay or non-approval of the drug); and (d) independent academic investigators whose major professional interest lies in the area of public health and epidemiology. The drug surveillance programmes at Shands Hospital in Florida and the Boston Collaborative Drug Surveillances Program are two internationally known examples. From the 1960s, the FDA has directly funded several other organizations such as the Kaiser-Permanente record linkage study and the Armed Forces Institute of Pathology Tissue Reactions to Drug Registry.

Details of the procedures used to monitor the adverse effects of marketed drugs in the United States have been considered in more detail by Jick et al. (1979).

Post-Marketing Surveillance in the United Kingdom

In 1961 in the Federal Republic of Germany, the pediatrician Lenz expressed concern about the sudden dramatic increase in the number of children referred to his clinic with phocomelia and other mesodermal defects. This was the first observation of what became known as the thalidomide disaster, and it soon became apparent that the epidemic had begun some 2 years earlier, 5 years after the drug had been marketed as a hypnotic frequently prescribed for pregnant women.

Following the thalidomide disaster, which had a major impact on British society, voluntary controls on the investigation and marketing of drugs were established. In 1963 the Committee on Safety of Drugs was established to review the evidence regarding the efficacy and safety of new drugs. By 1964 the Committee had established an adverse event report system under the auspices of the Subcommittee on Adverse Reactions. Under this scheme, physicians, dentists and coroners were invited to submity summary reports of a suspected adverse drug side effect to a central Register of Drug Reactions. These reports were provided by the physician on pre-paid business reply cards (so-called "yellow cards", because of their colour) and provided the machinery by which adverse drug effects could be detected.

The Medicines Act of 1968, implemented in 1971, converted a number of formerly voluntary procedures into compulsory ones. The Committee on Safety of Medicines (CSM) replaced the Committee on Safety of Drugs and required the pharmaceutical companies to submit reports on any adverse effects brought to their attention.

Several disadvantages were soon recognized in the voluntary method of reporting adverse drug side effects to the CSM, not the least of which was the low level of reporting with consequent delays in the detection of the drug hazards. In an attempt to improve the post-marketing surveillance system, the CSM developed the "Recorded Release" approach, based on the identification of patients and their physicians by means of prescriptions, all of which are handled for the National Health Service by a single agency, the Prescription Pricing Authority. From such data, the national monitoring centre can obtain all necessary information on a particular patient undergoing drug treatment. Event monitoring was introduced so that any change in the patient's condition, whether due to accident, disease, operation or drug administration, is classified as an "event", i.e. "event" may be positive or negative. The advantage of event monitoring is that it does not require physicians to render opinions about the possible cause of the event.

In 1980 an independent and non-regulatory Drug Surveillance Research Unit was established at the University of Southampton with financial support from both the government of the United Kingdom and the pharmaceutical industry. The major purpose of the Unit was to undertake prescription event monitoring. This provides an alerting function which allows the easy detection of unsuspected hazards and also establishes a cohort which allows estimates of the incidence and prevalence of side effects based on populations of at least 10000. Such a cohort permits long-term follow-up for the investigation of suspected adverse effects. It has been estimated that this system would have identified the potential adverse effects of both thalidomide and practolol much earlier in the marketing process had the procedure been implemented earlier (Inman 1981 a, b; Rawlins 1984).

Despite the advances that have been made in post-marketing surveillance in the United Kingdom in recent years, there are still major problems that arise in establishing causal connection between a drug and the reported adverse reaction. In summary, these problems are: (a) spontaneous reporting by the "yellow card" procedure is not systematic and relies heavily on the motivation of the clinician; (b) no precise definition of many adverse drug treatments is given when a report is made; and (c) insufficient manpower at the CSM and elsewhere for the collection, analysis, evaluation and reporting of the adverse effects data means that long delays may occur before the medical profession is informed of a potential problem.

Adverse Drug Reactions and Antidepressants

Suicidal thoughts are frequently experienced by the depressed patient and thereby predisposes such a patient to a greater risk of self-poisoning than occurs in the general population. Safety in overdose is therefore an important attribute of any drug which may be prescribed to treat depression. Despite the introduction of a number of novel non-tricyclic antidepressants during the past decade, tricyclic antidepressants are still the more widely prescribed form of medication. It has been estimated that this group of drugs comprise the single most important group that cause severe CNS and cardiac depression in overdose and account for the deaths of approximately 350 persons yearly in England and Wales alone (Proudfoot 1986). For the period 1977–1984 the percentage of deaths due to antidepressants remained at approximately 15% (OPCS 1977–1984). It is ironic that many of the antidepressant drugs currently available are toxic even in the case of a modest overdose and thereby provide the patient with an ideal means for successful suicide. Frommer et al. (1987) has estimated the incidence of significant clinical changes that occur following the overdose of a tricyclic antidepressant as follows: sinus tachycardia 51%; coma 35%; QRS prolongation 21%; hypotension 14%; seizures 8.4%; arrhythmias 6.2%; cardio-respiratory arrest 3.6%; and total fatalities 2.2%.

Cassidy and Henry (1987) in their investigation of the number of deaths in the United Kingdom from fatal poisoning using tricyclic antidepressants showed that there is wide variation in the toxicity of the various tricyclic antidepressants in common use. The position of the individual antidepressants in the toxicity table is similar to that reported by Leonard (1986), Montgomery and Pinder (1987) and Pinder (1988) and shown in Table 1.

It is apparent that the toxicity of all the more recently introduced antidepressants, including the novel tricyclic antidepressant lofepramine, is less than that of the older drugs. Data are also available on the adverse side effects of these drugs, together with an estimate of the number of fatal adverse reactions per million prescriptions (Pinder 1988).

It is apparent that there is a considerable disparity between the number of deaths resulting from acute overdose and those arising from a severe adverse

Table 1. Overdosage deaths in the United Kongdom (1975–1984) after antidepressants. (From Cassidy and Henry 1987)

Drug	Number of fatal poisonings	Number of deaths per million prescriptions
Tricyclic antidepressants		
Dothiepin	533	50
Amitriptyline	1181	46.5
Imipramine	278	28.4
Clomipramine	51	11.1
Lofepramine	0	0
Monoamine oxidase inhibitors		
Tranylcypromine	15	58.1
Phenelzine	24	22.8
Second-generation antidepressants		
Maprotiline	83	37.6
Trazodone	6	13.6
Mianserin	30	5.6
Nomifensin	3	2.5
All antidepressants	2551	34.9

Table 2. Approximate numbers of adverse drug reactions (ADRs) per million prescriptions. (From CSM Update 1985)

Drug	Year Introduced	Total ADRs	Fatal ADRs
Imipramine	1959	15–20	1–2
Amitriptyline	1961	10–15	<1
Trimipramine	1966	10–15	<1
Dothiepin	1969	20–30	<1
Clomipramine	1970	60–80	5
Maprotiline	1975	400	<1
Mianserin	1976	200	2–3
Nomifensin	1977	500	7
Zimelidine	1982	3500 [a]	50 [a]

[a] Estimate, abridged from Pinder (1988).

drug reaction at therapeutic doses. Thus the widely used tetracyclic antidepressant mianserin accounted for 5.6 overdose deaths per million prescriptions in comparison to three deaths from adverse side effects per million patients for the same period (OPCS 1984). By contrast, the figures for the widely used tricyclic antidepressants dothiepin and amitriptyline were 50 and 46.5, respectively, for overdose deaths and less than one in each case for deaths due to severe adverse side effects. Clearly antidepressant safety should be taken into account by the regulatory authorities when warnings are issued regarding the potentially dangerous side effects of new antidepressants. To date however, little consideration has been given to the safety of antidepressant overdose so that the more toxic tricyclic antidepressants continue to be widely prescribed, while less toxic newer antidepressants such as zimelidine and nomifensin are withdrawn because of their very rare, though severe, adverse effects.

Post-Marketing Surveillance and the Adverse Effects of Antidepressants

Speirs (1988) has used the example of the novel serotonin uptake inhibitor antidepressant zimelidine to illustrate how attention to the adverse side effects by the regulatory authorities, without taking into consideration the safety of the drug in overdose, can lead to the withdrawal of a useful drug. Following the release of zimelidine in Sweden in 1982, a flu-like syndrome was reported by general practitioners to occur some 7–14 days after commencement of treatment in a small number of patients. This was accompanied by a fever, general malaise, arthralgia, headache, nausea and raised serum transaminases, suggesting possible hepatotoxicity. Two cases of aseptic meningitis were also reported and later that year a case polyradiculitis associated with drug treatment. Being a very rare disease, it was assumed to have arisen by chance but as a result of the publication of a report by the Swedish drug regulatory authorities, information on a further eight cases was elicited. The annual incidence of Guillain-Barré syndrome is 2.5 per 100000; zimelidine exposure was estimated to have produced three times this incidence, and the drug was subsequently withdrawn. It should be emphasized that the pharmaceutical company chose to withdraw the drug on the opinion of their lawyers. Judgement was thus a combination of judicial opinion and public perception that nine severe neurological problems per 14000 patientyears of drug use outweighed the clinical advantages (i.e. lack of anticholinergic side effects, safety in overdose, tolerability) of the drug.

More recently, the novel non-sedative antidepressant nomifensin was abruptly withdrawn by the manufacturers following an increase in the incidence of haemolytic anaemia in patients taking the drug. It has been estimated that such severe adverse effects could account for up to seven deaths per million prescriptions (CSM Update 1985, 1986). A detailed analysis of the incidence of haemolytic anaemia attributable to nomifensin showed that this rose from approximately 0.1 cases per million in the period 1977–1981 and then rose exponentially nearly ten-fold by 1986. Detailed studies of the incidence of haemolytic anaemia in the Federal Republic of Germany, France and United Kingdom showed a similar trend to that exhibited worldwide, leading to an incidence of approximately 1.5, 0.7 and 2.5 cases per million in these countries in 1985, respectively. Precise figures for the incidence of causally related fever, hepatitis, alveolitis and haemolytic anaemia in the Federal Republic of Germany, France and United Kingdom from 1984 and 1985 are summarized in Table 3. Out of a total of 3614 adverse drug reactions to nomifensin reported worldwide, the number of cases of drug-related fever, haemolytic anaemia, hepatitis and alveolitis was 220, 242, 242 and 42, respectively. In addition, fever was associated with hepatitis in a further 191 cases, with alveolitis in 61 cases and with hepatitis and alveolitis in 29 cases each. Against these figures, it has been estimated that there were 2.5 fatal poisionings with nomifensin per million prescriptions in comparison to 50 for dothiepin and 46.5 for amitriptyline.

This analysis of the adverse drug reaction data for nomifensin is based on worldwide reports of all serious drug reactions that have been objectively assessed so that any event that may possibly be associated with nomifensin was

Table 3. Adverse drug reactions to nomifensin: number of reported cases in 1984 and 1985

	Federal Republic of Germany		France		United Kingdom	
	1984	1985	1984	1985	1984	1985
Fever	16	31	43	44	13	5
Hepatitis	9	17	24	21	10	7
Alveolitis	5	1	1	4	0	0
Haemolytic anaemia	8	18	9	14	12	22

Source: Hoechst internal report 1988.

included. Thus the rare, but potentially serious, immunological side effects of nomifensin must be assessed against the real therapeutic benefits of this drug. Such benefits, which were widely accepted in its 8–9 years of availability in many European countries and in the United States, include its greater tolerability than the tricyclic antidepressants, particularly in the elderly depressive. Furthermore, its lack of anticholinergic side effects, relative safety in overdose, lack of cardiotoxicity, lack of pro-convulsive activity and failure to produce psychomotor impairment are all factors that must be taken into account in making a costbenefit assessment of the drug. And yet nomifensin was withdrawn by the manufacturers worldwide in 1986. As with the withdrawal of zimelidine, judgement would appear to be based on a combination of judicial opinion and public perception that the rare incidence of haemolytic anaemia far outweighed the widely accepted clinical advantages of this drug.

The Use of Prescription Event Monitoring in Assessing the Adverse Drug Reactions to Antidepressants

A major problem that arises when interpreting the importance of adverse reactions data concerns the relevance of the findings of one drug when compared to a 'standard' drug which it may ultimately replace. Two examples were given in the previous section in which two novel antidepressants, zimelidine and nomifensin, were withdrawn from the market because of their rare, though serious, side effects. While this does not imply that the 'standard' antidepressants, against which such drugs are often compared, do not also produce rare but equally serious side effects, it is less likely that adverse side effects will be reported for any well-established drug than for a newly introduced drug. This is particularly the case when the regulatory authorities highlight the potentially adverse effects of the new drug. To obtain more objective assessment of the adverse effect profile of a drug the prescription event monitoring procedure was introduced in the United Kingdom. By this procedure, approximately 120000 requests for event monitoring may be sent to general practitioners for a specific drug. The general practitioner is asked to report any event, including the reason for stopping the drug, since the commencement of treatment. An event is any new diagnosis, accident, unexpected deterioration or improvement, cause of death or suspected adverse drug reaction that occurs to a particular patient. The general practitioner must also state whether the patient was referred to hospital and must also give the National Health Service number and date of birth of the patient. The analysis of these events can then be related either to a background risk of the event occurring or to the incidence of the event occurring with another drug. Alternatively, the number of events occurring during and following treatment can be objectively compared.

The application of prescription event monitoring may be illustrated by the comparison of the adverse drug reactions to the novel antidepressant mianserin with those to amitriptyline (Inman 1988). In this study, all prescriptions for mianserin and amitriptyline written by general practitioners in England in January in 1987 were sent to the Drug Safety Research Unit in Southampton. Approximately 180000 prescriptions were sorted by geographical area and general practitioner and the first six prescriptions for each drug written by any clinician were selected for the study. The clinicians were then contacted and asked whether any haematological disorder, other than iron deficiency anaemia, had occurred during treatment, and whether the patient had attempted suicide. A total of 26781 patients who had received mianserin and 42082 amitriptyline were then assessed. An analysis of the data showed that no cases of aplastic anaemia, agraulocytosis or leucopenia had occurred in either treatment group that was severe enough to endanger life. In each treatment group, two patients developed a blood dyscrasia which was causally related to the drug. Thus the incidence of drug-induced leucopenia was calculated to be in the range of 1:10000 to 1:100000. With regard to suicide attempts, 246 patients on amitriptyline and 92 on mianserin made attempts, of which four were successful in the amitriptyline group and none in the mianserin group. Of those attempting suicide with amitriptyline, 56 patients required treatment in an intensive care unit, whereas none of those on mianserin required such treatment. From such data, it would appear that the incidence of blood dyscrasias is extremely low for both antidepressants, but that mianserin is safer than amitriptyline in overdose.

It is of interest to contrast the results of this study by Inman (1988) with the summary of data on the causal relationship between blood dyscrasias and mianserin as indicated by the analysis of reported adverse reactions using the "yellow card" scheme. Since 1979, 137 cases of blood dyscrasias associated with mianserin were reported to the CSM of which in 87 cases, mianserin was the only drug prescribed. An analysis of the data showed 55 cases of agranulocytosis, 24 cases of leucopenia, 4 of aplastic anaemia and 4 of pancytopenia (CSM 1985). These blood dyscrasias were reported to occur mainly in elderly patients who, because of the greater tolerability of mianserin in such patients (due to the low incidence of anticholinergic side effects and cardiotoxicity) were more likely to be prescribed than antidepressants. Barrett and Farmer (1988) have concluded from their analysis of the suspected causal relationship between blood dyscrasias and mianserin that the incidence of such dyscrasias increases with age irrespective of drug treatment, and that such a factor must be taken into account when ascribing a causal relationship between mianserin and such adverse effects. Furthermore, a blood dyscrasia associated with an antidepressant would appear to be an idiosynacratic response. As a greater proportion of prescriptions for mianserin are to new patients (i.e. those who have not been exposed to the drug previously), this would lead to an apparent increase in the incidence of dyscrasias associated with the drug. Clearly this does not imply that mianserin does not cause blood dyscrasias in some individuals, but it does suggest that evidence from the "yellow card" data is insufficient to either confirm or refute that the drug is less safe than alternatives regarding adverse haematological changes.

Worldwide data on the incidence of white blood cell dyscrasia associated with mianserin show that leucopenia occurred in 141 patients (accounting for 11 deaths), aplastic anaemia in 22 cases (11 deaths) and agranulocytosis in 163 cases (13 deaths). In total, there were 326 cases of blood dyscrasias causally associated with mianserin for the period 1976–1982 accounting for a total of 35 deaths worldwide.

It may be concluded that voluntary returns made to the regulatory authorities by the "yellow card" system do not accurately reflect the extent of adverse effects. Undoubtedly, one of the main reasons for this is related to the preferential reporting of such data. For example, all clinicins know that commonly used tricyclic antidepressants cause dry mouth, blurred vision, tachycardia, etc., and it is well established that at least 17 different classes of drugs, varying from the sulphonamides, antiarrhythmics and diurectics to the phenothiazines and anticonvulsants, cause leucopenia and other blood dyscrasias. Unless an unexpected death occurs in a patient on such medication, such adverse effects are less likely to be reported than if the patient is being treated with a newly marketed drug whose side effects are likely to receive greater attention. An additional complication may arise regarding the evaluation of the effects of interacting medication on the frequency of the side effects of the new drug. Such factors serve to emphasize the need for more thorough and objective mechanisms of post-marketing surveillance by the regulatory authorities. Prescription event monitoring may offer at least a partial answer to these problems. However, in my opinion, it is also necessary to change the attitude of the regulatory authorities in many countries regarding the toxicity of antidepressants in addition to their safety when administered in therapeutic doses. A far greater concern would appear to be expressed in the very rare incidence of an idiosyncratic reaction to a new antidepressant than in the much more frequent, predictable and life-threatening consequence of an overdose of an older and well-established tricyclic antidepressant.

Conclusion

In this brief review of the various methods which have been used in the United States and the United Kingdom for post-marketing surveillance, it is apparent that while no completely satisfactory method has been developed, the prescription event monitoring system would appear to be the most objective to date. This method is inevitably limited by both the cost and manpower necessary to operate the scheme. Furthermore, it cannot cover all therapeutic agents but is usually restricted to a detailed investigation of one or two drugs that have been considered to be potentially hazardous. Inevitably this approach is biased against new drugs in that such drugs will probably have a higher therapeutic profile because of their relative novelty. By highlighting such drugs, clinicians will probably be more inclined to report any adverse effects of such a drug without considering the frequency of such side effects that may occur with the more standard drugs of the same therapeutic class. Fisher

(1987) has considered the difficulties and necessities for adequate post-marketing surveillance in his recent short review.

Regarding the post-marketing surveillance of antidepressants, it would seem essential that the regulatory agencies consider the safety and efficacy of these drugs in a far broader sense than is presently apparent. Thus acute toxicity in overdose must be taken into account as well as any idiosynchratic effects that the drug may have in therapeutic doses. Such facts should be considered not only for the new antidepressants but also for the well-established drugs so that an objective comparison may be made.

Acknowledgements. My sincere thanks are due to Dr. Karl Taeuber, Hoechst AG, Frankfurt, FRG, for supplying me with unpublished data on the adverse effects of nomifensin and Drs. Roger Pinder and Peter van Keep, Organon International B.V., Oss, Holland, for bringing to my attention details of the adverse effects data for mianserin.

References

Barrett, Farmer (1988) Submitted for publication.

Cassidy SL, Henry JA (1987) Fatal toxicity of antidepressant drugs in overdose. Br Med J 292:287–289

CMS (Committe on Safety of Drugs) Update (1985) Adverse reactions to antidepressants. Br Med J 291:1638

CSM (Committee on Safety of Drugs) Update (1986) Withdrawal of nomifensin. Br Med J 293:41

Fisher S (1987) Post-marketing surveillance of adverse drug reactions. In: Meltzer HY (ed) Psychopharmacology: the third generation of progress. Raven, New York, pp 1667–1673

Frommer DA, Kulig KW, Marx JA, Rumack B (1987) Tricyclic antidepressant overdose. JAMA 257:521–526

Hagler L, Luscombe F, Siegfried J (1987) A primer on post-marketing surveillance. Drug Inform J 21:699–701

Inman WHW (1981 a) Post-marketing surveillance of adverse drug reactions in general practise I. Search for new methods. Br Med J 282:1131–1134

Inman WHW (1981 b) Post-marketing surveillance of adverse drug reactions in general practise. II. Prescription event monitoring at the University of Southampton. Br Med J 282:1216–1218

Inman WHW (1988) Blood disorders and suicide in patients taking mianserin or amitriptyline. Lancet 2:90–93

Jick H, Walker AM, Spriet-Poura C (1979) Post-marketing follow-up. JAMA 242:2310–2314

Leonard BE (1986) Toxicity of antidepressants. Lancet 2:1105

Montgomery SA, Pinder RM (1987) Do some antidepressants promote suicide? Psychopharmacology (Berlin) 92:265–266

Office of Population Censuses and Surveys (1977–1984) Morality statistics: accidents and violence. Series DH4, table 10. Deaths from poisoning by solid or liquid substances. HMSO, London

Pinder RM (1988) The benefits and risks of antidepressant drugs. Hum Psychopharmacol 3:73–86

Proudfoot AT (1986) Acute poisoning with antidepressants and lithium. Prescribers J 26/4:1–10

Rawlins MD (1984) Post-marketing surveillance of adverse reactions to drugs. Br Med J 288:579–583

Speirs C (1988) Reporting the risks. In: Leonard BE, Parker SW (eds) Risk/benefits of antidepressants. Duphar Medical, Southampton, UK, pp 53–59

A General Perspective of Post-Marketing Surveillance

D. G. GRAHAME-SMITH [1]

Introduction

For 12 years I was a member of the Committee on Safety of Medicines (CSM) in the United Kingdom and latterly Chairman of a CSM Working Party on Post-Marketing Surveillance (PMS). It is from this general perspective that I approach the problem. There have been several excellent published discussions on PMS and related problems to which the reader is referred (Inman 1986; Mann 1987). Although there is special complex technology associated with the collection of information and its analysis in the various types of PMS, the most important matter is the education of the medical profession in the concepts and needs of PMS, without whose positive support no scheme of PMS can succeed.

It is important to appreciate that PMS is a phase of drug development. The problem begins with assessment of benefits versus risks in the establishment of effective and safe drug therapy. For example, if one considers a hypothetical drug for a very serious indication, such as heart failure, which has excellent efficacy with a very low incidence of adverse drug reactions (ADRs), the severities of which are trivial, the drug is said to have an excellent benefit:risk ratio, and it is accepted as being "very good" (Table 1). On the other hand, if the medical indications for the drug are trivial, say tension headache, its efficacy is poor, it has a high incidence of ADRs of a serious nature, it plainly has a poor benefit:risk ratio, and one would seriously question whether it should continue on the market for that indication. Between these two extremes there are all grades of benefit:risk ratio. The important point to emphasise is that in making practical decisions about drug therapy, whether it be at the level of the individual patient, at a population level, or in a regulatory context, the

Table 1. Factors in benefit versus risk assessment

Indications	Efficacy	Incidence of ADR	Severity of ADR
Serious	Excellent	High	Serious
Trivial	Poor	Low	Trivial

[1] MRC Unit and University Department of Clinical Pharmacology Radcliffe Infirmary, Oxford, United Kingdom.

Neuropsychopharmacology
Edited by Bunney/Hippius/Laakmann/Schmauß

concept of benefit versus risk should be kept in mind constantly. In this context one must consider the indications for the drug, its efficacy, the incidence of ADRs and their severity.

There are helpful practical applications of these concepts. In the United Kingdom, phenylbutazone has ceased to be available as a non-steroidal anti-inflammatory drug for muscular, skeletal or arthritic conditions other than ankylosing spondylitis, now the sole indication because of the risks of aplastic anaemia. Some drugs have been removed from the market because there has been a general perception that while efficacy was good, risks were greater than with other members of the therapeutic class. Perhaps nomifensin and zimelidine fall into this class. The immunological ADRs produced by these two drugs were particularly pernicious, and their relative benefit versus risk assessment against other drugs of the same therapeutic class therefore became an important consideration.

Fallability of Clinical Experience

It is part of traditional medical practice that the one-to-one physician-patient relationship is paramount, and the strength of this relationship emphasises in the practioner's mind anecdotal experience and tends to obscure appreciation of epidemiological factors in drug use. With certain treatments, for example, antihypertensive therapy in mild asymptomatic hypertension (even though the blood pressure *is* lowered), it is never within the personal experience of an individual physician to know whether the treatment really prevents stroke. The benefit at the population level may be appreciable, but it is of a degree insufficient to impinge on the physician's personal experience. The physician is absolutely reliant upon large-scale clinical trials for guidance in such therapeutic situations.

Similarly, infrequent ADRs, for example, aplastic anaemia caused by chlorampherical or phenylbutazone, do not often impinge on a physician's personal experience (and if they do, they produce a powerful negative anecdotal experience). But, it is not uncommon to hear individual physicians assert, "But I've never had any trouble with that drug!" Have they personally treated 30000 patients? Such attitudes die hard, and they influence the perception of ADRs and the approach of practitioners to the place of post-marketing surveillance. Active education of the medical professional in the epidemiological perspectives underlying PMS is very important.

The Influence of Intensive Marketing on ADR Perspective

There is a link between intensive post-marketing promotion and our perspective of the "importance" of ADRs for an individual drug. Let us suppose, for instance, that a drug is introduced with a serious ADR, having an incidence of one in 10000. In a simplistic view, if the prescribing rate is 10000 patients per year, it will take several years for the associated ADR to be appreciated. If the drug is very efficacious, it is quite likely to be "tolerated" by prescribing physicians. If the prescribing rate is 100 000 patients per year, and if the ADR is a serious and clear one, it is likely to become recognised in a year or so. However if intensive marketing techniques produce a prescribing rate of one million per year, then within 3 months 25 patients will have suffered. This will make a much greater impact on the regulatory authority, the pharmaceutical firm, the prescribers and on potential recipients – even though the *incidence* of the ADR is the same with the differing prescribing rates.

The Crucial Argument for PMS Studies

When a new drug is licensed, its safety will have been assessed in pharmacological and toxicological studies in animals and from the results of clinical trials in human patients – usually providing information, however, from only 1000–2000 patients. Whether or not ADRs come to light depends upon statistical evaluation of its incidence of the confounding effect of natural and spontaneous events which mimic the ADR (i.e. background noise), the number of patients receiving the drug and the diligence of observation and reporting.

These statistical aspects are put into perspective by Table 2, which accompanied the Report of the Working Party of the CSM on PMS and was prepared by Dr. Gerald Jones, the Senior Principal Medical Officer of the Medicines Division of the Department of Health and Social Security, United Kindom. Let us suppose (and these are not entirely unreasonable guesses), that the background non-drug related risk over the whole population of having a bleeding peptic ulcer is one in 10 000, and that the incidence of a bleeding peptic ulcer as an ADR to a non-steroidal inflammatory drug is one in 5000. As shown in Table 2, 67 400 patients would have to be exposed to detect this drug-related risk with statistical confidence. This is the sort of ADR with which we are all familiar, and that we accept as having a fairly high incidence, yet the number of patients which must be exposed in order to calculate the statistical risk involved is far beyond that which is ever likely to be achieved in pre-marketing clinical trials or to come within the anecdotal experience of individual physicians or a working group of physicians.

The aim of post-marketing surveillance is to measure the risks of ADRs and their severity sufficiently quantitatively so that one can go on to evaluate benefits versus risks. This is of vital importance in the assessment of drugs of comparable efficacy where differences in risk become increasingly important. A number of systems have been put forward for post-marketing surveillance:

- Spontaneous reporting
- Cohort studies (including prescription-based surveillance)
- Case control studies
- Record linkage
- Population statistics (e.g. death certificate data)

Table 2. The minimum number of patients who need to be exposed to a drug to detect a particular level of risk at varying levels of background incidence

Incidence (risk) of ADR be detected	Spontaneous background incidence of the adverse event	Minimum number of patients to be exposed
1 in 100	0	360
	1 in 10000	520
	1 in 1000	730
	1 in 100	2000
1 in 500	0	1800
	1 in 10000	3200
	1 in 1000	6700
	1 in 100	35900
1 in 1000	0	3600
	1 in 10000	7300
	1 in 1000	20300
	1 in 100	136400
1 in 5000	0	18200
	1 in 10000	67400
	1 in 1000	363000
	1 in 100	3255000

To detect an ADR occurring at the rate of 1 in 1000 (exposed) when the spontaneous background incidence is 1 in 1000 (in the absence of the drug) requires observations on at least 20300 patients taking the drug.

These figures were calculated from the normal approximation to the binominal distribution. The spontaneous background incidence was assumed to be known and fixed. A false-positive (α) error of 0.05 and a false-negative (β) error of 0.05 were assumed.

Source: CSM Working Party Report on Post-Marketing Surveillance 1985.

Spontaneous Reporting

The CSM in the United Kingdom decided that a spontaneous reporting system based upon physicians use of the "yellow card", whether written or computerised, is an essential PMS method for the foreseeable future. However, spontaneous reporting by means of this yellow card cannot meet all the information requirements. The system does have certain very positive attributes. These include the following:

- It operates as soon as the drug is marketed and provides a mechanism whereby a physician may report a reaction to a central, national point as soon as it is suspected.
- It is the only technique that collects information on all marketed drugs.
- It draws attention to previously unsuspected possible adverse effects of drugs.
- It provides confirmatory evidence in the form of further reports of the particular problem following first alerts in the literature.

- It can assist (although numerically imprecisely) in the assessment of the benefit: risk ratio of a drug compared with similar drugs.

Its drawbacks, on the other hand, are:

- The reports are observations of suspected association, and there is no control group. Merely plausible ADRs related in time to drug exposure tend to get reported.
- There is under-reporting. In any particular case the amount of this is unknown so that we have no good denominator for the number of ADR reports.
- There may be delay in submitting reports.
- Reports can be inaccurate or imprecise and without further enquiry difficult to validate.
- Reporting rates may be biased by publicity about ADR problems with a particular drug.
- There are problems analysing prescribing rates (repeat prescriptions, differences in quantities, doses prescribed).
- Similar drugs may be used in different types of patients, making comparison of ADR data difficult to comprehend.

Cohort Studies

In cohort studies the medical events occurring during follow-up of a cohort of patients using a drug are compared with those occurring in an appropriate control group not using the drug. Uncontrolled studies of cohorts are almost impossible to interpret because of the background incidence of events.

In principle, cohort studies can be designed and conducted as required to investigate specific drug safety risks. Large, specific cohort studies have been carried out on the adverse effects of oral contraceptives, hypertensive drugs and H_2-receptor antagonist drugs. Such special studies need to be large. They therefore take a long time to set up, are complex to analyse, but nevertheless fulfil a very special need. In my view, they are best used to achieve a definitive perspective on the qualitative and quantitative aspects of drug safety. But because of their very nature they are no use as a "fire-fighting" exercise.

We need to apply systems which allow one to estimate *quickly* the occurrence and incidence of reactions to drugs coming onto the market and provide clues as to the factors involved, e.g. age, sex, concurrent diseases, concurrent drug therapy and dosage problems. Systems in which patients who have received a drug can be identified from the prescription, i.e. prescription event monitoring, are finding favour. Once an event is identified, the prescribing physician can then be asked specific questions about suspected ADRs or asked to list any medical events which occurred before, during or after the treatment. The only general purpose prescription-based surveillance scheme operating in the United Kingdom at the present time is the prescription event monitoring (PEM) system developed by Prof. W.H. Inman at the Drug

Surveillance Research Unit, University of Southampton. This PEM system collects data about medical events rather than reports of suspected ADRs. It provides a reasonably precise denominator which allows a better estimate of risk than the yellow card system and enables physicians to be contacted directly about each patient in the cohort. In addition, under-reporting seems to be less of a problem.

The handling and interpretation of report forms is neither easy nor cheap, and expense rises with the size of the cohort. Inman's studies have been limited generally to cohorts of around 10000 patients, and this number may be insufficient to detect a low incidence of important ADRs. Professor Inman estimates that about 60% of physicians comply with his requests to complete reports. However, if the prescription-based surveillance scheme is extended to involve more and more drugs as they come onto the market, compliance in reporting is likely to fall as the demands on reporting physicians rise. Physicians do have other things to do than to report adverse drug reactions!

Case Control Studies

In case control studies patients who are affected by an ADR are identified, and their past medical and drug histories are compared with those of an unaffected controlled group. These studies are designed to test hypotheses about ADR and cannot be used to identify new, unsuspected ADRs. Additionally, they can only rarely provide an absolute estimate of risk. They can be smaller and easier to conduct than cohort studies and can be used to investigate uncommon or rare ADRs. An important example of the use of this type of study is the investigation of the relationships between drug use in pregnancy and congenital malformations.

Record Linkage

Record linkage systems bring together prescription records and hospital discharge records enabling investigation of possible links between drugs and disease. It therefore follows that it is necessary to (a) retrieve prescriptions and identify them; (b) retrieve hospital discharge records (having ensured recording of appropriate data on diagnosis and outcome); and (c) link them.

An increasing number of record linkage systems exist in the United States, where in geographically defined areas computerised methods of accounting identify prescriptions and link them with hospital attendances and diagnoses. In the United Kingdom, the most promising research is being carried out at the Universities of Dundee and Aberdeen under the aegis of the Medicines Evaluation and Monitoring Group (MEMO). Prescriptions for identified drugs written by general practitioners are identified by the Prescription Pricing Authority and passed to MEMO, who link them with hospital records. Without an identification number, the process of linking prescriptions to hospital records is exceedingly cumbersone, time wasting, fraught with errors and expensive. Thus, if record linkage is ever envisaged, it will be necessary to have a unique patient identification number used in all aspects of the patient's health care. We do not generally have this as yet in the United Kingdom.

Record linkage needs to be applied to a large population group of at most 5 million persons to allow identification of sufficiently large cohorts of medicine users of and control groups. However, if the linkage of prescriptions is to hospital records only, the technique would not identify ADRs which do not lead to hospitalisation. These would require a link to primary health care practice records, which would be extremely expensive and difficult to implement. The interpretation of confusing relationships between drugs prescribed and events leading to hospital treatment can be very difficult, indeed, and needs a sophisticated awareness of the tricks that record linkage can play.

Record linkage is able to investigate ADRs to new drugs once they have been on the market sufficently long to penetrate the market adequately. It also enables investigation of a large number of different drugs (provided the prescriptions can be identified) and would theoretically enable the investigation of links between drug prescription and long-latency diseases such as cancer.

Record linkage is extremely attractive for the overall monitoring of ADRs. However the technology is expensive to set up and run, is labour intensive on a national scale and requires "missionary zeal" to initiate it and to persuade governments to invest in it.

Population Statistics

In the United Kingdom the Office of Population Census and Surveys collects statistics on patterns of mortality from causes of death identified on death certificates. In certain instances these statistics provide useful indicators of patterns for mortality which may be drug related. However, even where trends of apparent association are suggested, it usually is not possible to establish a causal link with a drug. The data can, however, be useful in formulating hypotheses which can be examined in detail using other techniques.

The Current Need for PMS Studies

In the United Kingdom it has been recommended that post-marketing surveillance studies be carried out on most new chemical entities licensed which are likely to have widespread use. Such PMS studies would be requested under voluntary arrangements agreed between the regulation authorities and the pharmaceutical industry. The post-marketing surveillance technique used may vary from drug to drug. The pharmaceutical company in consultation with the CSM intended would decide on the appropriate nature of the studies. For drugs for widespread use, cohorts of at least 10 000 patients have been thought appropriate, and careful consideration must be given to the nature of control groups. Valuable new drug studies of this size using prescription-based surveillance techniques are currently being undertaken. One may criticise the number 10000, but a study of this size does give some indication of risk. That is, some upper limit of risk which in the phase after the introduction of a drug is an estimate, that is probably better than nothing. This is not to say that later studies will not establish a quantified risk of hazard in fewer than 10 000 subjects, but depending upon the penetration of the drug in the market, at least within the first 2 years, one may have established a rough upper limit of the risk, which can be balanced against perceived benefit.

Who Should Report ADRs?

I do not believe that patients should report their own ADRs because of the tremendous amount of useless "noise" that this would produce in the system.

The role of the pharmacist in reporting ADRs is a sensitive and difficult one. Hospital pharmacists are already often involved in operating drug information centres and work as members of teams investigating and reporting ADRs, but generally and traditionally it has been the physician's responsibility to report ADRs, although plainly the pharmacist can help formulate the details which go to make up such reports. In general it seems best that if the pharmacist spots an ADR or "event", it should be brought to the attention of the physician who prescribed the drug. The physician would then have to decide what action to take. I believe it would produce division between the two professions and their professional practice if pharmacists were to report ADRs directly to the regulatory authority, independently of physicians, and that this would be to the patients' detriment in the long run. The collaboration between the professions of pharmacy and medicine in the detection and reporting of ADRs needs more positive development, particularly in hospital practice.

Industry's Role in Reporting ADRs

The considerable resources that the pharmaceutical industry possess are not being harnessed sufficiently in the field of ADR reporting (in the United Kingdom at least). Non-medical management in the pharmaceutical industry needs to be made aware that ADRs are a natural consequence of innovative, biologically active new drugs, that the benefit:risk ratio is a fundamental concept in drug therapy, and that it does no good to dismiss, ignore or belittle the importance of ADRs. The industry at all levels must take a position of complete integrity toward ADR reporting. Bias towards benefits and against risks must not be allowed to cloud the issue. The problem must be faced squarely and honestly at all levels, throughout all the different disciplines in industry involved in drug development. Dr. R. N. Smith, in his Presidential Address to the Section of Experimental Medicine. delivered on 27 January 1986, made the point that there should be much more transnational interaction on ADRs, and that the information provided to the central regulatory authority of one nation ought to be automatically available to those of other nations.

Finally, I think the way forward is, in principle, quite clear. A spontaneous reporting system is necessary for PMS, such as the yellow card system or some computerised version of it. There should be the facility of ad hoc studies, either cohort studies or case control studies, as the situation demands. Prescription-based surveillance schemes for marketed new drugs are plainly attractive, recognising that this method may not be appropriate for some new drugs. Record linkage for ADR monitoring should be developed further and embrace some millions of the population. It will need great determination and lobbying to establish national or international routine working systems of this nature.

References

Inman WHW (1986) Monitoring for drug safety, 2nd edn. MTP Press, Lancaster, UK
Mann RD (1987) Adverse drug reactions. Parthenon, Lancaster, UK

Surveillance of Adverse Drug Reactions in the United States *

R. S. K. Young [1]

The postmarketing drug surveillance program of the United States Food and Drug Administration (FDA) is mandated by the Food, Drug and Cosmetic Act (FD & C). When first enacted by Congress in 1906, this law had no reporting provision for adverse drug reactions (ADRs) discovered in the course of selling a drug. The requirement that the party marketing a drug report such reactions was imposed when the statute was amended in 1962, principally in reaction to the adverse effects of thalidomide.

The FD & C is federal (national) legislation, and the FDA is a federal agency. As law, the FD & C is proscriptive, and those parties upon which obligations are imposed, such as a drug manufacturer, are subject to penalties if they fail to meet their responsibilities. On the other hand, no other parties have a legal obligation, although they may retain a professional or moral obligation. Thus the commercial distributor of a drug is obligated to report ADRs, whereas a treating physician who actually uncovers an ADR is under no legal obligation to report his observations to anyone other than his patient.

The FD & C is a product of the political system of the United States. The Congress and the President attempt to balance the perceived interests of a multitude of parties affected by standards imposed upon drugs administered to humans in the United States. Because compromise among the hundreds of members of Congress, the President's staff, drug manufacturers, consumers, medical professionals, etc. is frequently necessary to obtain some solution to a problem, legislative directives are not always clear. Lack of clarity in the law also sometimes arises because legislators, although theoretically well informed by their own staff and technical consultants, are not professional scientists or physicians. Furthermore, the judicial branch of government, which is generally composed of lawyers, also shapes food and drug laws through its interpretation of the various provisions of the FD & C. The FDA thus administers and functions within the confines of a law, which it did not write, and although it interprets its legislative mandate, definitive construction is rendered not by the agency itself but by the courts.

---

* The views expressed in this chapter are those of the author and not necessarily those of the Food and Drug Administration.

[1] Food and Drug Administration, HFD-344, 5600 Fishers Lane, Rockville, MD 20857, USA.

Neuropsychopharmacology
Edited by Bunney/Hippius/Laakmann/Schmauß

As errors which the FDA commits in carrying out its directive can be corrected by further legislation, the FDA is subject to congressional oversight, including public hearings on any of its actions. Given the great interest in and importance of matters of health, the FDA is also justly subjected to scrutiny in the press. As with many regulatory agencies, the actions taken by the FDA rarely pleases everyone, and usually manages to offend someone.

The provisions of the FD & C tend to be conservative. Generally they have been imposed because some specific catastrophe resulted in a perceived need to do something to avoid repetition of such an event. The initial 1906 legislation sought to inform consumers as to what ingredients are in the medicines that they use. The 1938 amendment imposed upon a drug manufacturer a premarket testing requirement to demonstrate that its drug is "safe," i.e., that it has no great propensity for being seriously, acutely toxic. It was the sale of a liquid preparation of sulfanilamide that caused the death of over 100 customers which prompted this change in standards. The product's solvent, diethylene glycol, which is nephrotoxic had not been tested for toxicity before the preparation went onto the market.

The 1962 amendment imposed upon drug manufacturers an obligation to report ADRs associated with marketed drugs. This represented a response to the thalidomide disaster in which a marketed product caused some 10000 malformations worldwide. This amendment also added the "effectiveness" provision and required that clinical investigations meet minimum scientific standards, i.e., testing in unbiased controlled studies.

New drug development is commonly divided into three segments: preclinical (animal), clinical (human), and postmarketing (commercial). The new drug provisions of the FD & C confer direct jurisdiction to the FDA only when drugs are administered to human beings, i.e., in the latter two segments. For convenience, the clinical segment is subdivided into phases I, II, and III, i.e., dose ranging, biological activity, and therapeutic usefulness studies, respectively. This experimental segment is commonly referred to as the IND (investigational new drug) segment whereas the marketing segment is denominated as the NDA (new drug application) segment. These acronyms are derived from the applications which must be submitted to the FDA and approved before human drug administration can legally begin.

On the average it takes 18 months to complete preclinical studies, 60 months for clinical trials, and 24 months for review of an application. On the average the number of subjects entered are 25 for phase I studies, 100 for phase II studies, and 1000 for phase III studies. The duration of drug administration in the controlled portion of a clinical trial may be short, and thereby only a small proportion of the duration of a chronic disease. For example, trials of drugs which control chronic diseases such as hypertension or rheumatoid arthritis symptomatically may be only 6–12 weeks long. As clinical experience with every new drug is quite limited, there is no expectation that all effects of a drug will be elucidated before a drug is marketed. Effects most likely to be missed are those which are rare, delayed, restricted to a peculiar group of patients, manifest only after cumulative doses larger than that achieved in the clinical trials, or the result of interaction with other drugs. Drug tolerance and resistance may also be discovered only after a drug is marketed. An efficient surveillance program which systematically collects information generated during marketing is essential to promptly discovering serious effects of a drug not uncovered in the clinical trials. Since at least one beneficial effect of a new drug must be demonstrated before marketing, most postmarketing efforts have been directed to uncovering the adverse or toxic effects of marketed drugs.

At present time, there are more than 35000 dosage forms of prescription drugs, e.g., Valium 2 mg, 5 mg, etc., being marketed by 3700 firms in the United States. The 100 most frequently prescribed drug entities, however, account for some 70% of all outpatient prescriptions. The United States domestic market is huge, the current population of the country being 240 million persons. Except for substances which may be addictive, drugs approved for marketing can be sold without restriction throughout the United States.

Responsibility for oversight of human drugs is located in eight FDA reviewing divisions, which are subdivided into groups according to therapeutic classes of drugs, e.g., anti-cancer, anti-inflammatory, anti-viral, endocrine. These divisions have complete responsibility for human drug use, i.e., in both the developmental (IND) and marketing (NDA) phases. Each drug product is assigned to a team of scientists that includes physicians, chemists, and pharmacologists. Based on data submitted by a manufacturer or researcher, they make the decision as to whether there is sufficient scientific evidence to justify clinical trials or general marketing of a drug. They also decide whether, in light of new information on a marketed drug, the sale of such drug should be restricted, curtailed, or stopped altogether.

Assisting the reviewing divisions are groups of consultants, such as biostaticians, pharmacokineticists, manufacturing and advertising experts, and medical epidemiologists. Consulting responsibility for postmarketing surveillance is centered in the Division of Epidemiology and Surveillance, which presently is composed of 50 professionals. This group was originally organized to evaluate ADR reports submitted to the agency. It has since added epidemiological activities to support and complement its ADR activities.

With its postmarketing monitoring system for ADRs, the FDA hopes not only to acquire the inevitable new information about a drug but also to acquire this information in a timely manner so that intelligent decisions about a drug's benefits may be tailored to and be in step with its adverse effects. For those drug products which are produced by only one manufacturer, this manufacturer is the primary collector and evaluator of ADR data. It is the goal of the FDA that this manufacturer also be the primary decision maker as to the appropriate course of action to be taken as new ADR information is accumulated about marketed products, e.g., adding or strengthening contraindications or warnings, modifying dosage or administration recommendations, and deleting misleading or unsupported claims of effectiveness.

The FDA employs an expanded definition of ADR, one which includes not only what is commonly considered as such an event, i.e., one which occurs in the course of the use of a drug, but also those which are the result of overdoses, drug abuse, drug withdrawal, and failure of the expected pharmacological action. A form, FDA 1639, has been developed to standardize reporting of data sought about an ADR, including demographic information on the patient, e.g., name, age, and sex; information on the drug, e.g., dose, route of administration; and information on the reaction, e.g., date, description, and outcome. Although all ADRs received by a manufacturer are forwarded to the FDA, serious unexpected ADRs are to be reported within 15 working days. A serious reaction is one that is life threatening or permanently disabling, and that requires hospitalization or drug therapy, e.g., death, congenital abnormalities, or cancer. An unexpected reaction is one not specifically listed in the package insert. Also to be reported promptly are increases in the rate of occurrence (reporting) of a particular adverse drug experience.

Because physicians who detect ADRs are under no legal obligation to report them, the ADRs which they do submit are "spontaneous" or voluntary. Other sources of ADRs are postmarketing clinical investigations, epidemiological/surveillance studies, and published and unpublished papers. Most physicians report ADRs to the manufacturer and not directly to the FDA. That there is serious underreporting of ADRs is highlighted in a recent survey (Rogers et al. 1988) in which 37% of the 3000 urban Maryland physicians sampled returned their questionaires; only 5% who stated they had detected an ADR had reported it. Also disturbing was the fact that only 57% of respondents claimed even to know of the FDA reporting system. The FDA is itself well aware that many ADRs go undetected, i.e., unrecognized, although it appears that those resulting in death or hospitalization are more frequently recognized and reported.

More than 50000 ADR reports are received annually, and the FDA's computerized data base contains almost 400000 reports. ADRs detected in investigational studies are not entered into the postmarketing surveillance data base. When an ADR report is received, it is first classified according to standardized key terms using a sign and symptom thesaurus – the Coding Thesaurus of Standardized Reaction Terms. An ADR report may be assigned a maximum of four reaction terms, the most serious of which characterizes it. Up to five drugs can be linked to a reaction, ranked in order of its index of suspicion for causing the reaction. Case reports are entered into the database without professional evaluation.

All serious, unlabeled reactions are immediately and individually referred to a health professional for evaluation. An on-line search of the file is conducted to determine whether similar reactions have been reported previously for the suspect drug. Several reports or one well-documented, unambiguous case report is denominated a monitored adverse reaction (MAR) and is currently evaluated by a team including physicians from the appropriate reviewing division, drug utilization experts, and epidemiologists. After their initial evaluation, MARs are categorized as annual or signal MARs. If no further reports are received, annual status MARs are formally reevaluated each year. Signal status MARs are accorded an ongoing investigation and evaluation including search of the scientific literature and drug marketing and epidemiological data bases. Special monitoring or postmarketing studies may be implemented to further define the reaction.

A myriad of uncontrolled factors confine the ADR reporting system to the somewhat unsatisfying but still important task of raising suspicions that a previously undescribed ADR is real and important. Causality cannot be ascribed. A given ADR may in fact be a misdiagnosis, a manifestation of the underlying disease, or caused by a concomitant drug. Only a reporting rate can be calculated, not the actual occurrence rate. Furthermore, the reporting rate is subject to marked distortion. Rates of reporting are higher for drugs newly on the market and for more serious ADRs, i.e., those resulting in hospitalization or death. Some classes of drugs, for example, nonsteroidal anti-inflammatory agents, have higher reporting rates than might be expected from population exposure data. Manufacturers differ as to their promotional, detailing, and reporting practices. Reports in the literature, regulatory action (e.g., an alerting letter or solicitation for reaction reports), and publicity also affect the reporting rate. Finally, the actual number of persons exposed and the amount/duration of exposure is unknown.

Because of the limitations associated with ADR reports, specific studies are generally needed to gather sufficient data upon which to base regulatory decisions. Field investigation, rapid systematic case finding and characterization, and the employment of cohort or case-control methodology are often required. A recent example of a previously unreported adverse reaction (flank pain syndrome) associated with a newly marketed drug (suprofen) which was detected by the ADR report system, evaluated, and acted upon has been published (Rossi et al. 1988). In order to better estimate drug exposure and changing patterns of drug use several data bases are followed including those provided by IMS America (Ambler, PA) and Medicaid.

A scientific approach to the collection and interpretation of postmarketing surveillance data is provided by epidemiological studies. Analytic methods such as stratifying, matching, etc. are used to control problems such as confounding and bias. The FDA may require a manufacturer to conduct a postmarketing study, conducts some studies itself, and conducts others by contract. It also collaborates with other investigators in research projects. For example, the FDA participates in a case-control surveillance study through the Boston Collaborative Drug Surveillance Program (Waltham, MA) and makes use of linked data bases through the Puget Sound Health Maintenance Organization (Seattle, WA), Mayo Clinic (Rochester, MN), and several state Medicaid systems (Michigan, Minnesota, and Tennessee).

In the United States, postmarketing surveillance requires a mix of programs and activities appropriate to the existing social and legal environment governing the use of drugs. The various programs of the FDA have only recently been restructered (Faich 1986) and have yet to be tested by a major pharmaceutic disaster. Although institutional safeguards have been set in place, it appears that much remains to be done to motivate the individual practitioner to contribute his singularly important observations to the system

(Edlavitch 1988) and to advance the process of identification of new ADRs beyond mere pattern recognition (gestalt).

Acknowledgement. The author thanks Charles Anello, D. Sc. for helping him obtain the material necessary to prepare this manuscript.

References

Edlavitch SA (1988) Adverse drug event reporting. Arch Intern Med 148:1499–1503

Faich GA (1986) Postmarketing surveillance of prescription drugs: current status. Clinical Research Institute, New York

Rogers AS, Israel E, Smith CR, Levine D, McBean AM, Valente C, Faich G (1988) Physician knowledge, attitudes, and behavior related to reporting adverse drug events. Arch Intern Med 148:1596–1600

Rossi AC, Bosco L, Faich GA, Tanner A, Temple R (1988) The importance of adverse reaction reporting by physicians. JAMA 259:1203–1204

15 Pharmacological Aspects of Sleep and Sleep Disorders

Sleep and Sleep Deprivation Studies in Patients with Premenstrual Depression

B. L. Parry[1,2], W. B. Mendelson[1], W. B. Duncan[1], D. A. Sack[1], and T. A. Wehr[1]

Sleep Studies in PMS Patients

Various sleep abnormalities such as decreased or increased sleep, fragmented sleep, shortened REM latency, phase advance of REM sleep, fragmentation of REM sleep, increased REM density, and decreased delta sleep have been described in depression (Gillin et al. 1984). Furthermore, sleep manipulations affect mood in many affective patients (Gillin 1983; Wehr et al. 1987). Specifically, sleep deprivation may mitigate depression, and sleep may promote it (in patients who respond to sleep deprivation). Since women sleep longer than men (Wever 1984; Wirz-Justice et al. 1984), and women are more likely to develop depression (Weissman and Klerman 1977), investigations of the effect of cyclic changes in the female neuroendocrine reproductive axis on sleep may increase our understanding of women's vulnerability to depression. Furthermore, since many depressed patients undergoing sleep studies are women, as a methodological issue it is important to know whether reproductive status or phase of the menstrual cycle affects sleep. We designed this study to investigate the effect of the menstrual cycle on the sleep of women with and without premenstrual affective changes.

Some women with premenstrual syndrome (PMS), more specifically described in the DSM-III-R as late luteal phase dysphoric disorder, have depressive symptoms during the luteal or premenstrual phase of their menstrual cycle. Since several studies (Halbreich and Endicott 1985; Endicott et al. 1981; Wetzel et al. 1975; Schuckit et al. 1975; MacKenzie et al. 1986; Hallman 1986) suggest that PMS may be related to the affective disorders, we sought to determine whether sleep disturbances that occur in depressed patients occur in PMS patients as well.

In rats, levels of motor activity and REM and non-REM sleep vary across the estrous cycle in a predictable way. Motor activity increases and REM sleep decreases during proestrus and estrus at the time of ovulation. Activity decreases and sleep increases during diestrus when gonadal hormones decline

[1] Clinical Psychobiology Branch, National Institute of Mental Health, 10/4S–239, 9000 Rockville Pike, Bethesda, MD 20205, USA.

[2] *Present address*: Department of Psychiatry, University of California, San Diego T-004, La Jolla, CA 92093, USA.

Neuropsychopharmacology
Edited by Bunney/Hippius/Laakmann/Schmauß

(Colvin et al. 1968; Yokoyama et al. 1966). These effects can be blocked by ovariectomy and can be reinstated with gonadal hormone replacement (Colvin et al. 1969; Branchey et al. 1971). It is unknown whether analogous changes occur across the normal human menstrual cycle.

In this study (Parry et al. 1989), we examined sleep across the menstrual cycle in patients with prospectively documented PMS and in age- and sex-matched control subjects without significant PMS. We hypothesized that (a) changes in REM and non-REM sleep, similar to those occurring across the estrus cycle in animals, occur across the menstrual cycle in normal women, and (b) disturbances in sleep similar to those which occur in major depressive disorders (MDD) occur during the premenstrual phase in women with PMS.

Sleep, temperature, and activity measurements in humans reflect the oscillations of endogenous pacemakers (Wever 1984; Aschoff 1979; Wehr and Wirz-Justice 1980). In some depressed patients, the timing or phase position of an oscillator controlling REM sleep and temperature has been hypothesized to be shifted abnormally earlier (phase advanced) relative to the timing of another oscillator controlling sleep and activity (Kripke 1978; Wehr and Goodwin 1983). We sought to determine whether similar chronobiologic disturbances occur in patients with PMS by measuring rectal temperature and wrist motor activity across the menstrual cycle in PMS patients and controls.

Subjects and Methods

Patients were referred from local gynecologists and psychiatrists, from an NIH information center, from a local community mental health center and women's group, and via an advertisement placed in a local newspaper requesting subjects for studies of mood and behavior changes during the menstrual cycle. Subjects completed screening questionnaires, and a psychiatrist obtained a medical and psychiatric history and performed a physical examination. Samples of blood were obtained for chemistry, blood counts, urinalysis, and thyroid tests. If, based on these screening procedures, the patient had no history of major medical, gynecologic or psychiatric illness (except affective illness), was having regular menstrual cycles, appeared to have premenstrual symptoms which were severe enough to disrupt social or occupational functioning, and was willing to endure the rigors of a long-term research study, she was admitted to a 2-month evaluation phase. This evaluation period consisted of twice daily ratings of mood, daily sleep logs, weekly mood inventories, activity monitoring using a wrist actometer (Colburn et al. 1976), and weekly clinic visits for a psychiatric rating (Hamilton Rating Scale for Depression, HRSD; Hamilton 1967).

Based on these 2-month prospective ratings, subjects were included in the study in whom the timing and severity of affective symptoms met DSM-III criteria for major depressive episode during the week prior to menses (excluding the 2-week duration criterion). Since we were interested in studying the relationship of PMS and MDD, an ongoing affective illness, but not a history of affective illness, was reason for exclusion from the study. The timing of patients' affective symptoms was such that the onset and peak intensity occurred during the week prior to menses with an offset of symptoms within a few days following the onset of menses. All subjects gave informed consent prior to participation in the study. At the time of the study, patients had been free of psychoactive medications for 2 months except for one patient who was maintained on thyroid supplement.

After a night of adaptation, subjects had sleep EEG recordings on an NIMH research ward 2 nights per week for the duration of one menstrual cycle. Subjects slept in a room by themselves and were asked to adhere to their normal sleep schedule. They were asked to complete daily sleep and mood ratings during the month of sleep studies. Subjects' clinical states were assessed in the evening before and the morning after the sleep studies by a specially trained nurse research team using a modified Bunney-Hamburg scale (Bunney and Hamburg 1963) with global ratings of depression, mania, anxiety, and psychosis. Subjects entered the study at different phases of their menstrual cycles to avoid sequencing effects. They were asked to abstain from alcohol and drugs, including aspirin, during the study and to adhere to a low-monoamine diet 2 days prior to each sleep recording. Serum collected the morning after each sleep recording was assayed using standardized radioimmunoassay techniques for estradiol, progesterone, follicle-stimulating hormone, luteinizing hormone, prolactin, growth hormone, and cortisol.

The onset of menses was used to calculate menstrual cycle length for each individual. Each subject's cycle was then divided into four equal phases in which phase 1 corresponds to the early follicular phase, phase 2 to the late follicular phase, phase 3 to the early luteal, and phase 4 to the late luteal or premenstrual phase of the menstrual cycle. This approach made it possible to compare individuals with different cycle lengths. A technician scored the sleep records using the criteria of Rechtschaffen and Kales (1968). The data were analyzed for group effects (patients versus controls), phase of the menstrual cycle effects (phase 1 versus 2 versus 3 versus 4), and interaction between these effects using a two-way analysis of variance (ANOVA) with repeated measures. Main effects were analyzed with post hoc *t* tests with the Bonferroni correction for multiple comparisons.

Results

Forty patients were screened. Eight patients and eight women without significant premenstrual mood disturbances (controls), who also underwent at least 1 month of evaluation, entered the study. The mean age for both patients and control subjects was 30 years (range, 26–45 years). The mean HRSD for patients during the premenstrual phase was 16.5 ± 6.3. The mean HRSD for patients during the follicular phase and for controls in both the follicular and the premenstrual phases needed to be less than 7 for admission to the study. A description of the symptom profile of women with and without prospective confirmation of mood changes is reported elsewhere (Roy-Byrne et al. 1987).

Sleep Studies. Values for the principal sleep variables were as follows. Patients had a significantly ($p < 0.05$) higher percentage of stage II sleep (59.68 ± 11.36) than controls (48.83 ± 8.99). There was a trend ($p < 0.06$) in the same direction in stage II minutes (patients, 223.41 ± 49.77; controls, 186.15 ± 43.24). In patients, REM sleep minutes (81.3 ± 23.57) and percentage (21.7 ± 6.10) were significantly ($p < 0.05$) lower than in controls (104.17 ± 34.83 and 27.48 ± 8.43, respectively). REM sleep latency was similar in patients (95.21 ± 56.73) and in controls (84.54 ± 48.10). There were no significant differences between groups in total sleep, delta sleep, REM density, or duration of the first and second REM periods. Significant menstrual phase effects ($F = 5.29, p < 0.01$) were found (a) in stage III minutes: phase 1, 35.41 ± 27.51; phase 2, 41.36 ± 23.70; phase 3, 44.68 ± 20.15; phase 4, 33.58 ± 22.30; (b) in stage III percentage ($F = 5.65$, $p < 0.01$): phase 1, 9.10 ± 7.01; phase 2, 11.05 ± 6.47; phase 3, 12.06 ± 5.73; phase 4, 9.02 ± 6.38; and (c) in intermittent wakefulness ($F = 4.19$, $p < 0.01$): phase 1, 10.94 ± 4.56; phase 2, 9.64 ± 3.98; phase 3, 8.82 ± 6.57; phase 4, 16.06 ± 14.66. However post hoc t tests showed no significant differences among cycle phases with respect to these parameters. There were no significant interaction effects of group (patients versus normals) and phase of the menstrual cycle.

Hormone Studies. Progesterone levels (> 5 ng/ml) and temperature values in the luteal phase of the menstrual cycle indicated that the subjects had ovulated. The levels of reproductive hormones were not abnormal in any of the subjects, although marked inter- and intrasubject variability was present. There were multiple correlations between levels of the hormones measured (estradiol, progesterone, follicle-stimulating hormone, luteinizing hormone, prolactin, growth hormone, and cortisol) and sleep stages. Of particular interest, given the relationship of REM sleep and estrogen in rats, guinea pigs, and rabbits (Colvin et al. 1968; Malven and Sawyer 1966; Kawakami and Sawyer 1959), when patients and normals were combined, there was a significant inverse correlation of estradiol and REM minutes ($r = -0.26$, $df = 54$, $p = 0.05$) and REM percentage ($r = -0.29$, $df = 54$, $p = 0.02$). Also, there was a significant inverse relationship of prolactin and delta sleep ($r = -0.26$, $df = 57$, $p = 0.04$).

Temperature and Activity Studies. Motor activity levels did not show a consistent pattern of variation across the menstrual cycle. The mean daily activity counts in patients were: phase 1, 5438 ± 1036; phase 2, 4893 ± 1456; phase 3, 5067 ± 1231; phase 4, 5125 ± 1216. The means for control subjects were: phase 1, 5189 ± 829; phase 2, 5081 ± 680; phase 3, 5374 ± 6037; phase 4, 5665 ± 910. Examining the data by ANOVA, the main effect for diagnosis (patient versus control) was nonsignificant ($F = 0.20$, df = 1,13), for menstrual cycle phase (1–4) significant ($F = 2.48$, df = 3,39, $p = 0.01$) and for interaction nonsignificant ($F = 1.72$, df = 3,39).

Mean temperature minima in patients and controls did not differ significantly for menstrual cycle phase. In five subjects (two controls and three patients) there were two time points per night for the temperature minima. The occurrence of "double" minima was not related to menstrual cycle phase. In these cases, the earlier of the two temperature minima was used for data analysis. Although the time of the temperature minima was earlier in patients versus controls at all phases of the menstrual cycle, ANOVA showed no significant effect of group (patients versus controls; $F=0.12$, df$=1,44$) or phase of the menstrual cycle (1–4; $F=2.42$, df$=3,44$) on timing of the temperature minima, and there were no significant interactions ($F=0.46$, df$=3,44$). Similar results of a nonsignificant phase advance of the temperature rhythm in PMS patients compared to controls at all menstrual cycle phases were obtained when second temperature minima were used in data analysis.

Discussion

Patients had more stage II percentage sleep and less REM sleep (minutes and percentage) than controls. Stage III sleep and intermittent awakening varied with menstrual cycle phase. Patients with PMS did not have sleep EEG abnormalities that are often found in patients with MDD. Furthermore, there were no significant differences in the timing of temperature minima or in levels of motor activity data between patients and controls, nor were there among different phases of the menstrual cycle.

Our findings with polygraphic sleep recording techniques are mostly negative, but they must be interpretated with caution, since schedules and procedures used in the sleep laboratory may mask patients' natural sleep patterns. Other differences between groups or among phases may have been present but not detected because of the small size of the sample (type II error). Furthermore, individual variability in the timing of symptoms in relation to the timing of the EEG recording may have obscured findings.

Our results failed to validate previous subjective reports of sleep changes during the menstrual cycle. For example, Patkai et al. (1974), in six normal women over two menstrual cycles, reported that the duration of sleep was longest (by 1 h) and most disturbed premenstrually (5 days preceding the onset of menses) and shortest at ovulation (12–16 days preceding onset of menses). Halbreich et al. (1983) found that women with premenstrual depression ($n=145$) reported more hypersomnia than insomnia, and Billiard et al. (1975) and Sachs et al. (1982) reported case histories of two adolescent females with periodic hypersomnia associated with menstruation.

No consistent findings emerge from the studies done to date on sleep during the menstrual cycle in normal individuals. In sleep EEG studies done once per week across three menstrual cycles, Hartmann (1966) found an increase in REM sleep (minutes and percentage) in the premenstrual period, which correlated with severity of "premenstrual tension" symptoms in four normal individuals and three inpatients with diagnoses including depression and schizophrenia. There were no changes in total sleep time or number of awakenings. However the fact that the subjects were taking medications, including oral contraceptives, dexadrine, and prolixin, compromises this study. Ho (1972) recorded the sleep of three normal women and three women on oral contraceptives on 2 consecutive nights at three different times in the menstrual cycle (premenses, menses, postmenses) and found an increase in slow-wave sleep (stages III and IV) during premenses in the ovulating women but a decrease during premenses in women taking oral contraceptives. A larger sample size in this study would lend more support to their findings. Henderson et al. (1970), in a similar design, found increased variability in latency to stage III sleep premenstrually. Cluydts and Visser (1980), in four female students whose sleep EEG was recorded on 8 nights over one menstrual cycle, found an increase in stage II and a decrease in delta sleep at the time of menses in the one subject who reported dysphoric mood premenstrually. The reliability of reading slow-wave sleep is generally better than the reliability of separating stage III and stage IV sleep. Thus, our findings of changes in stage III sleep without changes in total slow-wave sleep, should be interpreted with caution.

Our findings of increased stage II sleep in PMS patients agrees with that of Cluyats and Visser (1980). Our finding of decreased REM sleep in patients with PMS is opposite to that of Hartmann (1966). Ho (1972) found an effect of menstrual cycle phase on stage III sleep, as we did, but the pattern of phase-related changes in her study was different than the changes that we found.

Other investigators have obtained information about the effects of reproductive hormones on sleep from studies of the effect of estrogen replacement therapy on the sleep of postmenopausal women. Thomson and Oswald (1977) reported that estrogen treatment decreased wakefulness after sleep onset and increased REM sleep in a placebo-controlled study of perimenopausal women. In a placebo-controlled study of hypogonadal women, Regestein et al. (1981) found that estrogen (0.625 mg) decreased sleep latency, increased the percentage of REM sleep, but had no effect on wakefulness. They suggested estrogen was like a hypnotic that did not decrease REM sleep. Our finding of increased intermittent wakefulness in the premenstrual phase when estrogen and progesterone levels are declining parallels the findings of Thomson and Oswald (1977) and Regestein (1981) of increased wakefulness in women with low levels of gonadal hormones (perimenopausal or hypogonadal women). Heuser et al. (1967) gave 200 mg progesterone to five young adult subjects for 4–7 consecutive nights and found that REM sleep increased. The authors noted that progesterone, an anesthetic in high doses, did not decrease REM time as many sedatives do. Thus, it is possible that some complaints of sleep disturbance in women reflect an effect of the menstrual cycle on sleep, particularly on intermittent wakefulness. In perimenopausal or hypogonadal women, low levels of gonadal hormones may increase wakefulness. In women, disturbances in sleep partly may be caused by a decline in gonadal hormones. The same may be true for men. However, men may be even more sensitive to the effects of gonadal hormones on sleep. Although elderly women complain of more sleep disturbances than men, men have more diagnosable polysomnographic abnormalities than women (Reynolds et al. 1985; Williams et al. 1974).

Investigators have also obtained information about the effects of reproductive hormones on sleep from studies of sleep during pregnancy and the puerperium. The results of these studies (Petre-Quadens and Lee 1974; Roffwarg et al. 1968; Karacan et al. 1967) are inconsistent, but they suggest that stage IV sleep decreases prior to delivery, and that REM sleep decreases after delivery.

The hypothesis that REM sleep decreases and motor activity increases in normal women, as it does in rats, at the time of ovulation, with a rebound in REM sleep and decrease in activity after ovulation was not supported by our study. However, since we did not achieve high enough resolution in our endocrine measurements to document precisely the time of ovulation, we cannot specify accurately the timing of the sleep studies in relation to the timing of ovulation. Nonetheless, when patients and controls were combined, increased estradiol levels, usually seen in the late follicular phase (midcycle), correlated with a decrease in the amount of REM sleep (minutes and percentage), a finding which parallels results in some rat studies (Colvin et al. 1969). This result suggests that further investigation into the effects of hormones on sleep may be worthwhile.

We did not find sleep stage abnormalities in patients with premenstrual depression similar to those found in patients with MDD. We cannot exclude the possibility that the premenstrual depressive episodes were too short in duration to induce changes in sleep parameters, or they did not occur with sufficient severity during the month of study. However, our patients were young, and they had normal sleep durations. Other investigators have found that REM sleep latencies are normal in young depressives (Goetz et al. 1987; Puig-Antich et al. 1982) and in depressives with normal or increased duration of sleep (Taub et al. 1978; Hawkins et al. 1985; see review, Gillin 1984). Experiments in normal persons suggest that short REM latency in depression may be a correlate and a consequence of insomnia (Mullen et al. 1986).

In summary, in our longitudinal study of sleep in eight patients with prospectively confirmed premenstrual depressive changes and eight age- and sex-matched controls, we found that patients had more stage II percentage sleep and less REM sleep (minutes and percentage) than controls. Stage III sleep and intermittent awakening varied with menstrual cycle phase. We did not demonstrate abnormalities in sleep architecture similar to those seen in some patients with MDD. Our small sample size, the short duration of premenstrual depressive symptoms which may have occurred at a different time from that when we measured the EEG recordings, and the relatively young age of our patients may have obscured findings that might be detectable or more robust in a larger sample size. Our patients with premenstrual depression appear to have sleep patterns similar to those reported in young depressed patients whose sleep is not reduced. Finally, the effects of estrogen and progesterone on sleep may be a fruitful area for further research.

Therapeutic Effect of Sleep Deprivation in Patients with Premenstrual Depression

Total and partial sleep deprivation (TSD and PSD) temporarily alleviate symptoms in a majority of patients with MDD (Gillin 1983). PMS and affective disorders may be related illnesses (Hallbreich and Endicott 1985; Endicott et al. 1981; Wetzel et al. 1975; Schuckit et al. 1975). The possible antidepressant effects of manipulations of the sleep-wake cycle have not been investigated in PMS patients. In this pilot study (Parry and Wehr 1987), we examined the effects of total and partial sleep deprivation on the symptoms of women with premenstrual depression. We felt that the possible therapeutic effects of sleep deprivation in PMS patients would be of interest because (a) it would help to clarify the relationship between PMS and MDD, (b) an effective intervention with TSD or PSD would be consistent with current theories that implicate prolactin in the pathogenesis of PMS (Carroll and Steiner 1978) inasmuch as sleep deprivation profoundly lowers prolactin levels (Sassin et al. 1973; Parker et al. 1973), and (c) sleep deprivation might prove useful in the treatment of PMS. With regard to this last possibility, the clinical use of sleep deprivation in MDD has been limited by the short duration of its therapeutic effect; however in PMS depressive episodes are themselves short in duration and might therefore be treated effectively with one or several periods of PSD or TSD.

Subjects and Methods

Patients were screened as described in the section on sleep studies. Patients who met diagnostic criteria for late luteal phase dysphoric disorder, and who then began to develop affective symptoms (HRSD $\geqq 10$) during a premenstrual phase of the cycle were admitted to an inpatient research unit at the NIMH and totally deprived of sleep for 40 h (7 A.M. to 11 P.M. the following day). The HRSD score, excluding items relating to sleep (items 4–6), weight (item 16), and diurnal mood variation (item 18) was obtained by a non-blind psychiatrist the morning (7–9 A.M.) and evening (7–9 P.M.) before TSD, after TSD, and after a recovery night's sleep in the hospital. The mean of the two ratings for each day was used in data analysis. Since many premenstrual symptoms include those characteristic of atypical depressions that are not assessed by the HRSD, separate items (NE Rosenthal et al., unpublished data) to assess fatigue, social withdrawal, increase in appetite, and carbohydrate craving (maximum of 23 points), as well as a hypomania rating scale were added to the HRSD. In addition, patients completed self-ratings every 2 h from the time of admission to the time of discharge using a 100-mm visual scale. During the night of sleep deprivation, patients were checked every 15 min by nurses to ensure wakefulness.

In five of the patients who responded to total sleep deprivation, a random-order crossover trial of early PSD (PSD-E; sleep from 2 A.M. to 8 A.M.) versus late PSD (PSD-L; sleep from 8 P.M. to 2 A.M.) for 2 consecutive nights in each condition was undertaken in subsequent months. Results of previous studies with MDD patients (Sack et al. 1988) indicated that PSD-E (in contrast to PSD-L) was ineffective and therefore might be used as a possible sham treatment to control for nonspecific aspects of the intervention. A therapeutic response to TSD and PSD was defined as a decrease of five or more points on the HRSD.

Results

Forty patients were screened, and 10 entered the study. Their mean age was 30 years (range, 26–45 years). According to the criterion of reduced HRSD score by at least 5 points, eight of the ten women showed a positive response to TSD. HRSD scores before and after TSD were 18 ± 5 and 6 ± 5, respectively (paired t test, two-tailed: $t = 5.56$, $df = 9$, $p < 0.0001$). For the six patients in whom ratings were obtained after a recovery night's sleep, HRSD score was 3 ± 2 (paired t test, before versus recovery, two-tailed: $t = 8.09$, $df = 5$, $p < 0.001$). There was no significant difference between HRSD after TSD and after recovery sleep ($t = 1.31$, $df = 5$). The atypical item scores (fatigue, carbohydrate craving, social withdrawal) before and after TSD ($t = 2.91$, $df = 9$, $p < 0.05$) and after recovery sleep ($t = 2.0$, $df = 5$, NS) were 8 ± 5, 4 ± 4, and 5 ± 3, respectively. Differences between atypical ratings after TSD and after recovery sleep were nonsignificant ($t = 0.78$, $df = 5$). Although several patients reported feeling "high" with increased energy and euphoria, no patient was actually rated manic. In two patients, significant further improvement occurred after the recovery night's sleep; one patient reported improvement for 6 months thereafter. Patients with and without a prior history of affective disorder (five of ten patients) responded equally well to sleep deprivation.

The five patients who received PSD improved greatly when sleep deprivation occurred in the second half of the night (PSD-L) but very little in the first (PSD-E). Mean HRSD scores before and after PSD-L were 19 ± 3 and 6.5 ± 4.8, and those before and after PSD-E were 14 ± 3.65 and 10.9 ± 3.89, respectively (paired t tests delta change before and after PSD-L versus PSD-E; $t = 6.12$, $df = 4$, $p < 0.05$). In the three women whose baseline ratings revealed protracted premenstrual symptoms at least 1 week), a follow-up HRSD was done 1 week later. One patient who underwent PSD-L maintained her response (HRSD = 1); two patients undergoing PSD-E showed a relapse (HRSD 20 and 22). There was no consistent pattern of mood change across the day (morning versus evening HRSD) in responders versus nonresponders.

Discussion

In this study, eight of ten women with PMS (80%) responded to TSD with sustained improvement in their symptoms through the remainder of their premenstrual period. This response rate is consistent with or superior to that seen in endogenously depressed patients (Gillin 1983) and contrasts with the dysphoric response seen in normals (Gerner et al. 1979).

This study shares with most other clinical investigations of therapeutic sleep deprivation a significant methodological problem: neither raters nor patients were blind to the procedure when clinical assessments were made. The results of the study indicate simply that PMS patients' responses to TSD are similar to those of other types of depressed patients studied under similar conditions. In future studies, it may be possible to control for nonspecific aspects of sleep deprivation therapy. Results in this and other studies indicate that partial sleep deprivation in the first half of the night is ineffective compared with PSD in the second half of the night; therefore, PSD-E may serve as a sham treatment. The favorable responses of PMS patients to TSD in this uncontrolled study of ten patients and to PSD-L versus PSD-E in a subgroup of TSD responders suggest that a large-scale crossover comparison of PSD-L and PSD-E in PMS might be worthwhile. Furthermore, since PSD is as effective as TSD (Schilgen and Tolle 1980), repeated periods of PSD are more readily tolerated than repeated periods of TSD, and the duration of an untreated episode of PMS is short, repeated PSD may prove to be an effective and acceptable alternative or adjunct to the pharmacological treatment of PMS.

References

Aschoff J (1979) Circadian rhythms. General features and endocrinological aspects. In: Kruger DT (ed) Endocrine rhythms. Raven, New York, pp 1–61

Billiard M, Guilleminault C, Dement WC (1975) A menstruation-linked periodic hypersomnia. Neurology 25:436–443

Branchey M, Branchey L, Nadler RD (1971) Effects of estrogen and progesterone on sleep patterns of female rats. Physiol Behav 6:743–746

Bunney WE Jr, Hamburg DA (1963) Methods for reliable longitudinal observation of behavior. Arch Gen Psychiatry 9:280

Carroll BJ, Steiner M (1978) The psychobiology of premenstrual dysphoria: the role of prolactin. Psychoneuroendocrinology 3:171–180

Cluydts R, Visser P (1980) Mood and sleep. Effects of the menstrual cycle. Waking Sleeping 4:193

Colburn TR, Smith BM, Guarini J et al. (1976) An ambulatory activity monitor with solid state memory. ISA Trans 15:149–154

Colvin GB, Whitmoyer DI, Lisk RD, Walter DO, Sawyer CH (1968) Changes in sleep wakefulness in female rats during circadian and estrus cycles. Brain Res 7:173–181

Colvin GB, Whitmoyer DI, Sawyer CH (1969) Circadian sleep-wakefulness patterns in rats after ovariectomy and treatment with estrogen. Exp Neurol 25:616–625

Endicott J, Halbreich U, Schacht S, Nee J (1981) Premenstrual changes and affective disorders. Psychosom Med 43:519–529

Gerner RH, Post RM, Gillin JC, Bunney WE (1979) Biological and behavioral effects of one night's sleep deprivation in depressed patients and normals. J Psychiatr Res 15:21–40

Gillin JC (1983) The sleep therapies of depression. Prog Neuropsychopharmacol Biol Psychiatry 7:351–364

Gillin JC, Sitaram N, Wehr TA, Duncan WB, Post R, Murphy DL, Mendelson WB, Wyatt RJ, Bunney WE (1984) Sleep and affective illness. In: Post RM, Ballenger JC (eds) Neurobiology of mood disorders. Williams and Wilkins, Baltimore, pp 157–189

Goetz RR, Puig-Antich J, Ryan N et al. (1987) Electroencephalographic sleep of adolescents with major depression and normal controls. Arch Gen Psychiatry 44:61–68
Halbreich U, Endicott J (1985) Relationship of dysphoric premenstrual changes to depressive disorders. Acta Psychiatr Scand 71:331–338
Halbreich U, Endicott J, Nee J (1983) Premenstrual depressive changes. Value of differentiation. Arch Psychiatry 40:535–542
Hallman J (1986) The premenstrual syndrome – an equivalent of depression? Acta Psychiatr Scand 73:403–411
Hamilton M (1967) Development of a rating scale for primary depressive illness. Br J Soc Clin Psychol 6:228
Hartmann E (1966) Dreaming sleep (the D-state) and the menstrual cycle. J Nerv Ment Dis 143:406
Hawkins DR, Taub JM, Van de Castle RL (1985) Extended sleep (hypersomnia) in young depressed patients. Am J Psychiatry 142:905–910
Henderson A, Nemes G, Gordon NB, Roos L (1970) The sleep of regularly menstruating women and of women taking an oral contraceptive. Sleep Study Abstracts 337, September
Heuser G, Kales A, Jacobson A (1967) Human sleep patterns after progesterone administration. Assoc Psychophysiol Study Sleep Meeting 4:378
Ho MA (1972) Sex hormones and the sleep of women. PhD Thesis, Yeshiva University
Karacan R, Williams WB, Webb H, Agnew Ross J (1967) Sleep and dreaming during late pregnancy and postpartum. Assoc Psychophysiol Study Sleep Meeting 4:378 (Abstract)
Kawakmi M, Sawyer CH (1959) Neuroendocrine correlates of changes in brain activity thresholds by sex steroids and pituitary hormones. Endocrinology 65:668
Kripke DF, Mullaney DJ, Atkinson M, Wolf S (1978) Circadian rhythm disorders in manic depressives. Biol Psychiatry 13:335
MacKenzie TB, Wilcox K, Baron H (1986) Lifetime prevalence of psychiatric disorders in women with premenstrual difficulties. J Affective Disord 10:15–19
Malven PV, Sawyer CH (1966) Sleeping patterns in female guinea pigs; effects of sex hormones. Exp Neurol 15:229
Mullen PE, Linsell CR, Parker D (1986) Influence of sleep disruption and calorie restriction on biological markers for depression. Lancet 2 (8):1051–1052
Parker DC, Rossman LG, Vanderlaan EF (1973) Sleep related, nyctohemeral and briefly episodic variation in human plasma prolactin concentrations. J Clin Endocrinol Metab 36:1119–1124
Parry BL, Wehr TA (1987) Therapeutic effect of sleep deprivation in patients with premenstrual syndrome. Am J Psychiatry 144(6):808–810
Parry BL, Mendelson WB, Duncan WC et al. (1989) Longitudinal sleep EEG, temperature and activity measurements across the menstrual cycle in patients with premenstrual depression and in age-matched controls. Psychiatry Res (in press)
Patkai P, Johannson G, Post B (1974) Mood, alertness and sympathetic-adrenal medullary activity during the menstrual cycle. Psychosom Med 36:503–512
Petre-Quadens O, De Lee C (1974) Sleep-cycle alterations during pregnancy, postpartum, and the menstrual cycle. In: Ferin M, Halberg F, Richart R, Vande Wiele RL (eds) Biorhythms and human reproduction. John Wiley, New York, pp 335–353
Puig-Antich J, Goetz R, Hanlon C et al. (1982) Sleep architecture and REM sleep measures in prepubertal children with major depression. Arch Gen Psychiatry 39:932–939
Rechtschaffen A, Kales AA (1968) A manual of standardized terminology. Techniques and scoring system for sleep stages of human subjects. US Government Printing Office, Washington, DC
Regestein QR, Schiff I, Tulchinsky D, Ryan KG (1981) Relationships among estrogen-induced psychophysiological changes in hypogonadal women. Psychosom Med 43:147
Reynolds CF, Kupfer DJ, Taska LS et al. (1985) Sleep of healthy seniors: a revisit. Sleep 8(1):20–29
Roffwarg HP, Frantel B, Pessah M (1968) The nocturnal sleep pattern in pregnancy. Assoc Psychophysiol Study Sleep March (Abstract)

Roy-Byrne PP, Rubinow DR, Hoban C et al. (1987) Premenstrual changes: a comparison of five populations. Psychiatry Res 17:77–85

Sachs C, Persson HE, Hagenfeldt K (1982) Menstruation-related periodic hypersomnia: A case study with successful treatment. Neurology 32:1376–1379

Sack DA, Duncan W, Rosenthal NE et al. (1988) The timing and duration of sleep in partial sleep deprivation therapy of depression. Acta Psychiatr Scand 77:219–224

Sassin JF, Frantz AG, Kapen S et al. (1973) The nocturnal rise of human prolactin is dependent on sleep. J Clin Endocrinol Metab 37:436–440

Schilgen B, Tolle R (1980) Partial sleep deprivation as therapy for depression. Arch Gen Psychiatr 37(3):267–271

Schukit MA, Daly V, Herrman G, Hineman S (1975) Premenstrual symptoms and depression in a university population. Dis Nerv Syst 36:516–517

Taub JM, Hawkins DR, Van de Castle RL (1978) Electrographic analysis of the sleep cycle in young depressed patients. Biol Psychol 7:203–214

Thomson J, Oswald I (1977) Effect of oestrogen on the sleep, mood, and anxiety of menopausal women. Br Med J 2:1317

Wehr TA, Goodwin FK (1983) Biological rhythms in manic depressive illness. In: Wehr TA, Goodwin FK (eds) Circadian rhythms in psychiatry. Boxwood, Pacific Grove, Ca, pp 129–201

Wehr TA, Wirz-Justice A (1980) Internal coincidence model for sleep deprivation and depression. In: Sleep 1980. 5th European congress on sleep research, Amsterdam. Karger, Basel, pp 26–33

Wehr TA, Sack DA, Rosenthal NE (1987) Sleep reduction as a final common pathway in the geneses of mania. Am J Psychiatry 144:201–204

Weissman MM, Klerman GL (1977) Sex differences and the epidemiology of depression. Arch Gen Psychiatry 34:98–111

Wetzel RD, Reich T, McClure JN, Wald JA (1975) Premenstrual affective syndrome and affective disorder. Br J Psychiatry 127:129–221

Wever RA (1984) Properties of human sleep-wake cycles: parameters of internally synchronized free-running rhythms. Sleep 7:27–51

Williams RL, Karacan I, Hersch CJ (1974) Electroencephalography (EEG) of human sleep: clinical applications. Wiley, New York

Wirz-Justice A, Wever RA, Aschoff J (1984) Seasonality in free-running rhythms in man. Naturwissenschaften 71:316–319

Yokoyama A, Ramirez VD, Sawyer CH (1966) Sleep and wakefulness in female rats under various hormonal and physiological conditions. Gen Comp Endocrinol 7:10–17

Epidemiological Aspects of Insomnia Research

M. PARTINEN [1]

Insomnia is a common sleep disorder, and sleeping pills are commonly prescribed drugs. This chapter presents no new data on the prevalence of chronic insomnia or the incidence of transient insomnia but only a very short and fragmentary note about the quality of hypnotics research from a single point of view.

Hypnotic drugs should be used mainly for transient or short-term insomnia (CDC 1984). Most prescriptions are, however, written for chronic users. Why do 3%–15% (Partinen et al. 1985) of adults take hypnotics almost every evening before going to bed? Most persons take hypnotics because their physician have advised them to do so. Fortunately, most modern hypnotic drugs, for example, benzodiazepines, are relatively safe even in long-term use. However, various side effects have been reported with the use of hypnotics (CDC 1984; Goldenberg 1985). These side effects include daytime sedation, memory problems, anxiety, dizziness, and even confusion.

Pharmacologists have the key role in developing new drugs and in evaluating pharmacological effects of drugs. However, the dosage of hypnotics should not be based on pharmacological studies alone, and collaboration should be increased between pharmacologists working in laboratories, clinicians treating patients with insomnia on the field, and epidemiologists.

Insomnia is a symptom and not a disease. While we need drugs to relieve symptoms, especially in chronic insomnia the main aim should be etiological treatment of the cause. Is the etiology of insomnia taken into consideration in insomnia research? Are the studies on insomnia otherwise adequate? To answer this a literature search was made of the 40 most recent data sets using the Medline database with the following wording: "insomnia and double-blind and randomized." Ten references were randomly selected from the 40 publications (McClure et al. 1988; Nicholson and Stone 1987; Billiard et al. 1987; Anderson 1987; Allen et al. 1987; Castleden et al. 1987; Wheatley 1986; Simonoff and Stores 1987; Overstall and Oldman 1987; Autret et al. 1987). All the studies were done by experienced researchers, and all were perfectly adequate from the pharmacological point of view. However, the etiology of insomnia was specified in only two (McClure et al. 1988; Wheatley 1986) of the seven studies on chronic insomnia. Three studies (Nicholson and Stone 1987;

[1] Department of Neurology, University of Helsinki, 00290 Helsinki, Finland.

Neuropsychopharmacology
Edited by Bunney/Hippius/Laakmann/Schmauß

Billiard et al. 1987; Castleden et al. 1987) were performed in healthy subjects, and insomniacs were not included. None of the randomly selected studies dealt with transient insomnia, the main indication for hypnotics. The results were based on subjective evaluation in seven of the ten studies; objective sleep recordings were performed in three studies only (McClure et al. 1988; Nicholson and Stone 1987; Billiard et al. 1987). The sample sizes in the seven studies with subjective evaluation varied between 18 and 175 subjects; in the three studies (McClure et al. 1988; Nicholson and Stone 1987; Billiard et al. 1987) with objective measurement of sleep parameters the sample sizes were 8, 6, and 6, respectively. The power of these studies is quite low for sleep latency and other sleep parameters except those in which a difference was found. This does not matter when efficacy of hypnotics is concerned; only marked differences reach statistical significance. However, as regards side effects or complications, there is a high probability of missing important differences in side effects with such small sample sizes.

Clinicians need more information about the usefulness and side effects of hypnotics. In addition to subjective assessments, objective outcome parameters should be used in randomized studies. In addition, the sample size should be large enough, and calculations of statistical power should be used to estimate the needed sample sizes before starting any study. Clinical meaningfulness counts more than purely statistical significance of results. Inferences from all the above mentioned studies were based mainly on statistical significance. We should, however, base our inferences on the results and not to look solely at the value of the p statistic because of the risk of making wrong decisions when only this is used (Rothman 1986; Miettinen 1985). Confidence intervals should also be given (Bulbitt 1987; Gardner and Altman 1988).

Randomized clinical trials (RCT) form the basis for experimental epidemiological hypnotics research. Except for descriptive prevalence studies, nonexperimental epidemiological studies have rarely been used with insomnia. One reason for this could be the difficulty of nonexperimental epidemiological studies as compared to RCT. The validity of nonexperimental epidemiological studies rests on the same three features as RCT (Miettinen 1985): (a) comparability of effects (placebo or other drug in RCT); (b) comparability of populations (randomization in RCT); (c) comparability of information (blinding in RCT). In nonexperimental research comparability of effects is achieved by providing an appropriate reference category. Comparability of information means that in the absence of differences in effect, the outcomes of the compared populations could be expected to be identical (Miettinen 1985). The comparability of information may become a serious problem if the outcome information is based solely on routine documentation (Miettinen 1985).

Nonexperimental epidemiological research is difficult. However, case-control studies (Rothman 1986; Miettinen 1985; Schlesselman 1982), prospective cohort studies (Rothman 1986; Miettinen 1985; Kahn 1983), or so-called single-patient randomized clinical trials (McLeod et al. 1986) could be conducted on the side effects and complications of hypnotics. They could give valuable information to practitioners in addition to conventional pharmacological studies.

References

Allen RP, Mendels J, Nevins DB, Chernik DA, Hoddes E (1987) Efficacy without tolerance or rebound insomnia for midazolam and temazepam after use for one to three months. J Clin Pharmacol 27:768–775

Anderson AA (1987) Zopiclone and nitrazepam, a multicenter placebo controlled comparative study of efficacy and tolerance in insomniac patients in general practice. Sleep 10 (Suppl 1):54–62

Autret E, Maillard F, Autret A (1987) Comparison of the clinical hypnotic effects of zopiclone and triazolam. Eur J Clin Pharmacol 31:621–623

Billiard M, Besset A, de Lustrac C, Brissaud L (1987) Dose-response effects of zopiclone on night sleep and on nighttime and daytime functioning. Sleep 10 (Suppl 1):27–34

Bulbitt CJ (1987) Confidence intervals. Lancet 1:494–497

Castleden CM, Aleen JG, Altman J, St John-Smith P (1987) A comparison of oral midazolam, nitrazepam and placebo in young and elderly subjects. Eur J Clin Pharmacol 32:253–257

CDC (Consensus Development Conference) (1984) Drugs and insomnia. Consensus Development Conference, Summary, vol 4, no 10. US Department of Health and Human Services. National Institutes of Health

Gardner MJ, Altman DG (1988) Estimating with confidence. Br Med J 296:1210–1211

Goldenberg F (1985) Advantages and disadvantages of different benzodiazepines in chronic insomnia. In: Koella WP, Rüther E, Schulz H (eds) Sleep 84. Fischer, Stuttgart, pp 56–59

Kahn HA (1983) An introduction to epidemiologic methods. Oxford University Press, New York

McClure DJ, Walsh J, Chang H, Olah A, Wilson R, Pecknold JC (1988) Comparison of lorazepam and flurazepam as hypnotic agents in chronic insomniacs. J Clin Pharmacol 28:52–63

McLeod RS, Cohen Z, Taylor DW, Cullen JB (1986) Single-patient randomised clinical trial. Use in determining optimum treatment for patient with inflammation of Kock continent ileostomy reservoir. Lancet 1:726–728

Miettinen OS (1985) Theoretical epidemiology. Principles of occurrence research in medicine. Wiley, New York

Nicholson AN, Stone BM (1987) Efficacy of zopiclone in middle age. Sleep 10 (Suppl 1):35–39

Overstall PW, Oldman PN (1987) A comparative study of lormetazepam and chlormethiazole in elderly in-patients. Age Ageing 16:45–51

Partinen M, Eskelinen L, Tuomi K (1985) Epidemiology of insomnia: environmental factors. In: Koella WP, Rüther E, Schulz H (eds) Sleep '84. Fischer, Stuttgart, pp 42–44

Rothman KJ (1986) Modern epidemiology. Little, Brown, Boston

Schlesselman JJ (1982) Case-control studies. Design, conduct, analysis. Oxford University Press, New York

Simonoff EA, Stores G (1987) Controlled trials of trimeprazine tartrate for night waking. Arch Dis Child 62:253–257

Wheatley D (1986) Insomnia in general practice: the role of temazepam and a comparison with zopiclone. Acta Psychiatr Scand 332 (Suppl):142–148

Antidepressant Medication and Total Sleep Deprivation in Depressives

S. ELSENGA and R. H. VAN DEN HOOFDAKKER [1]

Introduction

Since the discovery of the antidepressant effects of total sleep deprivation (TSD) in depressives, the relevance of antidepressant medication (ADM) for the clinical effects of TSD has quite often been neglected. However, knowing to what extent, if any, the course of depression is influenced by the combination of ADM and TSD is of both practical and theoretical value (Post et al. 1987). The response of depression to ADM and TSD shows very different time courses. Unlike the more delayed and lasting effects of ADM, those of TSD are acute and short lived, that is, they are generally restricted to the period of wakefulness during and after TSD. Subsequent night sleep is, in general, almost always followed by a relapse (Van den Burg and Van den Hoofdakker 1975; Gerner et al. 1979).

This chapter considers the question of the extent to which the administration of ADM influences the course of depression during and after TSD. Do the effects of TSD change with the concurrent use of ADM, on the day following the TSD, and on the day subsequent to the next sleep night? What are the effects of ADM on repeatedly administered TSDs? The only study relevant in this respect is the comparison between the effects of a series of TSDs in depressed patients who received either placebo or the ADM clomipramine (Elsenga and Van den Hoofdakker 1983 a). It was found that clomipramine did not have an influence on the acute antidepressant effect of TSD, however the course of depression thereafter was changed quite dramatically by the drug. This paper analyzes the results of that study in more detail. In addition, the results of another study are used to investigate whether the results of this analysis can be replicated.

A large number of demographic, clinical, and diagnostic variables have been studied regarding their possible relationship with the acute response to TSD (for a review, see Kuhs and Tölle 1986). Two of these deserve special attention: the presence or absence of diurnal variation (DV) and that of psychotic features (Elsenga and Van den Hoofdakker 1987). It was found that DV is positively related to the antidepressant response to TSD under

[1] Department of Biological Psychiatry, Psychiatric University Clinic, Oostersingel 59, 9713 EZ Groningen, The Netherlands.

Neuropsychopharmacology
Edited by Bunney/Hippius/Laakmann/Schmauß

clomipramine conditions. Likewise, patients with psychotic features reacted more favorably than did nonpsychotics. DV predicts a better response to a traditional treatment regime without TSD (Carpenter et al. 1986). However, psychotic depression is associated with poor response to tricyclic ADM (Spiker et al. 1986), at least when the treatment is of insufficient duration (Quitkin et al. 1978; Howarth and Grace 1985). Psychotic depression is therefore often regarded as an indication for electroconvulsive treatment (Minter and Mandel 1979; Avery and Lubrano 1977) or for the combined use of antipsychotics and antidepressants (Spiker et al. 1985). In view of the above-mentioned findings (Elsenga and Van den Hoofdakker 1987) one may raise the question as to whether diurnality and psychoticism are of not only short-term but also long-term therapeutic relevance.

Thus, the main issues in this exploratory analysis regard the influence of ADM on the time course of response to TSD in depressives and the clinical usefulness of the combination of ADM and TSD. The distinctions between psychotic versus nonpsychotic depression and between the presence or absence of DV are emphasized.

Method

Study I. The three groups in the first study (Fig. 1) were treated with either the ADM clomipramine alone (CL; $n = 10$), a combination of TSD and CL (CL/TSD; $n = 10$), or a combination of TSD and placebo (PL/TSD; $n = 10$). The TSDs were carried out twice weekly. After the first and after the third TSD only one full night of sleep was allowed. Medication started on the day before the first TSD at 6:00 P.M. and was doubled the following day at 8:00 A.M. Further increases in dose were made on the 4th day at 12:00 A.M. and on the 6th day at 10:00 P.M. The dosage of 4 × 50 mg was maintained thereafter. No other

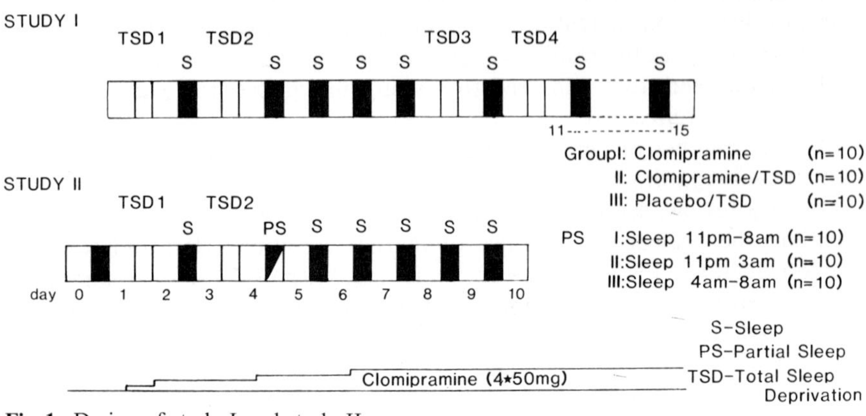

Fig. 1. Design of study I and study II

psychotropic drugs were allowed during the whole experimental period. Sleep deprivation was introduced as part of the treatment plan. Patients were engaged in several recreational activities; nurses took great care preventing patients from falling asleep. No sleep was allowed during daytime. Patients were drug free for at least 3 days before the first baseline day.

Study II. The first phase of the second study was similar to that of the former one except for the addition of an extra baseline day (day 0; Fig. 1). An analogous sleep-wake schedule and ADM treatment were used (until day 4; Fig. 1). During the night after the second TSD, however, patients were allowed to sleep between 11:00 P.M. and 8:00 A.M. ($n = 10$), between 11:00 P.M. and 3:00 A.M. ($n = 10$), or between 4:00 A.M. and 8:00 A.M. ($n = 10$). The differences in course of depression after this night of either partial or unlimited sleep were not significant (Elsenga and Van den Hoofdakker 1983 b).

Subjects. All subjects were hospitalized, endogenously depressed patients. The main criteria for entrance into the study were (a) depressed mood; (b) other endogenously depressed features, such as DV, loss of libido, loss of weight and appetite; (c) absence of life events adequately explaining the depression; and (d) a minimum score on the Hamilton rating scale for depression (HRSD; Hamilton 1967) of 15 and 20 for study I and study II, respectively. For more detailed information the reader is referred to Elsenga and Van den Hoofdakker (1983 a, 1988).

Measurements. For both studies self-ratings (SR) of depression (von Zerssen 1986) were obtained at about 9:00 A.M. and 5:00 P.M. and, additionally, for study II at 11:00 P.M. The scale score ranges from 0 to 56; the higher the score, the greater is the degree of depression. Interviews for the HRSD took place prior to the first TSD and at the end of the experimental period (study I, day 15; study II, day 10; see Fig. 1). The interviews were rated independently in both studies by the same two raters.

The main purpose of this report is to examine the influence of the administration of CL on the clinical effects of TSD. Therefore, in general, the results for the CL group from study I will not be dealt with here.

Results

Response to TSD

The course of depression before and after each of the four TSDs for study I is presented in Fig. 2. The effects of TSD and of subsequent sleep are examined in terms of the differences between the mean depression scores at the same time of day before and after TSD and sleep. Both the PL/TSD and the CL/TSD group showed a significant amelioration after the first TSD. The most marginal *p*

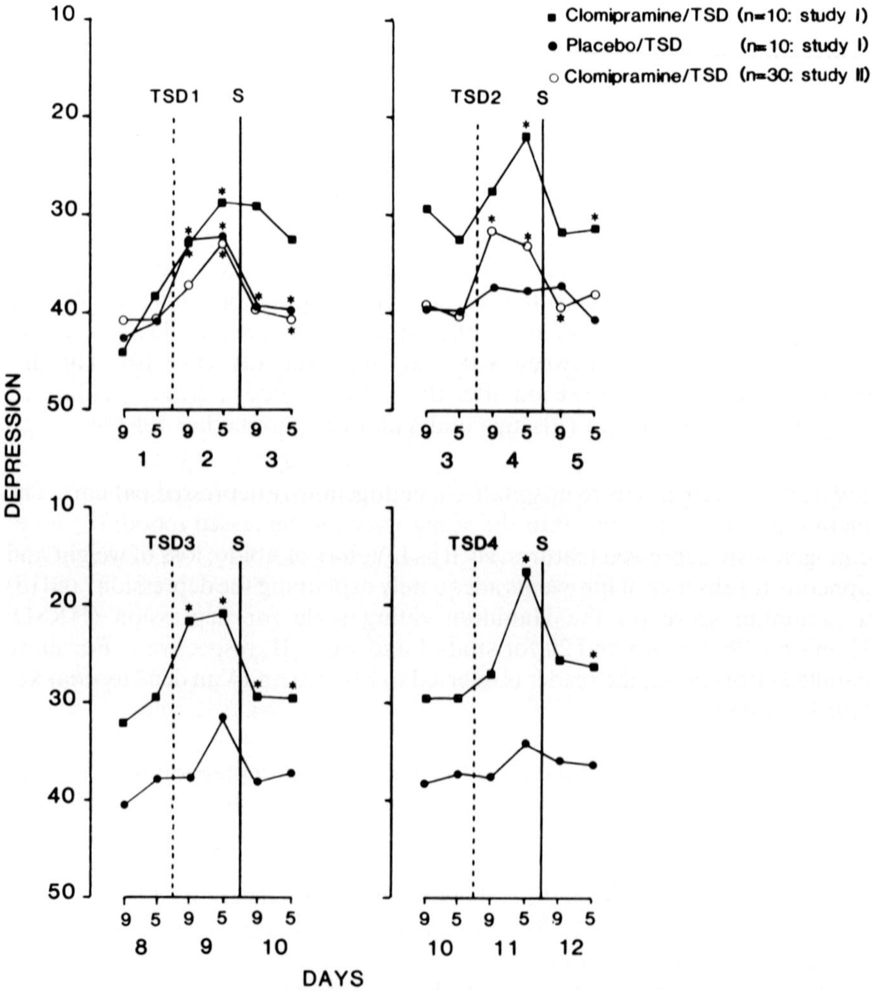

Fig. 2. The course of self-rated depression before and after the TSDs for study I (four TSDs; *upper*, *lower*), and study II (two TSDs; *upper*). *Asterisks*, significant difference from the measurement 24 h earlier ($\alpha = 0.05$)

value for the comparisons made for is obtained for the CL/TSD group at 9:00 A.M. ($t_9 = 3.09, p < 0.02$). In contrast to the CL/TSD group, the PL/TSD group showed a significant relapse after the night following this TSD (9:00 A.M. and 5:00 P.M.; $t_9 = -2.29, p < 0.05$), suggesting that the course of depression after a night of sleep following TSD is influenced by the use of CL.

In the PL/TSD group no significant responses to the second, third, or fourth TSD were found. The use of CL appeared to maintain the antidepressant efficacy of TSD. However, unlike the nightsleep after the first TSD, that after the second, third, and fourth TSD appeared to be followed by relapses equal to the prior antidepressant responses.

In study II only two TSDs were employed. The antidepressant efficacy was replicated (Fig. 2). The course of depression after the night following the first TSD, however, differed considerably from that in study I. The significant relapse at 5:00 P.M. ($p < 0.005$) indicates that the relapse preventing effect of CL could not be corroborated.

Response to TSD and Subsequent Sleep

The relationship between the response to the first TSD and that to the subsequent night sleep are shown in Fig. 3. Response to TSD was defined as the difference between the averaged morning and afternoon values before and after TSD. The general pattern was that the responses to TSD were outweighed by sleep. The majority of exceptions were found among the CL/TSD group of study I. Many patients did not relapse in this study whereas all patients did so in study II. These contradictory findings are the more puzzling because data of Loosen et al. (1976) and Philipp (1978) also suggest that an ADM may prevent the relapse usually observed in drug-free patients (Van den Burg and Van den

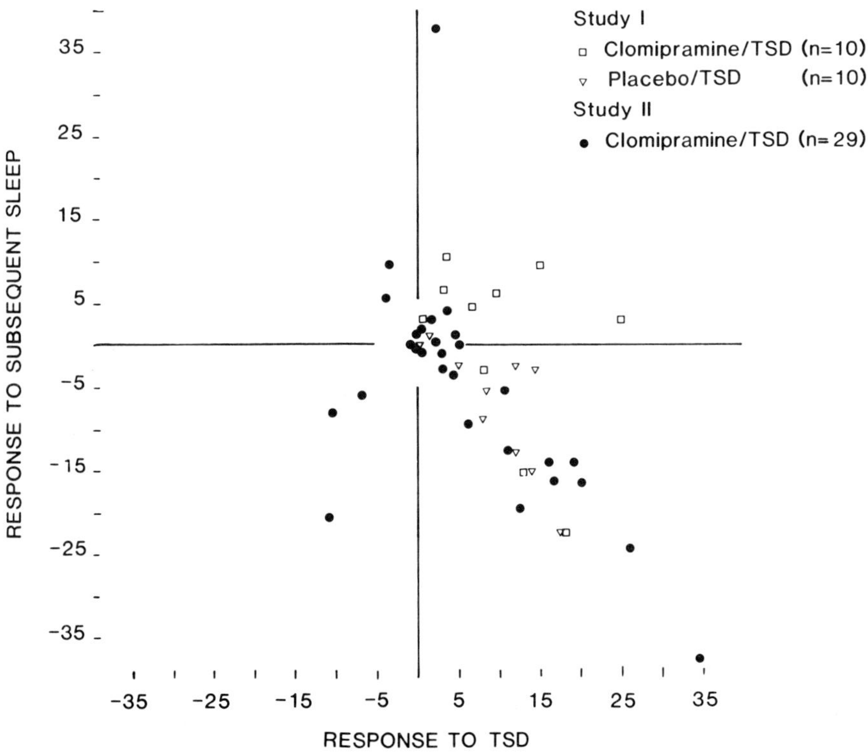

Fig. 3. Relationship between responses to the first TSD and responses to the subsequent night in both study I and study II

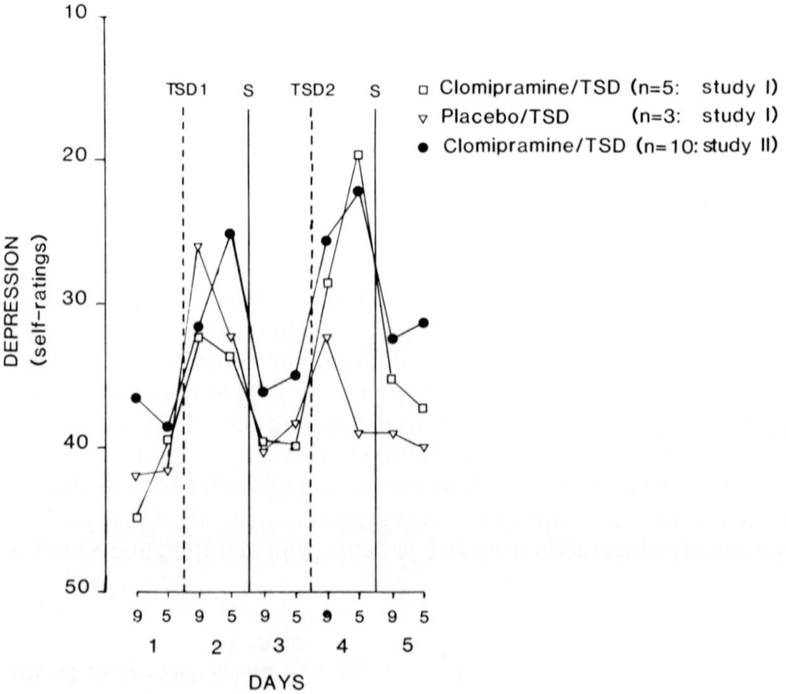

Fig. 4. Response to TSD among psychotic depressives in study I and study II (those from the PL/TSD group are added to the figure)

Hoofdakker 1975; Gerner et al. 1979). Thus, the question is whether those who relapse can be distinguished from those who do not.

A first factor to be considered regards the responsiveness to TSD. What is the course of depression among responders in either of the two CL/TSD groups? As can be deduced from Fig. 3, responsiveness cannot be a decisive factor because five out of the seven responders in the first study showed no relapse whereas all responders in the second study did so.

A second factor concerns the presence of psychotic features. Figure 4 demonstrates the remarkable result that the psychotic depressives in both studies show, on average, a large relapse following a night's sleep subsequent to the first TSD. Apparently, CL does not prevent the relapse in psychotic depressives in either study. Consequently, psychoticism may distinguish between those who relapse and those who do not, but it does not provide a plausible explanation for the difference between the two studies.

A different strategy to analyze the discrepancy is shown in Fig. 5. The patients were divided according to treatment condition into two groups: those who were improved on day 3 and those who were not. Improvement was defined as a score difference of at least 6 points between day 3 and day 1. The course of depression for the six day 3 improvers and the four nonimprovers in study I is shown in the upper part of the figure. The course for the day 3

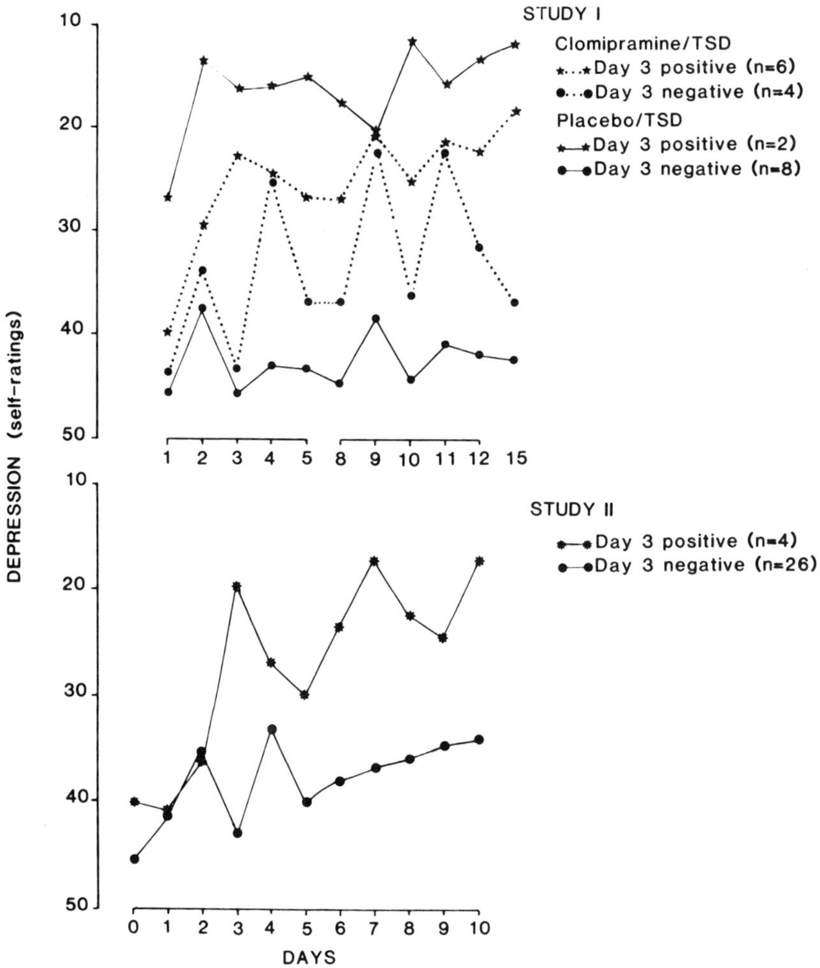

Fig. 5. The course of self-rated depression for subjects who had and who did not have an improvement of 6 points or more after 2 days of treatment with TSD and clomipramine. The groups presented are the CL/TSD and PL/TSD group of study I (*upper*), and the total group of study II (*lower*)

improvers is very different from that for the day 3 nonimprovers. Four of the six day 3 improvers of the CL/TSD group were also responders to the previous TSD, as were both day 3 improvers of the PL/TSD group. Improvement after the 2-week treatment period was significantly greater among the day 3 improvers than among the day 3 nonimprovers (SR, $t_8 = 2.10$, $p < 0.07$; HRSD, $t_8 = 2.62$, $p < 0.03$). Although the number of subjects with a positive response on day 3 was notably small in study II, the course of depression thereafter was nevertheless again positive (Fig. 5, lower part). The total group of day 3 improvers had, on average, a lower baseline HRSD score than the group who did not show this early improvement ($t_{48} = 2.49$, $p < 0.02$). In addition, none of the seven bipolar patients belonged to the group of day 3 improvers, while only four in this group were psychotic.

A possible explanation for the discrepancy between the results of studies I and II is that the practice of referral to the hospital had changed over the course of years, resulting in a more severely disturbed hospital population. Moreover, the minimum HRSD score as entrance criterion was higher in study II than in study I, i.e., 20 versus 15. When HRSD baseline values below 20 in study I are excluded, there is still a tendency towards increased mean baseline HRSD scores ($F_{1,50} = 3.17$, $p < 0.08$). Mean HRSD values for nonpsychotics changed from 29.8 in study I to 33.5 in study II and those for psychotics from 30.7 to 31.7, respectively. The less severe, nonpsychotic, unipolar depressives may be candidates for a quick, early, and lasting response to the combination of ADM and TSD, or perhaps even TSD alone.

Consistency of Response to TSD and Clomipramine

Results shown in Fig. 2 led to the conclusion that CL positively influences the response to repeated TSDs. The results in Fig. 6 show that there is some consistency between two successive TSDs ($r_{37} = 0.35$, $p < 0.04$). This consis-

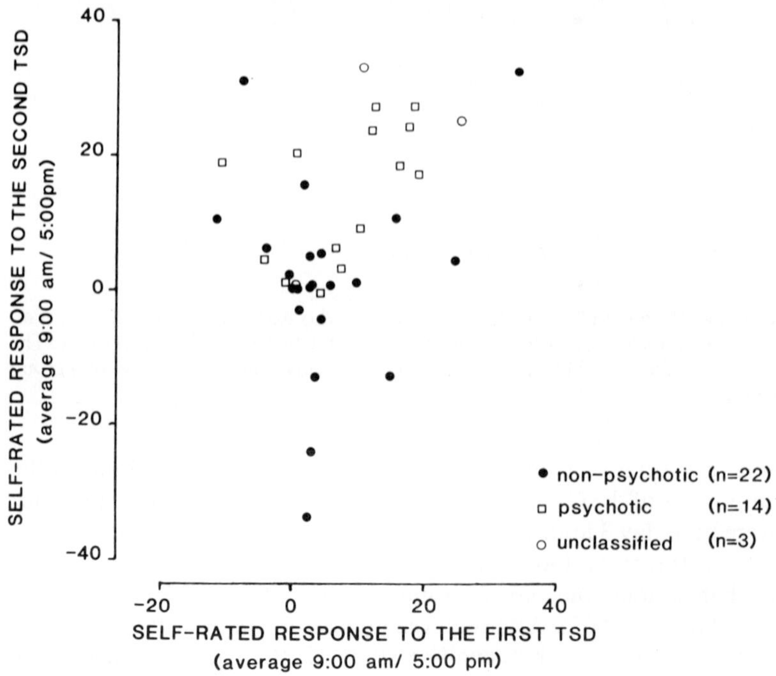

Fig. 6. Consistency of response to TSD in psychotic and nonpsychotic depressives treated with clomipramine. Classification was uncertain in this respect for three subjects; one other subject had missing data

tency in response is less likely to be attributed to the nonpsychotic ($r_{20} = 0.17$, $p < 0.45$) than to the psychotic depressives ($r_{12} = 0.48$, $p < 0.09$). (Note that three subjects could not be attributed with certainty to either class; one subject had missing data.)

The mean response to both TSDs in psychotic subjects has already been shown in Fig. 4. The low response to the second TSD for the PL/TSD group is in line with the conclusion drawn above that CL raises the probability of a positive response to continued TSD. Hence, the results indicate that a large *and* consistent response is obtained to continued TSD in psychotic depressives, and that this consistency is probably due to the use of CL.

TSD and the Continued Use of Clomipramine

In the second study the patients underwent only two TSDs. Thereafter, the course of depression was measured until the 11th day of the experiment (Fig. 1). As noted above, both DV and psychoticism predict a positive short-term response to TSD. The question is whether DV and psychoticism have predictive value for the course of depression in the long run.

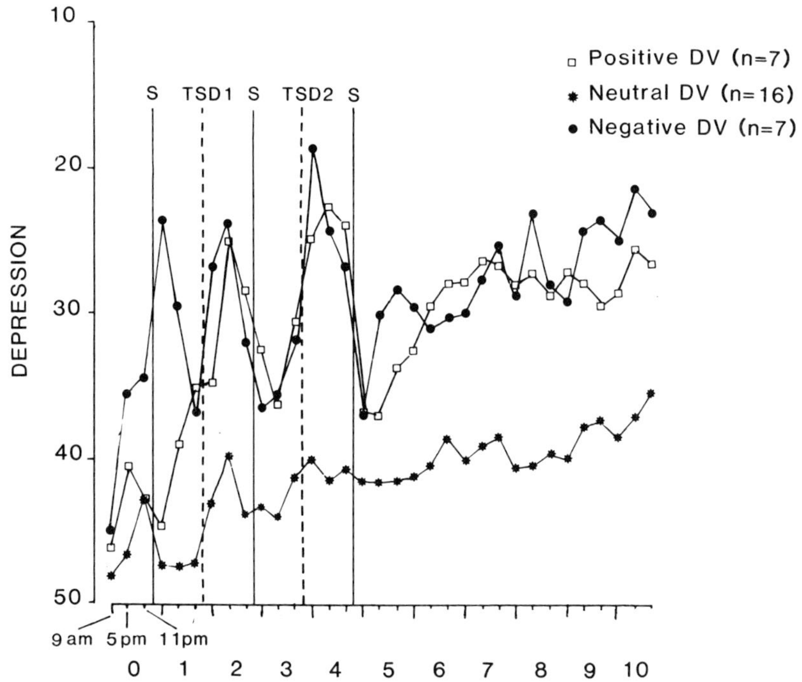

Fig. 7. The course of self-rated depression during the 11 experimental days of study II among subjects with positive, negative, and neutral DV on the day before the first TSD

DV on the day before the first TSD has been defined as the difference between self-rated depression at 9:00 A.M. and at 11:00 P.M. Three groups were formed: one in which on that day at least a 6-point decrease was measured on self-rated depression (positive DV), a second in which at least a 6-point increase was measured (negative DV), and a third in which less than a 6-point difference was found (neutral DV). After pretreatment with clomipramine and TSD, improvement was faster for those patients who initially showed DV, irrespective of the direction of DV (Fig. 7). As a consequence, groups could be formed according to the mere presence or absence of DV. The groups could be further subdivided on the basis of the presence or absence of psychotic features. The course of depression in the four resulting groups is represented in Fig. 8. Psychotic depressives who initially showed DV before the first TSD demonstrate, relative to the baseline value at day 0 (see Fig. 1), a significantly faster improvement than the other three groups ($F_{1,25} = 4.94$, $p < 0.04$). Hence, these observations suggest that DV and psychoticism are relevant predictors not only for a positive acute response to TSD but also for a positive long-term improvement afterwards. Although on the 11th day of the experiment no significant difference was found in favor of the psychotic/DV group in comparison to the other three groups in terms of HRSD ratings ($\alpha = 0.05$), it must be noted that HRSD scores of 10 points or less were obtained in four cases, three of which belonged to the psychotic/DV group.

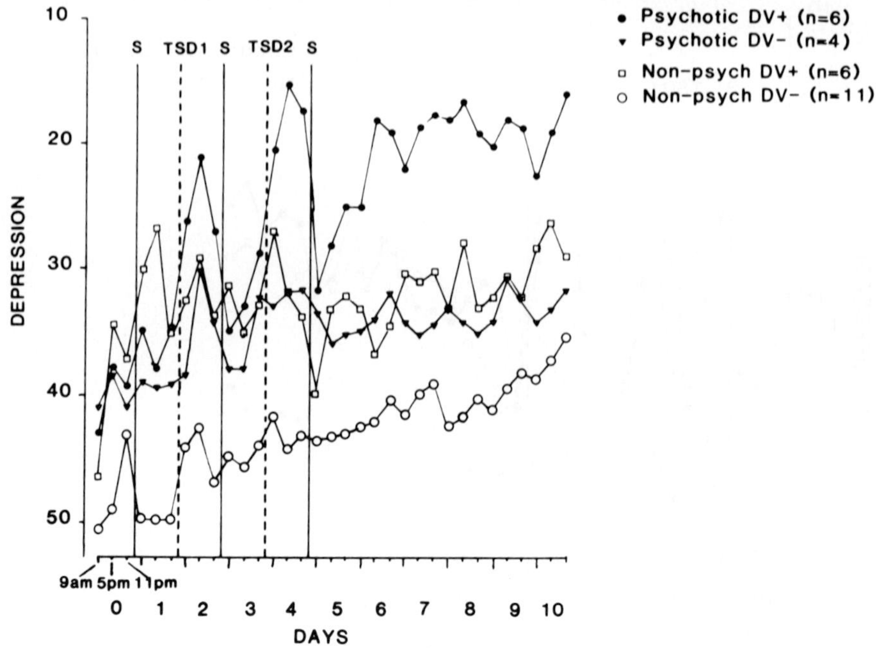

Fig. 8. The course of self-rated depression during the 11 experimental days of study II in subjects distinguished on the basis of presence or absence of DV and on that of psychotic features

Concluding Remarks

This chapter considers (a) the influence of ADM on the response to TSD and subsequent sleep and (b) the therapeutic usefulness of the combination of ADM with TSD.

Several observations have been made with respect to the first issue. As was shown in study I, the response to the first TSD was not different whether placebo or CL was used concurrently. The results of ensuing TSDs, however, did depend on the use of placebo or CL. Only small differences in depression were found for the PL/TSD group after the second, third, and fourth TSDs. In contrast, continued TSD used in combination with CL led to significant differences in depression. Hence, the use of ADM is likely to maintain the antidepressant efficacy of continued TSD. The results of study II supported the finding that TSD preserves its antidepressant potency when ADM is used concurrently. No doubt the close scheduling of two TSDs separated by only 1 night may have interfered with the antidepressant effects for the PL/TSD group. However, this reasoning does not affect the afore mentioned conclusion because both TSD groups were subjected to the same schedule. Moreover, the antidepressant effect of the third TSD (PL/TSD group) was also small. Of course, the effects of CL itself may have contributed to the antidepressant effects of repeated TSDs, but, as shown elsewhere (Elsenga and Van den Hoofdakker 1983a), these effects were variable and small.

Several observations were made with respect to the course of depression after sleep following TSD. As a general rule, it was found that response to sleep outweighs the previous response to TSD. A notable exception was found after the night following the first TSD (study I), where CL prevented the relapse. This result could not be replicated in study II. The most plausible conclusion might have been that the results from study I (CL/TSD group) were due to chance fluctuations, however, other data (of Loosen et al. 1976 and Philipp 1978) support the idea that ADM sustains the antidepressant effect of a TSD following 1 night's sleep. Possibly, selection of patients due to changing referral practices over the years may have influenced the results obtained. Mean HRSD values tended to increase between the studies, in particular for the nonpsychotic depressives. Perhaps, for the more severely depressed patients mental health and referral practices changed less than for the milder cases. Furthermore, prestudy use of ADM differed markedly between the psychotic and the nonpsychotic depressives. From the total of 50 subjects involved in the two studies, 3 of 18 psychotics and 14 of 28 nonpsychotics had been pretreated by ADM. (Only one patient had received a combination treatment of ADM and neuroleptics; one had missing data.) It is also of interest to note that among the day 3 improvers only a few psychotic depressives were found. The possibility that selection may have played a role is even more plausible in view of the finding that, in contrast to patients with psychotic features, those with less severe depression were more likely to respond to ADM alone (Croughan et al. 1988). Thus, the early responders to ADM/TSD might be those who are treated by a general practioner or in an outpatients' clinic rather than being referred to an inpatient setting, i.e., unipolar major depressives of intermediate severity.

The question of prolonged antidepressant effects of sleep deprivation procedures (Gillin 1983) with ADM or lithium (Baxter et al. 1986) is not only therapeutically but also theoretically important. This raises the further question of whether different mechanisms are involved in the way that improvement is effectuated by both interventions (Post et al. 1987; Roy-Birne et al. 1984). For a better understanding of these mechanisms the study of the effects of a variety of psychotropic drugs in combination with TSD is mandatory.

The second issue of this report concerns the course of depression after pretreatment by TSD and ADM. Carpenter et al. (1986) observed that the presence of DV predicts a better response to a traditional antidepressant treatment, regardless of whether patients felt worse in the morning or in the evening. Outcome was assessed after a long period of several months. The observations presented here indicate that in diurnal patients improvement may also start very early under the treatment regime used for the present studies. These data, however, suffer from the absence of a long-term follow-up. Interestingly, the results suggest that the presence of psychotic features in addition to the presence of DV may predict a fast and lasting improvement on ADM after TSD has been employed in the early stage of the treatment. No doubt this observation may merely be a result of chance. On the other hand, psychoticism and DV were chosen as predictors for the long-term course of depression under CL *because* these variables had already been found to predict response to TSD (Elsenga and Van den Hoofdakker 1987). Another source of explanation may be that depressive patients may show placebo responses. Spiker et al. (1988), however, have shown that placebo responses have a low probability in psychotic depression. Whether diurnality predisposes for placebo sensitivity is unclear. Another problem concerns the relative importance of the initial addition of TSDs to the drug treatment. The absence of an adequate comparison group treated with CL alone rules out a definite conclusion. Nevertheless, it should be noted that the psychotic depressives in study I treated with CL alone (group I; see Fig. 1) showed on average hardly any change in depression during the first 11 days of treatment (unpublished data). Whatever the explanation may be, a tentative conclusion may be that TSD in combination with ADM is a possible alternative treatment for diurnal psychotic depressives as opposed to electroconvulsive therapy (Minter and Mandel 1979) or the combined use of tricyclics and antipsychotics (Spiker et al. 1985).

In summary, ADM used concurrently with TSD (a) does not potentiate the antidepressant response to a first TSD, (b) is likely to maintain the antidepressant efficacy of repeated TSD, and (c) probably promotes a large and consistent response to continued TSD especially in psychotic depression. Further, the observation was made that pretreatment by TSD and ADM (i.e., clomipramine) is followed by a fast and lasting improvement, in particular in psychotic depressives who show diurnal variation prior to TSD.

References

Avery D, Lubrano A (1977) Depression treated with imipramine and ECT: the DeCarolis study reconsidered. Am J Psychiatry 136:559–562

Baxter LR, Liston EH, Schwartz JM, Altshuler LL, Wilkens JN, Richeimer S, Guze BH (1986) Prolongation of the antidepressant response to partial sleep deprivation by lithium. Psychiatry Res 19:17–23

Carpenter LL, Kupfer DJ, Frank E (1986) Is diurnal variation a meaningful symptom in depression? J Affective Disord 11:255–264

Croughan JL, Sekunda SK, Katz MM, Robins E, Mendels J, Swann A, Harris-Jarkin B (1988) Sociodemographic and prior clinical course characteristics associated with treatment response in depressed patients. J Psychiatr Res 22:227–237

Elsenga S, Van den Hoofdakker RH (1983a) Clinical effects of sleep deprivation and clomipramine in endogenous depression. J Psychiatr Res 17:361–374

Elsenga S, Van den Hoofdakker RH (1983b) Clinical effects of several sleep/wake manipulations on endogenous depression. Sleep Res 12:326

Elsenga S, Van den Hoofdakker RH (1987) Response to total sleep deprivation and clomipramine in endogenous depression. J Psychiatr Res 21:151–161

Elsenga S, Van den Hoofdakker RH (1988) Body core temperature and depression during total sleep deprivation in depressives. Biol Psychiatry 24:531–540

Gerner RH, Post RM, Gillin JC, Bunney WE (1979) Biological and behavioral effects of one night's sleep deprivation in depressed patients and normals. J Psychiatr Res 15:21–40

Gillin JC (1983) The sleep therapies of depression. Prog Neuropsychopharmacol Biol Psychiatry 7:351–364

Hamilton M (1967) Development of a rating scale for primary depressive illness. Br J Soc Clin Psychol 6:278–296

Howarth BG, Grace MGA (1985) Depression, drugs, and delusions. Arch Gen Psychiatry 42:1145–1147

Kuhs H, Tölle R (1986) Schlafentzug (Wachtherapie) als Antidepressivum. Fortschr Neurol Psychiatry 54:341–355

Loosen PT, Merkel U, Amelung U (1976) Combined sleep deprivation and clomipramine in primary depression. Lancet 2:156–157

Minter RE, Mandel R (1979) The treatment of psychotic major depressive disorder with drugs and electroconvulsive therapy. J Nerv Ment Dis 167:726–733

Philipp M (1978) Depressionsverlauf nach Schlafentzug. Nervenarzt 49:120–123

Post RM, Uhde TW, Rubinow DR, Huggins T (1987) Differential time course of antidepressant effects after sleep deprivation, ECT, and carbamazepine: clinical and theoretical implications. Psychiatry Res 22:11–19

Quitkin F, Rifkin A, Klein DJ (1978) Imipramine response in deluded depressive patients. Am J Psychiatry 135:806–811

Roy-Byrne P, Uhde TW, Post RM, Joffe RT (1984) Relationship of response to sleep deprivation and carbamazepine in depressed patients. Acta Psychiatr Scand 69:379–382

Spiker DG, Kupfer DJ (1988) Placebo rates in psychotic and nonpsychotic depression. J Affective Disord 14:21–23

Spiker DG, Weiss JC, Dealy RS, Griffin SJ, Hanin I, Neil JF, Perel JM, Rossi AJ, Soloff PJ (1985) The pharmacological treatment of delusional depression. Am J Psychiatry 142:430–436

Spiker DG, Dealy RS, Hanin I, Weiss JC, Kupfer DJ (1986) Treating delusional depressives with amitriptyline. J Clin Psychiatry 47:243–246

Van den Burg W, Van den Hoofdakker RH (1975) Total sleep deprivation on endogenous depression. Arch Gen Psychiatry 32:1121–1125

von Zerssen D (1986) Clinical self-rating scales (CSRS) of the Munich Psychiatric Information Systems (Psychis München). In: Sartorius N, Ban TA (eds) Assessment of depression. Springer, Berlin Heidelberg New York, pp 270–303

Pharmacology of New Sleep-Improving Drugs

J. M. Stutzmann, P. M. Laduron, and J. C. Blanchard[1]

Introduction

Our modern way of life with its high levels of stress and anxiety has increased the salience of problems associated with insomnia and consequently also the search for drugs to alleviate this symptom. This review presents the most recent pharmacological data on two types of new sleep-improving drugs: (a) new hypnotics, which have proven active in humans, and (b) sleep modulators, which represent a speculative but interesting approach to the treatment of sleep disorders. We describe here compounds representative of each in terms of pharmacological profile and biochemical characteristics.

Man has always tried to find drugs for the treatment of insomnia, and the number of compounds used for their sedative-hypnotic properties has increased steadily. Alcohol and opium were probably the two first compounds to be used widely as hypnotics during antiquity. In the nineteenth century, bromide was the first agent introduced specifically as a hypnotic, followed by chloral and its derivatives. The twentieth century, due to the development of modern biological chemistry, has seen the advent of many compounds with sedative-hypnotic properties. An important step was the discovery in 1903 of the chemical structure of barbiturates, leading to the development of potent drugs which dominated the class of hypnotics until the discovery in the early 1960s of a new family of drugs, the benzodiazepines (BZD). Over the past 20 years there has been a clear evolution in favor of the use of BZD at the expense of barbiturates, due not only to better efficacy but also to the larger safety margin in overdose, the reduced risk of dependence, and the lower degree of drug interaction (Hollister 1973; Marks 1980). Although used mainly as anxiolytics, some BZD, such as nitrazepam, flurazepam, flunitrazepam, and triazolam, are prescribed principally as hypnotics. During the past few years some new BZD such as brotizolam, quazepam, and midazolam have been employed exclusively as hypnotics.

---

[1] Rhône Poulenc Santé, Centre de Recherches de Vitry, 13 quai J. Guesde, 94403 Vitry Cedex, France.

Neuropsychopharmacology
Edited by Bunney/Hippius/Laakmann/Schmauß

New Nonbenzodiazepine Hypnotics

Zopiclone

A breakthrough in the field of hypnotics came with the recent discovery of new drugs which do not belong to the BZD family. We describe here the pharmacology of such a compound, zopiclone (RP 27267; Fig. 1), which belongs to the cyclopyrrolone family, and which in 1987 became the first non-BZD drug to be introduced as hypnotic since 1960.

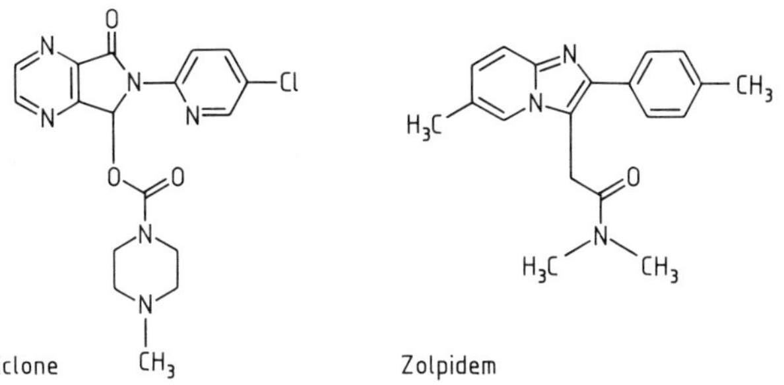

Fig. 1. Chemical structures of zopiclone and zolpidem

Behavioral Pharmacology. Due to the relative insensitivity of animal test procedures available in the psychotropic field it has been possible to define a compound as a hypnotic only after the study of its activity in a battery of tests. Thus the first question about a new hypnotic is: does it possess the pharmacological spectrum which chracterizes sedative-hypnotic drugs? The five main pharmacological properties of hypnotics, including barbiturates and BZD, are that they are anticonvulsant, myorelaxant, sedative-hypnotic, antiaggressive, and "anxiolytic." Qualitatively, zopiclone also possesses anticonvulsant, myorelaxant, sedative-hypnotic, and antiaggressive properties (Table 1). But, quantitatively, what is characteristic of zopiclone is its high sedative and anticonvulsant effects, mainly against pentylenetetrazol, in pharmacological spectrum which characterizes sedative-hypnotic drugs? The Moreover, in a conditioned conflict behavioral test adapted from Geller and Seifter (1960) and Cook and Davidson (1973), zopiclone possessed a clear "anxiolytic" effect, although lower than that of diazepam (Julou et al. 1983, 1985; Blanchard and Stutzmann 1988).

Electroencephalographic Studies. Besides the behavioral models used mainly to characterize the psychotropic profile of drugs, EEG studies can also be performed in animals to demonstrate hypnotic properties. These types of studies are able not only to show the possible qualitative modifications of EEG recordings but also to allow a better appreciation of the hypnotic properties of

Table 1. Pharmacological profile of zopiclone and zolipidem in comparison with benzodiazepines (mg/kg per os)

	Pharmacological properties				
	Anti-convulsant (PTZ; Rat; ED_{50})	Myorelaxant (Inclined screen; Rat; ED_{50})	Sedative hypnotic (Confinement motor activity; Rat; ED_{50})	Anti-aggressive (Foot shock; mouse; ED_{50})	Anxiolytic (Conflict; Rat; EC_{min})
Zopiclone	3	33	3.5	16	2.5[a]
Zolpidem	8	25	2	14	1[b]
Flunitrazepam	1.5	2	8	0.08	–
Triazolam	0.4	2.5	0.7	0.11	0.05[a]
Flurazepam	17.5	40	3.4	6	–

PTZ, Pentylenetetrazol.
[a] Cook test.
[b] Vogel test (from Zivkovic et al. 1988).

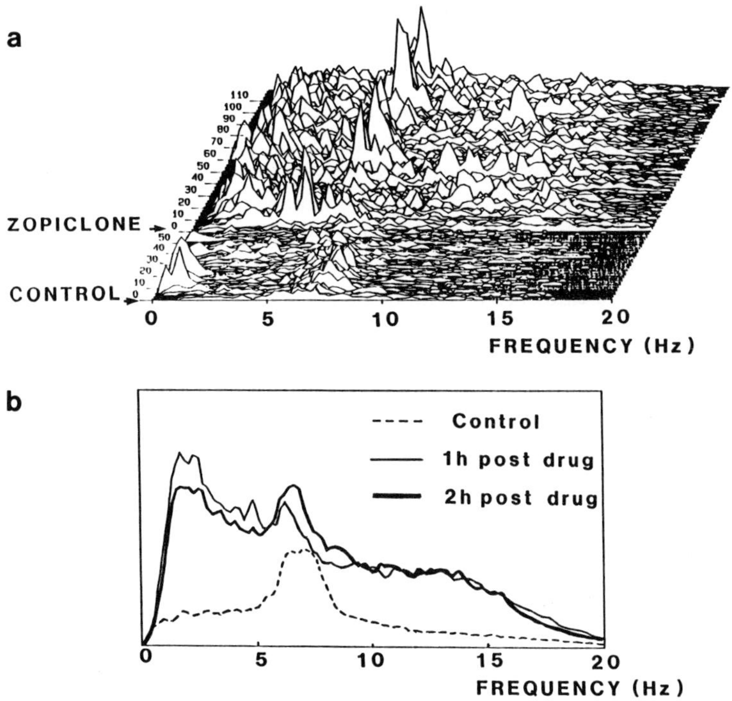

Fig. 2. Sequential (**a**) and average (**b**) spectral analysis of 20-s EEG epochs of the frontal cortex before (control) and after intraperitoneal administration of 2.5 mg/kg zopiclone in rat. In the sequential analysis: *x-axis*, frequency in hertz; *y-axis*, time in minutes; *z-axis*, energy in μvolt^2/Hz

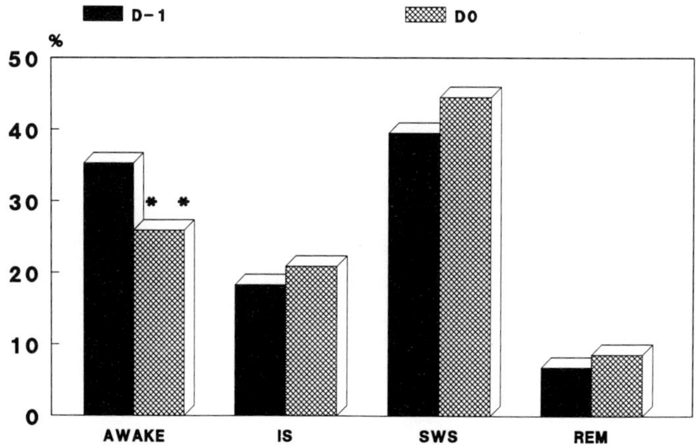

Fig. 3. Sleep-wakefulness stages the day before (*D-1*) and the day of intraperitoneal administration (*DO*) of 2.5 mg/kg zopiclone in rat ($n = 6$). All values are expressed as percentage of the total recording period (7 h). *IS*, intermediate sleep; *SWS*, slow-wave sleep; *REM*, rapid eye movement sleep; Comparison between treated and control periods was made using Student's t test for paired series *double asterisk*, $p < 0.01$

a drug. Two types of EEG studies can be performed. One is spectral analysis, which investigates the modification of energy as a function of frequency and time. The lowest dose at which zopiclone modified repartition in spectral analysis was 2.5 mg/kg, administered intraperitoneally. Figure 2 indicates that as early as 10 min following the administration of zopiclone an increase in energy occurred at very low frequencies (slow waves, D band: 1–4 Hz) as well as at high frequencies (B band: >12 Hz), which is a spectral profile characteristic of hypnotics such as barbiturates or BZD. The second type of EEG study is that of sleep-wakefulness stages in animals. In the rat, four basic stages of vigilance can be characterized in an EEG (Michel et al. 1961): awake, intermediate sleep, slow-wave sleep (SWS), and rapid eye movement sleep (REM). The major changes induced by zopiclone in these sleep-wakefulness stages after the low intraperitoneal dose of 2.5 mg/kg are illustrated in Fig. 3. One can see on the day of administration a significant decrease in wakefulness whereas, interestingly, SWS and REM were slightly increased.

Biochemical Results. A further question concerning any new hypnotic drug is: what is its mechanism of action? It is now generally agreed that the discovery in 1977 of specific high-affinity binding sites for BZD in rat and human brain tissues was a major breakthrough in understanding the mechanism of action of these drugs (Möhler and Okada 1977; Squires and Braestrup 1977). It is of prime importance to know whether non-BZD hypnotics recognize this so called BZD receptor, which belongs to the γ-aminobutyric acid (GABA) receptor complex. It was demonstrated as early as 1979 that zopiclone was able to recognize rat cortical BZD sites labeled with diazepam (Blanchard et al. 1979). This is proof that these sites are true receptors and not merely acceptor

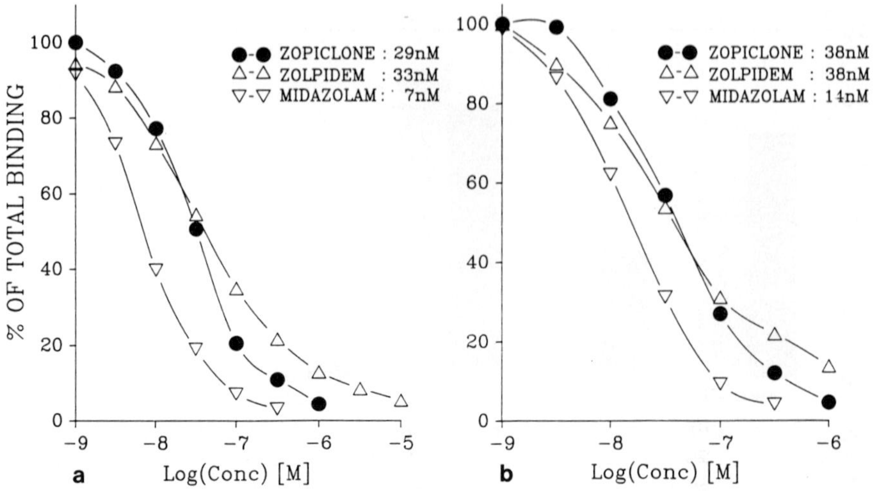

Fig. 4. Inhibition (IC_{50}) by zopiclone, zolpidem, and midazolam of [^{3}H]Ro 15-1788 specific binding to rat (**a**) and human (**b**) cortical receptors

sites. The affinity of zopiclone is specific for this type of receptor, and no other brain receptors, such as dopamine, serotonin (5-HT), acetylcholine, and even peripheral BZD sites, show affinity for zopiclone. Further, studies using zopiclone as a ligand revealed that its mode of interaction with receptors is different from that of BZD; zopiclone had a low photoshift and a low GABA shift (Snyder 1987; Blanchard et al. 1983a, 1983b). Zopiclone also showed a high affinity for receptors in human brain tissue; its affinity for the human receptor was similar to that found in the rat cortex (Fig. 4).

Zolpidem

Zolpidem, which belongs to the family of imidazopyridines (Fig. 1), has been described and developed by LERS as a hypnotic (Langer et al. 1985; Depoortere et al. 1986; Scatton et al. 1986). We present here results obtained with this compound in our laboratory (the compound used was synthesized in the Rhône Poulenc Chemistry Department).

Behavioral Pharmacology. Zolpidem shares the five main pharmacological properties listed above of sedative-hypnotics in animals. Its profile in terms of these properties is close to that of zopiclone (Table 1). However zolpidem, in contrast to zopiclone failed to produce any antipunishment activity in the conditioned conflict paradigm; an anticonflict effect of zolpidem could, on the other hand, be observed in the Vogel test (Zivkovic et al. 1988), a nonconditioned punished drinking test.

Electroencephalographic Studies. In freely moving rats, both zolpidem and zopiclone at an intraperitoneal dose of 2.5 mg/kg induced an increase in energy in sequential spectral analysis with a maximal activity at low frequencies (D band: 1–4 Hz) and high frequencies (Fig. 5). These EEG effects of zolpidem on slow-wave frequencies were previously reported in the curarized rat at an intraperitoneal dose of 0.3 mg/kg by Depoortere et al. (1988). Moreover, in rats recorded during the light period, zolpidem at 3 mg/kg per os significantly decreased the total duration of wakefulness (Depoortere et al. 1988).

Biochemical Results. Using the BZD antagonist Ro 15-1788 as a ligand, zolpidem, like zopiclone, recognized the BZD receptor in rat and in human tissue (Fig. 4). Since the discovery of high-affinity BZD binding sites in mammalian brain, evidence has accumulated for the existence of at least two subtypes of BZD receptors in the CNS: BZD_1 which predominate in the cerebellum and BZD_2 which are found in the spinal cord, putamen, and hippocampus. The cerebral cortex possesses a mixed population of BZD_1 and BZD_2 sites (Klepner et al. 1979; Braestrup and Nielsen 1981). It is tempting to associate pharmacological activity with the recognition of each subtype. CL 218 872 was the first drug shown to possess a higher affinity for BZD_1 than BZD_2 receptors and was pharmacologically described as a nonsedative

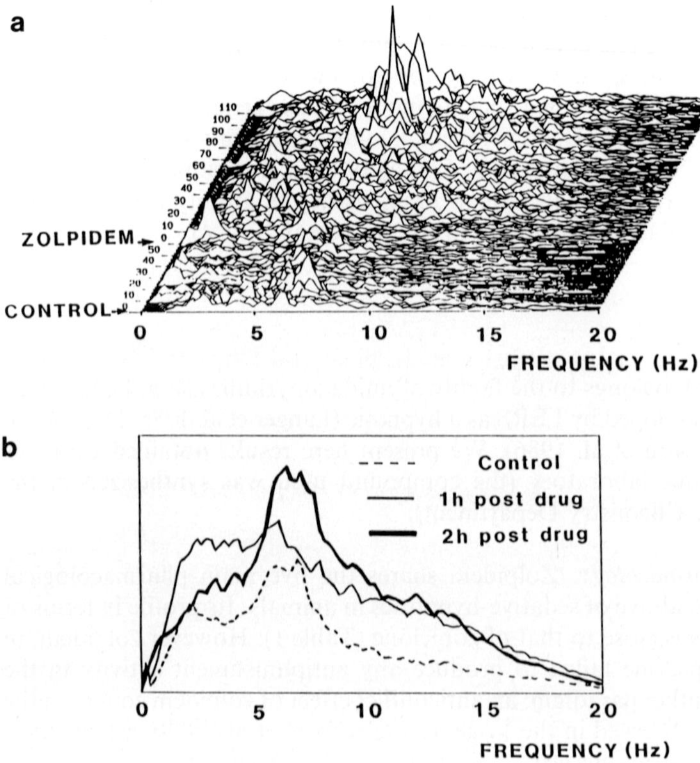

Fig. 5. EEG sequential (**a**) and average (**b**) spectral analysis before and after intraperitoneal administration of 2.5 mg/kg zolpidem. (See Fig. 2)

anxiolytic (Klepner et al. 1979; Lippa et al. 1982). In contrast to zopiclone, which recognized with the same affinity the receptor sites in cortex, putamen, and cerebellum, zolpidem possessed a higher affinity for BZD_1 sites (Table 2). It was proposed that this BZD_1 affinity could be responsible for its hypnotic activity. The fact that zolpidem does not possess a pharmacological profile different from that of zopiclone, which did not distinguish between BZD_1 and BZD_2 sites, questions the relevance of this interpretation; therefore the

Table 2. Inhibition of [^{3}H]Ro 15-1788 binding to human brain (0 °C; IC_{50}, nM)

	Cortex	Putamen	Cerebellum
Zopiclone	35	32	29
Zolpidem	42	41	17
CL 218 872	249	228	142
Midazolam	13	13	12
Diazepam	47	48	44

functional significance of the selective activation of BZD_1 or BZD_2 sites is still an open question. A new classification of the BZD receptors has recently been proposed by Langer and Arbilla (1988), designating as $\omega 1$ the formerly named BZD_1 site, $\omega 2$ the BZD_2 site and, $\omega 3$ the peripheral BZD site. This new nomenclature, the purpose of which seems to be to avoid the utilization of BZD receptor terminology, is in our view rather misleading since with recent progress in molecular biology, it has been demonstrated that the sedative-hypnotics which displace the BZD ligand bind in fact to the α subunit of the GABA receptor (Schofield et al. 1987). Thus, if we want to avoid BZD receptor terminology, we should preferentially adopt that of the GABA α subunit.

In addition to pharmacological, EEG, and biochemical properties, estimating the duration of action is of prime importance in the field of hypnotics. In in vivo binding studies using a dose of zopiclone, which occupies about 90% of sites at 0.5 h, it took 6 h to obtain a 50% displacement of ligand. This is in contrast with zolpidem, with which the same decrease in receptor occupancy was obtained after 3.5 h. These results fit very well with the half-life observed in man with these two drugs, zopiclone having a short half-life and zolpidem a shorter half-life.

New Sleep-Modulating Compounds

Another approach to insomnia treatment has led to the search for compounds which lack the pharmacological profile of hypnotics but present activities indicating that they could be of interest in the treatment of sleep disorders. These can be defined as sleep-modulating compounds. Recently an important step was made with the discovery by Janssen Laboratories that a $5\text{-}HT_2$ antagonist, ritanserin, improves sleep and thus belongs to the group of sleep-modulating drugs.

Ritanserin

Binding Studies. Ritanserin, a thiazolopyrimidine derivative (Fig. 6), is a drug which possesses high affinity for central $5\text{-}HT_2$ receptors ($IC_{50} = 1\ nM$; Table 3) but lacks affinity for the $5\text{-}HT_1$ site, as shown by Leysen et al. (1985), and does not recognize the BZD sites, as shown by J. L. Zundel (personnal communication).

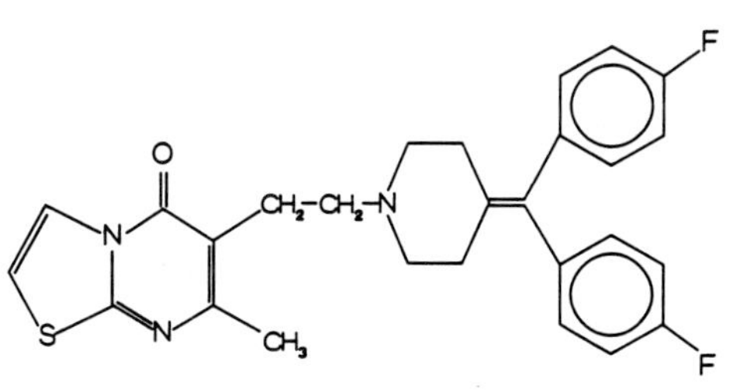

Fig. 6. Chemical structure of ritanserin

Table 3. In vitro receptor binding profile of ritanserin. (From Leysen et al. 1985)

Receptor site	Binding affinity (IC_{50}, n*M*)
5-HT_2	0.9
5-HT_1	>1000
α_1	97
α_2	150
D_2	70
H_1	35

Electroencephalographic Studies. Ritanserin, up to the dose of 2 mg/kg per os induced an increase in energy principally at low frequencies (<4 Hz), which corresponds to the SWS activity of the drug; its sequential spectral analysis is clearly different from that observed with the hypnotics described above because there is no increase at high frequencies (Fig. 7). In Sprague-Dawley rats, we have confirmed the SWS-improving effect of ritanserin at 0.5 mg/kg per os, as previously reported in Wistar rats at 0.63 and 2.5 mg/kg administered intraperitoneally (Dugovic and Wauquier 1987). Moreover, ritanserin prevented insomnia induced by DOM [(2,5-dimethoxy-4-methyl-phenyl)-2-aminopropane], a 5-HT_2 agonist, but not that induced by 8-OH-DPAT [8-hydroxy-2-(di-*n*-propylamino) tetralin] or RU 24969, which are 5-HT_1 agonists (Dugovic and Wauquier 1987). In sleep studies by Idzikowski et al. (1987) and Declerck et al. (1987), ritanserin significantly increased SWS in humans.

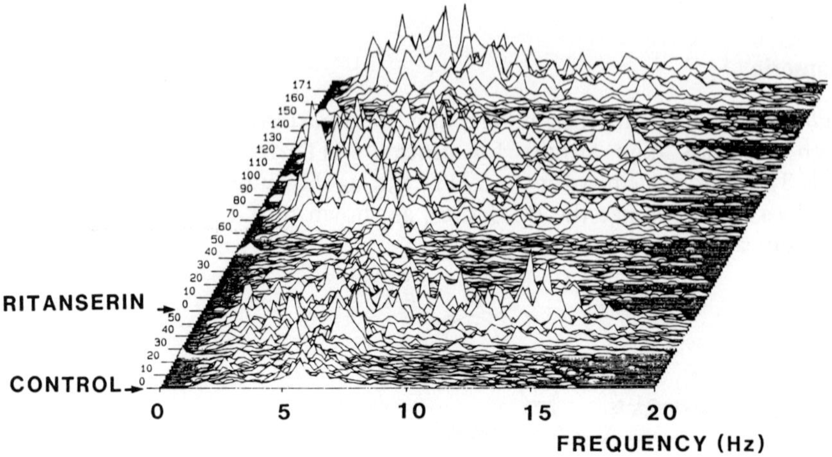

Fig. 7. EEG sequential spectral analysis before and after oral administration of 2 mg/kg ritanserin. (See Fig. 2)

Riluzole

Biochemical Studies. Riluzole (PK 26124 or RP 54274) is a benzothiazole derivative (Fig. 8). In biochemical models it antagonized in vitro the increase in cGMP levels in the cerebellum induced by glutamate or aspartate. It also decreased the release of dopamine induced by glutamate in the push-pull in cat striatum and the aspartate release stimulated by ibotenate in rodent cerebellar

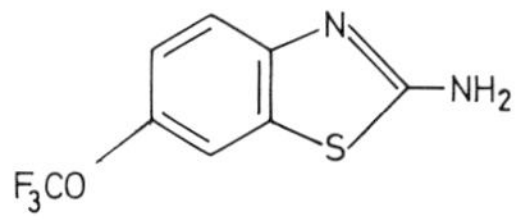

Fig. 8. Chemical structure of riluzole

cells (Benavides et al. 1985; Cheramy et al. 1986; Doble et al. 1987). Although riluzole does not bind to any of the glutamate receptors (or to other known binding sites), it interferes with glutamate neurotransmission. Moreover, riluzole does not bind to BZD or 5-HT receptors.

Behavioral Pharmacology. Riluzole protected rodents in different models of convulsions, including those induced by glutamate administered intracerebrovascularly in rats, by glutamic acid decarboxylase inhibitors administered intraperitoneally in mice and rats, and by maximal electroshock in mice. It also affected epileptogenic discharges in the kindling phenomenon in rats. But in contrast with BZD or barbiturates, it was ineffective against clonic seizures induced by pentylenetetrazole, bicuculline, or picrotoxin (Mizoule et al. 1985; Rataud et al. 1988). Moreover, in behavioral pharmacology, riluzole did not possess any myorelaxant, sedative, or antiaggressive activities (Fig. 9).

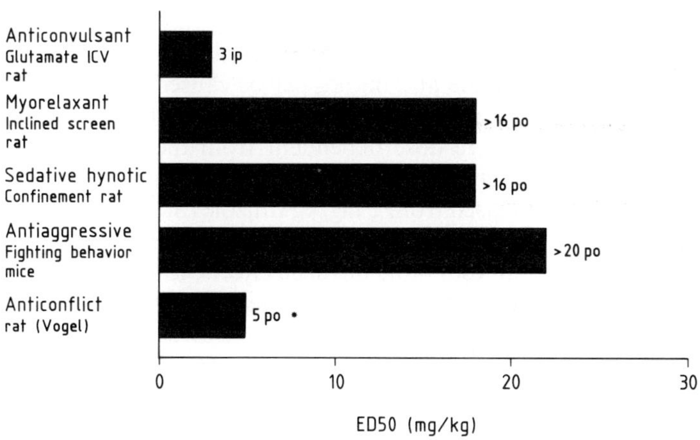

Fig. 9. Pharmacological profile of riluzole. Values are ED_{50} (mg/kg; *asterisk*, EC_{min})

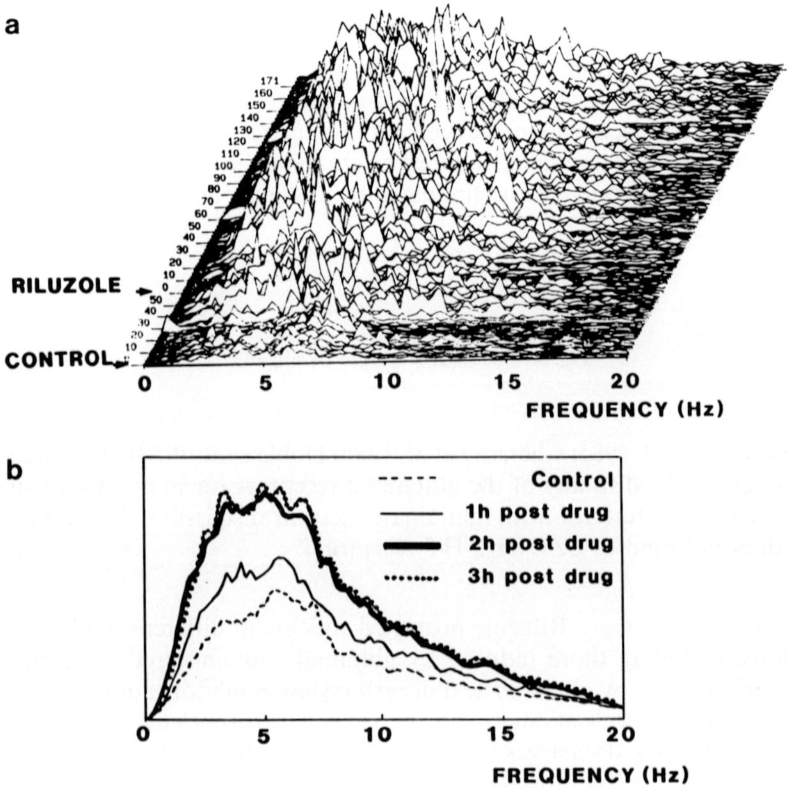

Fig. 10. EEG sequential (**a**) and average (**b**) spectral analysis before and after oral administration of 2 mg/kg riluzole. (See Fig. 2)

Electroencephalographic Studies. Energy at low frequencies (<4 Hz) was increased after 2 mg/kg riluzole per os (Fig. 10); this indicates an SWS effect of the drug. The lack of increased activity at high frequencies differentiates it from hypnotics. Administration or riluzole at 2 mg/kg per os caused a significant increase in SWS and REM at the expense of wakefulness; these effects could be observed for 6 h postdrug and were dose dependent from the low dose of 1 mg/kg per os (Fig. 11). Moreover, sleep latencies were significantly reduced and REM phase frequencies increased from 2 mg/kg riluzole (Stutzmann et al. 1988a). In the cat, riluzole at 2 mg/kg also increased SWS and REM for 3 and 7 h, respectively. In addition to studies of its intrinsic effects, riluzole has also been examined in insomnia models in rats. Various compounds with different mechanisms of action are able to induce wakefulness in a dose-dependent way; these include (a) caffeine, a methylxanthine adenosine antagonist; (b) FG 7142, an inverse agonist at the GABA-BZD receptor; (c) amphetamine, which increases the release of cathecholamines; and (c) DOI, [(2,5 dimethoxy-4-iodophenyl)-2-aminopropane] a 5-HT_2 agonist. Riluzole tended to prevent

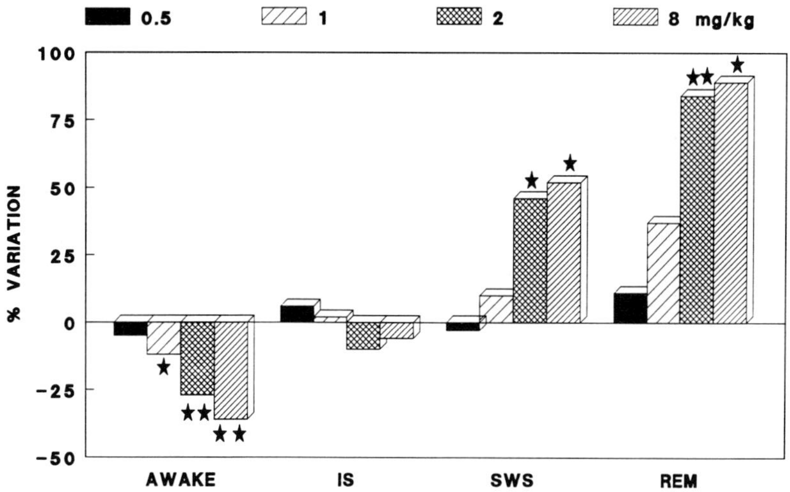

Fig. 11. Dose-response effects of riluzole on sleep-wakefulness stages in rat. All values are expressed as percentage of variation from the control period ($n = 5$; rats/dose). Comparison between treated and control periods were made using Student's t test for paired series; *single asterisk*, $p < 0.05$; *double asterisk*, $p < 0.01$

insomnia induced by caffeine and FG 7142 but not that observed under amphetamine or DOI (Stutzmann et al. 1988b).

Conclusion

Among the new sleep-improving drugs we have distinguished between those which have proven to be active in man, such as zopiclone (Billiard et al. 1987), and can be considered as true hypnotics and those with sleep-modulating activity, such as ritanserin or riluzole, which need further clinical investigation. The first group possesses the pharmacological, biochemical, and pharmacokinetic properties which seem necessary for a good hypnotic, and clinical results have proven the efficacy of these compounds against insomnia. Moreover, biochemical data obtained with these new drugs have confirmed the pharmacological importance of the GABA system in the control of sleep-wakefulness cycles.

The second group contains drugs which are characterized as sleep modulators because they do not possess the pharmacological profile of hypnotics but behave in certain models as sleep-inducing drugs. In this group, we have considered ritanserin, which acts through the serotoninergic system and allows reconsideration of the 5-HT theory of sleep (Jouvet 1983), and riluzole which probably acts through glutamatergic transmission. This raises the importance of glutamate in sleep-wakefulness regulation. Very few studies have been performed concerning the relationships between glutamate neurotransmission and sleep-wakefulness cycles in animals. Nevertheless, the release of glutamate was observed to be significantly decreased in genetically "long-sleep" mice in comparison to "short-sleep" ones (Disbrow and Ruth 1984). In cats and rabbits the increase in cortical glutamate release induced by electrical stimulation of different brain structures including the thalamus and reticular formation are correlated with electrocortigraphic desynchronization (Blagoeva et al. 1972; Jasper and Koyama 1969). Thus, the sleep-promoting effect of riluzole could be explained by possible modulation of the glutamatergic transmission. However, taking into account the results obtained with riluzole versus caffeine, one cannot exclude a participation of adenosine neurotransmission in the sleep-inducing effect of riluzole since adenosine, adenosine analogs, and adenosine deaminase increase not only SWS but also REM through interaction with adenosine A_1 receptors (Radulovacki et al. 1983).

The greatest difficulty in research on sleep modulators is the definition of a new predictive pharmacological profile for this type of compound. The use of electrophysiological studies, particularly the development of insomnia models associated with classical behavioral and biochemical studies, seems to be an interesting approach in this field.

Sleep-modulating compounds could be of prime importance in the future for the treatment of disorders associated with sleep disturbances. As proposed by Janssen (1988), these compounds might allow the restoration of energy functions during sleep, thus improving negative symptoms in psychiatric diseases.

Acknowledgement. We are grateful to J. Pratt for editing of the manuscript and critical comments.

References

Bénavides J, Camelin JC, Mitrani N, Flamand F, Uzan A, Legrand JJ, Gueremy C, Le Fur G (1985) 2-Amino-6-trifluoromethoxy benzothiazole, a possible antagonist of excitatory amino acid neurotransmission. II. Neuropharmacology 24:1085–1092

Billiard M, Besset A, De Lustrac C, Brissand L (1987) Dose-response effects of zopiclone on night sleep and on nightime and daytime functioning. Sleep 10 (Suppl) 1:27–34

Blagoeva P, Masi I, Scotti de Carolis A, Longo VG (1972) Amino acid release from the cerebral cortex of the rabbit, its relationship with the electrocorticogram. Physiol Behav 9:307–313

Blanchard JC, Stutzmann JM (1988) Zopiclone (Imovane) un nouvel hypnotique non benzodiazepinique: propriétés pharmacologiques et mécanisme d'action. Rev Sci Méd 2:65–81

Blanchard JC, Boireau A, Garret C, Julou L (1979) In vitro and in vivo inhibition by zopiclone of benzodiazepine binding to rodent brain receptors. Life Sci 24:2417–2420

Blanchard JC, Boireau A, Julou L (1983a) Brain receptors and zopiclone. Pharmacology 27 (Suppl) 2:59–69

Blanchard JC, Zundel JL, Julou L (1983b) Differences between cyclopyrrolones (suriclone and zopiclone) and benzodiazepines binding to rat hippocampus photolabelled membranes. Biochem Pharmacol 32:3651–3653

Braestrup C, Nielsen M (1981) [^{3}H]Propyl β-carboline-3-carboxylate as a selective radioligand for the BZD_1 benzodiazepine receptor subclass. J Neurochem 37:333–341

Chéramy A, Romo R, Godeheu G, Baruch P, Glowinski J (1986) In vivo presynaptic control of dopamine release in the cat caudate nucleus. II. Facilitory or inhibitory influence of L-glutamate. Neuroscience 19:1081–1090

Cook L, Davidson AB (1973) Effects of behaviourally active drugs in a conflict punishment procedure in rats. In: Garattini S, Mussini E, Randall LO (eds) The benzodiazepines. Raven, New York, pp 327–345

Declerck AC, Wauquier PHM, Van der Ham-Veltman, Gelders Y (1987) Increase of slow wave sleep in human volunteers by the serotonin S_2 antagonist ritanserin. Curr Ther Res 41:427–432

Depoortere H, Zivkovic B, Lloyd KG, Sanger DJ, Perrault G, Langer SZ, Bartholini G (1986) Zolpidem, a novel nonbenzodiazepine hypnotic. I. Neuropharmacological and behavioral effects. J Pharmacol Exp Ther 237:649–658

Depoortere H, Decobert M, Riou-Merle F, Granger P (1988) Pharmaco-EEG profile of zolpidem: an imidazopyridine hypnotic agent. In: Sauvanet JP, Langer SZ, Morselli PL (eds) Imidazopyridines in sleep disorders. Raven, New York, pp 81–96

Disbrow JK, Ruth JA (1984) Differential glutamate release in brain regions of long sleep and short sleep mice. Alcohol 1:201–203

Doble A, Hubert JP, Perrier ML (1987) The pharmacology of an excitatory amino acid receptor. Br J Pharmacol 91:23

Dugovic C, Wauquier A (1987) 5-HT_2 receptors could be primarily involved in the regulation of slow wave sleep in the rat. Eur J Pharmacol 137:145–146

Geller I, Seifter J (1960) The effects of meprobamate, barbiturates D-amphetamine and promazine on experimentally induced conflict in the rat. Psychopharmacology 1:482–492

Hollister LE (1973) Antianxiety drugs in clinical practice. In: Garettini S, Mussini E, Randall LO (eds) The benzodiazepines. Raven, New York, pp 367–377

Idzikowski C, Mills FJ, Glennard R (1986) 5-Hydroxytryptamine-2 antagonist increases human slow wave sleep. Brain Res 378:164–168

Janssen PAJ (1988) The relevance of pharmacological studies to sleep research in psychiatry. Pharmacopsychiatry 21:33–37

Jasper H, Koyama I (1969) Rate of release of amino acids from the cerebral cortex in the cat affected by brainstem and thalamic stimulation. Can J Physiol Pharmacol 47:889–905

Jouvet M (1983) Mecanismes des etats de sommeil. In: Benoit O (ed) Physiologie du sommeil. Masson, Paris, pp 1–18

Julou L, Bardone MC, Blanchard JC, Garret C, Stutzmann JM (1983) Pharmacological studies on zopiclone. Pharmacology 27:46–58

Julou L, Blanchard JC, Dreyfus JF (1985) Pharmacological and clinical studies of cyclopyrrolones: zopiclone and suriclone. Pharmacol Biochem Behav 23:653–659

Klepner CA, Lippa AS, Benson DI, Sano MC, Beer B (1979) Resolution of two biochemically and pharmacologically distinct benzodiazepine receptors. Pharmacol Biochem Behav 11:457–462

Langer SZ, Arbilla S (1988) Limitations of the benzodiazepine receptor nomenclature: a proposal for a pharmacological classification as omega receptor subtypes. Fundam Clin Pharmacol 2:159–170

Langer SZ, Depoortere H, Sanger D, George P, Zivkovic B, Arbilla S, Lloyd KG, Bartholini G (1985) Biochemical and pharmacological profile of SL 80.0759-23N, a new short acting hypnotic. J Neurochem 44:S179

Leysen JE, Gommeren W, Van Gompel P, Wynants J, Janssen PFM, Laduron P (1985) Receptor-binding properties in vitro and in vivo of ritanserin. Mol Pharmacol 27:600–611

Lippa AS, Jackson D, Wennogle LP, Beer B, Meyerson LR (1982) Non-benzodiazepine antagonists for benzodiazepine receptors. In: Usdin E, Skolnick P, Tallman JF, Greenblett D, Paul SM (eds) Pharmacology of benzodiazepines. MacMillan Press, London, pp 431–440

Marks J (1980) The benzodiazepine use and abuse. Arzneimittelforschung/Drug Res 30:388–390

Michel F, Klein M, Jouvet D, Valatx JL (1961) Etude polygraphique du sommeil chez le rat. C R Soc Biol (Paris) 155:2389–2392

Mizoule J, Meldrum B, Mazadier M, Croucher M, Ollat C, Uzan A, Legrand JJ, Guérémy C, Le Fur G (1985) 2-Amino-6-trifluoromethoxy benzothiazole, a possible antagonist of excitatory amino acid neurotransmission. I. Anticonvulsant properties. Neuropharmacology 24:767–773

Möhler H, Okada T (1977) Benzodiazepine receptor: demonstration in the central nervous system. Science 198:849–851

Rataud J, Bardone MC, Stutzmann JM, Mazadier M, Uzan A, Blanchard JC, Laduron P (1988) Riluzole (PK 26124) induces discriminative stimuli in rats. Psychopharmacology 96 (Suppl):373

Radulovacki M, Virus RM, Djuricic-Nedelson M, Green RD (1983) Adenosine analogs and sleep in rats. J Pharmacol Exp Ther 228:268–274

Scatton B, Claustre Y, Dennis T, Nishikawa T (1986) Zolpidem, a novel nonbenzodiazepine hypnotic. II. Effects on cerebellar cyclic GMP levels and cerebral monoamines. J Pharmacol Exp Ther 237:659–665

Schofield PR, Darlison MG, Fujita N, Burt DR, Stephenson FA, Rodriguez M, Rhee LM, Ramachadran J, Reale V, Glencorse TA, Seeburg PH, Barnard EA (1987) Sequence and functional expression of the $GABA_A$ receptor shows a ligand-gated receptor super-family. Nature 328:221–227

Snyder SH (1987) GABA-benzodiazepine receptor complex: focus on receptor subtypes and cyclopyrrolone drugs. Isr J Med Sci 23:145–152

Squires RF, Braestrup C (1977) Benzodiazepine receptor in rat brain. Nature 266:732–734

Stutzmann JM, Lucas M, Blanchard JC, Laduron PM (1988a) Riluzole, a glutamate antagonist, enhances slow wave and REM sleep in rats. Neurosci Lett 88:195–200

Stutzmann JM, Laduron PM, Blanchard JC (1988b) Sleep enhancing effect of riluzole in rats and cats. 9th European congress of sleep research, Jérusalem, Abstracts, p 207

Zivkovic B, Perrault G, Morel E, Sanger DJ (1988) Comparative pharmacology of zolpidem and other hypnotics and sleep inducers. In: Sauvanet JP, Langer SZ, Morselli PL (eds) Imidazopyridines in sleep disorders. Raven, New York, pp 97–110

16 Drug Effects and Morphological Investigations in Human Postmortem Tissue

Neurotransmitter Function in Post-Mortem Human Brain: An Overview

C. J. FOWLER[1], R. F. COWBURN[2], J. A. HARDY[3], P. WESTER[4], and B. WINBLAD[1]

Introduction

Use of post-mortem human brain samples in research is associated with a number of advantages and disadvantages. The two main advantages are (a) that the disease process in question can be studied per se instead of using animal models, the relevance of which are sometimes doubtful (for discussion, see Willner 1984; Fowler et al. 1988), and (b) that the observed neurochemical changes can be correlated with symptomatology. Disadvantages include the fact that autopsy samples represent the end point of the disease, where secondary symptoms may play an obfuscatory role. In addition, interpretation of findings is hindered by a number of factors, such as drug treatment, agonal state and post-mortal stability, that must be taken into account. Finally, the nature of the samples, and the necessity for their storage, rules out a number of assays (for further discussion, see Hardy and Dodd 1983; Perry and Perry 1983; Lee 1988).

Until recently, these limitations have largely restricted investigations in post-mortem tissue to assay of neurotransmitter and neurotransmitter metabolite levels, neurotransmitter-related enzyme activities and receptor recognition site densities (for recent reviews, see Mann et al. 1986; O'Neill et al. 1987; Lee 1988; Lloyd and Carter 1988; Morgan et al. 1988; Perry and Candy 1988; Young and Penney 1988). Whilst these studies have undoubtedly enhanced our understanding of the neurochemical pathology of the brain, there is a need for more "functional" data. In recent years, advances have been made allowing the assay of functional parameters such as neurotransmitter uptake and release. This area of research is the subject of the present chapter.

[1] Department of Geriatric Medicine, Karolinska Institutet, Huddinge Sjukhus, B56, 141 86 Huddinge, and Research and Development Laboratories, Astra Research Centre AB, 151 85 Södertälje, Sweden.

[2] Department of Geriatric Medicine, Karolinska Institutet, Huddinge Sjukhus, B56, 141 86 Huddinge, Sweden.

[3] Biochemistry Department, St. Mary's Hospital Medical School, London W2 1PG, United Kingdom.

[4] Departments of Internal Medicine and Pathology, University of Umeå, 901 87 Umeå, Sweden.

Neuropsychopharmacology
Edited by Bunney/Hippius/Laakmann/Schmauß

Post-Mortem Stability of Functional Neurochemical Parameters

A prerequisite for the assay of functional neurochemical parameters in post-mortem human brain tissue is that their post-mortem stability is good. Wester et al. (1985) reported that the post-mortal retention of metabolic activity of synaptosomal preparations was critically dependent upon agonal status. Thus, synaptosomal preparations from patients who had died after a short terminal phase, such as from acute myocardial infarction, retained good metabolic activity, assessed by measuring basal and veratrine-stimulated oxygen uptake, for death–autopsy delays of up to 12–15 h. On the other hand, cases with long terminal phases, such as in bronchopneumonia, rapidly lost metabolic activity, no oxygen uptake being found for post-mortem delays of 6 h or longer (Wester et al. 1985). Parallel with this, it was found that the brain samples from cases with long terminal phases were acidotic compared with the those of short terminal phase (Hardy et al. 1985). These studies indicate that functional parameters that are critically dependent upon retention of metabolic activity should be limited to autopsy cases with relatively short (i.e. less than 12 h) death–autopsy intervals and short terminal phases. This means considerable selection of samples, particularly in disease states such as dementia of Alzheimer type, in which the terminal phase is often long.

Stability Upon Storage of Functional Neurochemical Parameters

For practical purposes, it is important that storage methods are available that allow the functional parameter to be measured upon thawing. In some cases, such as those with vasoactive intestinal polypeptide and forskolin stimulated adenylate cyclase activity, simple freezing of the tissue at −80 °C is sufficient

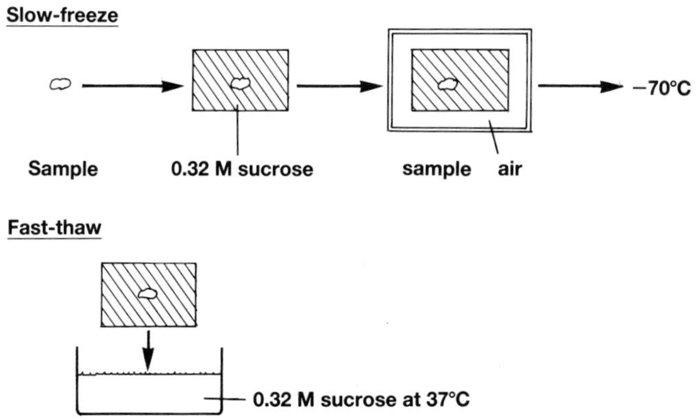

Fig. 1. Diagrammatic representation of the "slow-freeze – fast-thaw" method of Hardy et al. (1983). Using this procedure, the temperature of the tissue drops slowly. The temperature of a rat cerebral cortical sample was reduced from +10 °C at $t=0$ to 0 °C and $t=1$ h, −15 °C at $t \simeq 3$ h and −40 °C at $t=4$ h (Dodd et al. 1986)

(Westlind-Danielsson et al. 1987; Danielsson et al. 1988). Parameters requiring synaptosomal integrity, however, require methods of freezing that protect against freeze–thaw injury. Two such methods are the "slow-freeze – fast-thaw" method of Hardy et al. (1983; see Fig. 1 for diagrammatic representation, and Dodd et al. 1986 for further methodological studies) and freezing in the presence of dimethyl sulphoxide (Haan and Bowen 1981).

Such methods have allowed the measurement of several functional neurochemical parameters, such as monoamine and amino acid accumulation and release, in human post-mortem tissue. Since these studies have recently been reviewed (Dodd et al. 1988; Fowler 1988), the following section restricts itself to some selected examples.

Applications and Limitations – Some Selected Examples

In 1986 Hardy et al. reported that [^{3}H]γ-aminobutyric acid ([^{3}H]GABA) accumulated in human cerebral cortical synaptosomes prepared from tissue stored by the "slow-freeze – fast-thaw" technique in a manner that was both temperature and sodium dependent, and which could be prevented by osmotic shock of the synaptosomes. The K_M of the uptake was 10 μM, although the nonlinearity of the Hanes plot used to calculate the data suggested the presence of more than one uptake system. A more detailed analysis using human frontal

Table 1. Comparison of [^{3}H]γ-aminobutyric acid uptake in human and rat brain samples

	Human Cortex	Rat cerebral cortex
K_M (μM)	1.94/21/– [a]	1.34/48/2923 [a]
V_{max} (nmol min^{-1} mg protein^{-1})	0.15/0.78/– [a]	0.26/0.56/4.24 [a]
IC_{50} values (μM)		
Guvacine	13 [b]	8 [c]
Nipecotic acid	16 [b]	9 [c], 12 [d]
ACHC	65 [b]	62 [d]
Arecaidine	70 [b]	122 [c]
DABA	80 [b]	66 [e]
β-Alanine	1250 [b]	21000 [f]

K_M and V_{max} values represent high-, medium- and low-affinity components (–, not detected). ACHC, *cis*-3-aminocyclohexane carboxylic acid; DABA, L-2,4-diaminobutyric acid.

[a] Frontal cortical synaptosomes (from Sidhu et al. 1987).
[b] Cerebral cortical synaptosomes (from Hardy et al. 1986; assayed after storage of samples by the "slow-freeze – fast-thaw" method of Hardy et al. 1983).
[c] Cerebral cortical slices (from Johnson et al. 1975).
[d] Cerebral cortical slices (from Bowery et al. 1976).
[e] Cerebral cortical slices (from Harris et al. 1973).
[f] Cerebral cortical slices (from Iversen and Kelly 1975).

cortical synaptosomes found two sites, with K_M values of 1.94 and 21 μ*M* (Sidhu et al. 1987). A low affinity site found in rat cerebral cortical synaptosomes (K_M approximately 3 m*M*) was not found in the human samples (Sidhu et al. 1987).

The [^{3}H]GABA accumulation into the cerebral cortical synaptosomes was blocked by inhibitors of neuronal GABA uptake such as *cis*-3-aminocyclohexane carboxylic acid and nipecotic acid, whereas β-alanine, an inhibitor of the glial uptake (see Iversen and Kelly 1975; Bowery et al. 1976, for discussion), only weakly inhibited the uptake (Hardy et al. 1986). The IC_{50} values for a number of compounds towards [^{3}H]GABA uptake in human cerebral cortical synaptosomes and rat cerebral cortical slices are given in Table 1, where the similarities are apparent.

The pharmacological characteristics of functional neurochemical parameters in rat and human brain have been compared in several other studies. Thus, Harms (1983) reported that the inhibitory potencies of desipramine, fluvoxamine, fluoxetine and norzimeldine towards [^{3}H]noradrenaline uptake were similar in human post-mortem and rat cortical brain slices. Human and rat synaptosomal [^{3}H]D-aspartate uptake sites also appear to have similar sensitivities to inhibition by glutamate and a series of structural analogues (Cowburn et al. 1987). On the other hand, desipramine and fluoxetine (but not fluvoxamine or norzimeldine) appear more potent inhibitors of [^{3}H]5-hydroxytryptamine ([^{3}H]5-HT) uptake into human cortical brain slices than for rat brain slices (Harms 1983). Recently, the pharmacological properties of H_3 receptors controlling histamine release have been investigated in the human brain (albeit in neurosurgical rather than autopsy samples) and compared with the rat. Histamine inhibited the K^+-evoked release of tritium from slices prelabelled by incubation with [^{3}H]histidine, with similar potencies in man and rat (approximately 40 n*M*). This inhibition was reversed by the histamine H_3 antagonists thioperamide and impromidine with K_i values of 16 and 36 n*M*, respectively, for human cortical slices, and 7.6 and 65 n*M*, respectively, for rat cortical slices (Arrang et al. 1988).

From the data shown in Table 1, it is clear that the pharmacological properties of [^{3}H]GABA synaptosomal uptake can be studied in post-mortem brain samples that have been stored at −70 °C. Such good cryopreservation, however, is not always the case. Thus, for example, freezing of rat cerebral cortical samples by the "slow freeze – fast thaw" technique prior to assay results in a decreased [^{3}H]5-HT accumulation into miniprisms, an increased sensitivity to the releasing effects of K^+ and a reduction in the sensitivity of the K^+-evoked release of [^{3}H]5-HT to inhibition by 5-methoxy-*N*,*N*-dimethyltryptamine (see Fig. 2) compared with freshly prepared miniprisms (Fowler et al. 1989). Interpretation of functional data when comparing different disease states (see Hardy et al. 1987 for comparison of synaptosomal [^{3}H]GABA uptake in control and dementia of Alzheimer type autopsy cases) is also critically dependent upon the assumption that the post-mortem stability and cryopreservation of the neurochemical process under study is the same for the different groups.

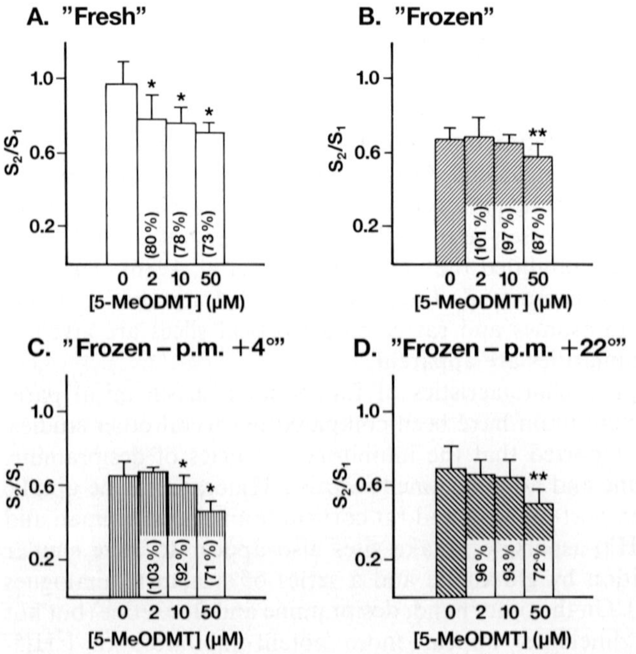

Fig. 2 A–D. Cryo- and post-mortem stability of the inhibitory effect of 5-methoxy-*N*,*N*-dimethyltryptamine (*5-MeODMT*) upon K^+ (25 m*M*) evoked release of tritium from rat cerebral cortical miniprisms preloaded with [^{3}H]5-hydroxytryptamine. 5-MeODMT was added after the first K^+ stimulation (S_1), and its effect upon a second K^+ stimulation (S_2) is given as S_2/S_1 (for details, see Fowler et al. 1989). Miniprisms were prepared from cerebral cortical samples used either immediately after dissection (**A**), after storage at −70 °C by the "slow-freeze – fast-thaw" method of Hardy et al. (1983; **B**), or after being left in situ for 5 h at either +4 °C (**C**) or +22 °C (**D**) after the animals were killed prior to storage at −70 °C. Storage time was 1–55 days. Values are means ±SD; $n = 4–5$; *, $p < 0.05$; **, $p < 0.01$ with respect to the corresponding values in the absence of 5-MeODMT (two-tailed paired *t* test); *values in parentheses* are the mean values as percentage of the corresponding mean values in the absence of 5-MeODMT. (From the data of Fowler et al. 1989)

Conclusions

In recent years it has become possible to study functional neurochemical parameters in post-mortem human brain samples. These studies have allowed both the pharmacological and kinetic characterization of, for example, neurotransmitter uptake sites and the determination of the effect of disease states on the uptake processes (for recent reviews, see Dodd et al. 1988; Fowler 1988). As indicated above, the methods are not universally applicable, and assumptions concerning similar post-mortem and cryostabilities must be made when comparing different disease groups. However, when used critically, these methods can greatly further our understanding of the functional neurochemistry of the human brain.

References

Arrang JM, Devaux B, Chodkiewicz JP, Schwartz JC (1988) H_3-receptors control histamine release in human brain. J Neurochem 51:105–108

Bowery NG, Jones GP, Neal MJ (1976) Selective inhibition of neuronal GABA uptake by *cis*-1,3-aminocyclohexane carboxylic acid. Nature 264:281–284

Cowburn RF, Dodd PR, Hardy JA, Johnston GAR (1987) A comparison of high affinity synaptosomal uptake of D-aspartate in rat and human brain. Neurochem Int 10:339–346

Danielsson E, Eckernäs SÅ, Westlind-Danielsson A, Nordström Ö, Bartfai T, Gottfries CG, Wallin A (1988) VIP-sensitive adenylate cyclase, guanylate cyclase, muscarinic receptors, choline acetyltransferase and acetylcholinesterase, in brain tissue afflicted by Alzheimer's disease/senile dementia of the Alzheimer type. Neurobiol Aging 9:153–162

Dodd PR, Hardy JA, Baig EB, Kidd AM, Bird ED, Watson WEJ, Johnston GAR (1986) Optimization of freezing, storage, and thawing conditions for the preparation of metabolically active synaptosomes from frozen rat and human brain. Neurochem Pathol 4:177–198

Dodd PR, Hambley JW, Cowburn RF, Hardy JA (1988) A comparison of methodologies for the study of functional transmitter neurochemistry in human brain. J Neurochem 50:1333–1345

Fowler CJ (1988) Validity of human brain autopsy samples for characterizing neurotransmitter function. Trends Pharmacol Sci 9:232–233

Fowler CJ, Cowburn R, Archer T, Mohammed AK, Cross AJ (1988) La fragilité des modèles animaux "cholinergiques" dans la maladie d'Alzheimer. Alzheimer Actualites 18:4–5

Fowler CJ, Thorell G, Fagervall I (1989) Postmortem- and cryostability of the potassium-evoked release of [^{3}H]5-hydroxytryptamine from rat cerebral cortical miniprisms. J Neural Transm 75:135–148

Haan EA, Bowen DM (1981) Protection of neocortical tissue prisms from freeze-thaw injury by dimethyl sulphoxide. J Neurochem 37:243–246

Hardy JA, Dodd PR (1983) Metabolic and functional studies on post-mortem human brain. Neurochem Int 5:253–266

Hardy JA, Dodd PR, Oakley AE, Perry RH, Edwardson JA, Kidd AM (1983) Metabolically active synaptosomes can be prepared from frozen rat and human brain. J Neurochem 40:608–614

Hardy JA, Wester P, Winblad B, Gezelius C, Bring G, Eriksson A (1985) The patients dying after long terminal phase have acidotic brains; implications for biochemical measurements on autopsy tissue. J Neural Transm 61:253–264

Hardy JA, Barton A, Lofdahl E, Cheetham SC, Johnston GAR, Dodd PR (1986) Uptake of γ-aminobutyric acid and glycine by synaptosomes from postmortem human brain. J Neurochem 47:460–467

Hardy J, Cowburn R, Barton A, Reynolds G, Dodd P, Wester P, O'Carroll AM, Lofdahl E, Winblad B (1987) A disorder of cortical GABAergic innervation in Alzheimer's disease. Neurosci Lett 73:192–196

Harms HH (1983) The antidepressant agents desipramine, fluoxetine, fluvoxamine and norzimelidine inhibit uptake of [^{3}H]noradrenaline and [^{3}H]5-hydroxytryptamine in slices of human and rat cortical brain tissue. Brain Res 275:99–104

Harris M, Hopkin JM, Neal MJ (1973) Effect of centrally acting drugs on the uptake of γ-aminobutyric acid (GABA) by slices of rat cerebral cortex. Br J Pharmacol 47:229–239

Iversen LL, Kelly JS (1975) Uptake and metabolism of γ-aminobutyric acid by neurones and glial cells. Biochem Pharmacol 24:933–938

Johnston GAR, Krogsgaard-Larsen P, Stephanson A (1975) Batel nut constituents as inhibitors of γ-aminobutyric acid uptake. Nature 258:627–628

Lee T (1988) Postmortem studies of dopamine receptors in schizophrenia. In: Sen AK, Lee T (eds) Receptors and ligands in psychiatry. Cambridge University Press, Cambridge, pp 11–28 (Intercellular and intracellular communication, vol 3)

Lloyd KG, Carter CJ (1988) Cholinergic neurons in Huntington's disease. In: Sen AK, Lee T (eds) Receptors and ligands in neurological disorders. Cambridge University Press, Cambridge, pp 1–24 (Intercellular and intracellular communication, vol 4)

Mann JJ, McBride PA, Stanley M (1986) Postmortem monoamine receptor and enzyme studies in suicide. Ann NY Acad Sci 487:114–121

Morgan DG, May PC, Finch CE (1988) Neurotransmitter receptors in normal human aging and Alzheimer's disease. In: Sen AK, Lee T (eds) Receptors and ligands in neurological disorders. Cambridge University Press, Cambridge, pp 120–147 (Intercellular and intracellular communication, vol 4)

O'Neill C, Marcusson J, Nordberg A, Winblad B (1987) The influence of age on neurotransmitters in the human brain. In: Govoni S, Battaini F (eds) Modification of cell to cell signals during normal and pathological aging. Springer, Berlin Heidelberg New York, pp 183–198 (NATO ASI series, vol H9)

Perry EK, Candy JM (1988) Cortical neurotransmitter receptors: distribution and involvement in Alzheimer's disease. In: Sen AK, Lee T (eds) Receptors and ligands in neurological disorders. Cambridge University Press, Cambridge, pp 98–119 (Intercellular and intracellular communication, vol 4)

Perry EK, Perry RH (1983) Human brain neurochemistry – some postmortal problems. Life Sci 33:1733–1743

Sidhu HS, Munoz DG, Wood JD (1987) γ-Aminobutyric acid (GABA) uptake systems in human frontal cortex. Brain Res 435:334–336

Wester P, Bateman DE, Dodd PR, Edwardson JA, Hardy JA, Kidd AM, Perry RH, Singh GB (1985) Agonal status affects the metabolic activity of nerve endings isolated from postmortem human brain. Neurochem Pathol 3:169–180

Westlind-Danielsson A, Undén A, Abens J, Andell S, Bartfai T (1987) Neuropeptide Y receptors and the inhibition of adenylate cyclase in the human frontal and temporal cortex. Neurosci Lett 74:237–242

Willner P (1984) The validity of animal models of depression. Psychopharmacology 83:1–16

Young AB, Penney JB (1988) Receptor mapping using autoradiographic techniques. In: Sen AK, Lee T (eds) Receptors and ligands in psychiatry. Cambridge University Press, Cambridge, pp 505–525 (Intercellular and intracellular communication, vol 3)

Modulation of Cholinergic Activity in Alzheimer Brains by Potential Drugs *

A. Nordberg [1] and L. Nilsson-Håkansson [2]

Introduction

Alzheimer's disease/senile dementia of Alzheimer's type (AD/SDAT) is a most prevalent disease causing a progressive dementia with gradual loss of intellectual abilities such as memory, abstract thinking, judgement and changes in personality and behavior. The prevalence of the disease is considered to be less than 0.5% for definite cases of dementia among those aged at least 65 years old but rises dramatically with increasing age and is about 35% at age 90 years.

The diagnostic hallmarks of AD/SDAT histopathologically are the presence of senile plaques and neurofibrillary tangles. For the definitive diagnosis of AD/SDAT both a clinical and a histopathological diagnosis is required. Neurochemical studies on AD/SDAT have been performed mostly in human brain tissue obtained at autopsy. Deficiencies in several transmitter systems such as acetylcholine (ACh), dopamine, serotonin, and some peptides have been observed (for review see Gottfries 1985; Hardy et al. 1985). The most consistent deficiency has been found for the cholinergic system (for review see Perry 1986). Neurochemical studies in human brain have until recently been restricted to analysis of neurotransmitter contents, enzyme activities, and number of neuroreceptor binding sites. There is now a growing body of evidence showing that metabolically and functionally active preparation can be obtained from human brain after considerable postmortem delay and can be used in in vitro functional neurotransmitter methods (for review see Dodd et al. 1988; Fowler et al., this volume). These new techniques will make it possible to measure presynaptic transmitter uptake and release as well as postsynaptic response to receptor stimulation in diseased versus normal states. The techniques will also enable measurements of drug effects.

Table 1 illustrates possible presynaptic and postsynaptic markers for cholinergic activity in human brain and the changes reported in some of these

* This research was supported by grants from the Swedish Medical Research Council, the Swedish Tobacco Company, Stiftelsen för Gamla Tjänarinnor, Stohne's Foundation, and Loo and Hans Osterman's Foundation.

[1] Department of Pharmacology, Uppsala University, Uppsala, Sweden; and Department of Geriatric Medicine, Karolinska Institute, Stockholm, Sweden.

[2] Department of Pharmacology, Uppsala University, Uppsala, Sweden.

Neuropsychopharmacology
Edited by Bunney/Hippius/Laakmann/Schmauß

Table 1. Possible presynaptic and postsynaptic markers for cholinergic activity in human brain and changes in normal aging and AD/SDAT

	Normal aging	AD/SDAT
Presynaptic markers		
ChAT activity	↓	↓↓
High affinity choline uptake		↓
ACh synthesis/release		↓↓
Muscarinic M_2 receptors (?)	→	↓?
Nicotinic N_1 receptors (?)	↓	↓↓
Postsynaptic markers		
Muscarinic M_1 receptors	↓	→↑
Muscarinic M_2 receptors	→	↓?
Nicotinic N_1 receptors	↓?	↓?
Nicotinic N_2 receptors		
Phosphoinositide hydrolysis		
cAMP formation		

markers in AD/SDAT brains (Nordberg et al. 1982; Nordberg and Winblad 1986a, b; Nordberg et al. 1986, 1987, 1988a). Additional muscarinic receptor subtypes (M_3; M_4) have recently been cloned (Bonner et al. 1987). Our interest has been to develop a technique to study the effect of drugs on functional cholinergic activity in human brain. We have therefore developed an in vitro method to study ACh release from human brain tissue slices.

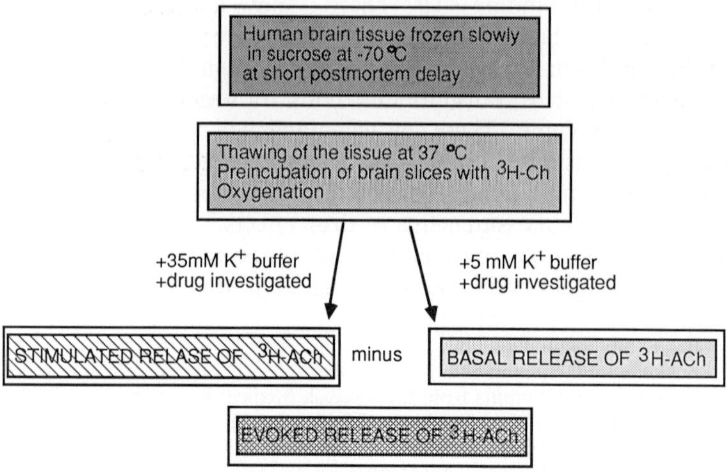

Fig. 1. Schematic presentation of method for in vitro ACh release in human postmortem brain tissue

ACh Release in Human Brain

By freezing autopsied human brain tissue slowly in an isosmotic solution, storing it at −70 °C and thawing it rapidly on the experimental day, metabolic and functional active synaptosomal preparations can be obtained after considerable postmortem delay (Hardy and Dodd 1983). Figure 1 summarizes our in vitro technique which allows measurement of synthesis and release of ACh from human brain slices (Nilsson et al. 1986). Thin brain tissue slices are incubated with labeled choline at high (35 m*M*) and low (5 m*M*) potassium concentrations. The calcium-dependent potassium-evoked release of labeled ACh can thereby be measured (Fig. 2). The ACh release is stable for more than 60 min. The agonal state of the tissue is, of course, of significant importance.

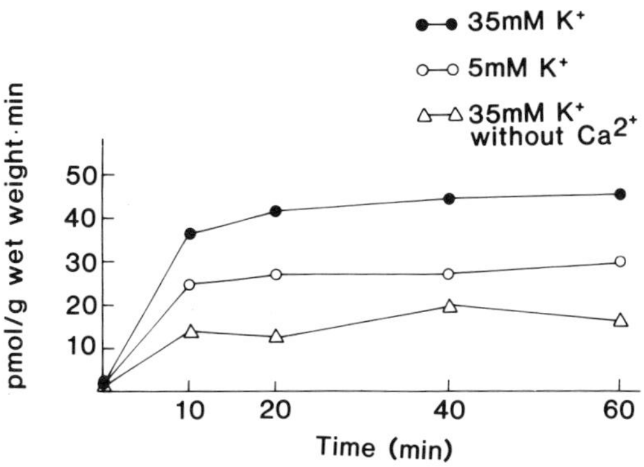

Fig. 2. In vitro release of [^{3}H]ACh in human control cortical brain tissue in the presence of 5 m*M* K^+, 35 m*M* K^+, and 35 m*M* K^+ without Ca^{2+}. Postmortem delay 6 h

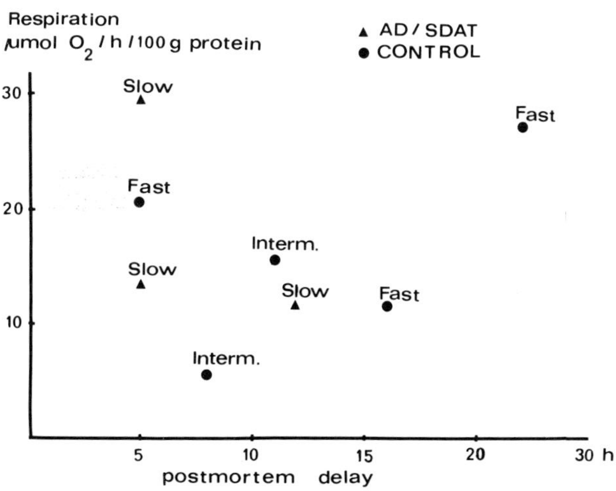

Fig. 3. Tissue respiration (µmol O_2/100 g protein per hour) in control and AD/SDAT cortical tissue with different postmortem delays

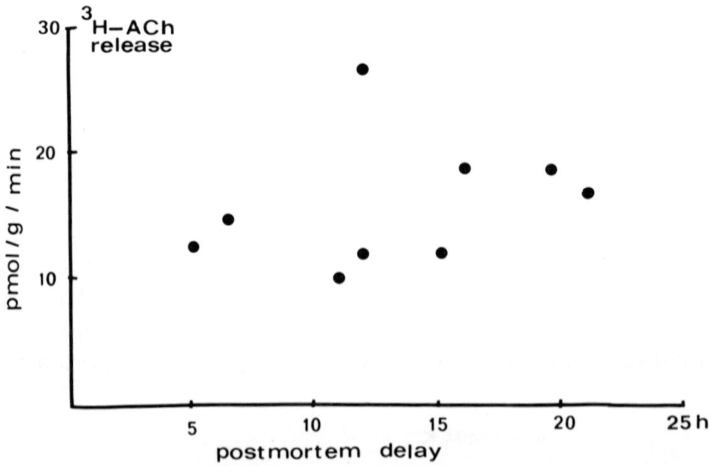

Fig. 4. Correlation between postmortem delay (hours) and [^{3}H]ACh release in human control cortical tissue (pmol/g per minute)

Normally, viable preparations from control human brain can be obtained up to 24 h postmortem if the subject had died suddenly. For AD/SDAT, in which death is often slow, the tissue is less viable, which means that the cell respiration declines faster in AD/SDAT tissue compared to control tissue (Wester et al. 1985). Figure 3 illustrates tissue respiration activity measured in control and AD/SDAT cortical tissue obtained with different postmortem delays and used in ACh release studies. The [^{3}H]ACh evoked release measured in human control frontal cortex seems to be rather stable when the postmortem delay is less than 24 h (Fig. 4).

A positive correlation between amount of potassium-induced in vitro ACh release and number of nicotinic or muscarinic receptors is observed in different human cortices (Fig. 5). As indicated in Fig. 5a, a parallel reduction in ACh release and number of [^{3}H]nicotine binding sites is measured in the frontal cortex of AD/SDAT brains compared to controls. No such parallel change can be observed for ACh release and number of muscarinic receptors. The potassium-evoked release of ACh is markedly diminished in AD/SDAT cortical tissue compared to control tissue (Fig. 6).

Effects of Drugs on ACh Release in Control and AD/SDAT Brains

In order to increase cholinergic activity in the brain several strategies are possible. Various therapeutic agents with various cholinergic effects have been tried in AD/SDAT (Fig. 7). The outcome of clinical trials has been modest except for those of cholinesterase inhibitors (for review see Giacobini and Becker 1988). Selective muscarinic receptor agonists are still lacking.

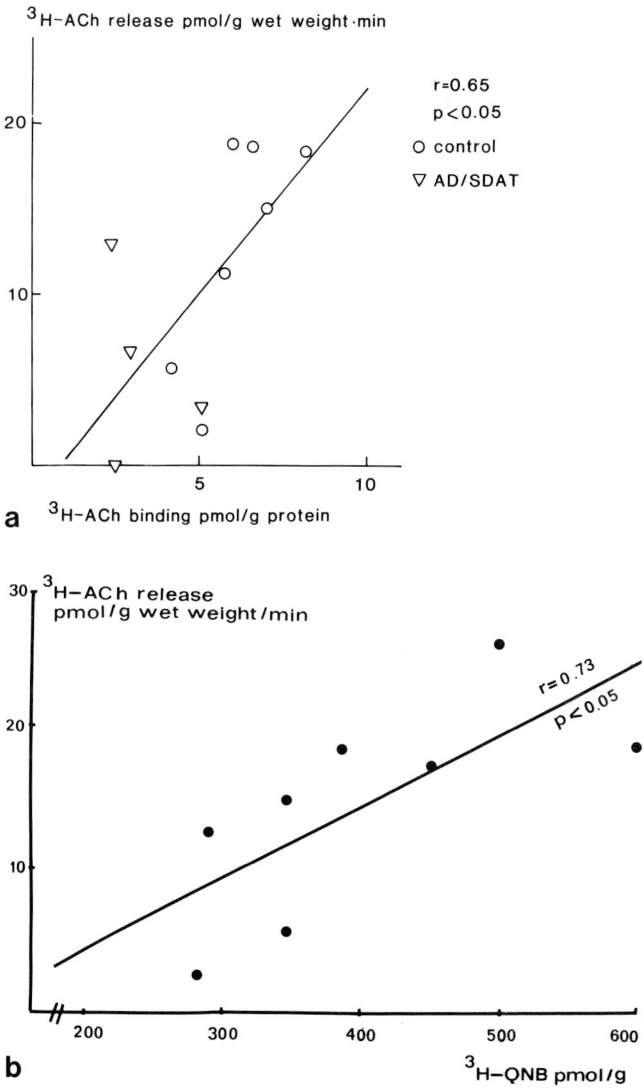

Fig. 5. a Correlation between number of nicotinic receptors (measured as [^{3}H]ACh binding) and [^{3}H]ACh release in control and AD/SDAT cortical tissue. **b** Correlation between number of muscarinic receptors (measured as [^{3}H]QNB binding) and [^{3}H]ACh release in control cortical tissue

In human control cortical brain tissue the cholinesterase inhibitors physostigmine and tetrahydroaminoacridine (THA; 10^{-4} M) reduce the potassium-evoked in vitro release of ACh while the muscarinic antagonist atropine (10^{-5} *M*) enhances it (Fig. 8). These opposite effects obtained by the drugs on ACh release can be explained by feedback mechanisms (negative and positive, respectively) induced via presynaptic muscarinic autoreceptors. This

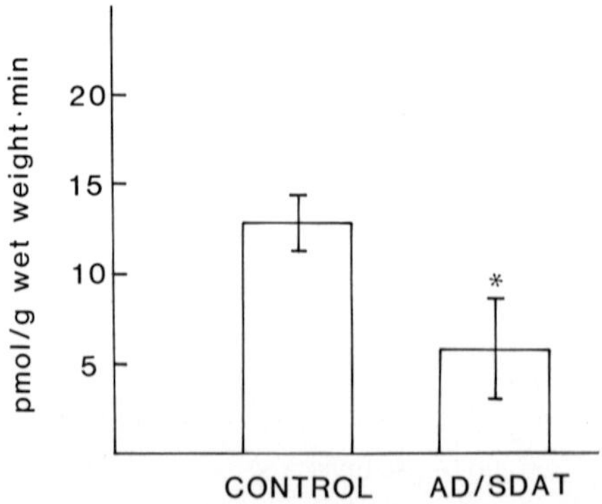

Fig. 6. In vitro release of [^{3}H]ACh in frontal cortical control and AD/SDAT tissue. *, $p < 0.05$

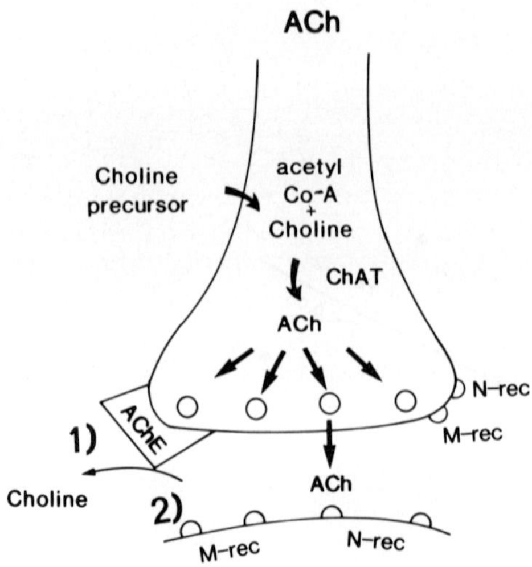

Fig. 7. Drugs with different modes of action in the cholinergic synapse. *1*), Cholinesterase inhibitors, physostigmine, THA; *2*), muscarinic agonists, bethanecol, oxotremorine, arecoline, RS86

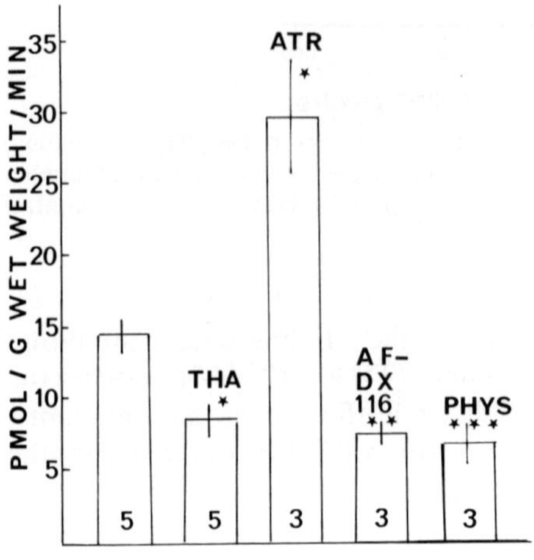

Fig. 8. Effect of physostigmine (*PHYS*), THA (10^{-4} *M*), atropine (*ATR*; 10^{-6} *M*) and AF-DX-116 (10^{-5} *M*) on potassium-evoked [^{3}H]ACh release in human control cortical tissue. *Leftmost bar*, no drug; *, $p < 0.05$; **, $p < 0.01$; ***, $p < 0.001$
n = number of experiments

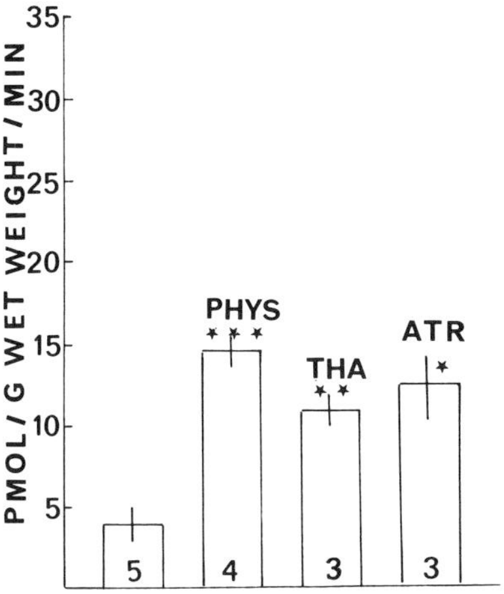

Fig. 9. Effect of physostigmine (*PHYS*), THA (10^{-4} *M*), and atropine (*ATR*; 10^{-6} *M*) on potassium-evoked ACh release in human AD/SDAT cortical tissue. *Leftmost bar*, no drug; *, $p < 0.05$; **, $p < 0.01$; ***, $p < 0.001$ n = number of experiments

phenomena is well known from animal studies (Szerb and Somogyi 1973; Marchi et al. 1981). Interestingly, the selective M_2 antagonist AF DX 116 (10^{-5} *M*) reduces in our model system the evoked ACh release in control tissue. In the presence of physostigmine or THA the release of ACh from AD/SDAT brain slices is restored to that in control slices (Fig. 9; Nilsson et al. 1987). Both in control tissue and in AD/SDAT tissue atropine (10^{-6} *M*) elicits enhanched ACh release, as an indication of preserved muscarinic autoreceptors in AD/SDAT tissue (Fig. 9).

Is it possible to reverse the effect of the cholinesterase inhibitors on ACh release in control and AD/SDAT cortical tissue? As indicated in Fig. 10, the increased release of ACh induced by THA in AD/SDAT tissue is prevented in the presence of the nicotinic antagonist mecamylamine (10^{-5} *M*). Interest-

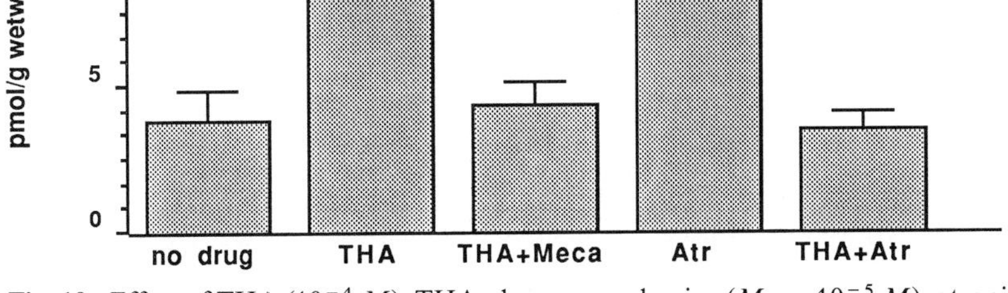

Fig. 10. Effect of THA (10^{-4} *M*), THA plus mecamylamine (*Meca*; 10^{-5} *M*), atropine (*Atr*; 10^{-6} *M*), and THA plus atropine on potassium-evoked release of [^{3}H]ACh release in AD/SDAT frontal cortex. **, $p < 0.01$; *, $p < 0.05$

ingly, mecamylamine does not counteract the effect of THA in control tissue. Both THA and atropine alone enhance the release of ACh in AD/SDAT tissue, but when added together in our release system, the effect on ACh release is abolished (Fig. 10). These findings indicate that both muscarinic and nicotinic receptors must be involved either directly or indirectly in the mechanism of action of acetylcholinesterase inhibitors such as THA; this is also supported by ligand binding studies (Nilsson et al. 1987; Nordberg et al. 1988b).

Future Vistas

We have presented here a technique by which human postmortem brain tissue can be used to study functional transmitter activity in pathological disorders such as AD/SDAT. Because neurosurgery is seldom carried out in patients with dementia, the amount of tissue obtained from biopsies will probably be rare, and the use of autopsy tissue will continue. Transmitter release and its regulation by receptor feedback mechanisms can be studied, in the future possibly also second messenger response. There is a great need for developing therapeutic agents in dementia. No reliable animal model is yet available. The different effects on ACh release by physostigmine, THA in control compared to AD/SDAT brain tissue clearly illustrate the importance of using AD/SDAT brain tissue instead of human control brain tissue or rodent brain tissue for studying the underlying mechanisms for the effect of potential therapeutic agents in neurodegenerative disorders such as Alzheimer's disease.

References

Bonner TI, Buckley NJ, Young A, Brann MR (1987) Identification of a family of muscarinic receptor genes. Science 237:527–532

Dodd PR, Hambley JW, Cowburn RF, Hardy JA (1988) A comparison of methodologies for the study of functional transmitter neurochemistry in human brain. J Neurochem 50:1333–1345

Giacobini E, Becker R (1988) Current research in Alzheimer therapy. Taylor and Francis, New York

Gottfries CG (1985) Alzheimer's disease and senile dementia biochemical characteristics and aspects of treatment. Psychopharmacology 86:245–252

Hardy JA, Dodd PR (1983) Metabolic and functional studies on post-mortem human brain. Neurochem Int 5:253–266

Hardy JA, Adolfsson R, Alafuzoff I, Bucht G, Marcusson J, Nyberg P, Perdahl E, Wester P, Winblad B (1985) Transmitter deficits in Alzheimer's disease. Neurochem Int 7:545–563

Marchi M, Paudice P, Raiteri M (1981) Autoregulation of acetylcholine release in isolated hippocampal nerve endings. Eur J Pharmacol 73:75–79

Nilsson L, Nordberg A, Hardy J, Wester P, Winblad B (1986) Physostigmine restores ^{3}H-acetylcholine efflux from Alzheimer brain slices to normal level. J Neural Transm 67:275–285

Nilsson L, Adem A, Hardy J, Winblad B, Nordberg A (1987) Do tetrahydroaminoacridine (THA) and physostigmine restore acetylcholine in AD/SDAT brains via nicotinic receptors? J Neural Transm 70:357–368

Nordberg A, Winblad B (1986a) Brain nicotinic and muscarinic receptors in normal aging and dementia. In: Fisher A, Hanin I, Lachman C (eds) Alzheimer's and Parkinson's disease: strategies for research and development, Plenum, New York, p 95. (Advances in behavioral biology, vol 29)

Nordberg A, Winblad B (1986b) Reduced number of ^{3}H-nicotine and ^{3}H-acetylcholine binding sites in the frontal cortex of Alzheimer brains. Neurosci Lett 72:115–119

Nordberg A, Adolfsson R, Marcusson J, Winblad B (1982) Cholinergic receptors in the hippocampus in normal aging and dementia of Alzheimer type. In: Giacobini E, Vernadakis A (eds) The aging brain: cellular and molecular mechanisms of aging in the neurons system, Raven, New York, p 231 (Aging, vol 20)

Nordberg A, Alafuzoff I, Winblad B (1986) Muscarinic receptor subtypes in Alzheimer's disease and mixed dementia type. Neurosci Lett 70:160–164

Nordberg A, Nyberg P, Adolfsson R, Winblad B (1987) Cholinergic topography in Alzheimer brains: a comparison with changes in the monoaminergic profile. J Neural Transm 69:19–32

Nordberg A, Adem A, Hardy J, Winblad B (1988a) Change in nicotinic receptor subtypes in temporal cortex of Alzheimer brains. Neurosci Lett 86:317–321

Nordberg A, Nilsson L, Adem A, Hardy J, Winblad B (1988b) Effect of THA on acetylcholine release and cholinergic receptors in Alzheimer brains. In: Giacobini E, Becker R (eds) Current research in Alzheimer therapy. Taylor and Francis, New York, p 247

Perry E (1986) The cholinergic hypothesis: ten years on. Br Med Bull 42:63–69

Szerb JC, Somogyi GT (1973) Depression of acetylcholine release from cortical slices by cholinesterase inhibition and by oxotremorine. Nature 241:121–122

Wester P, Bateman DE, Dodd PR, Edwardson JA, Hardy JA, Kidd AM, Perry RH, Singh GB (1985) Agonal status affects the metabolic activity of nerve endings isolated from postmortem human brain. Neurochem Pathol 3:169–180

Reduced Stimulated Adenylate Cyclase Activity in Postmortem Hippocampus of Demented Patients

T. G. OHM [1], J. BOHL [2], H. STEINMETZ [3], and B. LEMMER [4]

Introduction

Cognitive decline in dementia of the Alzheimer type is associated with the formation of neurofibrillary tangles and senile plaques. Both histopathological hallmarks represent probably irreversible endstages of an abnormal and disconnecting process in neuronal ageing. It is conceivable that functional changes parallel or even precede these alterations. Neurochemical studies, mainly on the cholinergic system, have documented a severe disturbance in synaptic signalling, indicated by a significant reduction in presynaptic and postsynaptic parameters. However, unaltered binding of receptor ligands does not necessarily imply unaltered receptor coupling to the elements involved in the second messenger formation.

The β-adrenoceptor mediated signal transduction is the best studied of all receptor systems. This system consists of at least five main components; the stimulatory β-adrenoceptor which is a transmembrane glycoprotein, the stimulatory guanine-binding regulatory protein which binds GTP and is tightly associated with the catalytic unit of the adenylate cyclase (AC), and AC responsible for the formation of the second messenger cAMP (Fig. 1). The catalytic unit of AC is a solitary transmembrane polypeptide carrying its catalytic site at the inner surface of the cell membrane. In addition, an inhibitory receptor and an inhibitory GTP-binding protein are associated with this multicomponent system (Levitzki 1988). However, it is now well established that other receptor systems are also able to stimulate or inhibit AC (Table 1). Thus, different receptors pertaining to the same cell can all couple to the same pool of AC. Recently, a study described an increased basal activity of vasoactive intestinal polypeptide stimulated AC in Alzheimer's disease (Danielsson et al. 1988).

[1] Zentrum der Morphologie, J.-W.-Goethe Universität, Theodor-Stern-Kai 7, 6000 Frankfurt, FRG.
[2] Abteilung für Neuropathologie, J.-Gutenberg Universität, 6500 Mainz, FRG.
[3] Psychiatrisches Krankenhaus Philippshospital, 6086 Riedstadt, FRG.
[4] Zentrum der Pharmakologie, J.-W.-Goethe Universität, Theodor-Stern-Kai 7, 6000 Frankfurt, FRG.

Neuropsychopharmacology
Edited by Bunney/Hippius/Laakmann/Schmauß

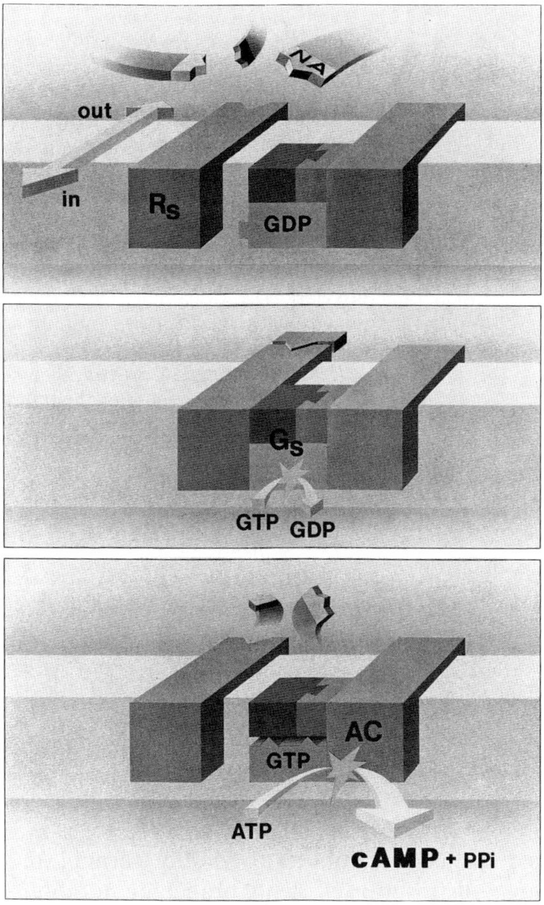

Fig. 1. The general mechanisms of β-adrenoceptor mediated transmembrane signalling. Molecules of noradrenaline (*NA*) link to the ligand binding site of the transmembrane β-adrenoceptor glycoprotein. This leads to a change in conformation with the consequence that a guanine nucleotide binding protein (G-protein; located at the inner surface of the membrane) is activated thus binding GTP. Consecutively the G-protein, probably the α subunit of the trimer, stimulates the transmembrane adenylate cyclase (*AC*) to form cAMP from ATP

Table 1. Signalling via cAMP

Stimulatory receptor systems	Inhibitory receptor systems
β-Adrenergic	α-Adrenergic
Vasoactive intestinal polypeptide	Muscarinic
Adenosine A_2	Adenosine A_1
Dopamine D_1	Somatostatin
Histamine H_2	Histamine H_1
Serotonin	μ-Opiate

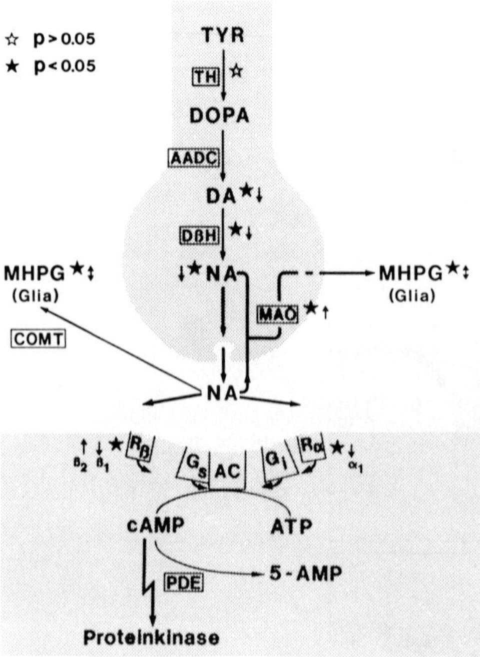

Fig. 2. Schematic representation of a synapse summarizing changes in the noradrenergic system in hippocampus in Alzheimer-type dementia. *Asterisks*, parameters which have been studied in AD/SDAT; *arrows*, increase of decrease of the examined parameter; *TYR*, tyrosine; *TH*, tyrosine hydroxylase; *DOPA*, dihydroxyphenylalanine; *AADC*, aromatic amino acid decarboxylase; *DA*, dopamine; *DβH*, dopamine-β-hydroxylase; *NA*, noradrenaline; *MAO*, monoamine oxidase; *MHPG*, 3-methoxy-4-hydroxyphenylglycol; *COMT*, catechol-*O*-methyltransferase; *AC*, adenylate cyclase; G_s, simulatory G-protein; G_i, inhibitory G-protein; R_β, β-adrenoceptor; R_α, α-adrenoceptor; *ATP*, adenosine triphosphate; *PDE*, phosphodiesterase; *5-AMP*, 5-adenosine monophosphate. (Data from Cross et al. 1981; Cross et al. 1983; Cross et al. 1984; Rossor et al. 1984; Shimohama et al. 1986; Shimohama et al. 1987)

Noradrenaline is considered to play an important role in learning and memory function. The widespread distribution of richly branching noradrenergic fibres seems to be inextricably linked to neuronal functions associated with an increased signal-to-noise ratio, thus enhancing information-processing capabilities of stimuli specific for these neurons (Saper 1987).

The density of β-adrenoceptors is very high in hippocampus of man (Reznikoff et al. 1986). Furthermore, quantitative autoradiography revealed in the hippocampus one of the highest densities of forskolin binding sites, which label the catalytic unit of AC (Gehlert et al. 1985). High levels of hybridization were seen in the human hippocampus using a cDNA probe complementary to an mRNA coding for a stimulatory G-protein (Mengod et al. 1988).

The hippocampal formation is one of the most frequently and severely altered structures in Alzheimer's disease as well as in the recently reported dementing syndrome displaying argyrophilic grains as its histological hallmark (Braak and Braak 1987). Reported changes in noradrenergic neurotransmission within the hippocampal formation are summarized in Fig. 2.

It was the aim of the present study to investigate in detail the steps involved in cAMP signal transduction in post-mortem hippocampal formation of demented patients and in age-matched controls.

Material and Methods

We examined AC activity in the middle portion of the post-mortem hippocampus of ten individuals who suffered from dementia of the Alzheimer type (AD/SDAT), one with argyrophylic grains syndrome, one with Down's syndrome and 15 age-matched controls. These diagnoses were established in accordance with clinical and histopathological criteria. Patients' characteristics in terms of sex, age, time of death, and post-mortem delay are presented in Table 2. There was no significant difference between controls and AD/SDAT patients concerning age ($t = 1.8$) or postmortem delay ($t = 0.42$). The characteristics of the patient with argyrophilic grains syndrome and the patient with Down's syndrome were comparable to those of the AD/SDAT patients. Concerning the causes of death we were careful to assure comparability between controls and the demented. The selected individuals died of bronchopneumonia, myocardial infarction, carcinoma, acute heart failure and lung embolia.

AC activity was determined as previously described (Lemmer et al. 1987) with the addition of an ATP-regenerating system. In brief, the tissue was homogenized at 37 °C in a buffer containing 50 m*M* Tris, 4 m*M* EDTA and 10 m*M* $MgCl_2$. After centrifugation the obtained pellet was resuspended in a buffer consisting of the phosphodiesterase inhibitor 1 m*M* isobutylmethylxanthine, 0.5 m*M* ATP, 10 m*M* phosphocreatine, and 0.1 mg/ml creatine phosphokinase. Each tissue homogenate was divided into four subsets for simultaneous determination of basal and drug-stimulated enzyme activity. This procedure allowed the use of identical tissue suspensions, thus minimizing methodical differences. AC was stimulated either (a) via the β-adrenoceptor by 0.1 m*M* isoprenaline, (b) via the G-protein by the nonhydrolyzable GTP analogue Gpp(NH)p at 0.1 m*M*, or (c) via mainly the catalytic unit stimulated by 0.1 m*M* forskolin (Lemmer and Witte 1988). Incubations were done at 37 °C for 6 min; linearity of the reaction was confirmed. The reaction was terminated by heating the incubation vials in a thermoblock at 120 °C. cAMP concentrations were determined in triplicates by radioimmunoassay with the protein binding-method (cAMP kit TRK 432, Amersham-Buchler, Braunschweig, FRG). cAMP concentrations in the tissues were calculated from competition curves by non-linear curve fitting. Protein content was determined in accordance with Lowry et al. (1951). AC activity was then expressed as picomoles cAMP formed per milligram protein per minute.

Results

The data on hippocampal AC of control and demented individuals are tabulated in Table 3. In controls the mean basal AC activity was 40.9 pmol mg^{-1} min^{-1}. Isoprenaline slightly increased AC activity while Gpp(NH)p elevated AC activity by about 50%. Stimulation by the diterpene

Table 2. Patients' characteristics

Patient number	Sex	Age (years)	Time of death (hours)	Post mortem delay (h)
Controls				
6	M	97	03:00	11.0
7	F	83	09:15	23.0
8	F	35	17:05	15.0
12	F	84	04:40	26.5
13	M	65	00:00	17.0
16	M	69	10:00	22.0
17	M	69	10:30	22.5
18	M	80	04:50	68.0
19	F	84	02:30	79.0
20	M	83	03:15	28.5
22	F	79	23:30	33.5
23	M	59	05:15	6.0
28	F	64	01:00	31.0
30	M	62	23:30	32.5
31	F	57	15:25	18.0
Mean		70.0		28.3
95% CL		62.5–77.5		17.1–39.4
AD/SDAT				
1	M	79	03:00	11.0
2	F	83	09:15	23.0
3	F	71	17:00	39.0
5	M	82	23:30	9.0
9	M	59	02:30	10.5
10	M	81	17:10	21.0
14	F	84	01:00	79.0
21	F	83	13:00	91.0
27	F	85	02:30	9.5
33	F	80	23:45	32.5
Mean		78.7		32.6
95% CL		73.0–84.4		11.4–53.7
Argyrophilic grains syndrome				
4	F	84	08:45	24.0
Down's syndrome				
32	M	65	23:00	15.0

forskolin revealed the most effective increase (about 6.5-fold). This rank order of stimulatory effects via the β-adrenoceptor, G-protein and the catalytic unit of AC in post-mortem human brain tissue is in good accordance with results established in animals.

Three major aspects result from comparison of these data with those obtained from demented patients. Firstly, in the cases with AD/SDAT basal as well as drug-stimulated AC activities were reduced; a mean reduction of about 50% was detected ($p < 0.01$; t test). Secondly, the rank order of stimulatory

Table 3. Adenylate cyclase activity (pmol mg^{-1} min^{-1})

Patient number	Basal	Isoprenaline	Gpp(NH)p	Forskolin
Controls				
6	15.0	25.1	31.1	165.8
7	25.1	45.5	30.6	219.4
8	35.2	61.8	95.1	387.0
12	31.6	57.6	87.3	318.5
13	35.3	54.3	83.8	382.0
16	62.2	66.7	75.7	293.0
17	53.8	58.5	63.0	228.7
19	66.8	83.2	94.3	306.3
18	46.7	56.9	62.1	233.1
20	57.9	65.9	77.6	260.1
22	46.4	54.9	64.8	273.0
23	39.3	44.1	51.2	242.1
28	34.6	46.9	50.7	195.9
30	37.5	55.6	68.7	209.4
31	25.5	26.4	32.0	169.5
Mean	40.9	53.6	64.5	258.9
95% CL	32.8–49.0	45.5–61.8	52.4–76.7	221.1–296.7
AD/SDAT				
1	41.0	52.1	58.8	268.0
2	17.6	22.7	23.3	96.3
3	10.5	13.1	11.6	62.0
5	13.1	17.9	18.0	51.3
9	17.6	28.1	33.4	100.7
10	17.4	23.3	27.4	78.7
14	23.9	37.3	59.3	162.9
21	27.3	31.9	36.7	132.1
27	29.6	40.8	47.6	191.3
33	21.6	23.3	34.1	133.4
Mean	22.0	29.0	35.0	127.7
95% CL	15.6–28.4	20.7–37.4	23.5–46.5	80.4–174.9
Argyrophilic grains syndrome				
4	17.3	17.3	24.7	89.6
Down's syndrome				
32	16.3	22.6	23.5	142.9

Analysis of variance among controls: $F_{3,56} = 115.1$, $p < 0.001$; among AD/SDAT patients: $F_{3,36} = 20.5$, $p < 0.001$. Student's t test between controls and AD/SDAT patients: basal, $p < 0.01$; isoprenaline, $p < 0.001$; Gpp(NH)p, $p < 0.01$; forskolin, $p < 0.001$.

effects was the same as in controls. Third, the results of the demented individual with Down's syndrome and the one who suffered from argyrophilic grains syndrome displayed generally similar effects.

Discussion

The present study demonstrates for the first time a pronounced reduction in cAMP signal transduction in brain tissue of demented patients. Basal and drug-stimulated cAMP formation were decreased by about 50% in post-mortem hippocampal tissue of patients with Alzheimer's disease, argyrophilic grains syndrome, and Down's syndrome when compared to controls. In contrast to the substantial information available on cholinergic neurotransmission in Alzheimer's disease, only little is known about the adrenergic system. In AD/SDAT β-adrenoceptor density has been reported to remain intact in hippocampal post-mortem tissue when studied with the non-selective ligand [^{3}H]dihydroalprenolol (Cross et al. 1984; Shimohama et al. 1987). Interestingly, examination of β-adrenoceptor subtypes demonstrated a reduction in β_1- and an increase in β_2-adrenoceptors in hippocampal tissue of AD/SDAT (Shimohama et al. 1987). However, receptor number is not the sole determining factor of neuronal responsiveness. Interactions between the receptor and G-proteins as well as interactions between the G-proteins and the catalytic subunit of AC may be of greater importance in modifying signal transduction. This assumption is supported by animal experiments in which an age-associated decrease in rat myocardial AC activity has been reported without changes in β-adrenoceptor number (O'Connor et al. 1983). Moreover, in rat brain tissue the change of β-adrenoceptors during ageing displays a region-specific behaviour either increasing, decreasing, or remaining stable (Scarpace and Abrass 1988).

Since in our study β-adrenoceptor number was not analysed we cannot contribute any information concerning this issue. However, our data clearly indicate that the main site of alteration in the β-adrenoceptor effector system of demented patients must be located at the postreceptor site. This is evidenced by the fact that not only β-adrenoceptor mediated stimulation of the AC but also stimulation via the G-protein by Gpp(NH)p and via the catalytic subunit by forskolin are reduced by about 50%. This fact excludes the occurrence of an alteration restricted to the receptor level. Furthermore, our data indicate that the crucial site must be the catalytic subunit of the AC because both G-protein activity and catalytic unit activity are reduced by the same amount. Since it is generally assumed that the G-protein is in excess relative to the catalytic unit, our data are in accordance with the hypothesis that a loss of the catalytic unit in demented patients accounts for the loss in AC activity. Furthermore, the reduction in AC activity is probably not caused by simple cell loss. This suggestion is supported by histological inspection and by the finding that total protein in both control and diseased brain probes showed comparable values, indicating that no significant cell loss occurred. Nevertheless, we cannot totally exclude the possibility that a quantitative loss of AC might still occur.

However, bearing in mind the multicomponent organization of the cAMP signalling system (see above), it cannot be ruled out that disease-induced changes in membrane composition and/or fluidity may contribute to an alteration in the coupling processes. Recent progress in molecular biology suggests that the Alzheimer amyloid contains a fragment cleaved from a membrane-associated molecule (Dyrks et al. 1988). Biophysical properties of neuronal membranes in Alzheimer hippocampus indicate an alteration in the structure of their superficial regions (Zubenko 1986). In vitro nuclear magnetic resonance spectroscopy detected a disturbed neuronal phospholipid metabolism in Alzheimer's disease consistent with a possible membrane dysfunction (Miatto et al. 1986) and the reduced phospholipase D activity in brain homogenates from AD/SDAT patients (Kanfer et al. 1986). Hippocampal membranes in Alzheimer's disease displayed consistently higher lipase activities when compared to controls (Farooqui et al. 1988). Interestingly, normal senescence is apparently not associated with reduced AC activity in brain tissue (Walker and Walker 1973; Nomura et al. 1984).

Hypotheses of transmembrane signalling frequently assume that some of the partners of signal transduction are laterally mobile, thus facilitating the signal transmission. Interestingly, direct measurements of β-adrenergic receptor mobility demonstrated that the receptor is immobile (Henis et al. 1982; see also Peters 1988). It has therefore been speculated that coupling mechanisms utilize a molecule (probably G-α) diffused in the aqueous compartment (Peters 1988). However, protein lateral mobility is strongly restricted at least in the red blood cell (Peters 1988).

Further studies are needed in order to evaluate whether the reduction in cAMP signal transduction is an age-dependent phenomenon which in Alzheimer's disease is only exaggerated. Finally, future studies should consider the fact that changes in cAMP signal transduction in humans may also be due to circadian variations, as has been shown in rat brain (Lemmer et al. 1987). Such circadian changes have been discussed in monoaminergic systems in human brain (Carlsson et al. 1980).

Acknowledgements. The technical assistence of K. Witte and T. Brühl is gratefully acknowledged. We are indebted to I. Szász for her excellent illustrations.

References

Braak H, Braak E (1987) Argyrophilic grains: characteristic pathology of cerebral cortex in cases of adult onset dementia without Alzheimer changes. Neurosci Lett 76:124–127

Carlsson A, Svennerholm N, Winblad B (1980) Seasonal and circadian monoamine variations in human brains examined post mortem. Acta Psychiatr Scand (Suppl 280]61:75–83

Cross AJ, Crow J, Perry EK, Perry RH, Blessed G, Tomlinson BE (1981) Reduced dopamine-beta-hydroxylase activity in Alzheimer's disease. Br Med J 282:93–94

Cross AJ, Crow TJ, Johnson JA, Joseph MH, Perry EK, Perry RH, Blessed G, Tomlinson BE (1983) Monoamine metabolism in senile dementia of Alzheimer type. J Neurol Sci 60:383–392

Cross AJ, Crow TJ, Johnson JA, Perry EK, Perry RH, Blessed G, Tomlinson BE (1984) Studies on neurotransmitter receptor systems in neocortex and hippocampus in senile dementia of the Alzheimer type. J Neurol Sci 64:109–117

Danielsson E, Eckernäs SA, Westlind-Danielsson A, Nordström Ö, Bartfai T, Gottfries CG, Wallin A (1988) VIP-sensitive adenylate cyclase, guanylate cyclase, muscarinic receptors, choline acetyltransferase and acetylcholinesterase, in brain tissue afflicted by Alzheimer's disease/senile dementia of the Alzheimer type. Neurobiol Ageing 9:153–162

Dyrks T, Weidemann A, Multhaup G, Salbaum JM, Lemaire HG, Kang J, Müller-Hill B, Masters CL, Beyreuther (1988) Identification, transmembrane orientation and biogenesis of the amyloid A4 precursor of Alzheimer's disease. EMBO J 7:949–957

Farooqui AA, Liss L, Horrocks LA (1988) Neurochemical aspects of Alzheimer's disease: involvement of membrane phospholipids. Metab Brain Dis 3:19–35

Gehlert DR, Dawson TM, Yamamura HI, Wamsley JK (1985) Quantitative autoradiography of ^{3}H forskolin binding sites in the rat brain. Brain Res 361:351–360

Henis YI, Hekman M, Elson EL, Helmreich EJM (1982) Lateral motion of β-receptors in membranes of cultured liver cells. Proc Natl Acad Sci USA 79:2907–2911

Kanfer JN, Hattori H, Orihel D (1986) Reduced phospholipase D activity in brain tissue samples from Alzheimer's disease patients. Ann Neurol 20:265–267

Lemmer B, Witte K (1988) Circadian rhythm in cAMP signal transmission in cardiac tissue. J Interdiscipl Cycle Res 19:189–190

Lemmer B, Bärmeier H, Schmidt S, Lang PH (1987) On the daily variation in the beta-receptor-adenylate cyclase-cAMP-phosphodiesterase system in rat forebrain. Chronobiol Int 4:469–475

Levitzki A (1988) Signal transduction in hormone-dependent adenylate cyclase. Cell Biophys 12:133–143

Lowry DH, Rosebrough NJ, Farr AL, Randall RJ (1951) Protein measurement with folin phenol reagent. J Biol Chem 193:265–275

Mengod G, Palacios JM, Probst A, Harris B (1988) Regional distribution of the expression of a human stimulatory GTP-binding protein α-subunit in the human brain studied by in situ hybridization. Mol Brain Res 4:23–29

Miatto O, Gilberto Gonzalez R, Buonanno F, Growdon JH (1986) In vitro ^{31}P NMR spectroscopy detects altered phospholipid metabolism in Alzheimer's disease. Can J Neurol Sci 13:535–539

Nomura Y, Makihata J, Segawa T (1984) Activation of adenylate cyclase by dopamine, GTP, NaF and forskolin in striatal membranes of neonatal, adult and senescent rats. Eur J Pharmacol 106:437–440

O'Connor SW, Scarpace PJ, Abrass IB (1983) Age-associated decrease in the catalytic unit activity of rat myocardial adenylate cyclase. Mech Ageing Dev 21:357–363

Peters R (1988) Lateral mobility of proteins and lipids in the red cell membrane and the activation of adenylate cyclase by β-adrenergic receptors. FEBS Lett 234:1–7

Reznikoff GA, Manaker S, Rhodes CH, Winocur A, Rainbow TC (1986) Localization and quantification of beta-adrenergic receptors in human brain. Neurology 36:1067–1073

Rossor MN, Iverson LL, Reynolds P, Mountjoy CQ, Roth M (1984) Neurochemical characteristics of early and late onset types of Alzheimer's disease. Br Med J 288:961–964

Saper CB (1987) Function of the locus coeruleus. TINS 10:343–344

Scarpace PJ, Abrass IB (1988) Alpha- and beta-adrenergic receptor function in the brain during senescence. Neurobiol Ageing 9:53–58

Shimohama S, Taniguchi T, Fujiwara M, Kameyama M (1986) Biochemical characterization of α-adrenergic receptors in human brain and changes in Alzheimer-type dementia. J Neurochem 47:1294–1301

Shimohama S, Taniguchi T, Fujiwara M, Kameyama M (1987) Changes in β-adrenergic receptor subtypes in Alzheimer-type dementia. J Neurochem 48:1215–1221

Walker JB, Walker JP (1973) Properties of adenylate cyclase from senescent rat brain. Brain Res 54:391–396

Zubenko G (1986) Hippocampal membrane alteration in Alzheimer's disease. Brain Res 385:115–121

Molecular Neuropathology: The Study of Transmitter and Receptor Expression in Human Postmortem Materials by In Situ Hybridization and Receptor Autoradiography

G. Mengod and J. M. Palacios [1]

Introduction

Progress in understanding how the brain works under both normal and pathological conditions is intimately related to the development of new techniques for analysis at the lowest anatomical and molecular levels. The application in the past three decades of biochemical techniques to the study of the brain has greatly increased our knowledge of the chemical make-up of the nervous system. The development of centrally acting drugs and the understanding of their mechanism of action are also closely related to these advances. Because of the high regional and cellular complexity of the brain and the limited resolution of classical biochemical techniques, histochemical methods have been developed to allow a cellular and subcellular analysis with a high degree of molecular specificity. Histochemical, immunohistochemical, and autoradiographical procedures take advantage of the development of antibodies and radioactive markers for brain molecules (Björklund and Hökfelt 1983).

Many of these molecules survive the postmortem conditions of the human brain and are amenable to analysis using biochemical or histochemical procedures (Bird and Iversen 1982; Palacios et al. 1986). The systematic study of samples from diseased brains and their comparison with control populations has led to the discovery of selective biochemical deficits in some diseases of the human brain. Classical examples are the dopamine deficit in Parkinson's disease (Hornykiewicz 1972) and the acetylcholine deficit in Alzheimer's disease (Rossor 1982). An extensive catalogue of biochemical alterations in these and other diseases is now available (Palacios et al. 1986).

In this chapter we review the use of two techniques which allow a quantitative or semiquantitative determination of receptors and neuropeptides expression with the resolution of the light microscope. These two techniques are in situ hybridization and receptor autoradiography. To illustrate the use of these techniques in neuropathology we review recent work in our laboratory focused on the human basal ganglia and associated areas. We selected these brain areas because of the wealth of information already available on their chemical, cellular, and regional organization (Graybiel and Ragsdale 1983;

[1] Preclinical Research, Sandoz Pharma Ltd., 4002 Basel, Switzerland.

Neuropsychopharmacology
Edited by Bunney/Hippius/Laakmann/Schmauß

Beal and Martin 1986; Gerfen et al. 1987a, b; Parent 1987), and because of the well-documented involvement of these regions in diseases such as Parkinson's disease, Huntington's chorea, and schizophrenia (Emson et al. 1986). The goal of our studies was to analyze how the expression of neuropeptides and neurotransmitter receptors is distributed and regulated as a consequence of the different types of neuronal degeneration characteristics of the diseases affecting the basal ganglia.

Neuropeptide Gene Expression in the Human Basal Ganglia: In Situ Hybridization

Several types of neurons have been recognized in the mammalian basal ganglia, including the human, on the basis of their morphological characteristics (Graveland et al. 1985). The majority of neurons (90% of the total) are medium-sized (10–20 μm); the rest compose a large group that can be further divided into five subsets of neurons. The main class (70%–80%) are medium-sized spiny neurons. A second class are the spiny type (10%). Aspiny neurons are divided into medium-sized and large and account for 10%–20% of the total. The fifth class is composed of small neurons and accounts for 1%–2% of striatal neurons.

Most projecting neurons of the striatum belong to the medium-sized spiny type, while local intrinsic circuits are made up by the aspiny neurons. Immunohistochemical studies have allowed the identification of the main transmitters used by these different neurons; they have also revealed a subnuclear organization of the striatum in two main compartments which have been named islands, striosomes, or patches and matrix. Several neuropeptides appear to be characteristic of these neuronal populations. Striatal spiny neurons contain enkephalin and substance P, while somatostatin and neuropeptide Y have been localized to aspiny neurons. Neuropeptides are also contained in afferents to the striatum, for example cholecystokinin.

Because of limitations on the application of immunohistochemistry in human postmortem materials – particularly difficulties associated with the visualization of the cell bodies that in the experimental animal requires the injection of colchicine – we decided to use the technique of in situ hybridization (Young 1986) to visualize the neurons which actively transcribe some neuropeptide genes.

We designed synthetic oligonucleotides complementary to selected regions of the human genes coding for the following: enkephalins (amino acids 133–141; Noda et al. 1982), cholecystokinin (amino acids 80–95; Takahashi et al. 1985), somatostatin (amino acids 88–98; Shen et al. 1982), and neuropeptide Y (amino acids 29–45; Minth et al. 1984). These peptides were chosen initially because of the reported localization to different cell types in the basal ganglia or to afferents to these nuclei.

We first examined the distribution of these peptide mRNAs in several control cases without reported neurological diseases. A heterogeneous distri-

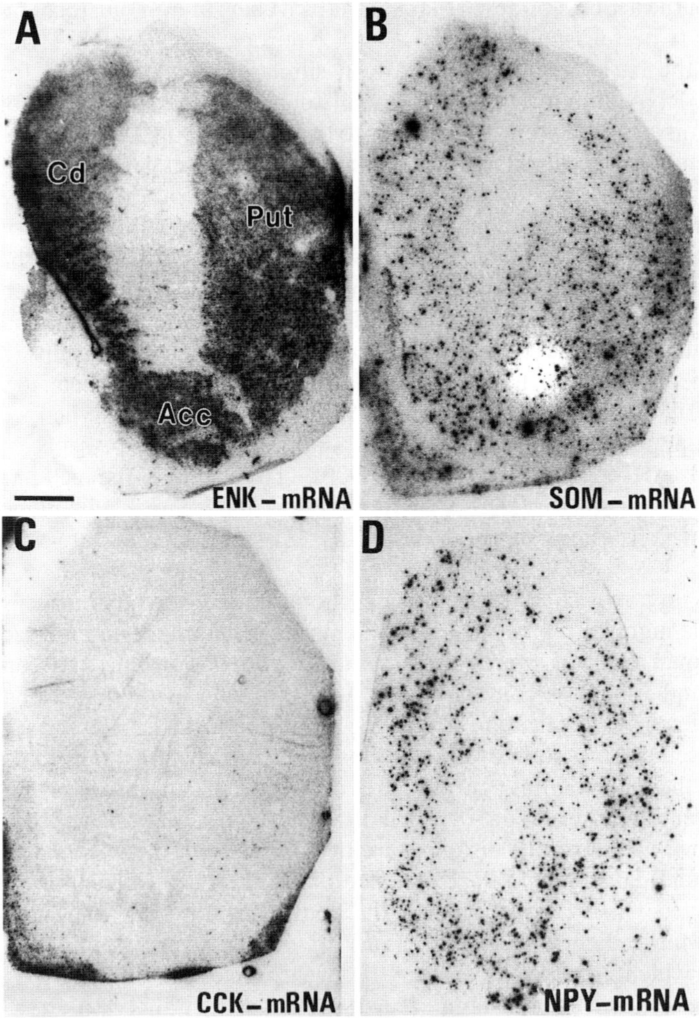

Fig. 1 A–D. Visualization of mRNAs for several neuropeptides in the human basal ganglia by in situ hybridization histochemistry. Photographs from film autoradiograms obtained by hybridizing sections from the same control case with ^{32}P-labeled oligonucleotides complementary to selective sequences from the mRNAs coding for: enkephalin (*ENK;* **A**); somatostatin (*SOM;* **B**); cholecystokinin (*CCK;* **C**); and neuropeptide Y (*NPY;* **D**). *Dark areas*, rich in the corresponding mRNA. See text for details. *Cd*, caudate nucleus; *Put*, putamen; *Acc*, nucleus accumbens; *bar*, 5 mm

bution of the expression of the mRNA for the neuropeptides was observed (Fig. 1). Enkephalin mRNA presented a patchy distribution overlapping with the distribution of acetylcholinesterase (AChE) activity. In contrast, cells expressing somatostatin mRNA were organized, in several striatal areas, around the patches of high enkephalin mRNA content. The distribution agrees well with that of the neuropeptides in the cat striatum using immunohistochemical techniques (Chesselet and Graybiel 1986). Neuropeptide Y mRNA was distributed in the basal ganglia in a pattern similar to that observed for somatostatin mRNA, in agreement with the histochemical demonstration of the colocalization of these two neuropeptides to the same neuronal population. This colocalization was particularly important in the basal ganglia but was not observed in other areas of the human brain examined, for example, the thalamus, where high levels of somatostatin mRNA contrasted with the lack of mRNA for neuropeptide Y. Cholecystokinin mRNA was not found in the striatum, indicating that striatal cholecystokinin immunoreactivity is localized to processes from cells extrinsic to this nucleus. While in the experimental animal, particularly in the rat, the colocalization of cholecystokinin in dopaminergic neurons has been demonstrated by both immunohistochemistry (Hökfelt et al. 1980) and in situ hybridization (Savasta et al. 1989), when we analyzed the human substantia nigra we were unable to show the presence of cholecystokinin mRNA (Palacios et al. 1989). To examine the cellular localization of these neuropeptides in the human striatum we took advantage of diseases in which lesions of the striatal afferents and efferents are well described.

Parkinson's disease is characterized by degeneration of dopaminergic cells of the substantia nigra. It represents a specific model of central dopaminergic denervation in man and is of interest for the study of the relationships between neuropeptides and dopamine-containing neurons. Such interactions have been shown in investigations on the corresponding animal model, the 6-hydroxydopamine induced degeneration of the rat dopaminergic ascending pathways. The levels of the enkephalin peptides are decreased in the striatum in Parkinson's disease (Agid and Javoy-Agid 1985). When basal ganglia from patients dying with Parkinson's disease were hybridized with the enkephalin probe, a pronounced decrease in the hybridization signal was observed for all the cases analyzed when compared with the control brains (Fig. 2). These results are in contradiction to those obtained with 6-hydroxydopamine lesioned rats, in which a marked increase in the level of enkephalin mRNA was observed on the lesioned side (Young et al. 1986; Savasta et al. 1989).

In contrast, somatostatin mRNA levels did not exhibit significant changes in the parkinsonian striatum. In the regions analyzed in our parkinsonian series for levels of cholecystokinin mRNA, we were unable to observe any difference. Finally, our preliminary studies on neuropeptide Y mRNA showed that the parkinsonian basal ganglia contained this mRNA, although no quantitative data are yet available. A differential regulation of somatostatin and neuropeptide Y mRNA levels by the ascending dopaminergic input has recently been documented immunohistochemically in the experimental animal (Kerkerian et al. 1986, 1988). The ability to analyze similar changes in Parkinson's disease at the mRNA level is now possible using in situ hybridization.

In Huntington's chorea some neurons of the caudate nucleus and putamen are selectively affected (Kowall et al. 1987), namely the spiny neurons. While the concentrations of a number of neurotransmitters which are known to be

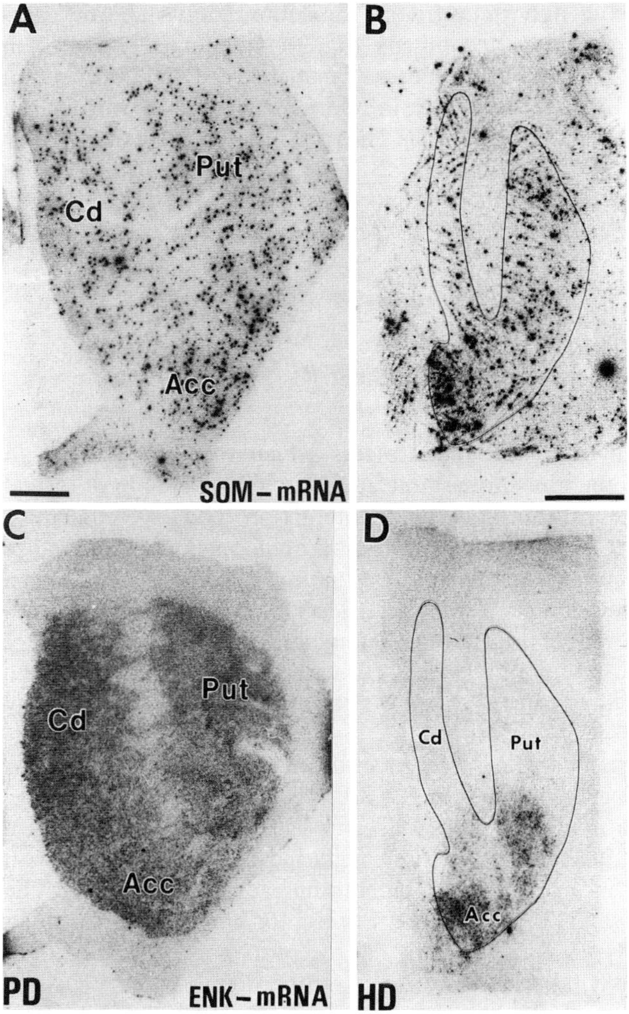

Fig. 2A–D. Alterations in the levels of neuropeptide mRNAs in Parkinson's disease (*PD*) and Huntington's chorea (*HD*). Levels of somatostatin mRNA were preserved in PD (**A**) and HD (**B**) while those of enkephalin mRNA were decreased in both PD (**C**) and HD (**D**). Because of the severe shrinkage of the basal ganglia in HD, the boundaries of these nuclei have been drawn over the autoradiograms. For a control see Fig. 1; other abbreviations and scale bar are as in Fig. 1

expressed by intrinsic cells projecting outside of the striatum are decreased – for example, acetylcholine, γ-aminobutyric acid (GABA), substance P, and enkephalins – other neurotransmitters such as dopamine, serotonin, and neurotensin, which are localized to extrinsic afferents, are preserved. Interestingly, some intrinsic transmitters, for instance, somatostatin and neuropeptide Y, and some cholinergic interneurons are also preserved. Using in situ hybridization we have observed a marked decrease in the levels of enkephalin mRNA in both caudate and putamen of the Huntington's chorea cases analyzed but little in the nucleus accumbens (Fig. 2). No alterations were seen in cholecystokinin mRNA content. In contrast, an increase in the hybridization signal was observed for both somatostatin and neuropeptide Y mRNAs in Huntington's chorea striatum (Fig. 2). The distribution of the neurons expressing somatostatin and neuropeptide Y was similar to that seen in controls. However, because of the marked shrinkage of the basal ganglia (Fig. 2), an apparent increase in the mRNA levels for these two neuropeptides was observed.

Imaging of Receptors in the Human Basal Ganglia

Receptors are specialized membrane proteins which recognize with high specificity and affinity the transmitter molecule and mediate the physiological effects triggered by the transmitter-receptor interaction. The development of high-affinity binding techniques and autoradiographic methods to visualize receptors in tissue sections has allowed the mapping of these receptors in human postmortem materials (Palacios et al. 1986). In correlation with studies on the expression of neuropeptides in the human basal ganglia, both in control and in pathological cases, we have also examined the distribution of the receptors for these neuropeptides using in vitro receptor autoradiography (Palacios et al. 1986).

In the human basal ganglia, receptors for neurotransmitters such as acetylcholine, dopamine, serotonin, and GABA and for neuropeptides such as enkephalin, somatostatin, cholecystokinin, neurotensin, and substance P are differentially enriched. These receptors show heterogeneous distributions with areas presenting a receptor binding higher than the background (Fig. 3). The distribution of these patches of high density of receptor binding varied among the different receptor types. This suggests that receptors present a differential localization to the two compartments of the striatum defined on the basis of immunohistochemical and histochemical studies (Graybiel and Ragsdale 1983; Beal and Martin 1986; Gerfen et al. 1987a, b; Parent 1987). Other receptors, such as those for substance P, present a more widespread distribution with high densities of binding localized to small areas more or less uniformly distributed.

Three types of alteration of receptor density and distribution have been observed in diseases of the human basal ganglia. One type is a decrease related locally to cell death. A second type is a distal change related either to denervation of an input to the basal ganglia, such as in the parkinsonian brain, or to hypersensitivity mechanisms in target areas which are denervated as a consequence of the death of striatal neurons. Finally, some receptor populations survive selectively pathological alterations in basal ganglia because they are probably localized to cell processes which are not affected by the diseases being studied. From the examination of a large number of receptors in several diseases it has been possible to gain information on the possible cellular

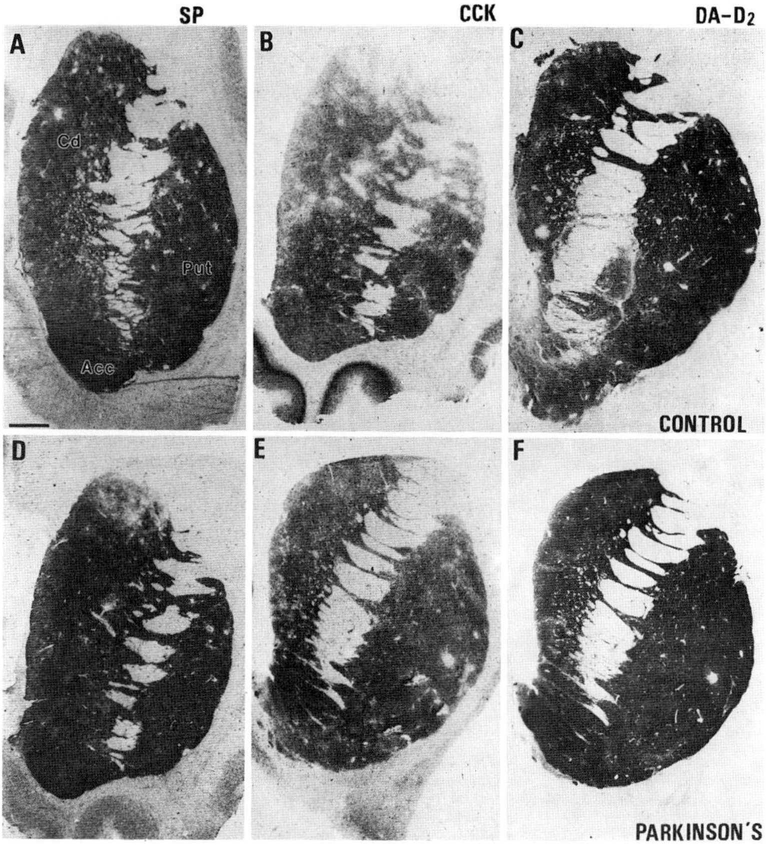

Fig. 3 A–F. The distribution of some neurotransmitter receptors visualized by autoradiography. **A, B, C** Control cases. **D, E, F** Parkinson's disease cases. **A, D** Substance P (*SP*) receptors with [^{125}I]-labeled Boulton-Hunter substance P. **B, E** Cholecystokinin (*CCK*) receptors with [^{125}I]-labeled Boulton-Hunter CCK. **C, F** Dopamine D_2 (*DA-D_2*) receptors with [^{125}I]iodosulpride. Other abbreviations and scale bar as in Fig. 1

localization of these receptors sites and to define possible therapeutic targets for the treatment of these diseases (Palacios et al. 1988 b).

In the population of parkinsonian brains examined we did not detect any significant alteration in the number of dopamine D_1 or D_2 receptors (Palacios et al. 1988 a). GABA receptors were also unchanged. These results contrast with those obtained in experimental animals and could be related to a different regulation or localization of receptors in the human basal ganglia. Of the neuropeptide receptors examined in the striatum we found a decrease in the levels of both somatostatin and neurotensin receptors. As mentioned above, somatostatin is expressed by interneurons of the striatum. In contrast, neurotensin appears to be localized to afferents to this nucleus. The levels of expression of both peptides remain unaltered in the parkinsonian brain (Agid

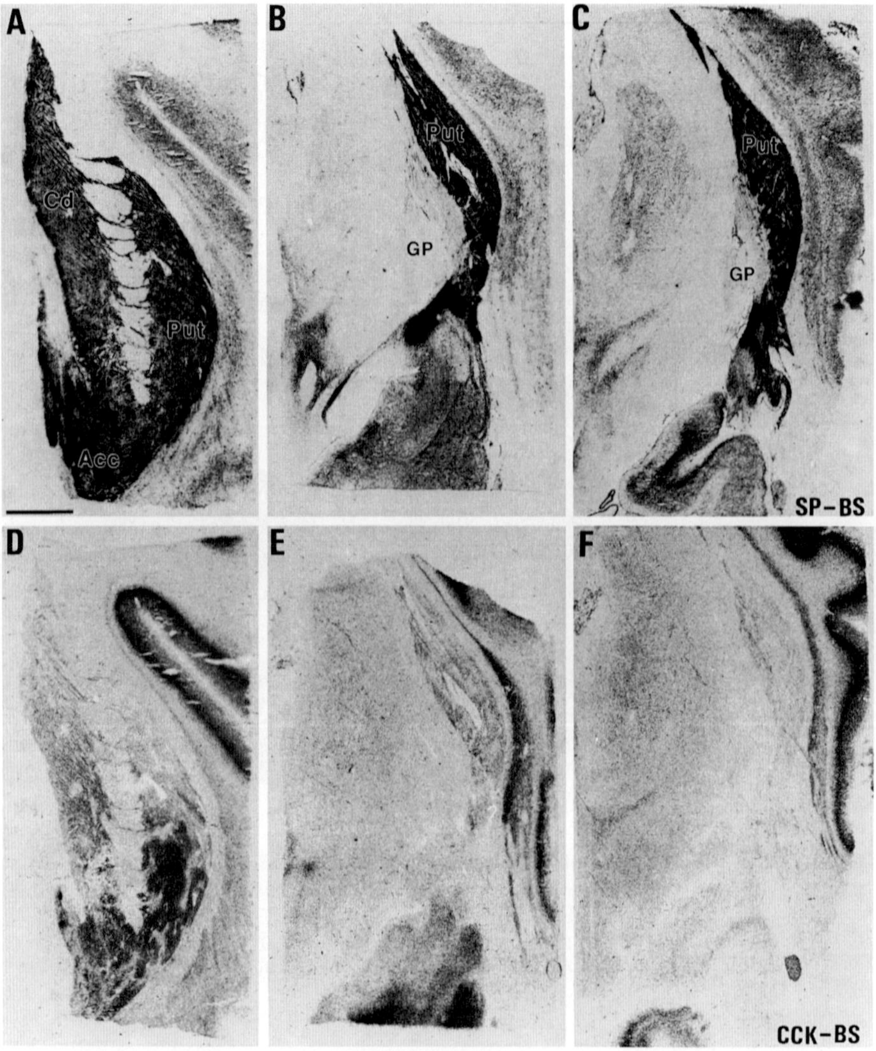

Fig. 4A–F. Alterations in neuropeptide receptor binding in the basal ganglia of a Huntington's chorea case. **A, B, C** Substance P binding sites (*SP-BS*) visualized at three different levels of the basal ganglia show densities comparable to those seen in control cases. **D, E, F** Cholecystokinin binding sites (*CCK-BS*), in contrast, are markedly reduced. *GP*, globus pallidus. Other abbreviations and scale bar as in Fig. 1

and Javoy-Agid 1985; Graybiel and Ragsdale 1983). It is difficult at the present moment to understand the down-regulation of neurotensin and somatostatin receptors in the parkinsonian brain; neurotensin receptors in the experimental animal are presynaptic, localized to the terminals and the cell bodies of the dopaminergic neurons (Quirion et al. 1985). The localization of somatostatin receptors in the striatum, however, is unknown. As discussed below, the decrease in somatostatin receptors in Huntington's chorea suggests that these receptors are expressed by cells intrinsic to the human striatum. Uhl et al. (1986) have described alterations in these peptide receptors in the parkinsonian substantia nigra, suggesting a presynaptic localization.

Many receptors have been found to be altered in the basal ganglia of the victims of Huntington's chorea. In general, these alterations were marked in the anterior and dorsal nucleus caudatus and the anterior putamen while receptor concentrations were less modified in the nucleus accumbens and ventral aspects of the caudatus and putamen. We found GABA and muscarinic receptors to be decreased. In the globus pallidus an increased density of GABA receptors was seen, probably due to a phenomenon of denervation hypersensitivity, in agreement with previous studies (Penney and Young 1982; Walker et al. 1984; Whitehouse et al. 1985). Receptors for several neuropeptides, such as somatostatin, cholecystokinin, and enkephalin, were decreased while substance P and neurotensin receptors were present in normal concentrations. Examples of these changes are illustrated in Fig. 4.

In both diseases alterations in receptors were not related to corresponding modification in the levels of endogenous peptides. For example, in Huntington's chorea the concentrations of neurotensin and cholecystokinin were normal, however neurotensin receptors were little affected, and cholecystokinin receptors were markedly decreased. Somatostatin levels were increased while somatostatin receptors were also markedly decreased. Finally, substance P concentration was decreased but substance P receptors were not altered. These findings question the role of the endogenous neurotransmitter in the regulation of receptor expression in disease states of the human brain. The status of the cell bearing the receptor appears to be more important. If the receptor is localized to a cell which degenerates in this disease, the receptor is lost in spite of the preservation of the transmitter. What physiological role the transmitter could have in the absence of the receptor is difficult to understand. In the opposite situation the presence of receptors could still serve a function, at least from the therapeutic point of view. A clear example of the therapeutic usefulness of these denervated receptors is provided by the use of dopamine receptor agonists in the treatment of Parkinson's disease. Similarly, drugs acting on some of the surviving receptors could be useful in the treatment of Huntington's disease.

Conclusions

The use of imaging techniques for the study of the human basal ganglia both at the pre- and postsynaptic levels has revealed a number of interesting features of these brain nuclei and of their modification in disease. First, we have seen that receptors and transmitters are heterogeneously distributed in these nuclei. There is not a good correlation between the distribution of the transmitter and that of the receptor. Furthermore, alterations in neurotransmitter levels are not always paralleled by compensatory receptor modifications. More studies are necessary to understand the mechanisms involved in the regulation of the expression of both neurotransmitters and receptors in the human basal ganglia.

For this the ability to visualize the expression of mRNA coding for these receptors by using in situ hybridization techniques will be of considerable help. Neurodegenerative diseases are slowly progressing diseases. To visualize the evolution of these biochemical parameters with the progress of the disease it is important to develop noninvasive methods such as positron emission tomography for the visualization of receptor and transmitter expression. The applicaton of these invasive and noninvasive techniques to the study of the basal ganglia will help in the understanding of diseases of the brain and the development or rational therapeutic approaches for the treatment of these diseases.

Acknowledgements. The authors gratefully acknowledge the collaboration of G. Chinaglia, M. Rigo, E. Ruberte, and M. Savasta in the experiments reported in the present work, as well as the invaluable help of K. H. Wiederhold with photography and image analysis. We also thank Prof. J. Ulrich and Dr. A. Probst from the Department of Neuropathology, Institute of Pathology, University of Basel, Switzerland, for providing control and Parkinson's disease tissues and Prof. E. Bird from the Brain Tissue Resource Center, McLean Hospital, Belmont, MA, USA, for kindly supplying the Huntington's disease specimens. This Center is supported in part by Public Health Service grant number MH/NS 31862.

References

Agid Y, Javoy-Agid F (1985) Peptides and Parkinson's disease. Trends Neurosci 1:30–35

Beal MF, Martin JB (1986) Neuropeptides and neurological disease. Ann Neurol 20:547–565

Bird ED, Iversen LL (1982) Human brain postmortem studies of neurotransmitter and related markers. In: Lajtha A (ed) Handbook of neurochemistry, vol 2. Plenum, London, pp 225–251

Björklund A, Hökfelt T (eds) (1983) Handbook of chemical neuroanatomy, vol. 1. Elsevier, Amsterdam

Chesselet MF, Graybiel AM (1986) Striatal neurons expressing somatostatin-like immunoreactivity: evidence for a peptidergic interneuronal system in the cat. Neuroscience 17:547–572

Emson PC, Rossor MN, Tohyama M (eds) (1986) Neuropeptides and neurodegenerative diseases. Elsevier Science, Amsterdam (Progress in brain research, vol 66)

Gerfen CR, Herkerham M, Thibault J (1987a) The neostriatal mosaic. II. Patch and matrix directed mesostriatal dopaminergic and non-dopaminergic systems. J Neurosci 7:3915–3934

Gerfen CR, Baimbridge KG, Thibault J (1987b) The neostriatal mosaic. III. Biochemical and developmental dissociation of patch-matrix mesostriatal systems. J Neurosci 7:3935–3944

Graveland GA, Williams RS, DiFiglia M (1985) A Golgi study of the human neostriatum: neurons and afferent fibers. J Comp Neurol 234:317–333

Graybiel AM, Ragsdale Jr CW (1983) Biochemical anatomy of the striatum. In: Emson PC (ed) Chemical neuroanatomy. Raven, New York, pp 427–504

Hökfelt T, Rhefeld JF, Skirboll L, Ivemark B, Goldstein M, Markey K (1980) Evidence for coexistence of dopamine and cholecystokinin in mesolimbic neurons. Nature 285:476–478

Hornykiewicz O (1972) Dopamine and its physiological significance in brain function. In: Bournes GM (ed) The structure and function of neurons systems, vol 6. Academic, New York, pp 367–415

Kerkerian L, Bosler O, Pelletier G, Nieoullon A (1986) Striatal neuropeptide Y neurons are under the influence of the nigrostriatal dopaminergic pathway: immunohistochemical evidence. Neurosci Lett 66:106–112

Kerkerian L, Salin P, Nieoullon A (1988) Pharmacological characterization of dopaminergic influence on expression of neuropeptide Y immunoreactivity by rat striatal neurons. Neurosci 26:809–817

Kowall NW, Perrante RS, Martin JB (1987) Patterns of cell loss in Huntington's disease. Trends Neurosci 10:24–29

Minth CD, Bloom SR, Polak JM, Dixon JE (1984) Cloning, characterization, and DNA sequence of a human cDNA encoding neuropeptide tyrosine. Proc Natl Acad Sci USA 81:4577–4581

Noda M, Teranishi Y, Takahashi H, Toyosato M, Notake M, Nakanishi S, Numa S (1982) Isolation and structural organization of the human preproenkephalin gene. Nature 297:431–434

Palacios JM, Probst A, Cortés R (1986) Mapping receptors in the human brain. Trends Neurosci 9:284–289

Palacios JM, Camps M, Cortés R, Probst A (1988a) Mapping dopamine receptors in the human brain. J Neural Transm 27:227–235

Palacios JM, Cortés R, Dietl M, Probst A (1988b) Receptors in human brain diseases: a use for receptor autoradiography in neuropathology. J Recept Res 8:509–520

Palacios JM, Savasta M, Mengod G (1989) Does cholecystokinin colocalize with dopamine in the human substantia nigra? Brain Res 488:369–375

Parent A (1987) Comparative neurobiology of the basal ganglia. Wiley, New York

Penney JB, Young AB (1982) Quantitative autoradiography of neurotransmitter receptors in Huntington's disease. Neurology 32:1391–1395

Quirion R, Chieueh CC, Everist HD, Pert A (1985) Comparative localization of neurotensin receptors on nigrostriatal and mesolimbic dopaminergic terminals. Brain Res 327:385–389

Rossor MN (1982) Dementia (neurotransmitters and CNS disease). Lancet 2:1200–1204

Savasta M, Ruberte E, Palacios JM, Mengod G (1989) The colocalization of cholecystokinin and tyrosine hydroxylase mRNAs in mesencephalic dopaminergic neurons in the rat brain examined by in situ hybridization. Neuroscience 29:363–369

Shen LP, Pictet RL, Rutter WJ (1982) Human somatostatin I: sequence of the cDNA. Proc Natl Acad Sci USA 79:4575–4579

Takahashi Y, Kato K, Hayashizaki Y, Wakabayashi T, Ohtsuka E, Matsuki S, Ikehara M, Matsubara K (1985) Molecular cloning of the human cholecystokinin gene by use of a synthetic probe containing deoxyinosine. Proc Natl Acad Sci USA 82:1931–1935

Uhl GR, Hackney GO, Torchia M, Stranov V, Tourtellotte WW, Whitehouse PJ, Tran V, Strittmatter S (1986) Parkinson's disease: nigral receptor changes support peptidergic role in nigrostriatal modulation. Ann Neurol 20:194–203

Walker FO, Young AB, Penney JB, Dovorini-Zis K, Shoulson I (1984) Benzodiazepine and GABA receptors in early Huntington's disease. Neurology 34:1237–1240

Whitehouse PJ, Trifiletti RR, Jones BE, Folstein S, Price DL, Snyder SH, Kuhar MJ (1985) Neurotransmitter receptor alterations in Huntington's disease: autoradiographic and homogenate studies with special reference to benzodiazepine receptor complexes. Ann Neurol 18:202–210

Young WS III (1986) In situ hybridization histochemistry and the study of the nervous system. Trends Neurosci 12:549–551

Young WS III, Bonner TI, Brann MR (1986) Mesencephalic dopamine neurons regulate the expression of neuropeptide mRNAs in the rat forebrain. Proc Natl Acad Sci USA 83:9827–9831

Further Cytoarchitectonic and Quantitative Studies in the Entorhinal Region of Schizophrenics and Normal Controls by Means of a Modified Nissl Technique *

H. HEINSEN and H. BECKMANN [1]

Introduction

The entorhinal region is located in the rostral third of the parahippocampal gyrus. In the clearest cases, especially in young individuals, the extent of the entorhinal region can be distinguished with the naked eye due to its rough, wartlike surface, which contrasts with the smooth pial surface of the rostrally located temporal pole, medial prepiriform cortex, periamygdaloid region, and the laterally and caudally ensuing fields of the temporal isocortex. In the human brain the entorhinal region with its rough surface has a size somewhat more than a thumb nail, that is, maximally 30 mm in rostrocaudal and 15 mm in mediolateral width. Rostrally the entorhinal region terminates in a conical manner; laterally it seems to disappear in the collateral sulcus.

Comparative anatomic, quantitative, and cytoarchitectonic aspects of the entorhinal region are extensively dealt with by Stephan (1975). Although representative of the allocortex, the lamination of the entorhinal region is very complicated in its central fields (Braak 1972); here up to 11 layers can be distinguished in pigment preparations. Furthermore, the entorhinal region is a progressive structure and reaches an extraordinary extent in primates and especially in man (Stephan 1975). From recent tracer studies in cat (Room and Groenewegen 1986a, b; Witter and Groenewegen 1986a, b; Witter et al. 1986) and monkey (Insausti et al. 1987a, b) the entorhinal region has been shown to represent an interface between cortical sensory inputs and the hippocampal formation. The connections between the entorhinal region and sensory and parasensory cortical areas are generally reciprocated, thus being interposed between the external and internal environments (Pandya and Yeterian 1985). It has been shown by Witter et al. (1986) that afferent and efferent fiber connections terminate or arise in circumscribed layers of the highly laminated entorhinal region and are furthermore arranged in dinstinct longitudinal and mediolateral zones. The most elaborate lamination in the human entorhinal cortex thus appears to represent an enormous increase in afferent, efferent and intrinsic connections compared with more primitive stages.

Recently it has been shown that the entorhinal cortex exhibits different pathological changes in various disease states. The nerve cells of the entorhinal

* Supported by a grant from the Deutsche Forschungsgemeinschaft (Be 602/6-1).

[1] Psychiatrische Klinik der Universität Würzburg, Füchsleinstr. 15, 8700 Würzburg, FRG.

Neuropsychopharmacology
Edited by Bunney/Hippius/Laakmann/Schmauß

cortex are afflicted in early stages of Alzheimer's disease (Hyman et al. 1984; Braak and Braak 1986; Heinsen et al. 1989). Likewise in Pick's disease, Jakob (1979) described nerve cell degeneration and gliosis in the entorhinal cortex, which in early states is confined to the third layer. Jakob and Beckmann (1986) emphasized circumscribed cytoarchitectonic disturbances in the rostral part of the entorhinal cortex in a large number of schizophrenics. The latter study prompted us to reinvestigate the entorhinal region in schizophrenics with a different method, allowing serial sections including preliminary quantitative studies.

Materials and Methods

Brains from schizophrenic patients and normal control cases without neurological or psychiatric diseases were fixed in 4% formalin within 24 h after death. The brains were fixed for at least 3 months in regularly changed formalin. According to Bauchot (1967), formalin fixation induces swelling of the brain tissue, which can attain a size of 130% of the initial volume. Three months after fixation brain tissue usually shrinks to about 95% of the initial volume. Prior to the removal of the meninges and larger brain vessels the fixed brain was subjected to gross neuropathological examination. After this examination we made cuts with two parallel razor blades fixed at a distance of 2 mm from one another into defined cortical gyri, including the medial frontal gyrus, medial temporal gyrus, and occipital gyri. The brains were then soaked in a cryoprotective solution (Rosene et al. 1987). Then the brain was embedded in gelatin; the gelatin was hardened in 4% formaldehyde in a refrigerator (4 °C), and again the embedded brain tissue together with a gelatin mantle was treated in an additional cryoprotective fluid. The gelatin block was then frozen in liquid isopentane (−60 °C), stored overnight in a regriferator (−80 °C), and cut the next day on a tetrander into serial sections about 600 µm thick. Sections this thick can be stored in formaldehyde solution until the staining procedures. After washing the sections for 1 h in running tap water and rinsing the slices in destilled water, sections were stained for 1–3 h in gallocyanin-chromalum (Einarson 1932). The stained sections were then washed in running tap water for another 1 h, and dehydrated in 70%, 80%, 96%, and 100% alcohol. The sections were cleared in a mixture of xylol-propanol and then in two changes of xylol. The sections were mounted in histological resins.

The staining and dehydrating procedures cause unpredictable swelling and shrinkage of the gelatin-embedded brain tissue. The parallel razor blade cuts which were applied prior to these procedures allow rapid and reliable assessment of the shrinkage factors during these procedures. The razor blades were 2 mm apart, and shrinkage of the brain tissue decreases the distance whereas swelling increases the distance. We have found that irrespective of age and disease the linear shrinkage factor of our brain tissues is only 5%. The section thickness was controlled by cutting small tissue blocks out from the brain slices and measuring the thickness of the small tissue fragments under the microscope with the aid of a calibrated ocular grid.

Since we had serially sectioned the brains, the volume of any confined structure could be calculated from the area of the structure in microscopic sections multiplied by section thickness and the distance between sections, which must be known in cases in which not all serial sections but only a representative sample was taken (Gundersen and Jensen 1987).

We prefer for our qualitative and quantitative investigations a modern stereo-zoom microscope. With the aid of this we are able to delineate the boundaries of the entorhinal region with a high degree of reproducibility.

The entorhinal region is composed of three parts: the lateral entorhinal area (Brodmann's area 28), the medial entorhinal area (Brodmann's area 34), and the perirhinal area (Brodmann's area 35). The latter field has been further subdivided by Braak (1972) and is collectively designated as area entorhinalis transitiva by this author. The perirhinal area usually occupies the walls and the depth of the collateral sulcus. In thick Nissl-stained sections the medial limit of the perirhinal area is characterized by a descending band of alpha pyramidal cells in the lamina principalis externa (PRE). Frequently the medial and the lateral entorhinal area are separated by a shallow sulcus, the sulcus inferior rhinencephali of Retzius. At the most rostral sites, where the latter sulcus is not as impressive, the medial and lateral entorhinal area can be distinguished by the generally smaller overall cell size of the medial entorhinal area. The main distinction between the prepiriform area and the entorhinal area is the appearance of a lamina dissecans in the latter. Especially in man, the lamina densocellularis of the prepiriform area tends to be arranged in nerve cell accumulations or nodules which are in general smaller than in the medial entorhinal region.

The area of the lateral entorhinal area was estimated by means of an ocular grid inserted into a stereomicroscope with tenfold magnification. With our optical equipment the depth of the field was rather low, and consequently we think that the bias introduced by the phenomenon of overprojection is negligible. The point number required in order to reduce the estimation error below 5% can be taken from Weibel (1979).

The relative volume, or volume density, indicates the quantitative composition of any regular or irregular structure. For example, a three-layered cortex in which the upper, middle, and lower lamina each have a relative volume of 33% is one composed of three lamina with exactly the same volume. In addition to the absolute volume of the lateral entorhinal area, we estimated the volumes of the lamina zonalis, PRE alpha, PRE beta, PRE gamma, lamina dissecans, and the layers of the lamina principalis interna (PRI). This was done with higher magnification (20×). Point counting methods are the most reliable methods here since the boundaries of the structures examined are highly irregular and cannot be outlined with digitizing instruments.

Results

Rostrocaudal Fields in the Lateral Entorhinal Area

In Nissl-stained sections we could distinguish a number of fields in the enthorinal region differing from one another by the width of the layers, by the basophilia of nerve cells, and by the width and number of cell-poor laminae dissecantes.

The most *rostral field* of the entorhinal region is characterized, in addition to the presence of the superficial lamina zonalis or molecularis, by a second layer consisting of nerve cell accumulations which are arranged in loosely interconnected nodules or glomeruli, the PRE alpha layer. The nerve cells of this second layer are intensely basophilic and rather large in Nissl-stained sections. They reside on the third layer, the PRE beta layer, which in its uppermost parts appears indented by conically shaped cell-poor clefts. The third layer, the PRE gamma layer, is difficult to distinguish from the more superficial PRE beta layer. A cell-poor transversally oriented band, the lamina dissecans, separates the PRE gamma layer from the deep PRI layers, which are also strongly basophilic and cannot be separated into alpha, beta, and gamma layers in Nissl-stained sections in the rostral parts of the entorhinal region. The PRI layers form a more or less compact band onto which the lamina cellularis profunda (Fig. 1 a, c) adjoins with its large, slightly basophilic nerve cells gradually intermingling with the central medullary gray.

In a more caudal direction, 3–5 mm from the rostral tip of the entorhinal region, i.e., topographically in an intermediate position, the PRE alpha nodules become larger (Fig. 1 a–c, thick arrows), and from the medial entorhinal area a cell-poor cleft begins to separate the large PRE alpha clusters from the PRE beta cell layer (Fig. 1 a–c, thin arrows). The cells of the PRE beta cell layer are now arranged in cell columns which are crowned by basophilic cell caps (Fig. 1 a–c, white asterisks). At variance to the PRE beta columns, the deep PRE gamma cell layer is a continuous layer abutting basally onto the lamina dissecans (Fig. 1 a, c). The layers from alpha through gamma are collectively designated as the lamina principalis externa (Fig. 1 a, c). The PRI layer (Fig. 1 a, c) clinging to the lamina dissecans can hardly be subdivided into sublayers alpha, beta, and gamma. The *intermediate field*, characterized by PRE beta cell columns with basophilic cell caps separated by a cell-poor cleft from PRE alpha nodules, can be distinguished in serial sections for a distance of 3–5 mm in rostro caudal direction.

Further caudally, in a *central position*, the PRE beta cell columns lose their basophilic caps, but this layer remains indented resulting in columnar arrangement of PRE beta cells. At these levels of sections the deeper layers, especially the PRI, becomes stratified by one or two small cell-poor streaks (Fig. 1 b, white arrow). These fields most probably correspond to Braak's (1972) central fields of the entorhinal region after pigment staining.

In the most *caudal planes*, the lamina dissecans usually disappears first, and the PRE alpha nodules tend to be arranged in adjacent sections as a continuous

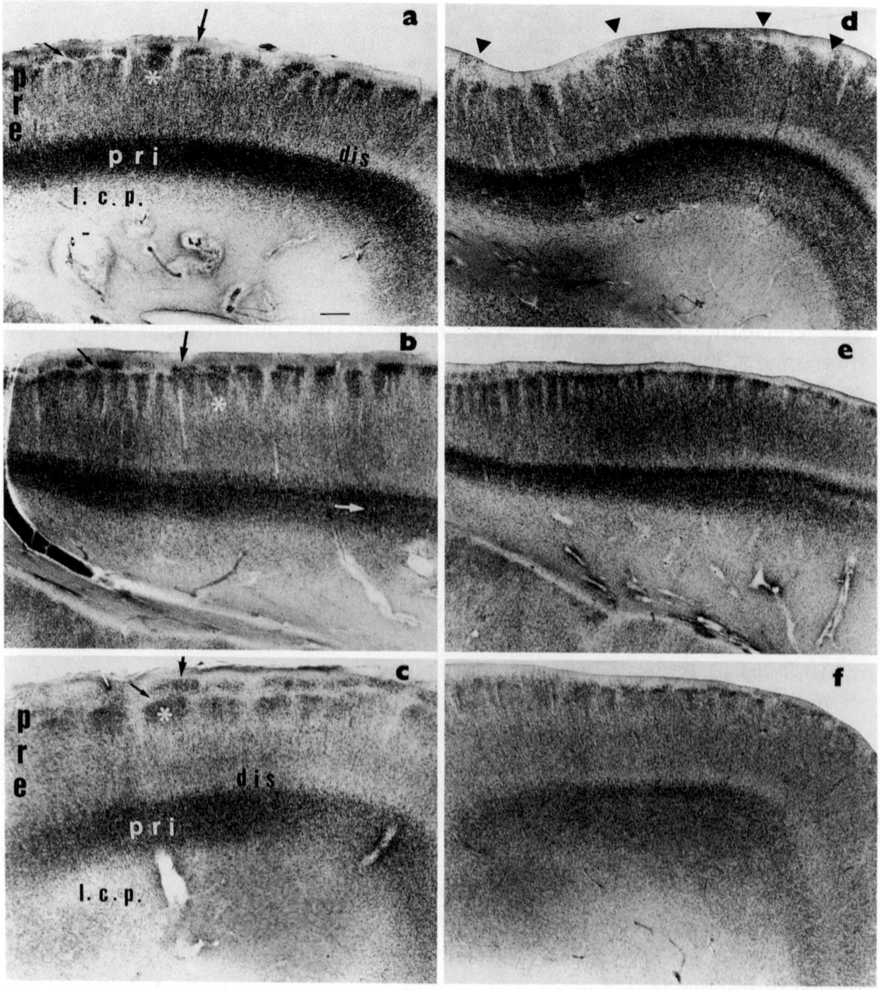

Fig. 1a–f. Nissl-stained sections of rostrocaudal fields in the lateral entorhinal area. **a**, **b**, **c** Control cases, **d**, **e**, **f** Schizophrenic cases. **a** Man, 35 years old; myocardial ischemia. **b** Woman, 79 years old; gastrointestinal hemorrhage. **c** Woman, 51 years old; pancreatitis. **d** Schizophrenic man, 31 years old; alcohol and drug intoxication. **e** Schizophrenic woman, 78 years old; myocardial infarct. **f** Schizophrenic woman, 59 years old; sepsis. *dis*, Lamina dissecans; *l.p.c.*, lamina cellularis profunda; *PRE*, lamina principalis externa; *pri*, lamina principalis interna; *thick black arrows*, pre alpha cell nodules; *thin black arrows*, pre beta cell layer; *white arrow*, cell-poor streak; *white asterisks*, basophilic cell caps; *black arrowheads*, absence of pre alpha cell nodules

cell band with decreasing nerve cell size and increasing nerve cell density. Isocortical layers indent to various degrees the allocortical layers resulting in complicated zones of transition.

Cytoarchitectonic Abnormalities in the Intermediate Field of the Entorhinal Area

In the control cases we could invariably observe PRE alpha cell nodules separated by a cell-poor cleft from the PRE beta cell columns with their basophilic cell caps (Fig. 1a–c, white asterisks). The fields with these cytoarchitectonic characteristics were encountered at the junction between the most rostral field, with a rather simple stratification, and the more caudally located central field, with a complicated lamination of the PRI.

Our age- and sex-matched schizophrenic cases were taken from identical planes of section (Fig. 1d–f). Prior to a description of the morphological changes in each case we give a brief account of the psychopathology.

Case 1. The case history from our first case (Fig. 1d) is that of a 31-year-old man who was raised by his parents, and who visited elementary school with moderate success. He first fell sick in 1980 and was admitted to a state psychiatric hospital. There he remained with one interruption until he died in 1988 from intoxication with alcohol and various psychotropic drugs. He frequently heard imperative and commenting voices, had ideas of reference, felt under the influence of his girlfriend by rays, and felt steered. His mood oscillated between dullness, flat affect, and panic-driven conditions with hostilities. Abuse of alcohol occurred frequently. The psychosis proceeded intermittently without clear remission. Diagnosis was:

ICD 9: paranoid hallucinatory schizophrenia, 295.3
DSM III: schizophrenia, paranoid type, subchronic course with acute exacerbations
Leonhard: affectful paraphrenia

This case is characterized by the absence of PRE alpha cell nodules over a wide distance (Fig. 1d, arrowheads). The PRE beta cell columns can be distinguished, as can also basophilic cell caps in some but not all of these columns.

Case 2. The second case, a 59-year-old woman, visited the elementary school with unknown performance. She had no profession, was housemaid in the household of her parents, and was unmarried. When she was 30 years old she became suspicious and dysphoric and behaved "uneducated." She could not keep track of ideas and was uncooperative. She had various hypochondric ideas: sometimes she had the feeling that her kidneys were being torn out; she could not eat meat or cheese since she had no air in her legs. She was completely withdrawn, negativistic, aggressive, and hostile with blunted affect. This symptomatology remained identical over the years until 1988, when she died from pneumonia. Her last medications were the neuroleptics levomepomazine, flupentixol, and haloperidol. In 1956 she had had approximately ten electroconvulsion treatments without any effect. Diagnosis was:

ICD 9: schizophrenia, hebephrenic type, 295.1
DSM III: schizophrenia, residual type, chronic course
Leonhard: hebephrenia, excentric type

In this case PRE alpha nodules and PRE beta cell columns are not separated by a cell-poor cleft but appear intermingled one with the other (Fig. 1e). In the medial entorhinal area (Fig. 1e, left side) the separation of laminae is complete, but it remains incomplete in the lateral entorhinal region for several millimeters caudally until the central fields of the entorhinal region where cytoarchitectonics appears undisturbed.

Case 3. The last case is that of a 78-year-old woman, the daughter of a farmer. She had visited the elementary school with unknown performance and was then housewife. No complete biography was available. She was 40 years old when she fell sick. She was dysphoric and aggressive toward her relatives and showed incoherence of thinking and various paranoid ideas toward the priest of the village, whom she accused of persecuting her. There was clear indication of hallucinations. Various paranoid ideas were uttered. Now she was more or less depressed without drive. The course of illness cannot clearly be stated. It was either chronic with acute exacerbations or in remission. Diagnosis was:

ICD 9: schizophrenia, paranoid hallucinatory type, 295.3
DSM III: schizophrenia disorganized type, 259.1
Leonhard: affectful paraphrenia

The level of section in this case and the control (Fig. 1f, c) is more rostral than that of the two preceding cases and controls. As in the preceding case, the PRE alpha nodules appear dysplastic, and PRE beta cell columns are virtually absent. In the adjoining caudal sections, 5–6 mm more caudal, the lamination did not differ from the control cases.

Quantitative Investigation

Absolute Volume of the Entorhinal Area. In the controls the total volume of the lateral entorhinal area varied considerably, with minimal values of 254 mm^3 and maximal volumes of 505 mm^3 (Fig. 2). There is probably a tendency to slight reduction in total lateral entorhinal area volume in the schizophrenic cases, with minimal volumes of 255 mm^3 and a maximal volume of 355 mm^3. We have not analyzed these data statistically since the number of cases is too low.

Relative Volume of the Individual Layers in the Lateral Entorhinal Area. Surprisingly, the relative volumes of the PRE alpha, PRE beta, PRE gamma, and the PRI alpha to gamma layers were greater in schizoprenics compared

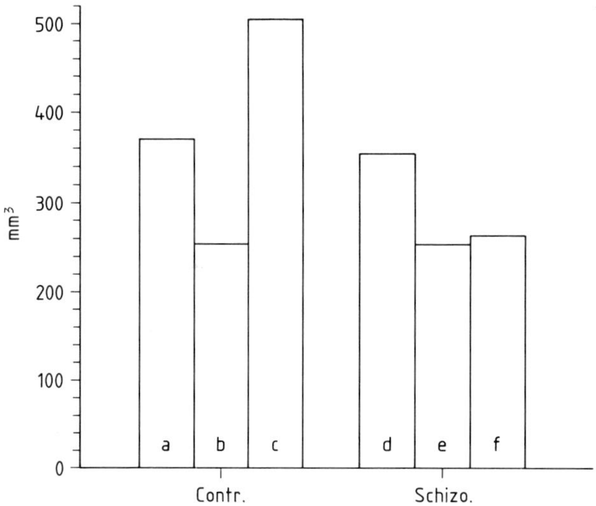

Fig. 2. Absolute volume in cubic millimeters of the lateral entorhinal area in controls (*CONTR.*) and schizophrenics (*SCHIZO.*). *Letters* correspond to the cases (panels) in Fig. 1

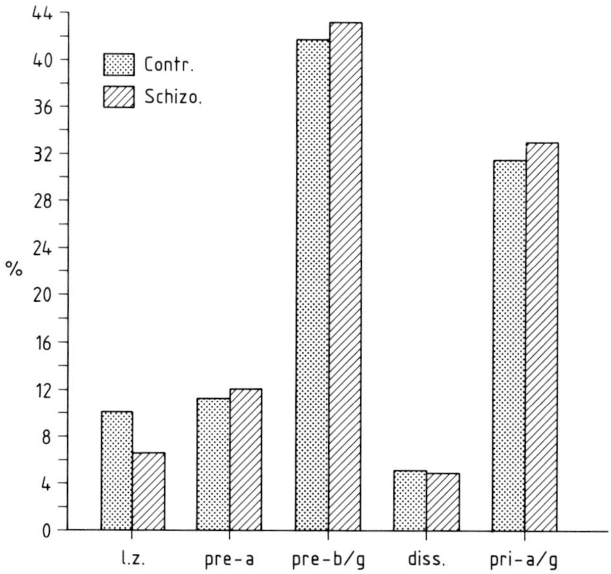

Fig. 3. Relative volume (percentage) of the layers in the entorhinal region in schizophrenics and controls. *l.z.*, Lamina zonalis (molecularis); *pre-a*, pre alpha; *pre-b/g*, pre beta/gamma; *diss.*, lamina dissecans; *pri-a/g*, pri alpha/gamma

with the control cases; differences between the individual layers are not as large, about 1 % for each lamina (Fig. 3). However, this does not imply that the layers of the PRE and PRI are also more voluminous in schizophrenics since one must multiply the relative volume of the individual layers by the absolute volume to obtain the mass of nervous tissue which contributes to the quantitative laminar composition. Since the absolute volume of the lateral entorhinal area is lower in schizophrenics, the quantitative laminar composition of the lateral entorhinal area in the latter does not differ from that in control cases, with the exception of the lamina zonalis – its volume and consequently also its thickness appears to be reduced in schizophrenia. But more cases are required to determine this definitely.

Discussion

Our present results are in good agreement with the findings of Jakob and Beckmann (1986) in a far larger number of schizophrenic cases. Their Fig. 2a and 3a can be directly compared with our Fig. 1e, f. The volume of the PRE alpha layer appears to be reduced and incompletely separated from PRE alpha cell columns. In agreement with Jakob and Beckmann (1986) we found these cytoarchitectonic disturbances exclusively in the intermediate fields of the entorhinal region (rostral field of Jakob and Beckmann 1986) with the more caudal fields being unchanged. At higher magnification we could exclude gliosis, circulatory disturbances, and, after staining with silver impregnation (Gallyas 1971), the existence of presenile and senile Alzheimer-type changes. Therefore, we designate the present changes as *dysplastic* rather than regressive. Dysplasia of the intermediate field of the lateral entorhinal area implies that the disturbances in the lamination of schizophrenic brains are probably due to prenatal developmental changes, including incomplete nerve cell migration or interconnection. The preliminary quantitative data support the view of Jakob and Beckmann (1986) and our own view that these dysplastic changes are confined to the rostral and intermediate parts of the lateral entorhinal area. More caudal regions do not show signs of disturbed lamination and appear unchanged. The quantitative data lead us to hypothesize that the caudal fields compensate the dysplastic rostral parts in schizophrenics, at least quantitatively.

A number of authors have subdivided the entorhinal region into various fields with up to 23 subfields (for review see Stephan 1975). It must be mentioned that there is hardly any agreement among the individual authors.

In a recent tracer study Insausti et al. (1987a) found the rostral parts of the entorhinal region in monkey interconnected with the frontal cortex. Compared with the frontal cortex in monkeys the prefrontal cortex in man has been enormously enlarged during evolution. According to Sgonina (1938) the entorhinal fields lambda 13 and lambda 15 are highly developed in man and are inconspicuous in apes. The cytoarchitectonic disturbances of the lateral entorhinal area coincide topographically with Sgonina's (1938) lambda 13 and lambda 15 fields. Together with the tracer studies in monkey (Insausti et al. 1987a), a dysplasia of the intermediate entorhinal field of the lateral entorhinal area could be indicative of an incomplete frontal cortical–lateral entorhinal area connection.

References

Bauchot R (1976) Les modifications du poids encéphalique au cours de la fixation. J Hirnforsch 9:253–283

Braak H (1972) Zur Pigmentarchitektonik der Großhirnrinde des Menschen. I. Regio entorhinalis. Z Zellforsch 127:407–438

Braak H, Braak E (1986) On areas of transition between entorhinal allocortex and temporal isocortex in the human brain. Normal morphology and lamina-specific pathology in Alzheimer's disease. Acta Neuropathol (Berl) 68:325–332

Einarson L (1932) A method for progressive selective staining of Nissl and nuclear substance in nerve cells. Am J Pathol 8:295–307

Gallyas F (1971) Silver staining of Alzheimer's neurofibrillary changes by means of physical development. Acta Morphol Hung 19:1–8

Gundersen HJG, Jensen EB (1987) The efficiency of systematic sampling in stereology and its prediction. J Microsc 147:229–263

Heinsen H, Beckmann H, Gallyas F, Heinsen YL, Haas S, Scharff G (1989) Laminar neuropathology in Alzheimer's disease by a modififed Gallyas impregnation. Psychiatry Res 29:463–465

Hyman BT, Hoesen GW van, Damasio R, Barnes CL (1984) Alzheimer's disease: cell-specific pathology isolates the hippocampal formation. Science 225:1168–1170

Insausti R, Amaral DG, Cowan WM (1987a) The entorhinal cortex of the monkey. II. Cortical afferents. J Comp Neurol 264:356–395

Insausti R, Amaral DG, Cowan WM (1987b) The entorhinal cortex of the monkey. III. Subcortical afferents. J Comp Neurol 264:396–408

Jakob H (1979) Die Picksche Krankheit. Monographien aus dem Gesamtgebiete der Psychiatrie 23. Springer, Berlin Heidelberg New York

Jakob H, Beckmann H (1986) Prenatal developmental disturbances in the limbic allocortex in schizophrenics. J Neural Trans 65:303–326

Pandya DN, Yeterian EH (1985) Architecture and connection of cortical association areas. In: Peters A, Jones EG (eds) Cerebral cortex, vol 4. Plenum, New York, pp 3–61

Room P, Groenewegen HJ (1986a) Connection of the parahippocampal cortex. I. Cortical afferents. J Comp Neurol 251:415–450

Room P, Goenewegen HJ (1986b) Connection of the parahippocampal cortex. II. Subcortical afferents. J Comp Neurol 251:451–473

Rosene DL, Roy NJ, Davis BJ (1986) A cryoprotection method that facilitates cutting frozen sections of whole monkey brains for histological and histochemical processing without freezing artifact. J Histochem Cytochem 34:1301–1315

Sgonina K (1938) Zur vergleichenden Anatomie der Entorhinal- und Präsubikularregion. J Psychol Neurol 38:56–113

Stephan H (1975) Allocortex. In: Bargmann W (ed) Handbuch der mikroskopischen Anatomie des Menschen, vol IV/9. Springer, Berlin Heidelberg New York

Weibel ER (1979) Stereological methods, vol 1. Academic, London

Witter MP, Groenewegen HJ (1986a) Connections of the parahippocampal cortex in the cat. III. Cortical and thalamic efferents. J Comp Neurol 252:1–31

Witter MP, Groenewegen HJ (1986b) Connections of the parahippocampal cortex in the cat. IV. Subcortical and thalamic efferents. J Comp Neurol 251:51–77

Witter MP, Room P, Groenewegen HJ, Lohmann AHM (1986) Connection of the parahippocampal cortex in the cat. V. Intrinsic connections; comments on input/output connections with the hippocampus. J Comp Neurol 252:78–94

The Dopaminergic and Glutamatergic Systems in Schizophrenia *

J. KORNHUBER, P. RIEDERER, and H. BECKMANN [1]

The Dopaminergic System

It is now well established that there is a proliferation of central dopamine D_2 receptors in postmortem brains of schizophrenic patients (Seeman 1987; Toru et al. 1988). However, controversy persists as to whether these changes are due to chronic neuroleptic drug treatment, which itself enhances B_{max} values of D_2 receptors (Owen et al. 1980; Mackenzie and Zigmond 1985). To pursue this question we investigated the time course of D_2 receptors after withdrawal of chronic neuroleptic treatment in human postmortem brain tissue (Kornhuber et al. 1989b). Furthermore, we studied the relationship between binding parameters of D_2 receptors and both psychopathology and presence of tardive dyskinesia prior to death.

Putamen samples from the left side of the brain were obtained at autopsy from 27 control patients and 27 schizophrenic patients (diagnostic criteria of Feighner et al. 1972). Histopathological examination was performed on all brains to rule out other abnormalities. Postmortem delay was less than 10 h in all but two cases (14 and 20 h, controls). For each brain sample a saturation analysis was performed using [^{3}H]spiperone as a ligand. B_{max} and K_d values were determined from Scatchard plots using linear regression. The presence or absence of tardive dyskinesia prior to death was recorded from case notes. Furthermore, two groups of patients were selected by retrospective analysis of case reports: one group exhibiting more positive schizophrenic symptoms at the time of death, such as hallucinations and delusions (corresponding to ICD 295.3), and one group exhibiting more negative symptoms, such as loss of volition and flattening of affect (corresponding to ICD 295.6). Patients were classified as drug-free when there had been no neuroleptic treatment within the last 3 months prior to death ($n = 9$). Data from case notes are presented in Table 1.

B_{max} values of patients treated with neuroleptics within a short time period prior to death were elevated compared to controls (Table 1; Fig. 1) and decreased as a function of drug-free time. B_{max} values in off-drug schizophrenic patients did not differ from control values. The K_d values were greatly elevated

* J. K. has received a scholarship grant from the Deutsche Forschungsgemeinschaft.

[1] Psychiatrische Klinik der Universität Würzburg, Füchsleinstr. 15, 8700 Würzburg, FRG.

Neuropsychopharmacology
Edited by Bunney/Hippius/Laakmann/Schmauß

Table 1. Case data and B_{max} and K_d values for [^{3}H]spiperone binding

	Controls	Schizophrenics		
		All	On drug	Off drug
n	27	27	18	9
Men/women	7/20	9/18	7/11	2/7
Age (years)	72.8 ± 15.4	70.6 ± 8.4	69.3 ± 8.5	73.3 ± 7.9
B_{max} (pmol/g tissue)	19.3 ± 7.1	23.0 ± 11.1	26.8 ± 11.2 [a]	15.3 ± 5.8
K_d (nM)	0.125 ± 0.062	0.475 ± 0.671 [b]	0.640 ± 0.775 [b]	0.144 ± 0.036

[a] $p < 0.05$ compared to controls.
[b] $p < 0.01$ compared to controls.

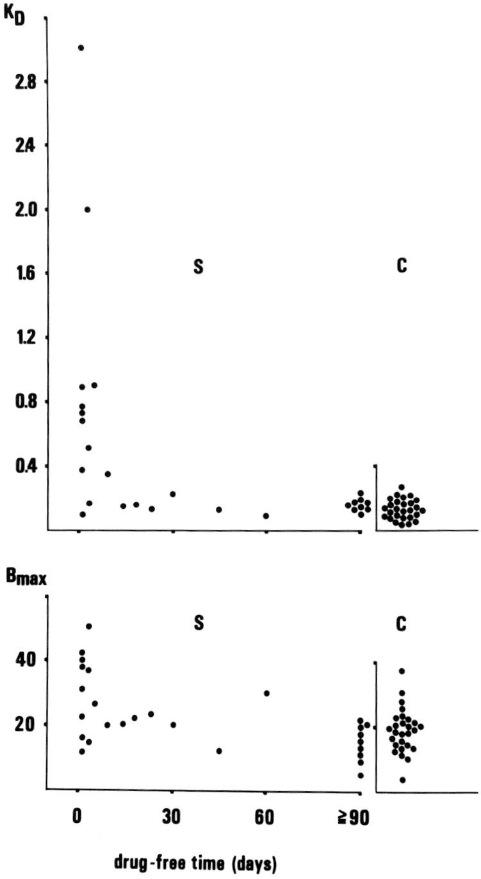

Fig. 1. Individual B_{max} (pmol/g tissue) and K_d (nM) values for [^{3}H]spiperone binding in postmortem putamen from schizophrenics (S) and controls (C). The neuroleptic drug-free time prior to death (day 0) is indicated

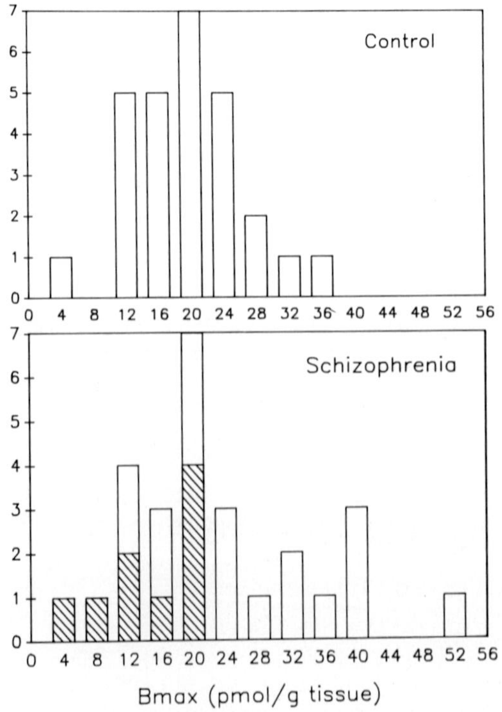

Fig. 2. Distribution of dopamine D_2 receptor densities in the putamen of control and schizophrenic patients. *Hatched areas*, patients who had been drug free for at least 3 months

in brain tissues from schizophrenics treated with neuroleptic drugs in the days before death and decreased to control values within 2 weeks after withdrawal of neuroleptic drugs (Fig. 1). It has been claimed that B_{max} values of D_2 receptors in schizophrenic patients have a bimodal distribution (Seeman et al. 1984). In the present study the D_2 receptor densities in the putamen of controls and schizophrenics did not differ significantly from a normal distribution (Kolmogoroff-Smirnoff test; Fig. 2). This may, however, be due to the smaller number of cases in the present investigation. B_{max} values showed a nonsignificant increase in patients with more positive schizophrenic symptoms (295.3: 29.15 ± 10.53 pmol/g tissue; 295.6: 20.93 ± 10.45 pmol/g tissue; $p > 0.05$). However, this seems to be related to the drug-free time interval, which was shorter in these patients (295.3: 4.2 ± 5.1 days; 295.6: 50.7 ± 41.3 days; $p < 0.05$). We found nearly identical dopamine receptor densities in putamen samples from schizophrenic patients who suffered from tardive dyskinesia prior to death compared to those who did not (22.97 ± 10.22 versus 22.69 ± 11.52 pmol/g tissue).

From our data we conclude that changes in B_{max} and K_d values in schizophrenics are entirely iatrogenic, and that there is no obvious relationship to abnormal movements or positive schizophrenic symptoms prior to death. These results are in agreement with the findings of Mackay et al. (1982) who found unchanged B_{max} values for [^{3}H]spiperone in the caudate nucleus and nucleus accumbens in drug-free schizophrenic patients. Furthermore, the results are in agreement with in vivo measurements with positron emission tomography using the selective D_2 antagonist [^{11}C]raclopride (Farde et al. 1987; but see also Wong et al. 1986).

The dopamine hypothesis of schizophrenia is based mainly on indirect pharmacological observations. However, the available biochemical data from schizophrenic patients may indicate that there is no absolute dopaminergic hyperactivity. The fundamental biochemical abnormality in schizophrenia may well be located therefore in another neurotransmitter system which is somehow linked to the dopaminergic neurones.

The Glutamatergic System

There are good reasons for a disturbance of the glutamatergic system in schizophrenia.

(1) Glutamate is one of the most excitatory substances present in the central nervous system, where it functions as a neurotransmitter. The distribution of glutamatergic neurones is quite extended (Fagg and Foster 1983; Iversen 1984; Storm-Mathisen and Ottersen 1988), and markers for glutamatergic neurotransmission are especially high in the entorhinal region, frontal cortex, and hippocampus (Fagg and Foster 1983). These are regions thought to be involved in the pathogenesis of schizophrenia. A dysfunction of the frontal and temporal regions in schizophrenia is likely and is observed in neuroradiological and neuropsychological studies (e.g., Shelton et al. 1988; Illowski et al. 1988). Recently, a disturbed structure of the second neuronal layer of the entorhinal region in schizophrenics has been found (Jakob and Beckmann 1986), suggesting a dysfunction of the glutamatergic perforant path, one of the main inputs to the hippocampus (e.g., Segal and Landis 1974) in schizophrenia.

(2) Phencyclidine (PCP) was first synthesized in 1926 in Germany (Kötz and Merkel 1926) and was later introduced by Parke Davis (United States) into clinical use as a general anesthetic agent. It is now widely abused as an euphoriant, frequently producing a schizophrenialike psychosis (Luby et al. 1959; Allen and Young 1978). The psychosis evoked by PCP is regarded as the best pharmacological model for schizophrenia available at the present time (Allen and Young 1978; Snyder 1980). The psychotomimetic action of PCP is not only faster and stronger than that of amphetamine, it also causes negative symptoms in addition to productive psychotic symptoms (Petersen and Stillman 1978). An existing schizophrenia may exacerbate under PCP (Luby et al. 1959). This psychotomimetic drug probably exerts its effects via the glutamatergic system. Some years ago it was reported (Anis et al. 1983) that PCP blocks responses of central neurones to *N*-methyl-D-aspartate (NMDA), which is a selective agonist of the NMDA receptor subtype of glutamate receptors, and it is becoming increasingly clear that PCP and related drugs (ketamine, MK-801) act as open channel blockers of the NMDA receptor coupled ion channel (Foster and Fagg 1987). Thus PCP behaves as a non

competitive glutamate antagonist. The possible usefulness of glutamate antagonists to produce an animal model for schizophrenia was first put forward by Kornhuber and Fischer (1982). The hypothesis that PCP produces its psychotomimetic effects via the NMDA receptor (Kornhuber et al. 1984; Lodge and Berry 1984; Kornhuber et al. 1986; Kim et al. 1986) has since then received much interest (e.g., Etienne and Baudry 1987).

(3) Direct investigations on the glutamatergic system in schizophrenia are rare. Cerebrospinal fluid glutamate levels were found to be reduced in schizophrenic patients by Kim et al. (1980) while other investigators did not find any differences (Perry 1982; Gattaz et al. 1982, Korpi et al. 1987). [^{3}H]MK-801 binding sites are increased in the putamen of schizophrenic postmortem brains (Kornhuber et al. 1989a). Furthermore, increases in [^{3}H]kainic acid binding sites in cortical regions have been found in the medial frontal cortex and eye movement area (Nishikawa et al. 1983; Toru et al. 1988) as well as in the orbital frontal cortex (Deakin et al. 1988). The functional meaning of these altered [^{3}H]kainic acid binding sites is not clear at present. However, Toru et al. (1988) have measured simultaneously the glutamate levels in brain tissue and found a negative correlation between glutamate levels in various subcortical regions and [^{3}H]kainic acid binding in the medial prefrontal cortex. This might indicate that enhanced [^{3}H]kainic acid binding sites are due to a denervation supersensitivity, thus supporting a glutamatergic hypofunction in schizophrenia.

The Glutamatergic–Dopaminergic Link

The glutamatergic and dopaminergic systems are tightly linked to each other, thus possibly explaining the therapeutic action of neuroleptic drugs (Kim et al. 1980; Kornhuber et al. 1984). Dopamine functionally antagonizes the glutamatergic system. For instance, activation of the dopaminergic system reduces glutamate release from corticostriatal terminals while neuroleptic drugs reconstitute the glutamate release (for review see Kornhuber and Kornhuber 1986). Direct and indirect glutamate antagonists such as DL-2-amino-5-phosphonovaleric acid, PCP, and MK-801 produce a stereotyped behavior in rats (Schmidt 1986; Koek et al. 1987) which is antagonized by haloperidol or clozapine (Schmidt 1986). On the other hand, MK-801 reverses the catalepsy induced by haloperidol (Schmidt and Bubser 1988). Furthermore, there is a negative correlation between dopamine metabolites and glutamate in human cerebrospinal fluid (Alfredsson et al. 1988).

Taken together, the glutamate hypothesis unifies the structural changes found in the cerebral cortex in schizophrenia, the psychotomimetic effects of PCP, and the therapeutic activity of dopamine antagonists in the treatment of schizophrenia. The glutamate hypothesis might provide a new pharmacological approach in the therapy of schizophrenia.

References

Alfredsson G, Wiesel FA, Tylec A (1988) Relationship between glutamate and monoamine metabolites in cerebrospinal fluid and serum in healthy volunteers. Biol Psychiatry 23:689–697

Allen RM, Young SJ (1978) Phencyclidine-induced psychosis. Am J Psychiatry 135:1081–1084

Anis NA, Berry SC, Burton NR, Lodge D (1983) The dissociative anaesthetics, ketamine and phencyclidine selectively reduce excitation of central mammalian neurons by *N*-methyl-aspartate. Br J Pharmacol 79:565–575

Deakin JFW, Simpson MDC, Gilchrist AC, Skan WJ, Slater P (1988) Cortical glutamate dysfunction in schizophrenia. Psychopharmacology 96S:108

Etienne P, Baudry M (1987) Calcium dependent aspects of synaptic plasticity, excitatory amino acid neurotransmission, brain aging and schizophrenia: a unifying hypothesis. Neurobiol Aging 8:362–366

Fagg GE, Foster AC (1983) Amino acid neurotransmitters and their pathways in the mammalian central nervous system. Neuroscience 9:701–719

Farde L, Wiesel FA, Hall H, Halldin C, Stone-Elander S, Sedvall G (1987) No D2 receptor increase in PET study of schizophrenia. Arch Gen Psychiatry 44:671–672

Feighner JP, Robins E, Guze SB, Woodruff RA, Winokur G, Munoz R (1972) Diagnostic criteria for use in psychiatric research. Arch Gen Psychiatry 26:57–63

Foster AC, Fagg GE (1987) Taking apart NMDA receptors. Nature 329:395–396

Gattaz WF, Gattaz D, Beckmann H (1982) Glutamate in schizophrenics and healthy controls. Arch Psychiatr Nervenkr 231:221–225

Illowski BP, Juliano DM, Bigelow LB, Weinberger DR (1988) Stability of CT scan findings in schizophrenia: results of an 8 year follow-up study. J Neurol Neurosurg Psychiatry 51:209–213

Iversen LL (1984) Amino acids and peptides: fast and slow chemical signals in the nervous system? Proc R Soc Lond [Biol] 221:245–260

Jakob H, Beckmann H (1986) Prenatal developmental disturbances in the limbic allocortex in schizophrenics. J Neural Trans 65:154–161

Kim JS, Kornhuber HH, Schmid-Burgk W, Holzmüller B (1980) Low cerebrospinal fluid glutamate in schizophrenic patients and a new hypothesis on schizophrenia. Neurosci Lett 20:379–382

Kim JS, Kornhuber HH, Kornhuber J, Kornhuber ME (1986) Glutamic acid and the dopamine hypothesis of schizophrenia. In: Chagass C, Josiassen RC, Bridger WH, Weiss HJ, Stoff D, Simpson GS (eds) Biological psychiatry 1985. Elsevier, Amsterdam, pp 1109–1111

Koek W, Woods JH, Ornstein P (1987) A simple and rapid method for assessing similarities among directly observable behavioral effects of drugs: PCP-like effects of 2-amino-5-phosphonovalerate in rats. Psychopharmacology 91:297–304

Kornhuber HH, Kornhuber J, Kim JS, Kornhuber ME (1984) Zur biochemischen Theorie der Schizophrenie. Nervenarzt 55:602–606

Kornhuber J, Fischer EG (1982) Glutamic acid diethyl ester induces catalepsy in rats. A new model for schizophrenia? Neurosci Lett 34:325–329

Kornhuber J, Kornhuber ME (1986) Presynaptic dopaminergic modulation of cortical input to the striatum. Life Sci 39:669–674

Kornhuber J, Mack-Burkhardt F, Riederer P, Hebenstreit GF, Reynolds GP, Andrews HB, Beckmann H (1989a) [^{3}H]MK-801 binding sites in postmortem brain regions of schizophrenic patients. J Neural Transm 77:231–236

Kornhuber J, Riederer P, Reynolds GP, Beckmann H, Jellinger K, Gabriel E (1989b) ^{3}H-Spiperone binding sites in post-mortem brains from schizophrenic patients: relationship to neuroleptic drug treatment, abnormal movements, and positive symptoms. J Neural Transm 75:1–10

Kornhuber ME, Kornhuber J, Zettlmeißl H, Kornhuber HH (1986) Phencyclidin und das glutamaterge System. In: Keup W (ed) Biologische Psychiatrie, Forschungsergebnisse. Springer, Berlin Heidelberg New York, pp 176–180

Korpi ER, Kleinman JE, Goodman SI, Wyatt J (1987) Neurotransmitter amino acids in post-mortem brains of chronic schizophrenic patients. Psychiatry Res 22:291–301

Kötz A, Merkel P (1926) Zur Kenntnis hydroaromatischer Alkamine. J Prakt Chem 113:49–79

Lodge D, Berry SC (1984) Psychotomimetic effects of sigma opiates may be mediated by block of central excitatory synapses utilizing receptors for aspartate-like amino acids. In: Bandler R (ed) Modulation of sensorimotor activity during alterations in behavioural states. Liss, New York, pp 503–518

Luby ED, Cohen BD, Rosenbaum G, Gottlieb JS, Kelley R (1959) Study of a new schizophrenomimetic drug – Sernyl. Arch Neurol Psychiatry 81:363–369

Mackay AVP, Iversen LL, Rossor M, Spokes E, Bird E, Arregui A, Creese I, Snyder SH (1982) Increased brain dopamine and dopamine receptors in schizophrenia. Arch Gen Psychiatry 39:991–997

Mackenzie RG, Zigmond MJ (1985) Chronic neuroleptic treatment increases D-2 but not D-1 receptors in rat striatum. Eur J Pharmacol 113:159–165

Nishikawa T, Takashima M, Toru N (1983) Increased ^{3}H-kainic acid binding in the prefrontal cortex in schizophrenia. Neurosci Lett 40:245–250

Owen F, Cross AJ, Waddington JL, Poulter M, Gamble SJ, Crow TJ (1980) Dopamine-mediated behaviour and 3H-spiperone binding to striatal membranes in rats after nine months haloperidol administration. Life Sci 26:55–59

Perry TL (1982) Normal cerebrospinal fluid and brain glutamate levels in schizophrenia do not support the hypothesis of glutamatergic neuronal dysfunction. Neurosci Lett 28:81–85

Petersen RC, Stillman RC (1978) Phencyclidine: an overview, In: Petersen RC, Stillman RC (eds) NIDA Research Monograph, vol 21, pp 1–17

Schmidt WJ (1986) Intrastriatal injection of DL-2-amino-5-phosphonovaleric acid (AP-5) induces sniffing stereotypy that is antagonized by haloperidol and clozapine. Psychopharmacology 90:123–130

Schmidt WJ, Bubser M (1988) Anti-cataleptic effects of the *N*-methyl-aspartate antagonist MK-801. Pharmacol Biochem Behav 32:621–623

Seeman P (1987) Dopamine receptors and the dopamine hypothesis of schizophrenia. Synapse 1:133–152

Seeman P, Ulpian C, Bergeron C, Riederer P, Jellinger K, Gabriel E, Reynolds GP, Tourtellotte WW (1984) Bimodal distribution of dopamine receptor densities in brains of schizophrenics. Science 225:728–731

Segal M, Landis S (1974) Afferents to the hippocampus of the rat studied with the method of retrograde transport of horseradish peroxidase. Brain Res 78:1–15

Shelton RC, Karson CN, Doran AR, Pickar D, Bigelow LB, Weinberger DR (1988) Cerebral structural pathology in schizophrenia: evidence for a selective prefrontal cortical defect. Am J Psychiatry 145:154–163

Snyder SH (1980) Phencyclidine. Nature 285:355–356

Storm-Mathisen J, Ottersen OP (1988) Localization of excitatory amino acid transmitter. In: Lodge D (ed) Excitatory amino acids in health and disease. Wiley, Chichester, pp 107–141

Toru M, Watanabe S, Shibuya H, Nishikawa T, Noda K, Mitsushio H, Ichikawa H, Kurumaji A, Takashima M, Mataga N, Ogawa A (1988) Neurotransmitters, receptors and neuropeptides in post-mortem brains of chronic schizophrenic patients. Acta Psychiatr Scand 78:121–137

Wong DF, Wagner HN, Tune LE, Dannals RF, Pearlson GD, Links JM, Tamminga CA, Broussolle EP, Ravert HT, Wilson AA, Toung JKT, Malat J, Williams JA, O'Tuama LA, Snyder SH, Kuhar MJ, Gjedde A (1986) Positron emission tomography reveals elevated D2 dopamine receptors in drug-naive schizophrenics. Science 234:1558–1563

17 AIDS

Peptide Intervention in Neuronal Death Caused by the HIV External Envelope Protein: Clinical Implications

D. E. BRENNEMAN [1]

Introduction

An early manifestation of acquired immunodeficiency syndrome (AIDS) infection is the occurrence of neuropsychiatric and neurological impairment (Snider et al. 1983; Ultmann et al. 1985; Navia and Price 1987). Neuropathological changes include infiltrates of macrophages and multinucleated cells and often white matter pallor and vacuolar myelopathy (Nielsen et al. 1984; Navia et al. 1986). In addition, neuronal cell death has been observed in the globus pallidus and substantia nigra (Rosenblum et al. 1988). However, very few brain cells have demonstrable human immunodeficiency virus (HIV) infectivity (Wiley et al. 1986). Furthermore, even in advanced stages of the disease, not all patients have evidence of secondary infections. The fundamental question remains: what is the mechanism of the CNS deficits when there is so little direct HIV infection? We have examined the possibility that the envelope protein, which is shed by HIV, plays a role in mediating the losses of neuronal function and survival.

HIV utilizes the CD4 receptor to gain entry into cells. This interaction is mediated by an interaction of the external envelope protein (gp120) with the CD4 receptor (Dalgleish et al. 1984; Klatzman et al. 1985). Invasion of the CNS is thought to occur via infected macrophages, which probably act as a reservoir for the virions (Gartner et al. 1986; Koenig et al. 1986).

The working model of AIDS-related neuronal deficits is based on two ideas: (a) the envelope protein, which is shed by virus-infected cells (Schneider et al. 1986; Gelderblom et al. 1987), causes neuronal death or functional impairment because of an interruption of glia-neuron interactions that are critical for neuronal function and survival; and (b) this interference is directed either at the vasoactive intestinal peptide (VIP), a substance of demonstrated action on neuronal survival in vitro (Brenneman et al. 1985, 1987; Brenneman and Eiden 1986; Brenneman and Foster 1987) or an endogenous growth factor stimulated by VIP. This hypothesis has a substantial basis in the observations of Pert and coworkers (1988) that a portion of the envelope protein (the peptide T region; Pert et al. 1986) has sequence similarity to the 7–

[1] Laboratory of Developmental Neurobiology, National Institute of Child Health and Human Development, National Institutes of Health, Bethesda, MD 20892, USA.

Neuropsychopharmacology
Edited by Bunney/Hippius/Laakmann/Schmauß

11 sequence of VIP (Ruff et al. 1987a). This is relevant in that peptide T has been shown to inhibit gp120 binding to human T cells and to inhibit viral infectivity under specified experimental conditions (Pert et al. 1986). These data support the conclusion that the VIP-like portion of the envelope protein is of importance in viral attachment to CD4-positive cells. Previous studies of the mechanism of action of VIP (Brenneman et al. 1987) suggest that interruption of neuron-glia communication is one possible way in which gp120 could cause neuronal death.

gp120-Induced Death in Neuronal Cell Culture

Hippocampal Assay System

Dissociated cell cultures from murine hippocampus (Forsythe and Westbrook 1988) were utilized for experiments in evaluating the potential toxic properties of gp120. This culture preparation was chosen for several reasons. The hippocampus has been shown to be rich in receptors relevant to gp120 and the peptides to be examined: the VIP receptor (Taylor and Pert 1979) and the T4 antigen (Pert et al. 1986; Hill et al. 1987). This receptor distribution combined with the clinical observation of early memory loss in AIDS supported the

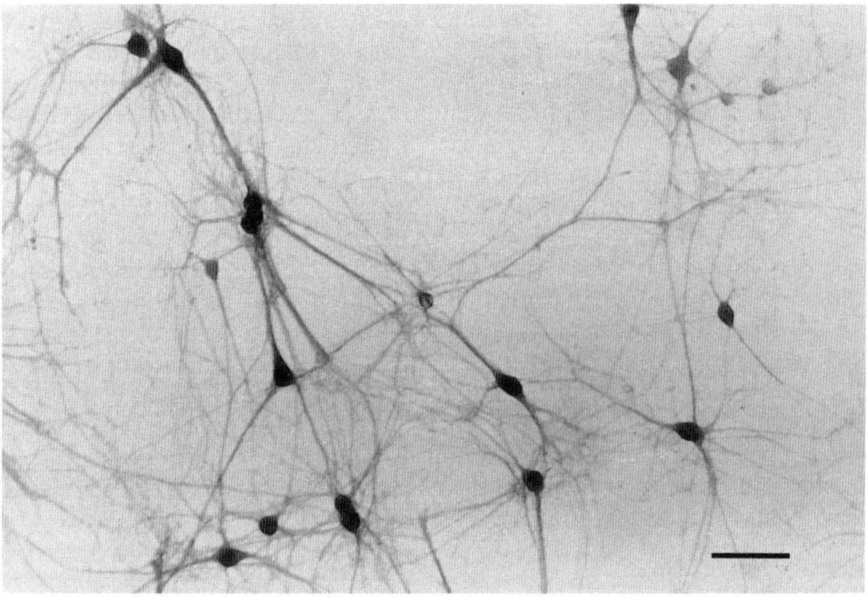

Fig. 1. Dissociated hippocampal cultures stained immunocytochemically with antiserum to neuron specific enolase. A control culture at the beginning of the test period (7 days in vitro) is shown. The number of somal bodies in 50 mm^2 was counted for the gp120/neuron killing assay. *Calibration bar*, 100 μm

decision to examine this brain region. Previous studies have indicated that mice do not become infected with HIV. However, it is not clear whether this is due to the inability of the envelope protein to interact with the mouse homologue of T4 or to a more distal mechanism related to viral entry or replication. The murine hippocampal test system has provided a means of testing for a receptor-mediated, pathological interaction between these brain cells and gp120, apart from considerations of infectivity.

The hippocampal cell culture model is a complex system composed of several recognized cell types. Neurons grow on top of a layer of nonneuronal cells comprised predominately of astroglia. Neurons appear phase bright with phase contrast optics, and these cells are routinely identified with antiserum to neuron-specific enolase (Schmechel et al. 1978). A typical control culture at the beginning of a treatment period is shown in Fig. 1. The neurons exhibit a heterogenous morphology with no mitosis. Neurons are synaptically linked, and the effects of the envelope protein are studied 1 week after plating, when the neurons have firmly attached to the astrocyte feeder layer.

Neuronal Loss After gp120

A variety of purified gp120 preparations were found to produce neuronal cell death in developing hippocampal cultures derived from the murine fetus (Fig. 2). The gp120 purified from three different HIV isolates had similar effects: neuronal killing at extraordinarily low concentrations. These studies also revealed that the neuronal cell loss was attenuated with amounts of gp120 greater than 10 p*M*. In subsequent time course studies, the neuronal deficits produced by the IIIB isolate of gp120 exhibited a slow, progressive effect to an observed maximal loss of 51% of control after 3 weeks of treatment. These data suggest that there may be neuronal specificity to these effects, since all neurons did not die during the chronic exposure to gp120.

In addition, a recombinant gp120 produced from encoding sequences from the lymphadenopathy-associated virus (LAV) isolate was also found to decrease neuronal survival when tested under the same experimental conditions. Identically prepared medium from parent cells infected with vaccinia virus without the gp120 construct had no detectable effect on neuronal survival when tested over the same range of concentrations (data not shown). A gp160 from recombinant baculovirus expressed in an insect cell (Rusche et al. 1987) was also tested and found to have no detectable effect on neuronal survival (Fig. 2). The reason for the absence of neuron-depleting activity from the insect-expressed protein is not clear, but altered tertiary structure due to differences in glycosylation and/or the presence of the gp41 sequence may be involved.

Receptor Mediation of gp120-Induced Death

To determine whether the neuronal death associated with gp120 is due to an interaction with the mouse homologue of CD4, L3T4 (Tourvieille et al. 1986),

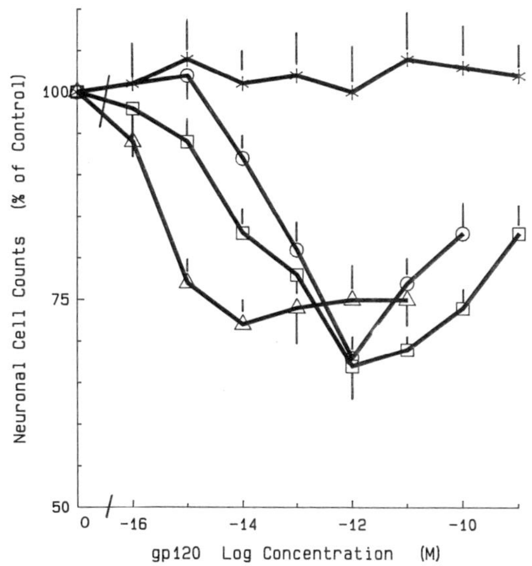

Fig. 2. HIV envelope protein produces neuronal cell death in dissociated hippocampal cultures from fetal mice. Recombinant gp120 (*triangles*) from the LAV-encoding sequences was compared to native gp120 purified (Robey et al. 1986) from two natural isolates, IIIB (*circles*) and RFII (*squares*). A recombinant gp160 from the IIIB encoding sequences was expressed in insect cells by recombinant baculovirus (*asterisks*). Significant decreases from control were observed at 0.01 p*M* for all gp120 preparations. No differences from controls were observed in cultures treated with the insect gp160 preparation. Control cultures had neuron counts that ranged from 750 to 1000 cells with standard errors that were less than 4% of the mean. Before treating with gp120, the cultures were given a complete change of medium. The duration of treatment was 5 days. (From Brenneman et al. 1988b)

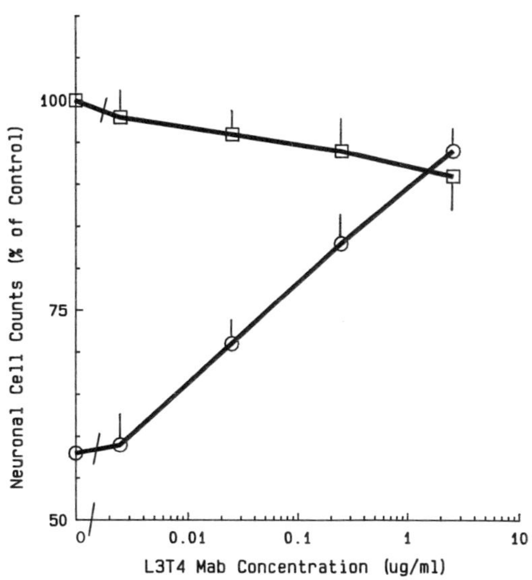

Fig. 3. A monoclonal antibody (GK1.5) against murine CD4 reduced gp120-induced neuronal death in dissociated hippocampal cultures. A comparison was made between cultures treated with antibody alone (*squares*) and antibody plus 1 p*M* gp120 (IIIB isolate; circles). In comparison to neuronal cell counts of cultures treated with gp120 alone, significant increases ($p < 0.01$) were observed with 0.02–2.5 µg/ml GK1.5. (From Brenneman et al. 1988b)

the effects of monoclonal antibodies directed against L3T4 were tested in gp120-treated cultures. The concentration effect curve for one of these antibodies (GK1.5) is shown in Fig. 3. This rat IgG2b produced a concentration-dependent protection against the neuronal death caused by gp120 (IIIB strain). Thus, a monoclonal antibody that was shown previously to inhibit the functional activity of mouse T cells (Dialynas et al. 1983) also effectively blocked the cell-killing action of gp120 in hippocampal neurons. Another monoclonal antibody against L3T4 (RL.172) was also found to prevent gp120-induced neuronal death, whereas control monoclonal antibodies from the same antibody class did not prevent neuronal death from gp120. These results support the conclusion that the neuronal death that occurs with gp120 treatment is the result of an interaction with the cell surface antigen L3T4 or a receptor with shared epitopes with L3T4.

Peptide Intervention in gp120-Induced Death

Vasoactive Intestinal Peptide

VIP and its receptors are present in brain and immune cells (Rostene 1984; O'Dorisio et al. 1980, 1981). This peptide was investigated for its ability to prevent gp120-induced death. The rationale for this study was: (a) the sequence similarity between the peptide T portion of the envelope protein and the 7–11 sequence of VIP, suggesting a possible competitive receptor-mediated mechanism; and (b) the demonstrated neurotrophic properties of VIP (Brenneman et al. 1985; Brenneman and Eiden 1986), with interference of this peptide perhaps

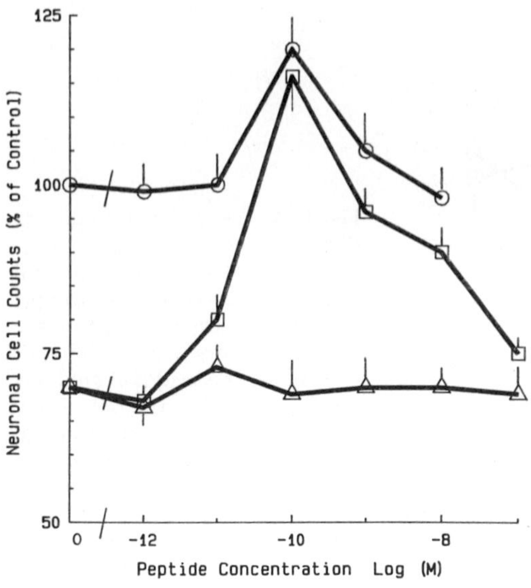

Fig. 4. VIP prevented gp120-induced neuronal cell death in hippocampal cultures. One-week-old cultures were treated for 5 days with VIP alone (*circles*), VIP plus 1 p*M* gp120 (*squares*), or secretin plus gp120 (*triangles*). Compared to cultures treated with gp120 alone, significant increases ($p < 0.02$) in the number of neurons were observed with the addition of 0.1–10 n*M* VIP plus gp120. The addition of 0.1 n*M* VIP plus gp120 resulted in neuronal cell counts that were not significantly different from cultures treated with 0.1 n*M* VIP alone. (From Brenneman et al. 1988b)

resulting in neuronal death. As shown in Fig. 4, the addition of low amounts (0.1 n*M*) of VIP prevented gp120-induced neuronal death whereas higher concentrations were not as effective. Secretin, a peptide of significant sequence homology to VIP, had no effect on neuronal death after gp120 treatment.

The mechanism of the protective action of VIP on gp120-induced neuronal death is not apparent from these initial studies. Previous work from our group has indicated that VIP exerts its neurotrophic effects indirectly through an interaction with nonneuronal cells (Brenneman et al. 1987). On the cellular level, the gp120 may be exerting its neuron-depleting action by interfering with the VIP-mediated communication between neurons and astroglia. VIP receptors have been demonstrated on cortical astrocytes in cell culture (Magistretti et al. 1983). Several lines of evidence support the conclusion that VIP and gp120 act at the same receptor: (a) antibodies to CD4 receptor inhibit VIP- and VIP fragment-stimulated chemotaxis of human monocytes (Sacerdote et al. 1987); (b) the CD4 receptor and one type of VIP receptor exhibit similar distribution patterns in brain sections (Pert et al. 1986; Hill et al. 1987); (c) there is sequence similarity between VIP and gp120, as discussed above; (d) VIP (7–11) potently displaces [^{3}H]peptide T binding (Smith et al. 1988). However, a direct toxic action of gp120 on neurons cannot be excluded from the present studies. The envelope protein may act to interfere with other growth factors that are stimulated by VIP. Regardless of the mechanism, these studies suggest that the VIP protection of gp120-induced death may give important clues as to the cause and the prevention of AIDS-related neuropathology.

Peptide T

Peptide T, an octapeptide found in the external envelope protein of the AIDS-associated retrovirus isolate of HIV, was investigated for its action in preventing neuronal death associated with gp120. Hypothesizing that attachment sequences are conserved among viruses (Pert et al. 1986), peptide T was deduced from computer-assisted comparisons of all known amino acid sequences of HIV with other viral envelope proteins. Previous reports indicated that peptide T inhibited gp120 binding to human T cells and inhibited human T cell infectivity from HIV (Pert et al. 1986). In addition, peptide T binding is potently displaced by gp120 (Ruff et al. 1987a). Incubation of the hippocampal cultures with the free acid or the amide of D-Ala-peptide T prevented gp120-mediated neuronal death (Fig. 5). Both peptide drugs had similar dose-response relationships at low concentrations; but with higher amounts the free acid of peptide T, like VIP, exhibited an attenuation of the survival-enhancing activity whereas the amide of peptide T remained active up to 0.1 μ*M*. The core pentapeptide sequence (TTNYT) also prevented gp120-induced death at concentrations similar to that of the octapeptide drug. Structure activity studies revealed that if the L-tyrosine, which occurs in the fourth position of all 20 HIV isolates, is substituted by D-tyrosine, the peptide is inactive. These

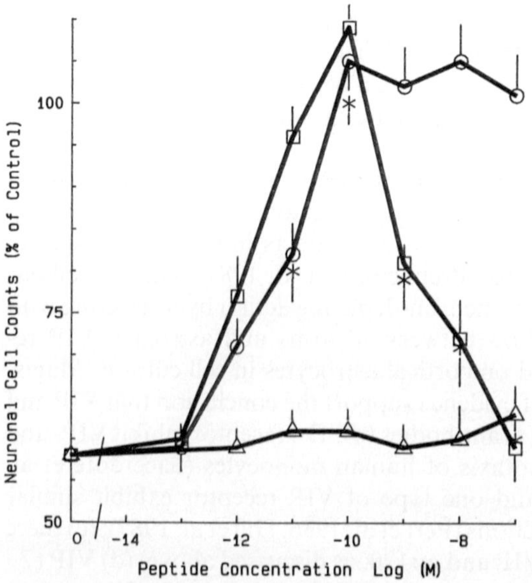

Fig. 5. Peptide T derivative prevents gp120-induced neuronal death in hippocampal cultures. A comparison was made of D-Ala-peptide T amide (*circles*), D-Ala-peptide T (*squares*), TTNYT (*asterisks*) and TTNdYT, containing a D-isomer of tyrosine (*triangles*). (From Brenneman et al. 1988a)

studies indicate that the various forms of peptide T have a significant and potent action in preventing neuronal death caused by gp120.

Summary

What relationship does the gp120/neuron killing assay have to AIDS neuropathology? What is the clinical significance of the observations that VIP and peptide T prevent the lethal action of gp120 in developing hippocampal cultures? Obtaining the definitive answers to these questions will require examining the action of gp120 and the peptide drugs in animal and human studies. Nevertheless, the observations of the killing effects of gp120 and the protection produced by peptide drugs provide strong impetus to continue testing the basic hypotheses proposed in this study. A substance (gp120) that is capable of killing neurons in picomolar amounts, and that is known to be released from infected cells must be given consideration as a candidate in the etiology of neurological and neuropsychiatric impairments in AIDS. Importantly, in recent open phase I trials of peptide T, AIDS patients showed significant improvement (Bridge et al. 1988; Wetterberg et al. 1987). Although these early results are promising, only expanded human trials of peptide T and related drugs will resolve the question of the relevancy of the gp120/neuron killing assay and the therapeutic value of the peptide drugs suggested by the in vitro studies.

References

Brenneman DE, Eiden LE (1986) Vasoactive intestinal peptide and electrical activity influence neuronal survival. Proc Natl Acad Sci USA 83:1159–1162

Brenneman DE, Foster (1987) Structural specificity of peptides that influence neuronal survival during development. Peptides 8:687–694

Brenneman DE, Eiden LE, Siegel RE (1985) Neurotrophic action of VIP on spinal cord cultures. Peptides 6 (Suppl):35–39

Brenneman DE, Neale EA, Foster GA, d'Atremont SW, Westbrook GL (1987) Nonneuronal cells mediate neurotrophic action of vasoactive intestinal peptide. J Cell Biol 104:1603–1610

Brenneman DE, Buzy JM, Ruff MR, Pert CB (1988a) Peptide T prevents gp120-induced neuronal cell death in vitro: relevance to AIDS dementia. Drug Dev Res 15:361–369

Brenneman DE, Westbrook GL, Fitzgerald SP, Ennist DL, Elkins KL, Ruff MR, Pert CB (1988b) Neuronal cell killing by the envelope protein of HIV and its prevention by vasoactive intestinal peptide. Nature 335:639–642

Bridge TP, Heseltine P, Parker ES, Eaton E, Baron D, Johnson W, Goodwin FK (1988) Phase I testing of peptide T in AIDS patients and controls. IV International Conference on AIDS 1:245

Dalgleish AG, Beverley PCL, Clapham PR, Crawford DH, Greaves MF, Weiss RA (1984) The CD4 (T4) antigen is an essential component of the receptor for the AIDS retrovirus. Nature 312:763–766

Dialynas DP, Wilde DB, Marrack P, Pierres A, Wall KA, Havran W, Otten G, Loken MR, Pierres M, Kappler J, Fitch FW (1983) Characterization of the murine antigenic determinant, designated L3T4a, recognized by monoclonal antibody GK1.5: expression of L3T4a by functional T cell clone appears to correlate primarily with class II MHC antigen-reactivity. Immunol Rev 74:29–56

Forsythe ID, Westbrook GL (1988) Slow excitatory postsynaptic currents mediated by *N*-methyl-D-aspartate receptors on cultured mouse central neurons. J Physiol (Lond) 396:515–533

Gartner S, Markovits P, Markovitz DM, Kaplan MH, Gallo RC, Popovic M (1986) The role of mononuclear phagocytes in HTLV-III/LAV infection. Science 233:215–219

Gelderblom HR, Hausmann E, Ozel M, Pauli G, Koch MA (1987) Fine structure of human immunodeficiency virus (HIV) and immunolocalization of structural proteins. Virology 156:171–176

Hill JM, Farrar WL, Pert CB (1987) Autoradiographic localization of T4 antigen, the HIV receptor, in human brain. Int J Neurosci 32:687–693

Klatzman D, Champagne E, Chamaret S, Gruest J, Guetard D, Hercend T, Gluckman JC, Montagnier L (1985) T-lymphocyte T4 molecule behaves as the receptor for human retrovirus LAV. Nature 312:767–768

Koenig S, Gendelman HE, Orenstein JM, Dal Canto MC, Pezeshkpour GH, Yungbluth M, Janotta F, Aksamit A, Martin MA, Fauci AS (1986) Detection of AIDS virus in macrophages in brain tissue from AIDS patients with encephalopathy. Science 233:1089–1093

Magistretti PJ, Manthorpe M, Bloom FE, Varon S (1983) Functional receptors for vasoactive intestinal peptide in cultured astroglia from neonatal rat brain. Regul Pept 6:71–80

Navia BA, Price RW (1987) The acquired immunodeficiency syndrome dementia complex as the presenting and sole manifestation of human immunodeficiency virus infection. Arch Neurol 44:65–69

Navia BA, Cho ES, Petito CK, Price RW (1986) The AIDS dementia complex II. Neuropathology. Ann Neurol 19:525–535

Nielsen SL, Petito CK, Urmacher CD, Posner JB (1984) Subacute encephalitis in acquired immune deficiency syndrome: a postmortem study. Am J Clin Pathol 82:678–682

O'Dorisio MS, O'Dorisio TM, Cataland S, Balcerzak SP (1980) Vasoactive intestinal polypeptide as a biochemical marker for polymorphonuclear leukocytes. J Lab Clin Med 96:666–672

O'Dorisio MS, Hermina ND, O'Dorisio TM, Balcerzak SP (1981) Vasoactive intestinal polypeptide modulation of lymphocyte adenylate cyclase. J Immunol 127:2551–2554
Pert CB, Hill JM, Ruff MR, Berman RM, Robey WG, Arthur LO, Ruscetti FW, Farrar WL (1986) Octapeptides deduced from the neuropeptide receptor-like pattern of antigen T4 in brain potently inhibit human immunodeficiency virus receptor binding and T-cell infectivity. Proc Natl Acad Sci USA 83:9254–9258
Pert CB, Smith CC, Ruff MR, Hill JM (1988) AIDS and its dementia as a neuropeptide disorder: role of VIP receptor blockade by human immunodeficiency virus envelope. Ann Neurol 23 (Suppl):S71–S73
Robey WG, Arthur LO, Matthews TJ, Langlois A, Copeland TD, Lerche NW, Oroszlan S, Bolognesi DP, Gilden RV, Fischinger PJ (1986) Prospect for prevention of human immunodeficiency virus infection: purified 120-kDa envelope glycoprotein induces neutralizing antibody. Proc Natl Acad Sci USA 83:7023–7027
Rosenblum M, Brew B, Cardle K, Schect A, Price R (1988) Pallidoingral degeneration in AIDS: implications for HIV-related neuronal damage. IV International Conference on AIDS, Stockholm, June 12–16, 1988. 1:204
Rostene WH (1984) Neurobiological and neuroendocrine functions of the vasoactive intestinal peptide (VIP). Prog Neurobiol 22:103–129
Ruff MR, Hallberg PL, Hill JM, Pert CB (1987a) Peptide T (4–8) is core HIV envelope protein sequence required for CD4 receptor attachment. Lancet 2(26):751
Ruff MR, Martin BM, Ginns EI, Farrar WL, Pert CB (1987b) CD4 receptor binding peptides that block HIV infectivity cause human monocyte chemotaxis. Relationship to vasoactive intestinal peptide. FEBS Lett 211:17–22
Rusche JR, Lynn DL, Robert-Guroff M, Langlios AJ, Lyerly HK, Carson H, Krohn K, Ranki A, Gallo R, Bolognesi DP, Putney SD, Matthews TJ (1987) Humoral immune response to the entire human immunodeficiency virus envelope glycoprotein made in insect cells. Proc Natl Acad Sci USA 84:6924–6928
Sacerdote P, Ruff MR, Pert CB (1987) Vasoactive intestinal peptide (1–12): a ligand for the CD4 (T4)/human immunodeficiency virus receptor. J Neurosci Res 18:102–107
Schmechel D, Marangos PJ, Zis AP, Brightman M, Goodwin FK (1978) Brain enolases as specific markers of neuronal and glial cells. Science 199:313–315
Schneider J, Kaaden O, Copeland TD, Oroszlan S, Hunsmann G (1986) Shedding and interspecies type sero-reactivity of the envelope glycopolypeptide gp120 of the human immunodeficiency virus. J Gen Virol 67:2533–2538
Smith CC, Williams P, Hallberg P, Sternberg EM, Pert CB, Ruff MR (1988) Tritiated D-Ala peptide T binding to the CD4 receptor in rat hippocampus and human T cell line. Drug Dev Res 15:371–379
Snider WD, Simpson DM, Nielsen S, Gold J, Metroka CE, Posner JB (1983) Neurological complications of acquired immune deficiency syndrome: analysis of 50 patients. Ann Neurol 14:403–418
Taylor DP, Pert CB (1979) Vasoactive intestinal polypeptide: specific binding to rat brain membranes. Proc Natl Acad Sci USA 76:660–664
Tourvieille B, Gorman SD, Field EH, Hunkapiller T, Parnes JR (1986) Isolation and sequence of L3T4 complementary DNA clones: expression of T cells and brain. Science 234:610–614
Ultmann MH, Belman AL, Ruff HA, Novick BB, Cone-Wesson B, Cohen HJ, Rubinstein A (1985) Developmental abnormalities in infants and children with acquired immune deficiency syndrome and AIDS-related complex. Dev Med Child Neural 27:563–571
Wetterberg L, Alexius B, Saaf J, Sonnerborg A, Britton S, Pert CB (1987) Peptide T in treatment of AIDS. Lancet 1(17):159
Wiley CA, Schrier RD, Nelson JA, Lampert PW, Oldstone BA (1986) Cellular localization of human immunodeficiency virus infection within the brains of acquired immune deficiency syndrome patients. Proc Natl Acad Sci USA 83:7089–7093

AIDS as a Neuropeptide Disorder: Does HIV Bind to a VIP Receptor?

J. M. Hill [1], A. I. Kook, and A. Harris [2]

Introduction

By mimicking the molecular structure of the binding site of a neurotransmitter or other endogenous ligand, viruses are known to bind to the receptor of that neurotransmitter and, by subsequent steps, infect the receptor-bearing cells. Toxic effects may also occur to cells when shed viral proteins, although not infectious, bind to a receptor site and block the functions of the endogenous ligand (see recent review by Lentz 1988).

Human immunodeficiency virus (HIV) infection is frequently characterized by central nervous system (CNS) complications including behavioral, cognitive, and motor deficits apparently due to the presence of HIV in the brain (Navia et al. 1986). However, these global and sometimes severe impairments occur despite the low numbers of HIV particles and infected cells found in the brain and the observation that the infected cells are primarily of macrophage origin (Price et al. 1988). One explanation for this apparent anomaly is that HIV and shed viral glypoproteins bind throughout the brain to the receptor of some neuroactive substance, and although the receptor-bearing cells may not have the necessary machinery to permit infection, the occupation of the receptor site can induce a variety of biological effects.

Peptide T, the proposed binding site of HIV (Pert et al. 1986) contains a pentapeptide sequence which is homologous with TDNYT, amino acids 7–11 of the vasoactive intestinal peptide (VIP). VIP is a neuropeptide with a multitude of functions in the CNS, immune system, and gut (Said and Mutt 1970; Fahrenkrug and Emson 1982; Rostène 1984). This paper outlines several kinds of evidence which support the idea that HIV binds to a receptor for VIP or some VIP-like peptide. VIP has several receptor subtypes, and perhaps one of these is CD4, the surface protein identified as the HIV receptor (Dalgleish et al. 1985).

CD4 in Brain

Molecular Evidence. The T4-lymphocytes are targeted by HIV because the viral external envelope protein gp 120 binds to CD4 (T4), a surface protein

[1] LDN, NICHD, NIH, 9000 Rockville Pike, Bethesda, MD 20892, USA.
[2] Section on Brain Biochemistry, Clinical Neuroscience Branch, National Institute of Mental Health, NIH, Bethesda, 20892, USA.

Neuropsychopharmacology
Edited by Bunney/Hippius/Laakmann/Schmauß

which is abundant on these cells. We have shown that CD4 is abundant in brain. Iodinated gp 120 was specifically bound to membranes from human T cells and human, monkey, and rat brain membranes. All three preparations yielded a radiolabeled cross-linking product of 180 kDa (Pert et al. 1986). These results show that ^{125}I-labeled gp 120 can be coupled to a 60-kDa protein, the approximate molecular weight of CD4 (Ruscetti et al. 1988), on human, monkey, and rat brain, which is indistinguishable from the molecule on human T cells. In addition, a 60-kDa protein was precipitated by OKT4, a monoclonal antibody to CD4, on monkey brain and human T4 T cells (Pert et al. 1986; Ruscetti et al. 1988).

Brain Distribution. Two methods were used to determine the location of the CD4 in the brain. Using autoradiography with gp 120 and the radioimmunohistochemical methods for fresh tissues and OKT4, the monoclonal antibody to CD4 (Hil et al. 1986), the distribution of CD4 in the brain was mapped. Figure 1 compares these two methods on adjacent sections of rat brain. The pattern of binding is similar with both methods; intensive binding takes place in the cortex and hippocampus. However, differences occur in the dentate gyrus where OKT4 binds to the molecular layer and ^{125}I-labeled gp 120 to the granule cell layer. In addition, gp 120 shows greater binding to deep brain structures including the superior colliculus superficial gray, thalamus, and mammillary nuclei. These differences may occur because the CD4 epitope which is recognized by OKT4 may not be equally available in all sites, and

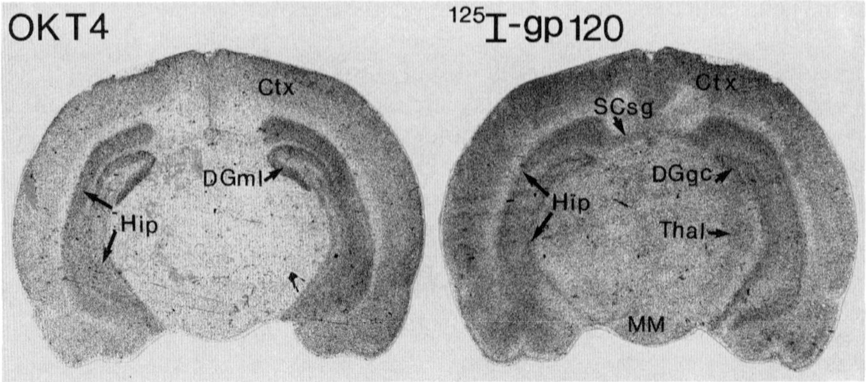

Fig. 1. A comparison of radioimmunohistochemistry with OKT4 (method of Hill et al. 1986) and autoradiography with ^{125}I-labeled gp 120 on adjacent sections of rat brain. For ^{125}I-labeled gp 120 autoradiography, gp 120 was iodinated by the lactoperoxidase method. Rat brain slices preincubated 2 × 5 min in phosphate-buffered saline (PBS) were incubated in PBS, with ^{125}I-labeled gp 120 0.1% aprotinin, 30 μg phenylmethylsulfonyl fluoride per milliliter, and 0.1% bovine serum albumin for 1 h at 37 °C. Sections were then rinsed in several changes of 0 °C PBS, dried quickly, and apposed to LKB Ultrofilm. *Ctx*, Cortex; *DGgc*, dentate gyrus granule cell layer; *DGml*, dentate gyrus molecular layer; *Hip*, hippocampus; *MN*, mammillary nuclei; *Thal*, thalamus; *SCsg*, superficial colliculus superficial gray

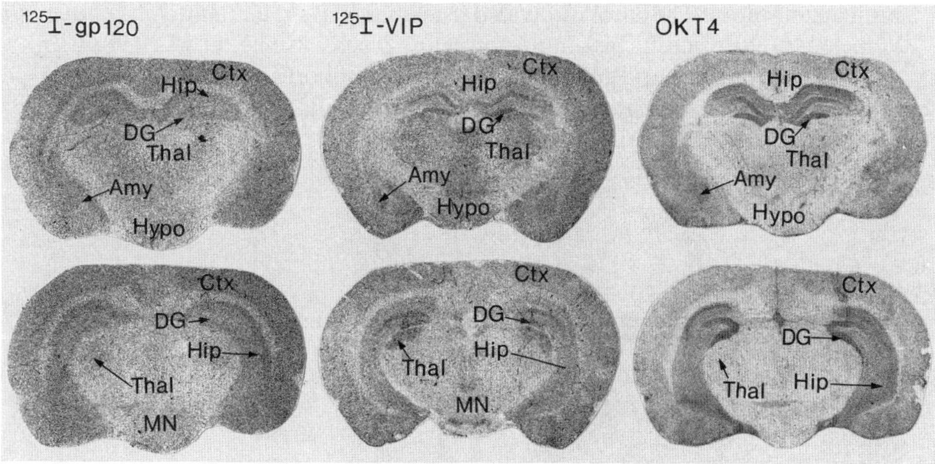

Fig. 2. A comparison of autoradiography with ^{125}I-labeled gp120 (see method Fig. 1). ^{125}I-labeled (Tyr 22) VIP (Amersham; method of Shaffer and Moody 1986), and radioimmunohistochemistry (method of Hill et al. 1986) in two regions of rat brain. *Amy*, Amygdala; *CG*, central gray; *Ctx*, cortex; *DG*, dentate gyrus; *Hip*, hippocampus; *Hypo*, hypothalamus; *MN*, mammillary nuclei; *Thal*, thalamus

OKT4 may cross-react with the dentate gyrus molecular layer VIP receptor (Fig. 2) which is not recognized by ^{125}I-labeled gp 120.

Comparison with VIP Distribution. Figure 2 compares ^{125}I-labeled gp 120 binding, ^{125}I-labeled VIP binding, and OKT4 binding at two sites in the rat brain. The similarity in binding pattern, especially between ^{125}I-labeled gp 120 and ^{125}I-labeled VIP is especially evident. There is extensive cortical binding, notably in superficial and deep layers. The amygdala, thalamus, hypothalamus, central gray, and mammillary nuclei have similar binding patterns. The VIP receptor in the dentate gyrus molecular layer is also a binding site for the related peptide secretin, which displaces VIP binding at this site (J. M. Hill, unpublished observations). This receptor is apparently recognized by OKT4 but not by gp 120. The similarity in binding patterns between gp 120 and VIP supports the idea that gp 120 binds to a receptor recognized by VIP.

The HIV Envelope Protein and VIP Binding

Competition Studies and SDS Gel Electrophoresis. The optimal conditions for binding VIP to brain and lymphocyte membranes have not yet been established. However, under some experimental conditions (5 mg tissue in 200 µl 50 mM Hepes KOH pH 7.4 with 5 mM $MgCl_2$ and 0.1% BSA at 37 °C for 30 min) peptide T (10^{-6} M) displaces about 44% of ^{125}I-labeled VIP from brain membranes. The corollary is also true, that VIP at 10^{-6} *M* displaces over 90% of [^{3}H]peptide T binding to human T cells (Smith et al., 1988). In addition, sodium dodecyl sulfate (SDS) gel electrophoresis of ^{125}I-labeled VIP bound to brain membranes produces a band at 60 kDa, the molecular weight of CD4 (Fig. 3). These results support the hypothesis that HIV envelope protein binds to a 60-kDa receptor which is also recognized by VIP.

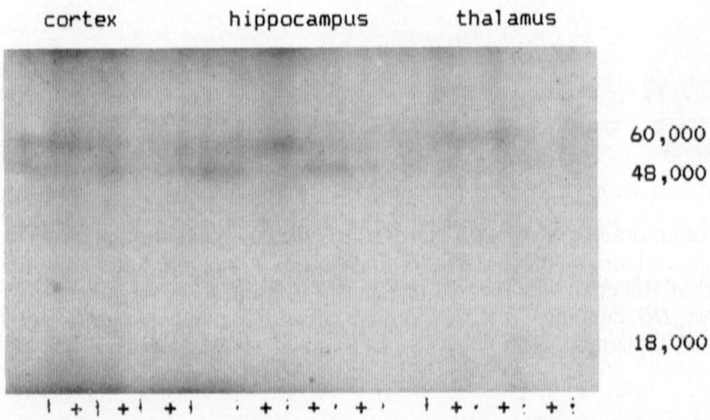

Fig. 3. SDS gel electrophoresis of ^{125}I-labeled VIP (New England Nuclear) bound to cortical, hippocampal, and thalamus membranes (see method Fig. 1) and cross-linked with 0.5 m*M* sulfodisuccinimidyl suberate 0.75 m*M*. *Lanes*, competition of VIP binding with various cold peptides

Chemotaxis Studies. An in vitro human monocyte chemotaxis assay has been used to characterize the interaction between VIP and the HIV receptor (Sacerdote et al. 1987; Ruff et al. 1987). In these studies OKT4a was able to inhibit the chemotaxis of monocytes to VIP. In addition, not only did TTNYT, the active pentapeptide sequence within peptide T, have chemotactic activity, but the effect of TTNYT plus VIP was also not greater than either of these active peptides alone. A combination of TTNYT and cholecystokinin was greater than each alone because each binds to a different receptor.

Hippocampal Culture Studies. In addition to the several types of evidence described above, a large body of work using a hippocampal culture assay system (Brenneman et al. 1988a, b; see also Brenneman, this volume) has produced results consistent with the hypothesis proposed here. In this in vitro system VIP demonstrated a growth-promoting activity, and gp120 was neurotoxic. However, both VIP and peptide T reverse the neuron-killing effect of gp120, presumably by blocking the attachment of the viral envelope protein to the CD4 receptor.

Summary and Conclusions

The diverse kinds of data presented here support the hypothesis that HIV and HIV viral products, i.e., gp 120, bind to a VIP receptor or a receptor for some VIP-like endogenous peptide. There is a pentapeptide sequence within VIP which is homologous with the proposed attachment site of gp 120, and in brain the binding patterns of gp 120 and VIP are the same. In preliminary experiments peptide T displaced VIP binding on brain membranes, and VIP bound to a 60-kDa protein (the molecular weight of CD 4). Also, VIP displaced peptide T in membrane-binding studies. OKT4a, a monoclonal antibody to CD 4, prevents chemotaxis of monocytes to VIP and the peptides TTNYT and VIP; both have chemotactic activity but together are not additive since they both use the same receptor. Finally, the neuronal cell death induced by gp 120 can be reversed by the addition of VIP or peptide T, presumably by binding to a receptor recognized by all three.

A multitude of CNS, immune system, and digestive system disorders characterize AIDS. Many of these may be due to opportunistic infections or direct infection with HIV. However, a substantial number of these symptoms may be due to gp 120, the HIV envelope protein which is shed in abundance by HIV (Pahwa et al. 1985; Gelderblom et al. 1987), binding to VIP receptors throughout the brain and body and causing either cell death or interfering with the normal VIP functions at these sites. Peptide T prevents lymphocyte infection by blocking HIV binding to CD 4 (Pert et al. 1986), however it may play an additional role in the treatment of AIDS patients by reducing gp 120-induced pathology by the same mechanism.

Acknowledgement. We gratefully acknowledge Deborah Lambie for excellent technical assistance.

References

Brenneman DE, Buzy JM, Ruff MR, Pert CB (1988a) Peptide T prevents gp 120 induced neuronal cell death in vitro: relevance to AIDS dementia. Drug Dev Res 15:361–369

Brenneman DE, Westbrook GL, Fitzgerald SF, Ennist DL, Elkins KL, Ruff MR, Pert CB (1988b) Neuronal cell killing by the envelope protein of HIV and its prevention by vasoactive intestinal peptide. Nature 335:639–642

Dalgleish AC, Beverly DCL, Clapham PR, Crawford DH, Greaves MF, Weiss RA (1985) The CD 4 (T4) antigen is an essential component of the receptor for the AIDS retrovirus. Nature 312:763–767

Fahrenkrug J, Emson PC (1982) Vasoactive intestinal polypeptide: functional aspects. Br Med Bull 38:265–270

Gelderblom HR, Hausman EH, Ozel M, Pauli G, Koch MA (1987) Fine structure of human immunodeficiency virus (HIV) and immunolocalization of structural proteins. Virology 156:171–176

Hill JM, Farrar WI, Pert CB (1986) Localization of the T4 antigen/AIDS virus receptor in monkey and rat brain: prominence in cortical regions. Psychopharmacol Bull 22:686–694

Lentz LL (1988) Binding of viral attachment protein to host-cell receptor: the Achilles heel of infectious viruses. TIPS 9:247–252

Navia BA, Jordan BD, Price RW (1986) The AIDS dementia complex. I. Clinical features. Ann Neurol 19:517–524

Pahwa S, Pahwa R, Saxinger C, Gallo RC, Good GA (1985) Influence of the human T-lymphotropic virus/lymphadenopathy-associated virus on functions of human lymphocytes: evidence for immunosuppressive effects and polyclonal B-cell activation by banded viral preparations. Proc Natl Acad Sci USA 82:8198–8202

Pert CB, Hill JM, Ruff MR, Berman RM, Robey WG, Arthur LO, Ruscetti FW, Farrar WL (1986) Octapeptides deduced from the neuropeptide-like pattern of antigen T4 in brain potently inhibit human immunodeficiency virus receptor binding and T cell infectivity. Proc Natl Acad Sci USA 83:9254–9258

Price RW, Sidtis J, Rosenblum M (1988) The AIDS dementia complex: some current questions. Ann Neurol 23(Suppl):S27–S33

Rostène WH (1984) Neurobiological and neuroendocrine functions of the vasoactive intestinal peptide (VIP). Prog Neurobiol 22:103–129

Ruff MR, Martin BM, Ginns EI, Farrar WL, Pert CB (1987) CD4 receptor binding peptides that block HIV infectivity cause human monocyte chemotaxis: relationship to vasoactive intestinal polypeptide. FEBS Lett 211:17–22

Ruscetti FW, Hill JM, Pert CB (1988) Visualization of the human helper lymphocyte related antigen (T4) in primate brain: implications for HTLV-III/LAV infection. Peptides 9:97–104

Sacerdote P, Ruff MR, Pert CB (1987) Vasoactive intestinal peptide 1–12: a ligand for the CD4 (T4)/human immunodeficiency virus receptor. J Neurosci Res 18:102–107

Said SI, Mutt V (1970) Polypeptide with broad biological activity: isolation from small intestine. Science 169:1217–1222

Shaffer MM, Moody TW (1986) Autoradiographic visualization of CNS receptors for vasoactive intestinal peptide. Peptides 7:283–288

Smith CC, Sacerdote P, Hallberg P, Sternberg E, Martin BM, Pert CB, Ruff MR (1988) Tritiated D-Ala^1-peptide T binding: a pharmacologic basis for the design of drugs which inhibit HIV receptor binding. Drug Dev Res 15:371–379

Neuropsychiatry of AIDS: Clinical Presentation and Treatment Research

T. P. Bridge, L. J. Ingraham, and F. K. Goodwin [1]

Introduction

Considerable progress has been made in the understanding of human immunodeficiency virus I (HIV I) infection during this decade since the initial description of the disorder (Gottlieb et al. 1981). While etiologic formulations for this disorder, now known as acquired immunodeficiency syndrome (AIDS), eluded initial investigators, all were impressed with the profound immunodysregulation that characterizes AIDS. Initial investigations focused upon T-cell function and modes of transmission. Critical to the development of effective treatments for AIDS, HIV I was identified as the etiologic agent for AIDS (Gallo et al. 1984). Based upon a decade of retrovirology, virologic studies identified the CD4 receptor as the entry protein for HIV I (Dalgleish et al. 1984). Emerging data then described monocyte/macrophage modes of transmission (Gartner et al. 1986), which are now believed central for the transmission of HIV I to the nervous system.

Initial descriptions of the nervous system signs and symptoms associated with HIV I infection were believed secondary either to the emotional reactions secondary to the knowledge of being infected with a fatal illness without known treatments or to the opportunistic infections and space-occupying lesions in the nervous system following the immune dysregulation of HIV I infection (Horowitz et al. 1982; Snider et al. 1983). Subsequently, many AIDS researchers became convinced that the clinical CNS manifestations observed in AIDS were due to the presence of HIV I in the nervous system. It was posited that HIV I directly infected the CNS, producing the cognitive, behavioral, and motoric symptoms now known as HIV I encephalopathy or AIDS dementia complex (Navia et al. 1986). HIV I is structurally similar to other lentiviruses, principally the visna virus, known to be both neurotropic and productive of a dementialike syndrome, contributing to the rapid acceptance that HIV I could directly produce nervous system disease (Gonda et al. 1985). At the same time, it was reported that the CD4 receptor was present in brain (Pert et al. 1986). These findings proved critical to the development of effective treatments for HIV I nervous system infection.

[1] National Institute of Mental Health, Intramural Research Program, 9000 Rockville Pike, Bethesda, MD 20892, USA.

Neuropsychopharmacology
Edited by Bunney/Hippius/Laakmann/Schmauß

Based on initial clinical reports by Navia and Price (1986) that noted the appearance of dementia in HIV I seropositive individuals who were otherwise immunologically asymptomatic, a codification of a diagnostic schema for HIV I encephalopathy was developed (Centers of Disease Control 1987). The diagnosis of AIDS can now be made by the presence of dementia in a seropositive individual without the previously requisite opportunistic infection or Kaposi's sarcoma.

As described by Navia and Price (1987), the early signs of this disorder may include psychomotor retardation, impaired cognition, ataxia, pyramidal tract signs, weakness, and/or tremor. Late in the course of the disorder, dementia is nearly universal, as are psychomotor retardation and ataxia. Other common signs can include mutism, organic psychosis, ataxia, hypertonia, incontinence, tremor, frontal release signs, motor weakness, myoclonus, and/or seizures. When present, HIV I encephalopathy can follow two distinct clinical courses. The more common is a slow, insidious decline, which can demonstrate a subacute acceleration. Less commonly, these patients have an acute onset of cognitive impairment leading to death within 6 months.

Although considerably fewer in number, data from pediatric HIV I patients make clear that the disease is neuropsychiatrically perhaps more incapacitating in them than it is in adults (Epstein et al. 1985).

HIV I Neurotropism

Although neuropathologic data do not demonstrate the intraneuronal presence of HIV I, and thus make the commonly used term of neurotropism for HIV I questionable, CSF data from HIV I infected patients document the presence of HIV I during the earliest stages of the infection (Marshall et al. 1988). HIV I is thought to be transmitted to the nervous system by HIV I infected monocytes. HIV I antibody, antigen, and viral recovery by culture is seen in the earliest stages of HIV I infection. CSF abnormalities, including increased protein, IgG, and white cells are associated with HIV I systemic infection (Hollander and Levy 1987; McArthur et al. 1988).

Cognitive and Neuromotor Changes in HIV I Infection

Because of the data that HIV I enters the nervous system early in the course of infection, it was reasoned that cognitive neuromotor abnormalities could possibly be observed in the early stages of HIV I infection. Several studies report a variable degree of nervous system disability in the earlier stages of HIV I infection, compared to seronegative, at-risk controls. While methodologic questions remain regarding these studies, these data do provide preliminary evidence of cognitive and neuromotor abnormalities across all phases of HIV I infection.

In a study of CDC class III HIV I patients, Janssen and colleagues found that these patients were significantly more likely to report cognitive, affective, and neurologic signs and symptoms than seronegative matched controls (Janssen et al. 1988). After removing subjects from the study who had neurobehavioral risk factors for impaired cognitive and neuromotor performance (e.g., childhood dyslexia, diagnosed history of nonintravenous substance abuse), there remained a statistically significant difference between the patients and controls. A recent replication of this study in the San Francisco hepatitis cohort found evidence for decrements in cognitive and neuromotor performance only among CDC class IVa, not class III patients (Janssen et al. 1989). In contrast, Grant and colleagues found evidence of statistically significant worsened neuropsychological performance among AIDS patients compared to seronegative, homosexual controls (Grant et al. 1987). This study also found a trend toward decrements of neuropsychological performance among CDC class II, III, and IVa HIV I infected patients. A replication of this study (Grant et al. 1988) found impairment in 5 of 14 HIV-seropositive individuals compared to 1 of 5 seronegative controls, consistent with the initial observation of early impairment following HIV infection. After controlling for mood and knowledge of serostatus Riccio et al. (1988) compared the cognitive performance of 60 seronegative and seropositive attendees to a London HIV clinic. HIV seropositive individuals' performance on the Wisconsin Card Sort Test and the Trail Making Test, Form B, was significantly poorer than that of seronegative controls, although better than of the CDC class IVa individuals and AIDS patients in the sample. Ollo and Pass (1988) compared 12 HIV-seropositive individuals to 12 controls infected with Lyme disease (a chronic CNS infection). After controlling for depression, they observed significantly poorer performance among HIV-seropositive individuals on tests of visual memory and psychomotor speed.

Investigators from the Multicenter AIDS Cohort Study (MACS) did not find significant decrements in neuropsychological performance compared to seronegative controls from the same cohort sample (McArthur et al. 1989). This cohort consists principally of CDC class II and III, with a few IVa patients. Selnes and his colleagues assessed 96 seropositive and 81 seronegative subjects over the course of 1 year and found no association between HIV I serostatus and change in neuropsychological measurements (Selnes et al. 1988a).

Other studies with similar findings to those of the MACS report include that of Poser and colleagues (1988). They found cognitive decrements in later stages of HIV infection but unimpaired performance on tests of intelligence and memory in CDC class II patients (Poser et al. 1988). Rubinow et al. (1988) reported using a broader battery for neuropsychological assessment and found no significant differences between 9 seropositive individuals and 6 healthy controls, but significantly reduced scores in 13 AIDS patients in tests of vocabulary, motor speed, and concentration. Tross et al. (1988b) compared 20 HIV-seronegative controls, 16 asymptomatic seropositive patients, 44 newly diagnosed AIDS patients, and 40 patients referred for neurologic consultation.

All AIDS patients had significantly more neuropsychiatric impairment compared to seronegative or CDC class II individuals. Catalan et al. (1988b) followed 25 hemophiliac patients for 2.5 years following precisely identified seroconversion; although seropositive patients reported increased hopelessness and depression, no differences in performance on neuropsychologic tests (including Trails-B) were seen compared to seronegative hemophiliac patients.

It is not possible at present therefore to conclude what the likelihood of neuropsychological deficits in CDC class II and class III HIV I infected persons is in comparison to appropriate controls. The impact of these findings on job function or activities of daily living is presently also not known.

Mood Disorders in HIV I Infection

Several studies have documented what would be intuitively expected: HIV I infected patients have increased incidence of affective disorder, ranging from transient adjustment reactions to major depressive disorder (Joffe et al. 1986; Grant et al. 1987; McArthur 1988). Past history of affective disorder may also be more common among HIV I infected patients (Joffe et al. 1986). The relationship of these changes in mood state to variant courses of HIV I infection is presently unknown but is under investigation. Further, it is unclear whether the presence of affective disorder is a prodrome to other neuropsychiatric manifestations for HIV I infection.

Several studies have shown hypothalamic-pituitary-adrenal (HPA) axis abnormalities, principally secondary to cytomegalic adrenal destruction described postmortem (Kalin et al. 1987). Adrenal insufficiency was also observed during suramin therapy in 13 of 48 patients tested for adrenal function (Levine et al. 1986). Unfortunately, observation of mood state in these patients was not reported. While the association of such neuroendocrine abnormalities to mood disorders is relatively well described, few studies of HIV I patients to date have focused on the description of these abnormalities in association with affective state or the neuroendocrine response of these patients to antidepressant therapy. Such studies would also need to attend to the relevance of potential increased prevalence of depressive disorder within at-risk groups and the relationship of this observation to disease course.

Neuropsychopharmacologic Therapeutics Research in HIV I Infection

No antiviral agent has yet demonstrated widely applicable efficacy in the treatment of HIV I CNS infection. As described in other chapters in this volume, HIV I may produce the observed nervous system symptomatology directly or indirectly by producing toxic products within the nervous system

(Hill et al., this volume; Brenneman, this volume). These findings are consistent with the absence of cytotoxic effects of HIV I observed in postmortem examination of HIV I dementia patients (Koenig et al. 1986; Stoler et al. 1986). Thus, any agent which either reduces the presence of HIV I or reduces the production/impact of HIV I toxic products could potentially lead to a reduction in nervous system symptomatology. Hence, the inclusion of CNS outcome measures across a broad range of anti-HIV I agents in HIV I patients with demonstrable neurobehavioral abnormalities is critical. Important outcome measures to the testing of these anti-HIV I therapeutics include: (a) demonstrated penetration of the nervous system by the agent under testing; (b) functional impact of the therapeutic on physiologic correlates of HIV I infection including CSF abnormalities and brain imaging; and (c) impact of the therapeutic on assessment of cognitive and neuromotor measures.

The relationship, if any, between the appearance of these abnormal nervous system signs and symptoms in HIV I infected persons and the onset of diagnosable HIV I encephalopathy is not established. Thus the selection of appropriate control group(s) will be necessary for many of the studies of drug efficacy in preventing or retarding the onset of this disorder.

Encouraging preliminary results from an open study of azidothymidine (AZT) in HIV I encephalopathy support the proposal that anti-HIV drugs may have beneficial effects in HIV I nervous system disease (Yarchoan et al. 1987). Penetration of the nervous system by any potential anti-HIV I therapeutic for efficacy against neurocognitive effects of HIV I would seem intuitively obvious. AZT has been clearly shown to penetrate the CSF when given peripherally. After 4–13 weeks of testing, AZT was reported to reduce nervous system signs and symptoms in HIV I encephalopathy. Normalization of nervous system outcome measures included brain imaging (positron emission tomography) and repeat measure instruments such as the Trails-B, subscales of the Wechsler Adult Intelligence Scale, and tests of motor skills were observed (Yarchoan et al. 1987). In another open test of a drug shown to penetrate the CSF, peptide T has been shown to be associated with normalization of results from magnetic resonance imaging in four near-terminal AIDS patients (Wetterberg et al. 1987). In an additional study of peptide T, cognitive and neuromotor performance on some measures was reported to demonstrate an increment of approximately 1 standard deviation during 30 days of testing in AIDS patients with dementia (Bridge et al. 1988). Most importantly, these studies indicate that the enormously disabling signs of HIV I encepathopathy may be reversible, and after relatively brief periods of drug therapy. Thus, these drugs may be reversing the effects of toxic HIV I products and may be able to do so in relatively short periods of time.

It is known, however, that HIV I infected patients demonstrate hypersensitivity to psychotropic medications. The etiology for these reactions is unknown, but reduced doses are clearly indicated in the treatment of affective disorder in HIV I infected patients and in the utilization of psychotropics in the treatment of nausea or behavioral control of psychotic states (Edelstein and Knight 1987; Bernstein and Scherokman 1986). The potential for adverse neuropsychiatric side effects of nonpsychotropic medications in HIVI patients exists as well. Recently reported were hypomanic reactions associated with AZT therapy in two patients without a history of bipolar disorder (Maxwell et al. 1988).

Summary

HIVI enters the nervous system early in the course of the infection. Without effective treatment within the nervous system, the brain remains a reservoir for continual reinfection of susceptible cells, i.e., those with the CD4 or OKT4 receptor. Thus we must expect that a therapeutic or a combination of therapeutics used for the treatment of HIVI infection must penetrate the nervous system and must do so in effective concentrations which can kill the virus or render it nontoxic. Without such therapies it is speculative as to whether continuous antiviral treatments to arrest immune dysfunction will in fact produce cognitive and neuromotor benefit in HIVI patients.

References

Bernstein WB, Scherokman B (1986) Neuroleptic malignant syndrome in a patient with acquired immunodeficiency syndrome. Acta Neurol Scand 73:636–637

Bridge TP, Heseltine P, Parker ES, Eaton E, Baron D, Johnson W, Goodwin FK (1988) Phase I testing of peptide T in AIDS patients and controls. IVth International conference on AIDS, Stockholm, Sweden, June 1988

Catalan J, Klimes I, Bond A, Garrod A, Day A, Rizza C (1988) Psychosocial and neuropsychiatric assessment of haemophiliacs with HIV infection: controlled investigation. IVth international conference on AIDS, Stockholm, Sweden, June 1988

Centers for Disease Control (1987) Revision of the CDC surveillance case definition for acquired immunodeficiency syndrome. Morbidity Mortality Weekly Rep 36:1S–14S

Dalgleish AG, Beverley PCL, Clapham PR (1984) The CD4 (T4) antigen is an essential component of the receptor for the AIDS retrovirus. Nature 312:763–767

Edelstein H, Knight RT (1987) Severe parkinsonism in two AIDS patients taking prochlorperazine. Lancet 2:341–342

Epstein LG, Sharer LR, Joshi VV (1985) Progressive encephalopathy in children with acquired immune deficiency syndrome. Ann Neurol 17:488–496

Gallo RC, Salahuddin SZ, Popovic M (1984) Frequent detection and isolation of cytopathic retroviruses (HTLV-III) from patients with AIDS. Science 224:500–502

Gartner S, Markovits P, Markovitz DM (1986) The role of mononuclear phagocytes in HTLV-III/LAV infection. Science 233:215–219

Gonda MA, Wong-Stall F, Gallo RC (1985) Sequence homology and morphologic similarity of HTLV-III and visna virus, a pathologic lentivirus. Science 227:173–177

Gottlieb MS, Schoff R, Schanker HM (1981) Pneumocystis carinii pneumonia and mucosal candidiasis in previously healthy homosexual men. N Engl J Med 305:1425–1431

Grant I, Atkinson JH, Hesselink JR, Kennedy CJ, Richmon DD, Spector SA, McCutchon JA (1987) Evidence for early central nervous system involvement in the acquired immunodeficiency syndrome (AIDS) and other human immunodeficiency virus (HIV) infections. Ann Intern Med 107:828–836

Grant I, Hesselink J, Jernigan T, Heaton RK, Atkinson JH, Weinrich J, Richman DD, Spector S, McCutchan AJ, Ostrow D (1988) Neuropsychology and magnetic resonance

imaging in HIV infection. IVth International conference on AIDS, Stockholm, Sweden, June 1988
Hollander H, Levy JA (1987) Neurologic abnormalities and recovery of human immunodeficiency virus from cerebrospinal fluid. Ann Intern Med 106:692–695
Horowitz SL, Benson DF, Gottlieb MS, Davos I, Benton JR (1982) Neurological complications of gay-related immunodeficiency disorder. Ann Neurol 12:80
Janssen RS, Saykin AJ, Cannon L (1989) Neurological and neuropsychologic manifestations of HIV I infection: association with AIDS related complex but not asymptomatic HIV I infection. Ann Neurol (in press)
Janssen RS, Saykin AJ, Kaplan JE, Spira TJ, Pinsky PF, Sprehn GC, Hoffman JC, Mayer B, Schonberger LB (1988) Neurological complications of human immunodeficiency virus infection in patients with lymphadenopathy syndrome. Ann Neurol 23:49–55
Joffe RT, Rubinow DR, Squillace K (1986) Neuropsychiatric aspects of AIDS. Psychopharmacol Bull 22:684–688
Kalin MF, Poretsky L, Seres DS, Zumoff B (1987) Hyporeninemic hypoaldosteronism associated with acquired immunodeficiency syndrome. Am J Med 82:1035–1038
Koenig S, Gendelman HE, Orenstein JM (1986) Detection of AIDS virus in macrophages in brain tissue from AIDS patients with encephalopathy. Science 213:1089–1093
Levine AM, Gill PS, Cohen J, Hawkins JG, Formenti SC, Aguilar S, Meyer PR, Krailo M, Parker J, Rashed S (1986) Suramin antiviral therapy in the acquired immunodeficiency syndrome. Ann Int Med 105:32–37
Marshall DW, Brey RL, Cahill WT, Houk RW (1988) Spectrum of cerebrospinal fluid findings in various stages of human immunodeficiency virus infection. Arch Neurol 45:954–958
Maxwell S, Scheftner WA, Kessler HA, Busch K (1988) Manic syndrome associated with zidovudine treatment. JAMA 259:340–347
McArthur JC, Cohen BA, Farzedegan H, Cornblath DR, Selnes OA, Ostrow D, Johnson RT, Phair J, Polk BF (1988) Cerebrospinal fluid abnormalities in homosexual men with and without neuropsychiatric findings. Ann Neurol 23 (Suppl):S34–S37
McArthur JC, Cohen BA, Selnes OA, Kumar AJ et al. (1989) Low prevalence of neurological and neuropsychological abnormalities in otherwise healthy HIV I-infected individuals: results from the multicenter AIDS cohort study. Ann Neurol (in press)
Navia B, Price RW (1987) AIDS dementia complex as the presenting sole manifestation of HIV infection. Ann Neurol 44:65–69
Navia BA, Jordan BD, Price RW (1986) The AIDS dementia complex I. Clinical features. Ann Neurol 19:517–524
Ollo C, Pass H (1988) Effect of depression on cognitive function in HIV disease. IVth International conference on AIDS, Stockholm, Sweden, June 1988
Pert CB, Hill JM, Ruff MR, Berman RM, Robey WG, Arthur LO, Ruscetti FW, Farrar WL (1986) Octapeptides deduced from the neuropeptide receptor-like pattern of antigen T4 in brain potently inhibit human immunodeficiency virus receptor binding and T-cell infectivity. Proc Natl Acad Sci USA 83:9254–9258
Poser S, Luer W, Eichenlaub D, Pohle HD, Weber T, Jurgens S, Felgenhauer K (1988) Chronic HIV encephalitis II. Clinical aspects. Klin Wochenschr 66:26–31
Riccio M, Thompson C (1987) AIDS and dementia. Br J Hosp Med 38:11
Riccio M, Wilson B, Hawkins D, Thompson C (1988) Neuropsychiatric manifestations of early HIV disease. IVth International conference on AIDS, Stockholm, Sweden, June 1988
Rubinow DR, Berrettini CH, Brouwers P, Lane C (1988) Neuropsychiatric consequences of AIDS. Ann Neurol 23 (Suppl):S24–S26
Selnes OA, McArthur JC, Munoz A, Cohn S, Gordon B, McArthur JH, Johnson RT, Polk BF (1988a) Longitudinal neuropsychological evaluation of healthy HIV I infected men: the Multicenter AIDS Cohort Study (MACS). IVth International conference on AIDS, Stockholm, Sweden, June 1988 (Abstract 8561)
Selnes OA, Miller EN, Becker JT, Cohen BA, McArthur JC, Visscher B, Gordon B, Satz P, Ginzburg HM, Polk BF (1988b) Normal neuropsychological performance in healthy

HIV I infected homosexual men: the Multicenter AIDS Cohort Study (MACS). IVth International conference on AIDS, Stockholm, Sweden (Abstract 8562)

Snider WD, Simpson DM, Nielson S, Gold JWM, Metroks CE, Posner JB (1983) Neurological complications of acquired immune deficiency syndrome: analysis of 50 patients. Ann Neurol 14:403–418

Stoler MH, Eskin TA, Benn S (1986) HTLV-III infection of the central nervous system. JAMA 256:2360–2364

Tross S, Abdul-Quader A, Friedman SR, Bartelme S, Garber J, Des Jarlais DC, Marmor M (1988a) Lack of neuropsychological impairment in HIV seropositive asymptotic drug users. IVth International conference on AIDS, Stockholm, Sweden, June 1988 (Abstract 8564)

Tross S, Price RW, Navia B, Thaler HT, Gold J, Sidtis JJ (1988b) Neuropsychological characterization of the AIDS dementia complex: a preliminary report. AIDS 2:81–88

Wetterberg L, Alexius B, Saaf J, Sonnerborg A, Britton S, Pert C (1987) Peptide T in treatment of AIDS. Lancet 1:159

Yarchoan R, Brouwers P, Spitzer AR (1987) Response of HIV associated neurological disease to 3′-azido-3′-deoxythymidine. Lancet 1:132–135

Psychiatric Symptoms and Neuropsychological Deficits in HIV Infection

D. Naber [1], C. Perro [1], U. Schick [1], M. Schmauss [2], A. Erfurth [1], D. Bove [1], F. D. Goebel [3], and H. Hippius [1]

Introduction

The frequent cerebral infestation of patients suffering from human immunodeficiency virus (HIV) infection or from AIDS is well documented in neuropathological and clinical studies. Neurological abnormalities occur in 30%–60% of AIDS patients and are the first clinical symptoms in 10% of patients (Jürgens et al. 1985; Navia and Price 1987; Pulst 1984). Discovery of the neurotropism of HIV helped researchers to understand the early intrathecal production of HIV antibodies (Lüer et al. 1988) and the manifestation of neuropsychiatric symptoms in patients with no signs of internal diseases (Faulstich 1987; Fenton 1987; Rundell et al. 1988).

Most patients with symptoms of organic psychoses such as paranoid-hallucinatory behavior, delirious states, mania, dementia, or depression are in late stages of the infection (Buhrich et al. 1988; Jones et al. 1987; Kermani et al. 1984, 1985; Koppell et al. 1985; Loewenstein and Sharpstein 1984; Nurnberg et al. 1984; Ochitill et al. 1984; Rundell et al. 1986; Schmidt and Miller 1988; Thomas et al. 1985; Thomas and Szabady 1987). However, some case reports show psychotic symptomatology already in early stages without secondary infections (Beckett et al. 1987; Gabel et al. 1986; Halevie-Goldman et al. 1987; Halstead et al. 1988; Maccario and Scharre 1987). In some HIV-positive patients psychotic symptoms may be (a) psychogenic, the reaction to knowledge of the diagnosis, (b) induced by drugs, or (c) first episodes of endogenous psychosis in patients who coincidentally are HIV positive. Nevertheless, a causal relationship between the neurotropic HIV and psychosis must be assumed in the majority of patients (Vogel-Scibilia et al. 1988).

Incidence, type, and severity of psychiatric symptoms in HIV-infected or in AIDS patients have not yet been systematically investigated. According to the sparse literature that exists, symptoms of depression seem to be most frequent (Dilley et al. 1985; Diederich et al. 1988; Perry and Tross 1984). The degree varies from a minor transient depression to despair and suicidal behavior (Marzuk et al. 1988). Very similar to depression is a syndrome of neurasthenia including fatigue, apathy, and reduction in memory and concentration. These

[1] Psychiatrische Klinik der Universität München, Nußbaumstr. 7, 8000 München 2, FRG.
[2] Bezirkskrankenhaus Augsburg, Dr.-Mack-Straße 1, 8900 Augsburg, FRG.
[3] Medizinische Poliklinik der Universität München, Nußbaumstr. 7, 8000 München 2, FRG.

Neuropsychopharmacology
Edited by Bunney/Hippius/Laakmann/Schmauß

nonspecific symptoms may be either psychogenic as a reaction to the life-threatening infection or somatogenic as the first symptoms of cerebral infestation, the subacute HIV encephalitis.

Marked neuropsychological deficits of AIDS patients have been observed, but data on incidence and severity are controversial. Navia and coworkers (1986), who coined the misleading and psychopathologically undifferentiated term AIDS dementia complex, reported that the majority of patients suffer from progressive dementia. However, neuropsychological studies revealed marked cognitive deficits only in 47% (Grant et al. 1987), 31% (Ayers et al. 1987), or in one of 16 patients (Bruhn 1987). Patients in early stages of HIV infection have also been reported to suffer from cognitive impairment. Several studies showed that asymptomatic HIV-positive patients performed worse than HIV-negative controls on tests measuring abstract thinking, learning, memory, and speed of information processing (Grant et al. 1987; Rubinow et al. 1988; Silberstein et al. 1987; Tross et al. 1988). However, there is also one investigation which did not show a cognitive deficit in HIV-positive subjects (Stieglitz et al. 1988). These studies do not reveal strong conclusions since they deal mostly with a small number of subjects. An organic etiology – a causal relationship between the neurotropic HIV and reduced functioning – is assumed in most studies, but they often do not fully consider other factors which may also be responsible for neuropsychological impairment, such as education, neuropsychiatric history, drug abuse, and depression.

Subjects and Methods

A total of 156 HIV-positive subjects were investigated. Of these, 24 had to be excluded because of insufficient knowledge of German, lack of education (elementary school not finished), or history of neuropsychiatric illness with somatic etiology (meningitis, epilepsy, brain trauma). Moreover, one chronic schizophrenic patient did not participate because of lack of motivation. For the statistical analysis there remained 132 patients (110 men, 22 women; age, 32 ± 7 years). They had known of their HIV infection for 17 ± 12 months. All gave their informed consent to participate. Subjects were either in- or outpatients of the Department of Internal Medicine or Dermatology ($n = 84$) or inmates of Bavarian prisons ($n = 48$). These prisoners, arrested for drug trafficking, did not differ from nonarrested drug addicts with regard to age or history of drug abuse. Bias in selection was not apparent since in both groups of subjects, patients and prisoners, those who refused participation (5%–10%) were without obvious psychopathological or intellectual abnormalities. Among the patients 45 were asymptomatic, 55 suffered from lymphadenopathy syndrome (LAS), 16 from AIDS-related complex (ARC), and 16 from AIDS. Among these subjects 62 were intravenous drug addicts, 65 bi- or homosexuals, and 5 heterosexual partners of drug addicts.

Psychiatric exploration, including documentation of history, was performed according to a semistructured interview. Psychopathology was rated by means of the AMDP system (Arbeitsgemeinschaft für Methodik und Documentation in der Psychiatrie; Angst et al. 1969). Self-rating tests were used for depression (Self-Rated Depression Scale, SDS; Zung and Durham 1965), anxiety (State-Trait Anxiety Inventory, STAI; Spielberger et al. 1970, and other mood states (Profile of Mood States, POMS; McNair et al. 1971).

Psychiatric history aside from drug abuse consisted of major depression with suicidal behavior in eight patients and manic-depressive illness, schizophrenia, and agoraphobia in one patient each. At the time of investigation, no patient was under continuous psychopharmacological treatment or, as evaluable, took other psychotropic drugs. Drug addicts had been free of opiates for at least 3 months.

The neuropsychological examination, which took 45–60 min, included eight tests: vocabulary (Merz et al. 1975): education, intelligence; similarities (Wechsler 1964): abstract thinking; digit-symbol (Wechsler 1964): visuomotor speed, visuoassociative memory; color-word interference (Golden 1976): cognitive functions of learning and naming; maze (Chapuis 1959): visual orientation and visuomotor speed; Benton test (Benton 1981): short-term memory, visuomotor reproduction; trail-making (Gordon 1972): concentration, visual orientation; and auditory verbal learning (Lezak 1983): short-term memory. For this study, only the recall after the third repetition was used.

A control group of 100 HIV-negative subjects (85 men, 15 women; age, 34 ± 11 years) underwent the same neuropsychological tests. This group consisted of 58 patients who were treated in the Department of Internal Medicine for minor diseases (no endocrinopathy, CNS illness, or drug abuse), 34 convicted intravenous drug addicts (drug free for at least 3 months) and 8 homosexual men. Controls did not differ from HIV-positive subjects with regard to sex, age, education, or percentage of prisoners; only the percentage of intravenous drug addicts was lower (34% versus 47%).

If the test result of a HIV-positive subject showed a reduction of more than 1 SD (compared to the mean of controls), function was classified as "slightly reduced;" if the difference was more than 2 SD, it was considered "markedly reduced." Aside from the eight tests, a neuropsychological total score was calculated: the sum of "slightly" (=1 point) and "markedly" (=2 points) reduced tests. If this score was 0–2, cognitive functioning was classified as "normal," 3–5 "slightly impaired," and over 6 "markedly impaired."

Results

Among the patients, 49% reported symptoms of depression when they learned of their HIV status; 5% had suicidal ideas; one patient took a high dosage of tranquilizers to commit suicide. Psychiatric exploration and self-rating of the actual mood state revealed in a high correlation (between AMP depression and SDS, $r = 0.573$, $p < 0.0005$), a clinically relevant depression in 27% (SDS > 48 points), and symptoms of major depression (SDS > 55 points) in 8%; 24%

Table 1. Neuropsychological functioning in HIV-positive patients and HIV-negative controls: individual scales

	Vocabulary (IQ points)	Similarities (points)	Digit-symbol (points)	Color-word interference (T value)	Maze (raw value)	Auditory verbal learning (raw value)	Trail making (T value)	Benton (difference from expected value)	Total score
HIV-negative ($n = 100$)	111 ± 11 (21/2)	12.3 ± 1.8 (13/3)	12.2 ± 2.4 (18/1)	52 ± 8 (17/2)	33 ± 13 (24/6)	11.5 ± 2.2 (13/4)	55 ± 11 (16/4)	0.2 ± 1.8 (12/1)	1.4 ± 1.7
HIV-positive, asymptomatic ($n = 45$)	106 ± 12 (29/9)	12.0 ± 1.8 (27/4)	11.2 ± 2.4 (29/7)	49 ± 7 (36/7)	38 ± 20 (24/9)	10.7 ± 2.6 (20/7)	60 ± 9 (33/7)	0.1 ± 1.7 (18/2)	2.5 ± 2.1
HIV-positive, LAS ($n = 55$)	105 ± 11 (29/2)	11.5 ± 2.2 (22/7)	11.4 ± 2.7 (22/5)	49 ± 10 (24/5)	37 ± 24 (13/4)	10.8 ± 2.2 (27/7)	57 ± 11 (22/9)	−0.3 ± 18 (22/2)	2.0 ± 2.3
HIV-positive, ARC ($n = 16$)	108 ± 14 (25/0)	11.9 ± 1.9 (19/6)	10.6 ± 2.4 (44.6)	48 ± 12 (50/25)	41 ± 27 (25/6)	9.2 ± 1.6 (56/13)	62 ± 3 (50/6)	−0.4 ± 1.3 (13/0)	3.6 ± 2.3
HIV-positive, AIDS ($n = 16$)	109 ± 17 (13/6)	11.7 ± 2.1 (25/13)	10.5 ± 3.1 (25/25)	48 ± 13 (3/10)	41 ± 16 (13/0)	9.5 ± 2.9 (50/19)	62 ± 10 (38/19)	−1.5 ± 2.7 (25/13)	3.2 ± 3.1
One-way analysis	n.s.	n.s.	$F = 2.51^{a}$	n.s.	n.s.	$F = 4.46^{c}$	$F = 3.89^{c}$	$F = 2.49$	$F = 4.67^{c}$
t Test: HIV-negative versus HIV-positive	$t = 2.67^{c}$	$t = 3.03^{c}$	$t = 3.92^{e}$	$t = 3.58^{d}$	$t = 2.40^{b}$	$t = 3.87^{d}$	$t = 3.31^{d}$	n.s.	$t = 3.62^{d}$
t Test: HIV-negative versus early stages	$t = 3.26^{b}$	$t = 2.39^{a}$	$t = 2.34^{a}$	$t = 2.65^{b}$	n.s.	$t = 2.15^{a}$	$t = 2.43^{a}$	n.s.	$t = 2.86^{c}$
t Test: HIV-negative versus late stages	n.s.	n.s.	$t = 2.67^{b}$	n.s.	n.s.	$t = 4.22^{e}$	$t = 3.52^{d}$	$t = 2.05^{a}$	$t = 3.65^{d}$

Means ± SD. Total score = sum of slightly reduced (= 1) and markedly reduced (= 2) test results. Values in parentheses, percentage with deficits: slightly reduced scores (difference from mean of controls > 1 SD; numerator) and markedly reduced scores (difference > 2 SD; denominator). Early stages, asymptomatic plus LAS cases; late stages, ARC plus AIDS cases.

[a] $p < 0.05$; [b] $p < 0.01$; [c] $p < 0.005$; [d] $p < 0.001$; [e] $p < 0.0005$.

Table 2. Neuropsychological functioning in HIV-positive patients and HIV-negative controls: total scores

	Normal	Slight impairment	Marked impairment
HIV-negative ($n = 100$)	81 (81%)	15 (15%)	4 (4%)
HIV-positive ($n = 132$)	84 (64%)	32 (24%)	16 (12%)
No symptoms ($n = 45$)	29 (65%)	11 (24%)	5 (11%)
LAS ($n = 55$)	42 (76%)	8 (15%)	5 (9%)
ARC ($n = 16$)	5 (31%)	8 (50%)	3 (19%)
AIDS ($n = 16$)	8 (50%)	5 (31%)	3 (19%)

suffered from marked anxiety (STAI > 54 points). One patient had psychotic symptoms such as auditory hallucinations and paranoid delusion; these symptoms had been known for at least 5 years, when chronic schizophrenia was diagnosed. The four groups of HIV-positive patients, classified according to the stage of the infection (asymptomatic, LAS, ARC, AIDS) did not differ in any of the psychiatric or self-rating scales.

In 55% of patients there was a subjective impression of reduced cognitive functioning. Mostly they reported disturbances of memory and concentration as well as fatigue. Objective evaluation, the results of eight neuropsychological tests, are presented in Table 1. Compared to HIV-negative controls, most tests showed a significant deficit in patients' functioning. A particular deterioration was revealed by the digit-symbol, auditory verbal learning, trail-making, and Benton tests.

Evaluation of neuropsychological functioning in terms of total score is presented in Table 2. Cognitive deficits characterized 29% of asymptomatic and LAS patients and 54% of patients with ARC or AIDS. The clinical relevance of these deficits was minor in most patients since their social and occupational functioning was mostly undisturbed. Only 3% of patients in early stages (8% in late stages) fulfilled DSM III diagnostic criteria of dementia.

Relationships between affective states and neuropsychological functioning showed numerous significant correlations (Table 3). Especially the results of digit-symbol, color-word interference, auditory verbal learning and trail-making tests correlated highly significantly with symptoms of depression or anxiety. Stage of illness correlated significantly only with the Benton test results ($r = 0.17$, $p < 0.05$); duration of drug abuse correlated with no neuropsychological test results.

Table 4 shows the incidence of marked depression, drug abuse, and late stage of HIV infection in different categories of neuropsychological functioning. Depression and late stages occur more often in patients with neuropsy-

Table 3. Relationship between neuropsychological functioning and psychopathy (Pearson product-moment correlations; $n = 132$)

	Similarities	Digit-symbol	Color-Word Interference	Maze	Auditory Verbal	Trail making	Benton	Total Score
Depression (AMDP)	n.s.	-0.31^{e}	-0.35^{e}	-0.27^{c}	-0.23^{b}	-0.22^{b}	-0.24^{b}	-0.39^{e}
Depression (SDS)	-0.17^{a}	-0.38^{e}	-0.18^{a}	n.s.	-0.21^{a}	-0.30^{d}	n.s.	-0.28^{d}
Anxiety (STAI)	n.s.	-0.36^{e}	-0.17^{a}	n.s.	-0.26^{c}	-0.26^{b}	n.s.	-0.28^{d}
Depression (POMS)	n.s.	-0.31^{e}	-0.15^{a}	n.s.	-0.21^{b}	-0.23^{b}	n.s.	-0.22^{c}
Fatigue (POMS)	n.s.	n.s.	n.s.	n.s.	n.s.	n.s.	n.s.	n.s.
Vigor (POMS)	n.s.	0.18^{a}	n.s.	n.s.	n.s.	n.s.	n.s.	n.s.
Anger (POMS)	n.s.	-0.24^{c}	-0.28^{d}	-0.24^{c}	-0.27^{d}	-0.27^{c}	n.s.	-0.29^{d}

[a] $p < 0.05$; [b] $p < 0.01$; [c] $p < 0.001$; [d] $p < 0.001$; [e] $p < 0.0005$.

Table 4. Incidence of depression (SDS > 48), intravenous drug abuse, and late stages of HIV infection (ARC, AIDS) at different levels of neuropsychological impairment

	Normal ($n = 84$)	Slight impairment ($n = 32$)	Marked impairment ($n = 16$)
Depression ($n = 36$)	16 (19%)	11 (34%)	9 (56%)
Intravenous drug abuse ($n = 62$)	38 (45%)	18 (56%)	6 (38%)
HIV infection, late stages ($n = 32$)	13 (15%)	13 (41%)	6 (38%)
No depression, no intravenous drug abuse, asymptomatic or LAS ($n = 20$)	16 (19%)	4 (13%)	0 (0%)

Percentages refer to neuropsychological functioning.

chological deficits; drug abuse is evenly distributed. Of the 16 patients with marked deficit, none was in an early stage and free of depression or drug abuse.

To evaluate the influence of drug abuse and imprisonment, patients and controls with drug abuse were excluded in one statistical analysis. Another analysis was done after exclusion of HIV-positive and HIV-negative prisoners. In neither analysis did they differ essentially from the total groups (analysis of variance, *t* test, Pearson product-moment correlations).

Discussion

The results of this study are in agreement with the findings of others regarding depression and anxiety in HIV infected patients (Diederich et al. 1988; Faulstich 1987; Fenton 1987; Marzuk et al. 1988; Navia et al. 1986; Perry and Tross 1984; Rubinow et al. 1988; Rundell et al. 1988). Other marked psychopathological symptoms were observed in only one patient; with regard to this long-known diagnosis of schizophrenia, a causal relationship between HIV infection and psychosis is unlikely for this patient. The lack of psychotic symptoms in the other patients agrees with the findings of most studies (Perry and Tross 1984) and our own experience in psychiatric consultation of AIDS patients (Erfurth et al. 1989). Although some patients reported marked fluctuations in mood states, mean scores of affective disturbances were independent of the clinical stage of HIV infection, probably reflecting the continuous threat of the illness. Unfortunately, there are no other data on the relationship between clinical (internal or immunological) status and symptoms of affective disorders.

Neuropsychological examination shows that tests highly sensitive for organic alterations and affective disturbances, such as the digit-symbol, auditory verbal learning, trail-making, and Benton tests (Benton 1981; Gordon 1972; Lezak 1983; Wechlser 1964), reveal a significant deficit even in asymptomatic patients. Most of the other tests also demonstrate significant changes. However, results of the vocabulary and similarities tests correlated highly significantly with education. The reduced scores on these tests may be more related to differences in education or premorbid intelligence among the subgroups of HIV-positive subjects than to HIV infection itself. These neuropsychological results, indicating a significant reduction already in early stages, are similar to four other investigations (Grant et al. 1987; Rubinow et al. 1988; Silberstein et al. 1987; Tross et al. 1988); only one recent study did not show a difference between HIV-infected patients and controls (Stieglitz et al. 1988). The clinical relevance of cognitive deficits, detected by sensitive neuropsychological tests, is individually very different and depends on social and other variables. Only a small minority of patients with documented impaired functioning fulfilled the criteria of dementia. The term "AIDS-dementia complex" describes a triad of dementia and motor and behavioral dysfunction (Price et al. 1988). However, there are numerous reports of psychotic patients with no signs of dementia and vice versa (Buhrich et al. 1988; Gabel et al. 1986; Halevie-Goldman et al. 1987). From a psychiatric perspective, the psychopathologically undifferentiated inclusion of three rather independent abnormalities is misleading, and the term of "AIDS-dementic-complex" is therefore of dubious usefulness.

The data suggest that drug abuse does not markedly influence neuropsychological abilites. This is an agreement with most studies testing heroin addicts without another neuropsychiatric illness but with normal education (Guerra et al. 1987; Rounsaville et al. 1982). Nevertheless, an effect of opiate abuse on neuropsychological functioning cannot be excluded individually. A major difference between patients and controls is naturally the affective state, due to the burden of a unique life-threatening illness with enormous social implications. It is doubtful whether patients suffering from cancer or another fatal disease are more suitable as controls. As regards the etiology of neuropsychological deficits, this study can give preliminary data only. The numerous significant correlations between psychopathology and cognitive performance do not prove causal relationships, but they indicate that affective disturbances and neuropsychological deficits are closely related. Cross-sectional studies hardly allow the differentiation between psychogenic and somatogenic components.

Regarding possible sources of selection bias and the small number of subjects in some subgroups, this study will be continued as a prospective investigation with repeated measurements of psychopathology and neuropsychological functioning. Initial data on 57 patients reexamined after 6 months show no psychopathological and only one neuropsychological change, a significant reduction in performance on the trail-making test. Moreover, examination of most patients includes a neurological evaluation with lumbar puncture and computed tomographic scan of the head (Naber et al., manuscript in preparation). The collection of psychiatric and neurological data will result in valuable information relevant for our understanding of the incidence, severity, etiology, and prognosis of psychiatric symptoms in HIV-infected subjects. This knowledge should help physicians to follow sound medical recognition rather than individual, social, or political opinions when they treat patients suffering from this devastating disease.

References

Angst J, Battegay R, Bente D, Berner P, Broeren W, Cornu F, Dick P, Engelmeier MP, Heimann H, Heinrich K, Helmchen H, Hippius H, Pöldinger W, Schmidlin P, Schmitt W, Weiss P (1969) Das Dokumentationssystem der Arbeitsgemeinschaft für Methodik und Dokumentation in der Psychiatrie (AMP). Arzneimittelforschung/Drug Res 19:399–405

Ayers MR, Abrams DI, Newell TG, Friedrich F (1987) Performance of individuals with AIDS on the Luria-Nebraska neuropsychological battery. Int J Clin Neuropsychol 9:101–105

Beckett A, Summergrad P, Manschreck T, Vitagliano HL, Henderson M, Buttolph ML, Jenike M (1987) Symptomatic HIV infection of the CNS in a patient without clinical evidence of immune deficiency. Am J Psychiatry 144:1342–1344

Benton AL (1981) Der Benton-Test. German Version. Huber, Stuttgart

Bruhn P (1987) AIDS and dementia: a quantitative neuropsychological study of unselected Danish patients. Acta Neurol Scand 76:443–447

Buhrich N, Cooper DA, Freed E (1988) HIV infection associated with symptoms indistinguishable from functional psychosis. Br J Psychiatry 152:649–653

Chapuis F (1959) Der Labyrinth-Test. Huber, Stuttgart

Diederich N, Karenberg A, Peters UH (1988) Psychopathologische Bilder bei der HIV-Infektion: AIDS-Lethargie und AIDS-Demenz. Fortschr Neurol Psychiatr 56:173–185

Dilley JW, Ochitill HN, Perl M, Volberding PA (1985) Findings in psychiatric consultations with patients with acquired immune deficiency syndrome. Am J Psychiatry 142:82–86

Erfurth A, Naber D, Goebel FD (1989) AIDS-Erkrankung und Psychopathologie – Beobachtungen aus dem psychiatrischen Konsiliardienst in einer internistischen Klinik. Fortschr Neurol Psychiatr 57:469–473

Faulstich ME (1987) Psychiatric aspects of AIDS. Am J Psychiatry 144:551–556

Fenton TW (1987) AIDS-related psychiatric disorder. Br J Psychiatry 151:579–588

Gabel RH, Barnard N, Norko M, O'Conell RA (1986) AIDS presenting as mania. Compr Psychiatry 27:251–254

Golden CJ (1976) Identification of brain disorders by the Stroop Color and Word Test. J Clin Psychol 32:621–630

Gordon HG (1972) The Trail Making Test in neuropsychological diagnosis. J Clin Psychology 28:167–169

Grant I, Atkinson JH, Hesselink JR, Kennedy CJ, Richman DD, Spector SA, McCutchan JA (1987) Evidence for early central nervous system involvement in the acquired immunodeficiency syndrome (AIDS) and other human immunodeficiency virus (HIV) infections. Ann Intern Med 107:828–836

Guerra D, Sole A, Cami J, Tobena A (1987) Neuropsychological performance in opiate addicts after rapid detoxification. Drug Alcohol Depend 20:261–270

Halevie-Goldman BD, Potkin SG, Poyourow P (1987) AIDS-related complex presenting as psychosis. Am J Psychiatry 144:964

Halstead S, Riccio M, Harlow P, Oretti R, Thompson C (1988) Psychosis associated with HIV infection. Br J Psychiatry 153:618–623

Jones GH, Kelly CL, Davies JA (1987) HIV and onset of schizophrenia. Lancet 1:982

Jürgens R, Thun F, Ackermann R (1985) Erstmanifestation des "Acquired Immundeficiency Syndrome" (AIDS) am Nervensystem. Nervenarzt 56:603–607

Kermani E, Drob S, Alpert M (1984) Organic brain syndrome in three cases of acquired immune deficiency syndrome. Compr Psychiatry 25:294–297

Kermani E, Borod JC, Brown PH, Tunnell G (1985) New psychopathologic findings in AIDS: case report. J Clin Psychiatry 46:240–241

Koppel BS, Wormser GP, Tuchmann AJ, Maayan S, Hewlett D, Daras M (1985) Central nervous system involvement in patients with AIDS. Acta Neurol Scand 71:337–353

Lezak MD (1983) Neuropsychological assessment. Oxford University Press, New York

Loewenstein RJ, Sharpstein SS (1984) Neuropsychiatric aspects of acquired immune deficiency syndrome. Int J Psychiatry Med 13:1983–1984

Lüer W, Poser S, Weber T, Jürgens S, Eichenlaub D, Pohle HD, Felgenhauer K (1988) Chronic HIV encephalitis. I. Cerebrospinal fluid diagnosis. Klin Wochenschr 66: 21–25

Maccario M, Scharre DW (1987) HIV and acute onset of psychosis. Lancet 2:342

Marzuk PM, Tierney H, Tardieff K, Gross EM, Morgan EB, Hsu MA, Mann JJ (1988) Increased risk of suicide in persons with AIDS. JAMA 259:1333–1337

McNair DM, Lorr M, Doppleman LF (1971) The profile of mood states (POMS). San Diego

Merz J, Lehrl S, Galster JV, Erzigkeit H (1975) MWT-B – ein Intelligenzkurztest. Psychiat Neurol Med Psychol (Leipz) 27:423–428

Naber D, Perro C, Schick I, Einhäupl K, Schielke E, Goebel FD (1989) Relationships between psychiatric, neuropsychological and neurological variables in HIV-infected patients. (submitted for publication)

Navia BA, Price WR (1987) The acquired immunodeficiency syndrome dementia complex as the presenting or sole manifestation of human immunodeficiency virus infection. Arch Neurol 44:65–69

Navia BA, Jordan BD, Price RW (1986) The AIDS dementia complex. I. Clinical features. Ann Neurol 19:517–524

Nurnberg HG, Prudic J, Fiori M, Freedman EP (1984) Psychopathology complicating acquired immune deficiency syndrome (AIDS). Am J Psychiatry 141:95–96

Ochitill HN, Perl M, Dilley J, Volberding P (1984) Case reports of psychiatric disturbance in patients with acquired immune-deficiency syndrome. Int J Psychiatry 14:259–263

Perry SW, Tross S (1984) Psychiatric problems of AIDS inpatients at the New York Hospital: preliminary report. Public Health Rep 99:200–205

Price RW, Brew B, Sidtis J, Rosenblum M, Scheck AC, Cleary P (1988) The brain in AIDS: central nervous system HIV-I infection and AIDS dementia complex. Science 239:586–592

Pulst SM (1984) Neurologische Komplikationen bei erworbenem Immundefekt-Syndrom (AIDS). Nervenarzt 55:146–152

Rounsaville BJ, Jones C, Novelly RA, Kleber H (1982) Neuropsychological functioning in opiate addcits. J Nerv Ment Dis 170:209–216

Rubinow DR, Berrettini CH, Brouwers P, Lane HC (1988) Neuropsychiatric consequences of AIDS. Ann Neurol 23 (Suppl):24–26

Rundell JR, Wise MG, Ursano RJ (1986) Three cases of AIDS-related psychiatric disorders. Am J Psychiatry 143:777–778

Rundell JR, Paolucci SL, Beatty DC, Boswell RN (1988) Psychiatric illness at all stages of human immundeficiency virus infection. Am J Psychiatry 145:652–653

Schmidt U, Miller D (1988) Two cases of hypomania in AIDS. Br J Psychiatry 152:839–842

Silberstein CH, McKegney FP, O'Dowd MA, Selwyn PA, Schoenbaum E, Drucker E, Feiner C, Cox CP, Friedland G (1987) A prospective longitudinal study of neuropsychological and psychosocial factors in asymptomatic individuals at risk for HTLV-III/LAV infection in a methadone program: preliminary findings. Int J Neurosci 32:669–676

Spielberger CD, Gorsuch RL, Lushene RE (1970) STAI, Manual for the State-Trait-Anxiety Inventory. Palo Alto

Stieglitz RD, Albrecht J, Lundt A, Pittlik V, Hedde HP (1988) Psychopathometrie bei HIV-infizierten Patienten. Nervenarzt 59:330–336

Thomas CS, Szabadi E (1987) Paranoid psychosis as the first presentation of a fulminating lethal case of AIDS. Br J Psychiatry 151:693–695

Thomas CS, Toone BK, Komy AE, Harwin B, Farthing CP (1985) HTLV-III and psychiatric disturbances. Lancet 2:395–396
Tross S, Price RW, Navia B, Thaler HT, Gold J, Hirsch DA, Sidtis JJ (1988) Neuropsychological characterization of the AIDS dementia complex: a preliminary report. AIDS 2:81–88
Vogel-Scibilia SE, Mulsant BH, Keshavan MS (1988) HIV infection presenting as psychosis: a critique. Acta Psychiatr Scand 78:652–656
Wechsler D (1964) Die Messung der Intelligenz Erwachsener. Huber, Bern
Zung WWK, Durham NC (1965) A self-rating depression scale. Arch Gen Psychiatry 12:63–70

Appendix

SYMPOSIUM
Molecular Biology in Neuropsychopharmacology

Chair: G. Racagni, Italy, and J. Mendlewicz, Belgium

TU.01.01 **Brain genetic structures (neurogens) and recombinant DNA technology**
M. E. Vartanian, USSR

TU.01.02 **Molecular biological approaches to brain region- and cell-specific molecules**
J. G. Sutcliffe, H. P. Ottiger, J. B. Watson, J. Bernal, M. B. Brennan and G. H. Travis, USA

TU.01.03 **The molecular biology of the $GABA_A$ receptor**
P. H. Seeburg, P. R. Schofield, D. B. Pritchett, S. Ymer, A. Draguhn, H. Sontheimer, M. Köhler, P. Werner, H. Kettenmann, B. D. Shivers and B. Sakmann, Fed. Rep. of Germany

TU.01.04 **Characterization and localization of human diazepam binding inhibitor gene**
I. Mocchetti, USA

TU.01.05 **Molecular biology of adrenergic receptors**
S. Cotecchia, R. J. Lefkowitz and M. G. Caron, USA

TU.01.06 **From the clonidine-growth hormone stimulation test to the alpha 2-noradrenergic receptor gene**
M. R. Hoehe, W. H. Berrettini and E. S. Gershon, USA

TU.01.07 **Protein phosphorylation in rat cerebral cortex after desipramine treatment: Possible modulation of transcription activity**
J. Perez, D. Tinelli, I. Zucchi and G. Racagni, Italy

SYMPOSIUM
Long-Term Treatment of Schizophrenia

Chair: H. Y. Meltzer, USA, and B. Woggon, Switzerland

TU.02.01 **Neuroendocrine and behavioural response to pharmacologic probes as predictors of outcome in maintenance treatment**
J. M. Kane and J. Lieberman, USA

TU.02.02 **Clozapine in the long term treatment of schizophrenia**
H. Y. Meltzer, USA

TU.02.03 **Duration of maintenance treatment**
D. A.W. Johnston, United Kingdom

TU.02.04 **Practical problems during treatment with long acting neuroleptics and also after withdrawal**
B. Wistedt, Sweden

TU.02.05 **Early intervention with neuroleptic drugs to prevent relapse in schizophrenia**
A. Pietzcker, W. Gaebel, W. Köpcke, M. Linden, P. Müller, F. Müller-Spahn and J. Tegeler, Fed. Rep. of Germany

TU.02.06 **Methodological issues in long-term treatment studies**
B. Woggon, Switzerland

SYMPOSIUM

Alpha-Adrenoceptor Activity in Depression and in Antidepressant Mechanisms

Chair: N. Matussek, Fed. Rep. of Germany, and J. Maj, Poland

TU.03.01 **Antidepressant drugs given repeatedly and α_1-adrenoceptors**
J. Maj, Poland

TU.03.02 **Role of alpha receptors in the regulation of beta-adrenoceptors by antidepressants**
N. Brunello, M. Riva, A. C. Rovescalli and G. Racagni, Italy

TU.03.03 **The effect of phenylethanolamine-N-methyltransferase inhibitor on locomotor activity in rats: The role of central α_2-adrenoceptor and PNMT activity**
M. Nakagawara, Japan

TU.03.04 **Neuroendocrine studies of the mechanism of action of antidepressant drugs**
S. A. Checkley, E. Palazidou, A. Papadopoulos, C. Franey and J. Arendt, United Kingdom

TU.03.05 **Neuroendocrinological and pharmacotherapeutic effects of NA-reuptake inhibition**
G. Laakmann, A. Hinz, H. Neuhauser, M. Ortner, U. Voderholzer and R. Meissner, Fed. Rep. of Germany

TU.03.06 **Levoprotilin-clinical therapeutic efficacy and tolerability**
G. Wendt, Fed. Rep. of Germany

TU.03.07 **α_2-adrenoceptors, opiate receptors, and serum-N-methyltransferase activity in depression and hypertension**
N. Matussek, Fed. Rep. of Germany

SYMPOSIUM

Possibilities and Limitations to Accomplish Regeneration and Restoration of Function in the CNS

Chair: H. Thoenen, Fed. Rep. of Germany, and G. Toffano, Italy

---

TU.04.01 **Spatial memory impairments and cholinergic neuron atrophy in aged rats: Effects of nerve growth factor**
A. Björklund, W. Fischer and F. H. Gage, Sweden

TU.04.02 **Regulation of nerve growth (NGF) synthesis: Comparison between the peripheral and central nervous system**
H. Thoenen, D. Lindholm, C. Bandtlow, B. Hengerer, R. Heumann, M. Meyer and M. Spranger, Fed. Rep. of Germany

TU.04.03 **Activation of beta-adrenergic or prostaglandin receptor increases NGF mRNA content in C6-2B astrocytoma cells**
R. Dal Toso, G. Toffano, I. Mocchetti, M. A. De Bernardi, A. M. Szekely and E. Costa, Italy

TU.04.04 **Factors influencing post-lesion axonal reelongation of adult retina ganglion cells**
S. Thanos, Fed. Rep. of Germany

TU.04.05 **Oligodendrocytes and myelin inhibit growth of neurites in the mammalian CNS**
M. E. Schwab, T. Savio and P. Caroni, Switzerland

Final remarks
G. Toffano, Italy

SYMPOSIUM

New Approaches to the Treatment of Anxiety and Anxiety Disorders

Chair: W. Haefely, Switzerland, and M.-H. Thiébot, France

TU.05.01 **Animal models of anxiety: How predictive are they for anxiolytic activity?**
M.-H. Thiébot and P. Soubrié, France

TU.05.02 **The concept of benzodiazepine receptor partial agonists: Imidazobenzodiazepinones**
W. Haefely, Switzerland

TU.05.03 **Benzodiazepine receptor partial agonists: β-carbolines**
D. N. Stephens, J. Bondo Hansen, J. Andrews and R. Schmiechen, Fed. Rep. of Germany

TU.05.04 **Imidazoquinolines and pyrimidines: Benzodiazepine receptor ligands with different separations of anxiolytic and CNS depressant effects**
C. R. Gardner, United Kingdom

TU.05.05 **Unique pharmacological profile of ritanserin, the first thymosthenic agent with anxiety reducing properties**
C. J. E. Niemegeers, T. F. Meert, F. Awouters, A. A. H. P. Megens and P. A. J. Janssen, Belgium

TU.05.06 **The potential anxiolytic activity of 5-HT receptor agonists and antagonists**
B. J. Jones, United Kingdom

SYMPOSIUM
PET Imaging in Neurosciences and Psychiatry

Chair: G. C. Sedvall, Sweden, and M. S. Buchsbaum, USA

TU.06.01 **D2-dopamine receptor binding in drug naive schizophrenics**
L. Farde, F.-A. Wiesel, H. Hall, C. Halldin, A.-L. Nordström and G. C. Sedvall, Sweden

TU.06.02 **Dopamine metabolism in brain studied with PET**
K. Leenders, Switzerland

TU.06.03 **Strategies for in vivo quantification of human neuroreceptors by PET**
D. F. Wong, USA

TU.06.04 **Imaging of neuroreceptor functions in opiate GABA transmission by PET**
J. Frost, USA

TU.06.05 **PET analysis of pre- and post-synaptic variables in dopamine transmission**
E. S. Garnett, Canada

TU.06.06 **PET imaging of D-2 receptors in the living baboon or human brain in normal and pathological conditions using 76Br-bromolisuride**
B. Mazière, C. Loc'h, P. Hantraye, O. Stulzaft, J. L. Martinot, A. Syrota and M. Mazière, France

TU.06.07 **Positron emission tomography with 18-F-deoxyglucose in schizophrenia**
M. S. Buchsbaum, J. C. Wu, K. Nuechterlein, S. G. Potkin and W. E. Bunney, USA

SYMPOSIUM
Pharmacological Aspects of Sleep and Sleep Disorders

Chair: E. Rüther, Fed. Rep. of Germany, and P. Laduron, France

TU.08.01 **Sleep intensification by physiological and pharmacological procedures**
A. A. Borbély, Switzerland

TU.08.02 **Sleep and sleep deprivation studies in patients with premenstrual depression**
B. L. Parry, W. B. Mendelson, D. A. Sack, W. B. Duncan and T. A. Wehr, USA

TU.08.03 **Individual differences and hypnotics**
I. Oswald and K. Adam, United Kingdom

TU.08.04 **Some epidemiological aspects of hypnotic research**
M. Partinen, Finland

TU.08.05 **Depression, circadian rhythms and trimipramine**
E. Rüther, Fed. Rep. of Germany

TU.08.06 **The influence of clomipramine on the antidepressant effects of sleep deprivation**
R. van den Hoofdakker and S. Elsenga, The Netherlands

TU.08.07 **Pharmacology of new sleep-improving drugs**
J. M. Stutzmann, P. M. Laduron and J. C. Blanchard, France

SYMPOSIUM
Definition and Phamacological Treatment of Atypical Depression

Chair: D. Klein, USA, and E. S. Paykel, United Kingdom

TU.09.01 **Introduction: The concept of atypical depression**
E. S. Paykel, United Kingdom

TU.09.02 **Moclobemide and diazepam in atypical depression**
J. W. G. Tiller, I. Schweitzer, K. P. Maguire and B. M. Davies, Australia

TU.09.03 **The role of antidepressants and monoamine oxidase inhibitors in the treatment of anxiety and panic**
N. Seivewright and P. J. Tyrer, United Kingdom

TU.09.04 **Multivariate classification of depression and response to MAO-I's**
J. R. T. Davidson, M. Woodbury, S. Zisook and E. Giller, USA

TU.09.05 **Differential response to the MAO-I phenelzine during acute, continuation, and maintenance treatment of depression**
D. S. Robinson, S. Lerfeld, D. Laux and B. Bennett, USA

TU.09.06 **Discontinuing antidepressants in atypical depressives**
M. R. Liebowitz, W. Harrison, J. Stewart, P. McGrath, S. Wager, E. Nunes, E. Tricamo and F. Quitkin, USA

TU.09.07 **The limits of atypical depression**
D. F. Klein and F. Quitkin, USA

SYMPOSIUM

Recent Progress in the Treatment of Epilepsy – Experimental and Clinical Aspects

Chair: A. Delini-Stula, Switzerland, and M. Sato, Japan

TU.10.01 **New trends in the development of antiepileptic drugs**
R. Porter, USA

TU.10.02 **Experimental models of epilepsy: Trends and rationale**
M. Schmutz, V. Baltzer, R. Bernasconi, K. Klebs and H. R. Olpe, Switzerland

TU.10.03 **Ecitatory amino acids and kindling**
M. Sato and K. Morimoto, Japan

TU.10.04 **Epilepsy and affective disorders – is there a relationship?**
M. R. Trimble and M. M. Robertson, United Kingdom

TU.10.05 **Cognitive functions and epilepsy – current progress in psychological testing**
W. C. J. Alpherts, A. P. Aldenkamp, The Netherlands

TU.10.06 **Optimization of the therapy with antiepileptic drugs**
G. Krämer, Fed. Rep. of Germany

General discussion and conclusions
A. Delini-Stula, Switzerland

SYMPOSIUM
Molecular Biology in Neurology and Psychiatry

Chair: J. Mendlewicz, Belgium, and G. Racagni, Italy

TU.16.01 **Comparative mapping in mouse of DNA markers from the vicinity of 2 disease loci, Huntington Chorea and familial Alzheimer's disease**
S. V. Cheng and J. F. Gusella, USA

TU.16.02 **Genetic linkage analysis in familial Alzheimer's disease**
C. van Broeckhoven, J. Gheuens, J. J. Martin and A. Vandenberghe, Belgium

TU.16.03 **Molecular genetics of catecholamines as an approach of the biochemistry of manic-depression**
J. Mallet, France

TU.16.04 **Molecular genetic approach in affective illness**
J. Mendlewicz, Belgium

TU.16.05 **Molecular genetic studies of affective disorders**
M. Baron, USA

TU.16.06 **Linkage and association studies in manic-depressive illness and schizophrenia**
E. S. Gershon, S. Detera-Wadleigh, M. R. Hoehe and W. H. Berrettini, USA

TU.16.07 **Localization of a single major locus involved in the genetic aetiology of schizophrenia**
H. M. D. Gurling, R. Sherrington, J. Brynjolfsson and H. Petursson, United Kingdom

SYMPOSIUM
Anti-Schizophrenic Drugs – Long-Term-Effects and Alternative Strategies

Chair: C. A. Marsden, United Kingdom, and C. A. Tamminga, USA

TU.17.01 **Sigma, PCP and glutamate sites as novel targets for antipsychotic drugs**
S. M. Stahl, United Kingdom

TU.17.02 **Schizophrenia, long-term neuroleptic treatment and mechanism of late-onset side effects**
J. L. Waddington, E. O'Callaghan and C. Larkin, Ireland

TU.17.03 **Dopamine D-1 vs D-2 receptor antagonists in schizophrenia. Relation to therapeutic effect and acute/tardive dyskinesia**
J. Gerlach and H. Lublin, Denmark

TU.17.04 **Studies of neuroleptic non-response**
B. Angrist and A. Wolkin, USA

TU.17.05 **Dopamine agonists in the treatment of schizophrenia**
C. A. Tamminga and G. K. Thaker, USA

TU.17.06 **Modulation of mesolimbic dopamine function by neurotensin**
C. A. Marsden, A. P. D. Ford and G. W. Bennett, United Kingdom

TU.17.07 **Acute and subchronic effects of low-dose bromocriptine in haloperidol-treated schizophrenics**
W. F. Gattaz, W. Rost, C. v. K. Hübner and K. Bauer, Fed. Rep. of Germany

SYMPOSIUM
New Reversible MAO-Inhibitors

Chair: G. D. Burrows, Australia, and M. Da Prada, Switzerland

---

TU.18.01 **An overview of monoamine oxidase inhibitors**
G. D. Burrows, T. R. Norman, I. M. McIntire and F. K. Judd, Australia

TU.18.02 **Preclinical profiles of the novel reversible MAO-A inhibitors moclobemide and brofaromine: Comparison with irreversible inhibitors**
M. Da Prada, R. Kettler, H. H. Keller and W. Burkard, Switzerland

TU.18.03 **Tyramine potentiation during treatment with MAO inhibitors: Brofaromine and moclobemide vs irreversible inhibitors**
P. R. Bieck and K. H. Antonin, Fed. Rep. of Germany

TU.18.04 **Brofaromine (MAO-A-inhibitor): Summary of dosefinding studies in major (endogenous) and other (non-endogenous) depressions**
W. Schiwy, A. Delini-Stula and W. R. Heath, Switzerland

TU.18.05 **Moclobemide and maprotiline in the treatment of inpatients with major depressive disorder**
G. Laux and H. Beckmann, Fed. Rep. of Germany

TU.18.06 **Monoamine oxidase, monoamine oxidase inhibitors and panic disorders**
T. R. Norman, G. D. Burrows, F. K. Judd and I. M. McIntyre, Australia

TU.18.07 **Moclobemide, imipramine and placebo in the treatment of outpatients with major depressive disorders (DSM III-R)**
M. Versiani, F. Mundim, A. Nardi and A. Alves, Brazil

TU.18.08 **Review of comparitive clinical trials. Moclobemide vs other antidepressants and vs placebo in depressive states**
M. Stabl and K. Bizière, Switzerland

TU.18.09 **The effects of moclobemide on cognition**
K. A. Wesnes, P. M. Simpson, L. Christmas, R. Anand and G. R. McClelland, United Kingdom

TU.18.10 **Possible trends for therapeutic and clinical research**
K. Bizière, Switzerland

SYMPOSIUM
Calcium as a Second Messenger and Calcium Antagonists

Chair: D. Ploog, Fed. Rep. of Germany, and M. Trabucci, Italy

---

TU.19.01 **The role of calcium-dependent processes in psychic disorder**
J. B. Aldenhoff, Fed. Rep. of Germany

TU.19.02 Withdrawn

TU.19.03 **Calcium channels and protein kinase C in central neurotransmitter release**
D. J. Dooley, USA

TU.19.04 **Calcium channels and calcium antagonists in neural systems**
H. Glossmann, J. Striessnig, H. G. Knaus and G. Zernig, Austria

TU.19.05 **Anaesthetic-potentiating actions of dihydropyriodines**
G. Hempelmann, Fed. Rep. of Germany

TU.19.06 **Types and pharmacological properties of neuronal Ca channels**
H. D. Lux, Fed. Rep. of Germany

TU.19.07 **The action of calcium antagonists on neuronal behaviour, relevance for epileptogenic features**
E. J. Speckmann, J. Walden and D. Bingmann, Fed. Rep. of Germany

TU.19.08 **In vitro and in vivo modulation of dihydropyridine receptors**
M. Trabucci, S. Govoni and M. Parenti, Italy

SYMPOSIUM

Anxiety and Anxiety Disorders – Clinical Research

Chair: G. L. Klerman, USA, and G. B. Cassano, Italy

TU.20.01 **Diagnosis and nosology of anxiety disorders**
A. Jablensky, Bulgaria

TU.20.02 **Neuroanatomical correlates of lactate-induced panic and anticipatory fear**
E. M. Reiman, M. E. Raichle, E. Robins, M. Fusselman, M. Mintun, P. Fox and J. Price, USA

TU.20.03 **Combined behavioural and pharmacological treatments of panic/agoraphobia**
M. R. Mavissakalian, USA

TU.20.04 **Drug treatment of panic disorder: Comparative efficacy of alprazolam, imipramine and placebo**
Sir Martin Roth, United Kingdom

TU.20.05 **Pharmacological and biochemical approaches to panic and anxiety disorders**
M. Ackenheil, M. Albus, B. Bondy and R. Engel, Fed. Rep. of Germany

Discussant
J. Costa e Silva, Brazil

SYMPOSIUM

Topographic EEG- and EP-Mapping in Neuropsychopharmacology

Chair: B. Saletu, Austria, and D. Lehmann, Switzerland

TU.21.01 **Mapping and analysis of ERP and EEG spectral power data**
D. Lehmann, Switzerland

TU.21.02 **On some approaches to quantifying EEG effects in multilead recordings**
R. Coppola, W. M. Herrmann and J. Röhmel, USA

TU.21.03 **Quantitative pharmaco electroencephalography and topographic mapping in evaluation of mild psychotropic property**
M. Saito, T. Kinoshita, O. Okajima, A. Saito and K. Nobuhara, Japan

TU.21.04 **Topographic brain mapping of EEG in diagnosis and treatment of MID and SDAT**
B. Saletu, P. Anderer, E. Paulus, J. Grünberger, L. Wicke, P.K. Fischhof, G. Wagner, G. Litschauer, R. Hatzinger and R. Dittrich, Austria

TU.21.05 **Mapping of evoked potentials in psychosis and dementia and their treatment**
K. Maurer, T. Dierks and R. Ihl, Fed. Rep. of Germany

TU.21.06 **Neurometric analysis of drugs effects in schizophrenic patients**
E. R. John, L. S. Prichep, J. Volavka and T. Essig-Peppard, USA

TU.21.07 **Correlative application of EEG and rCBF mapping in human neuropsychopharmacology**
G. Rosadini, G. Rodriguez and W. G. Sannita, Italy

TU.21.08 **Multimodal imaging with PET, MRI and EEG: Impact on psychiatry**
M. S. Buchsbaum, J. C. Wu and S. Guich, USA

SYMPOSIUM
The Thyroid Axis in Basic and Clinical Research

Chair: A. J. Prange, USA, and G. Laakmann, Fed. Rep. of Germany

---

TU.22.01 **Thyroid hormones in endogenous depression: Metabolism and the levels in cerebrospinal fluid**
C. Kirkegaard, A. Kørner and J. Faber, Denmark

TU.22.02 **TRH-induced TSH response in psychiatric patients**
P. T. Loosen, USA

TU.22.03 **The TSH-response to TRH: What does it tell us?**
G. Schönbeck, R. Hatzinger, G. Koinig and G. Langer, Austria

TU.22.04 **The simultaneous use of four releasing factors: Practical and theoretical issues**
G. Laakmann, A. Hinz, H. Neuhauser, O. A. Müller, O. Voderholzer, C. Linnenkohl, C. Daffner and M. Winkelmann, Fed. Rep. of Germany

TU.22.05 **Thyroid axis function and rapid cycling bipolar disorder**
P. C. Whybrow and M. Bauer, USA

TU.22.06 **Alcoholism and the thyroid axis**
J. C. Garbutt and A. J. Prange, USA

TU.22.07 **Subclinical hypothyroidism in psychiatric patients: Do small changes make big differences?**
J. J. Haggerty and A. J. Prange, USA

TU.22.08 **Antithyroid antibodies: Behavioural significance**
V. I. Reus, USA

SYMPOSIUM

GABA-Receptors – Structure, Function, Modulation

Chair: A. Guidotti, USA, and H. Möhler, Switzerland

TU.23.01 **Molecular mechanisms underlying GABA receptor function in the mammalian central nervous system**
J. Bormann, Fed. Rep. of Germany

TU.23.02 **The pre- and postsynaptic actions of baclofen may involve different $GABA_B$ receptor subtypes**
R. A. Nicoll and P. Dutar, USA

TU.23.03 **The molecular biology of the $GABA_A$ receptor**
P. H. Seeburg, P. R. Schofield, D. B. Pritchett, S. Ymer, A. Draguhn, H. Sontheimer, M. Köhler, P. Werner, H. Kettenmann and B. D. Shivers, Fed. Rep. of Germany

TU.23.04 **Molecular pharmacology of the $GABA_A$/benzodiazepine receptor**
H. Möhler, Switzerland

TU.23.05 **Modulation of (γ-aminobutyric acid) GABA receptors**
E. Costa, USA

TU.23.06 **Changes in the function of GABA dependent chloride channel after in vivo inhibition of GABAergic synapses**
G. Biggio, Italy

SYMPOSIUM

Disentagling Emotions, Neurochemistry and Specificity of Drug Treatment in the Affective Disorders

Chair: M. M. Katz and S. H. Koslow, USA

TU.24.01 **Tricyclic drug plasma concentrations and associations with specific affect components in depression**
M. M. Katz, S. H. Koslow, J. W. Maas, A. Frazer, J. Kocsis, J. Secunda, C. L. Bowden and R. C. Casper, USA

TU.24.02 **Linkage between depression, emotions, catecholamines and treatment with tricyclic antidepressants**
S. H. Koslow, J. W. Maas, C. Bowden, P. Stokes, J. Davies and M. M. Katz, USA

TU.24.03 **Functional versus nosological specificity of biological variables in behavioural disorders**
H. M. Praag, USA

TU.24.04 **Dementia disorders and depression in the elderly. Biochemical aspects**
C. G. Gottfries, Sweden

Discussant
P. Kielholz, Switzerland

SYMPOSIUM
Endogenous Ligands for Psychotropic Drug Receptors

Chair: A. Herz, Fed. Rep. of Germany, and M. Barbaccia, USA

WE.01.01 **Opioid peptides as endogenous ligands for opioid receptors**
A. Herz, Fed. Rep. of Germany

WE.01.02 **Motivational properties of opioid peptides**
T. S. Shippenberg, Fed. Rep. of Germany

WE.01.03 **Mechanisms of interaction of endogenous and exogenous phencyclidine (PCP) receptor ligands with the N-methyl-D-aspartate receptor/channel complex**
S. R. Zukin and D. C. Javitt, USA

WE.01.04 **Putative endogenous modulators of $GABA_A$/benzodiazepine receptors**
A. Guidotti, USA

WE.01.05 **Endogenous modulations of cocaine binding sites in caudate nucleus**
I. Hanbauer, M. Grilli and E. Sanna, USA

WE.01.06 **Endogenous ligands for imipramine recognition sites**
M. L. Barbaccia, USA

SYMPOSIUM

Biochemical and Morphological Research in Schizophrenia – Recent Advances and New Theories

Chair: A. Carlsson, Sweden, and P. Rakic, USA

Introductory remarks
A. Carlsson, Sweden

WE.02.01 **Genetic and epigenetic regulation of cortical development**
P. Rakic, USA

WE.02.02 **Cortical networks and higher brain function: Relevances to schizophrenia**
P. Goldman-Rakic, USA

WE.02.03 **In vivo physiological and anatomical studies of brain pathology in schizophrenia: A neurodevelopmental perspective**
D. R. Weinberger, USA

WE.02.04 **Clinical perspectives on the mechanism of neuroleptic action**
D. Pickar, USA

WE.02.05 **Regional cerebral metabolic response to PCP receptor stimulation: Delineation of psychosis pathway(s) in schizophrenia**
C. A. Tamminga, H. Kaneda, S. Kuo and G. Thaker, USA

WE.02.06 **Role of dopamine in the interaction between cortical and subcortical mechanisms**
A. Carlsson, Sweden

Concluding remarks
P. Rakic, USA

SYMPOSIUM

Monoamine Transporters as Targets for Antidepressant Drugs

Chair: S. Z. Langer, France, and I. Kopin, USA

WE.03.01 **Characterization of the serotonin (5-HT) transporter and its interaction with antidepressant drugs**
S. Z. Langer, C. Lee and D. Graham, France

WE.03.02 **Light-dark related changes in 5-HT-uptake/^{3}H-imipramine binding molecular complex in rat brain: Involvement in antidepressant mode of action**
A. C. Rovescalli, M. Brunello, M. Riva, R. Galimberti and G. Racagni, Italy

WE.03.03 **Drug structure as a determinant of specificity among uptake inhibitors: Emphasis on fluoxetine and tomoxetine**
R. W. Fuller and D. T. Wong, USA

WE.03.04 **Long-term activation of the [^{3}H]IMI site induces a desensitization of terminal 5-HT autoreceptors**
C. de Montigny, Y. Chaput and P. Blier, Canada

WE.03.05 **Serotonin uptake and imipramine binding in major depression and suicide**
F. J. Nash, R. C. Arora, P. Ambrosini and H. Y. Meltzer, USA

WE.03.06 **GABAergic/monoaminergic interactions and depression**
K. G. Lloyd, P. Pichat, B. Scatton, B. Zivkovic, P. L. Morselli and G. Bartholini, France

SYMPOSIUM
Neurobiology of Aging (in Relation to Alzheimer's Disease)

Chair: C. G. Gottfries, Sweden, and D. Perl, USA

WE.04.01 **Neocortical morphology and morphometry in normal aging and Alzheimer's disease**
R. D. Terry, USA

WE.04.02 **Etiologic mechanisms of Alzheimer's disease: A discussion of current concepts**
D. P. Perl, USA

WE.04.03 **Mechanisms of neuronal degeneration in cerebral aging and degenerative dementia of Alzheimer type**
S. Hoyer, Fed. Rep. of Germany

WE.04.04 **Fibroblast lactate and glycolitic enzymes in familial Alzheimer's disease**
L. Amaducci, S. Sorbi, S. Tonini, S. Piacentini and C. Fani, Italy

WE.04.05 **Monoamine oxidase activities in relation to normal aging and states of dementia**
L. Oreland, Y. Hiraga, S. S. Jossan, B. Regland and C. G. Gottfries, Sweden

WE.04.06 **Neurotransmitter changes in the normally aged brain in relation to AD/SDAT**
C. G. Gottfries, Sweden

WE.04.07 **The human hypothalamus in aging and Alzheimer's disease**
D. F. Swaab, E. Goudsmit and M. A. Hofman, The Netherlands

WE.04.08 **Hopes and limitations in geriatric psychopharmacology**
C. Giurgea, Belgium

SYMPOSIUM
New Findings with Anxiolytic Drugs

Chair: S. Gershon, USA, and J. Bruinvels, The Netherlands

WE.05.01 **Animal models for anxiety and response to serotonergic drugs**
C. L. E. Broekkamp and F. Jenck, The Netherlands

WE.05.02 **The new generation of serotonergic anxiolytics and their possible clinical roles**
M. S. Eison, USA

WE.05.03 **Serotonin-Ia agonists: An overview of anxiolytic activity**
J. P. Feighner and W. F. Boyer, USA

WE.05.04 **Serotonergic (5-HT) anxiolytics and treatment of depression**
D. S. Robinson, J. E. Copp, R. C. Shrotriya and D. L. Roberts, USA

WE.05.05 **Interrelationship of anxiety: Serotonin and alcoholism**
G. D. Tollefson, USA

WE.05.06 **Buspirone in the treatment of alcoholic patients**
F. Bruno, Italy

WE.05.07 **Serotonergic anxiolytics in the treatment of panic disorder**
R. Pohl, R. Balon, V. K. Yeragani and S. Gershon, USA

WE.05.08 **Serotonin uptake inhibitors and agonists in the treatment of panic disorder**
H. G. M. Westenberg and J. A. Den Boer, The Netherlands

SYMPOSIUM
WHO Multicentre Studies

Chair: P. Kielholz, Switzerland, and N. Sartorius, WHO

WE.06.01 **WHO collaborative activities in the field of biological psychiatry and psychopharmacology: 20 years of experience**
L. Prilipko, Switzerland

WE.06.02 **Chronobiological aspects of affective illness: A WHO collaborative study**
J. Mendlewicz, Belgium

WE.06.03 **Substance use (alcohol and drugs): Psychopathological and biological aspects**
C. N. Stefanis and I. Yamashita, Greece

WE.06.04 **Lithium prophylaxis: Situational analysis and perspectives**
M. E. Vartanian, E. Mellerup and D. Moussaoui, USSR

WE.06.05 **The validity of platelet ^{3}H-imipramine binding as a marker in depression**
S. G. Potkin, S. Z. Langer and E. Mellerup, USA

WE.06.06 **Treatment strategies in ICD-10 acute delusional disorder**
M. Maj, J. R. de la Fuente and D. Kemali, Italy

SYMPOSIUM

Biological Markers of Affective Disorders – Impact of Basic Neuroendocrine and Sleep Research

Chair: F. Holsboer, Fed. Rep. of Germany, and D. J. Kupfer, USA

WE.07.01 **Sleep-physiologic characteristics as potential biological markers in the affective disorders**
D. J. Kupfer, E. Frank and C. L. Ehlers, USA

WE.07.02 **The cholinergic-noradrenergic imbalance hypothesis of affective disorders**
M. Berger, D. Riemann, W. Müller, W. F. Gattaz and P. Fleckenstein, Fed. Rep. of Germany

WE.07.03 **Clinical implications of altered neurohormonal regulation in the affective disorders**
F. Holsboer, Fed. Rep. of Germany

WE.07.04 **Differential effects of adrenal steroids as modulators of central nerve cell function**
E. R. De Kloet, The Netherlands

WE.07.05 **The role of corticotropin-releasing factor (CRF) in the pathogenesis of depression**
C. B. Nemeroff, M. J. Owens and G. Bissette, USA

WE.07.06 **Molecular mechanisms controlling POMC expression and ACTH release**
T. Reisine, N. Margolis and K. Thermos, USA

SYMPOSIUM
D-1 and D-2 Dopamine Receptor Motor Effects

Chair: D. Casey, USA, and D. Hornykiewicz, Austria

WE.08.01 **Multiple forms of functional interactions between D-1 and D-2 dopamine receptor systems in the regulation of motor behaviour**
J. L. Waddington and A. M. Murray, Ireland

WE.08.02 **EEDQ-induced inactivation of dopamine D-1 or D-2 receptors in rats differentially inhibits stereotyped behaviour mediated by D-1/D-2 receptor interaction**
J. Arnt and J. Hyttel, Denmark

WE.08.03 **D-1 and D-2 dopamine receptor-mediated effects on basal ganglia output: Single unit recording studies**
J. Walters and B. G. Weick, USA

WE.08.04 **D-1 and D-2 agonist and antagonist motor effects in nonhuman primates**
D. E. Casey, USA

WE.08.05 **Effects of dopamine (DA) receptor agonists and antagonists in MPTP-pretreated and haloperidol-sensitized Rhesus monkeys**
G. Schingnitz, Fed. Rep. of Germany

WE.08.06 **Effects of B-HT 920 on pre- and postsynaptic dopamine receptors**
N.-E. Andén, Sweden

SYMPOSIUM
Therapeutic Issues in Biopolar Disorder

Chair: T. Silverstone, United Kingdom, and J. Angst, Switzerland

WE.09.01 **Switch rates from depression to mania in Switzerland from 1900–1980**
J. Angst, K. Angst and A. Graf-Nold, Switzerland

WE.09.02 **Thyroid function and susceptibility to relapse**
J. C. Cookson, United Kingdom

WE.09.03 **Lithium non-responders**
T. R. Silverstone and N. Coxhead, United Kingdom

WE.09.04 **Calcium and calcium antagonists in mania**
T. Dinan, Ireland

WE.09.05 **The switch process**
M. Haag, Fed. Rep. of Germany

WE.09.06 **Changing sensitivity to drugs in bipolar illness**
R. M. Post, S. R. B. Weiss and L. Altshuler, USA

SYMPOSIUM

Peripheral Cells as Pharmacological Models in Psychiatry Research

Chair: M. Ackenheil, Fed. Rep. of Germany, and E. T. Mellerup, Denmark

---

WE.16.01 **Lymphozyte cholinergic receptor changes in Alzheimer's disease**
A. Adem, Sweden

WE.16.02 **Clinical subtype of Alzheimer's disease identified by altered platelet membrane fluidity**
G. S. Zubenko, USA

WE.16.03 **Characterization of a D-1 dopamine receptor in cell membranes from fresh human lymphocytes and EBV-transformed lymphoblastoid cells: Stereospecific, saturable and high-affinity binding of [125 I]SCH 23982**
R. Ebstein, Israel

WE.16.04 **^{3}H-spiperone binding to lymphocytes in neuropsychiatric disorders**
B. Bondy, W. Oertel and M. Ackenheil, Fed. Rep. of Germany

WE.16.05 **Platelet binding sites for serotonin uptake inhibition**
P. Plenge and E. T. Mellerup, Denmark

WE.16.06 **Beta adrenergic receptors in manic-depressive illness: Functional and molecular genetic studies with peripheral cells**
W. A. Berrettini, M. R. Hoehe, K.-U. Lentes, L. R. Goldin, J. C. Venter and E. S. Gershon, USA

WE.16.07 **Receptors on blood cells: Changes in depression, mania and panic attack**
B. E. Leonard, Ireland

WE.16.08 **Platelet monoamine receptor binding and tricyclic antidepressant treatment**
P. J. Cowen, United Kingdom

SYMPOSIUM
Noradrenergic Function in Schizophrenia

Chair: D. P. van Kammen, USA, and D. Kemali, Italy

WE.17.01 **Selective beta-blockade in akathisia. Clonidine treatment of schizophrenia**
B. Angrist, L. Adler, T. Kim, E. Duncan, E. Peselow and J. Rotrosen, USA

WE.17.02 **Behavioural neuronal and chemical determinants of locus coeruleus activity: Functional implications**
G. Aston-Jones, M. Ennis, V. Pieribone and M. Shipley, USA

WE.17.03 **Possibilities for involvement of brain noradrenaline in schizophrenia**
O. Hornykiewicz, Austria

WE.17.04 **Peripheral NE, alpha-adrenergic receptor sensitivity and their relation to psychotic schizophrenic states**
R. Müller-Spahn, M. Ackenheil, M. Albus, B. Bondy and G. Kurtz, Fed. Rep. of Germany

WE.17.05 **Noradrenalin in the cerebrospinal fluid of schizophrenics and healthy controls**
W. F. Gattaz, P. Riederer, G. P. Reynolds and H. Beckmann, Fed. Rep. of Germany

WE.17.06 **Factors associated with increased noradrenaline levels in cerebrospinal fluid of schizophrenic patients**
D. Kemali, M. Maj, S. Galderisi and M. G. Ariano, Italy

WE.17.07 **Elevated CSF NE in schizophrenia: Cause or effect of relapse?**
D. P. van Kammen, J. Peters, K. Goetz, W. B. van Kammen, D. Shaw and J. Yao, USA

SYMPOSIUM
Novel Antidepressants – Methyl Donors and Reuptake Inhibitors

Chair: S. G. Potkin and A. Frazer, USA

WE.18.01 **S-adenosylmethionine: Overview of clinical and pharmacological effects**
S. G. Potkin and K. M. Bell, USA

WE.18.02 **S-adenosylmethionine in the treatment of depression**
K. M. Bell and S. G. Potkin, USA

WE.18.03 **Pharmacology of S-adenosylmethionine in central nervous system**
G. Stramentinoli and V. Olgiati, Italy

WE.18.04 **Clinical efficacy of serotonin receptor inhibitors**
K. Rickels, USA

WE.18.05 **Preclinical pharmacology of selective serotonin uptake inhibitors: A new generation of antidepressants**
J. Heym and B. K. Koe, USA

WE.18.06 **Electrophysiological determination of the efficacy of 5-HT neurotransmission following repeated 5-HT reuptake blocker treatment**
C. de Montigny, P. Blier and Y. Chaput, Canada

WE.18.07 **Effect of antidepressant drugs on subtypes of central beta adrenoceptors: A quantitative autoradiographic study**
A. Frazer, C. Gambarana and G. A. Ordway, USA

SYMPOSIUM
New Drugs in Memory and Learning

Chair: L. Maitre, Switzerland, and G. Pepeu, Italy

WE.19.01 **The effects of nootropics on memory**
C. Mondadori, F. Petschke and A. Haeussler, Switzerland

WE.19.02 **Long term potentiation and memory mechanisms: Effects of cognition-enhancing agents**
Y. Ben-Ari, France

WE.19.03 **Experimental evidences of oxiracetam direct activity on memory mechanisms**
F. Ponzio, O. Pozzi, S. Banfi and L. Dorigotti, Italy

WE.19.04 **The relationship between the behavioural effects of cognition enhancing drugs and brain acetylcholine**
G. Pepeu, G. Spignoli, M. G. Giovannini and M. Magnani, Italy

WE.19.05 **Neurotropic factors in cellular, functional and cognitive repair of adult brain**
S. Varon, USA

WE.19.06 **Effects of phosphatidylserine administration on age-related changes of the septo-hippocampal system in the rat**
M. G. Nunzi, F. Milan, D. Guidolin, P. Polato and G. Toffano, Italy

WE.19.07 **Pharmacological treatment strategies in dementia disorders**
C. G. Gottfries, Sweden

SYMPOSIUM
Psychopharmacology of Aggression

Chair: M. Sandler, United Kingdom, and B. Eichelman, USA

WE.20.01 Withdrawn

WE.20.02 **Alcohol-hormonal mechanisms of aggressive behaviour**
J. de Bold, USA

WE.20.03 **Drugs of abuse and aggressive behaviour**
K. Miczek, USA

WE.20.04 **A new nosology for human destructive (aggressive) behaviour**
B. Eichelman, USA

WE.20.05 **Use of beta blockers to treat destructive behaviour**
J. Ratey, USA

Discussant
M. Sandler, United Kingdom

SYMPOSIUM
Prediction of Response to Psychotropic Agents

Chair: B. Müller-Oerlinghausen, Fed. Rep. of Germany, and G. Simpson, USA

WE.21.01 **Neuroleptic drugs as maintenance therapy**
J. M. Kane, USA

WE.21.02 **Clinical, pharmacokinetic and neurophysiological predictors of acute response to neuroleptic drugs**
W. Gaebel, A. Pietzcker, G. Ulrich, J. Schley and B. Müller-Oerlinghausen, Fed. Rep. of Germany

WE.21.03 **Trial with high neuroleptic plasma concentrations in chronic schizophrenia**
S. J. Dencker, Sweden

WE.21.04 **Akathisia as a predictor of outcome in neuroleptic treatment**
G. M. Simpson, D. F. Levinson, H. Singh, M. J. Stephanos and K. G. Yadalam, USA

WE.21.05 **Prediction of acute response towards antidepressant drug treatment**
H. J. Möller, Fed. Rep. of Germany

WE.21.06 **Prediction of benefit from stabilizing lithium treatment**
P. Grof and E. Grof, Canada

SYMPOSIUM
Acetylcholine and Muscarinic Receptors

Chair: D. Janowsky, USA, and M. Berger, Fed. Rep. of Germany

WE.22.01 **Are shortened REM latencies in depression a consequence of muscarinic receptor supersensivity?**
M. Berger, D. Riemann, C. Benz and P. Fleckenstein, Fed. Rep. of Germany

WE.22.02 **Neurobiologic effects of bright artificial light**
S. C. Dilsaver, USA

WE.22.03 **Neurochemical imbalances in lines of rats differing in cholinergic sensitivity**
A. D. Crocker and D. H. Overstreet, Australia

WE.22.04 **Modulation of central transmitter release by subtypes of muscarinic presynaptic receptors**
M. Raiteri, M. Marchi, P. Boccieri and L. Garbarino, Italy

WE.22.05 **ACH supersensivity: A genetic risk factor for depression?**
S. Dube, USA

WE.22.06 **Acetylcholine and stress, clinical studies**
D. Janowsky, USA

WE.22.07 **Muscarinic receptor, plasticity and aging**
W. E. Müller, Fed. Rep. of Germany

SYMPOSIUM
Central and Peripheral Dopamine Receptor Mechanisms

Chair: P. F. Spano, Italy, and M. Karobath, Switzerland

WE.23.01 **Peripheral DA receptors**
L. I. Goldberg, USA

WE.23.02 **Electrophysiological studies of dopamine autoreceptor/ postsynaptic D-2 receptor differences**
J. Walters, D. A. Bergstrom, M. Beninato, H. S. Pan and J. H. Carlson, USA

WE.23.03 **Transduction mechanisms of central and peripheral dopamine receptors**
P. F. Spano, M. Pizzi, C. Missale, A. Valerio, L. Castelletti and M. Memo, Italy

WE.23.04 **Partial brain dopamine D-2 receptor agonists**
M. Karobath, Switzerland

WE.23.05 **Distribution and cellular localization of dopamine receptors in the animal and human brain studied by autoradiography**
J. M. Palacios, Switzerland

WE.23.06 **Effects of the atypical neuroleptics clozapine and fluperlapine on the in vivo DA-release in the dorsal striatum and in the prefrontal cortex**
A. Imperato and L. Angelucci, Italy

WE.23.07 **PET examination of human D-1 and D-2 dopamine receptor characteristics**
L. Farde, F.-A. Wiesel, A.-L. Nordström and G. C. Sedvall, Sweden

SYMPOSIUM
Obsessive Compulsive Disorder

Chair: J. J. López-Ibor, Spain, and S. A. Montgomery, United Kingdom

---

WE.24.01 **What biological treatment teaches about the psychopathology of obsessive-compulsive disorders**
J. J. López-Ibor, Spain

WE.24.02 **Clomipramine, self-exposure and therapists-aided exposure for obsessive-compulsive rituals**
I. M. Marks, P. Lelliott, M. Basoglu, H. Noshirvani, W. Monteiro, D. Cohen and Y. Kasvikis, United Kingdom

WE.24.03 **A multi-center trial of anafranil (clomipramine) in obsessive compulsive disorder (OCD)**
J. DeVeaugh-Geiss, R. Katz and P. Landau, USA

WE.24.04 **Serotonergic challenges in obsessive-compulsive disorders**
D. Murphy, USA

Discussant
E. Cuenca, Spain

SYMPOSIUM
Brain Transplants in Neurology and Psychiatry

Chair: R. J. Wyatt, USA, and A. Björklund, Sweden

TH.01.01 **Experience with adrenal medulla autografts to Rhesus monkey striatum**
R. J. Wyatt, USA

TH.01.02 **Transplantation of fetal substantia nigra into striatum of MPTP treated parkinsonian monkeys normalizes dopamine measures and behavioural function**
D. E. Redmond, J. R. Taylor, J. R. Sladek, J. D. Elsworth, T. J. Collier, V. O. Lewis, P. N. Foster, J. P. Blount and R. H. Roth, USA

TH.01.03 **Long term (more than one year) evolution of patients with adrenal medullary grafts to the caudate nucleus for the treatment of Parkinson's disease**
I. Madrazo, R. Drucker-Colin, C. Torres, F. Ostrosky and R. E. Franco-Bourland, Mexico

TH.01.04 **Neural grafting in an animal model of Huntington's disease**
A. Björklund, K. Wictorin and O. Isacson, Sweden

TH.01.05 **Use of human fetal substantia nigra for grafting in patients with Parkinson's disease**
O. Lindvall, P. Brundin and A. Björklund, Sweden

SYMPOSIUM
New Drugs in the Treatment of Schizophrenia – Pharmacological Aspects

Chair: S. Bischoff, Switzerland, and J. Gerlach, Denmark

TH.02.01 **The dopamine D-1 receptor: A potential target for antipsychotic drugs**
P. H. Andersen and E. B. Nielsen, Denmark

TH.02.02 **Drugs interacting with presynaptic DA receptors**
A. Carlsson, Sweden

TH.02.03 **Savoxepine, a novel antipsychotic agent highly selective for hippocampal dopamine (DA) receptors**
S. Bischoff, Switzerland

TH.02.04 **Potential antischizophrenic activity of serotonin antagonists**
B. Costall, A. M. Domeney, M. E. Kelly and R. J. Naylor, United Kingdom

TH.02.05 **CI-943: A potential antipsychotic agent without dopamine receptor blocking properties**
L. T. Meltzer, T. Heffner, D. Downs, T. Pugsley and L. Wise, USA

TH.02.06 **Isolation and characterization of an endogenous PCP- and sigma-like ligand from porcine and human brains**
P. C. Contreras and D. A. Di Maggio, USA

TH.02.07 **Drugs with desinhibitory properties as potential candidates for treatment of negative symptoms in schizophrenia**
A. J. Puech and S. Ravard, France

Concluding remarks
J. Gerlach, Denmark

SYMPOSIUM
Mood Stabilizing Drugs – Basic Mechanisms

Chair: A. Geisler, Denmark, and R. M. Post, USA

TH.03.01 **The use of anticonvulsants as mood-stabilizers in affective disorders: Psychopharmacological aspects**
H. M. Emrich, M. Dose, R. Wolf, A. Wendl and J. Zihl, Fed. Rep. of Germany

TH.03.02 **Mode of action of lithium on brain adenylate cyclase: In vitro versus ex vivo effects**
A. Mørk and A. Geisler, Denmark

TH.03.03 **Inhibition by lithium of adenylate cyclase may be mediated by lithium inhibition of GTP binding to G protein**
R. H. Belmaker, S. Avissar, G. Schreiber and A. Danon, Israel

TH.03.04 **Effects of lithium treatment on the metabolism of phosphoinositides in human granulocytes**
W. Greil and D. van Calker, Fed. Rep. of Germany

TH.03.05 **Carbamazepine: Mechanisms of action**
R. M. Post and S. R. B. Weiss, USA

TH.03.06 **Protein kinase C in the CNS: A possible site of action for lithium**
R. H. Lenox, D. D. Hendley, Y. Ehrlich and J. Ellis, USA

SYMPOSIUM
The Brain-Immune System Interactions

Chair: A. Pletscher and H. O. Besedovsky, Switzerland

TH.04.01 **Neuroendocrine immunoregulation**
H. O. Besedovsky, Switzerland

TH.04.02 Withdrawn

TH.04.03 **Autonomic nervous system in immunoregulation**
D. L. Felten, USA

TH.04.04 **Brain effect on immune processes**
M. Stein, USA

TH.04.05 **Neurotransmitters and neuropeptide receptors in the immune system**
H. Ovadia, Israel

TH.04.06 **Interconnection between the brain and the immune system**
C. J. Heijnen, A. Kavelaars and R. E. Ballieux, The Netherlands

SYMPOSIUM
Benzodiazepines: Long-Term Treatment Dependency and Alternatives

Chair: M. H. Lader, United Kingdom, and H. Helmchen, Fed. Rep. of Germany

---

TH.05.01 **Behavioural and biochemical aspects of benzodiazepine dependence in the rat**
S. E. File and H. A. Baldwin, United Kingdom

TH.05.02 **Clinical aspects of new anxiolytics**
M. H. Lader, United Kingdom

TH.05.03 **Consequences of long-term benzodiazepine abuse**
C. Schmauss, J.-C. Krieg, S. Apelt and H. M. Emrich, USA

TH.05.04 **Differences between imidazopyridines and benzodiazepines on omega receptor selectivity: Relevance to the effects on long-term administration**
S. Z. Langer, S. Arbilla, D. J. Sanger and B. Zivkovic, France

TH.05.05 **Long-term treatment and abuse problems in patients of doctors in domiciliary practice**
D. Ladewig, Switzerland

TH.05.06 **Who gets benzodiazepines why in private practice?**
M. Linden and B. Geiselmann, Fed. Rep. of Germany

SYMPOSIUM

Implications of Neuroadaptive Responses to Psychotropic Drug Therapy

Chair: D. G. Grahame-Smith, United Kingdom, and Z. Votava, Czechoslovakia

---

TH.06.01 **Neuroadaptive responses to antidepressants and ECT**
A. R. Green, United Kingdom

TH.06.02 **Neuroadaptive responses to lithium**
D. G. Grahame-Smith, United Kingdom

TH.06.03 **Adaptive responses to benzodiazepines in mouse and man**
D. J. Nutt, United Kingdom

TH.06.04 **Neuroadaptive responses to alcohol**
H. Little, United Kingdom

TH.06.05 **Neuroadaptive responses to neuroleptics**
J. L. Waddington, Ireland

TH.06.06 **Clinical manifestation of neuroadaptive responses to psychotropic drugs**
P. J. Cowen, United Kingdom

SYMPOSIUM

Neuropeptides – Basic Research

Chair: W. Zieglgänsberger, Fed. Rep. of Germany, and A. Rossi, Italy

---

TH.07.01 **Neuropeptides 20 years on**
J. Hughes, Switzerland

TH.07.02 **Regulation of opioid peptide gene expression**
V. Höllt, K. Feasey, N. Kley, J. P. Loeffler and B. Morris, Fed. Rep. of Germany

TH.07.03 **Biosynthesis of opioid peptides**
J. Rossier, France

TH.07.04 **VIP neurons and their role in local cortical energy metabolism**
P. Magistretti, P. R. Hof, J.-L. Martin and T. Stoyanov, Switzerland

TH.07.05 **How neuropeptides alter neuronal excitability**
G. R. Siggins, USA

SYMPOSIUM
Lipo- and Cyclo-Oxigenase Derivatives – Role in the CNS

Chair: R. Paoletti, Italy, and F. Dray, France

TH.08.01 **Formation and role of eicosanoids in the central nervous system of rodents**
G. Hertting and A. Seregi, Fed. Rep. of Germany

TH.08.02 **Lipid mediators of cell signal transduction in experimental epilepsy**
N. G. Bazan, USA

TH.08.03 **Lipoxygenase metabolites of arachidonic acid are second messengers of presynaptic inhibition in aplysia sensory neurons**
A. Volterra, S. A. Siegelbaum, D. Sweatt and E. R. Kandel, USA

TH.08.04 **Release of arachidonic acid and its oxygenated derivatives in brain ischemic/hypoxia and recovery: Pharmacological interventions**
C. Galli, A. Petroni, A. Bertazzo and S. Sarti, Italy

TH.08.05 **Roles of CO and LO products in the modulation of neurosecretion in brain**
F. Dray, France

SYMPOSIUM
New Research in Chronobiology of Psychotropic Drugs incl. Melatonin

Chair: A. Wirz-Justice, Switzerland, and T. Wehr, USA

TH.09.01 **What does a chronobiological strategy offer neuropsychopharmacological research?**
A. Wirz-Justice, Switzerland

TH.09.02 **Phase-shifting the circadian clock with short acting benzodiazepines**
F. W. Turek and O. Van Reeth, USA

TH.09.03 **Imipramine treatment affects the circadian pacemaker of the suprachiasmatic nucleus**
J. H. Meijer, The Netherlands

TH.09.04 **Methamphetamine and periodic food restriction; SCN independent circadian oscillations**
S. Honma and K. Honma, Japan

TH.09.05 **Methamphetamine, lithium and light: Modification of circadian rhythms, metabolism and structure of the rat retina**
C. Remé, J. Pfeilschifter and A. Wirz-Justice, Switzerland

TH.09.06 **Therapeutic potential of melatonin**
D. J. Skene, M. E. Aldhous and J. Arendt, United Kingdom

SYMPOSIUM

Drugs Effects and Morphological Investigations in Human Post Mortem Tissue

Chair: H. Beckmann, Fed. Rep. of Germany, and B. Winblad, Sweden

---

TH.16.01 **Neurotransmitter function in post mortem human brain: An overview**
C. Fowler, R. Cowburn, J. Hardy, P. Wester and B. Winblad, Sweden

TH.16.02 **Modulation of cholinergic activity in Alzheimer brains by potential drugs**
A. Nordberg and L. Nilsson, Sweden

TH.16.03 **Reduced stimulated adenylate cyclase activity in post mortem hippocampus of demented patients**
T. G. Ohm, J. Bohl, H. Steinmetz and B. Lemmer, Fed. Rep. of Germany

TH.16.04 **Quantitative autoradiographic studies of peptide and receptor expression in human post mortem materials**
J. M. Palacios, G. Mengod, E. Ruperte, M. Savasta and A. Probst, United Kingdom

TH.16.05 **Post mortem investigation of neurochemical and neuropeptidergic hypotheses of depression**
I. N. Ferrier, R. H. Perry, A. F. Fairbairn, I. G. McKeith, A. Leake and M. Yates, United Kingdom

TH.16.06 **Further cytoarchitectonic and quantitative studies in the entorhinal region of schizophrenics and normal controls by means of a modified Nissel-technique**
H. Heinsen and H. Beckmann, Fed. Rep. of Germany

TH.16.07 **Glutamate and dopamine receptors in schizophrenia**
J. Kornhuber and H. Beckmann, Würzburg

TH.16.08 **Post mortem investigations of dopamine systems in schizophrenia**
G. Reynolds and C. Czudek, United Kingdom

SYMPOSIUM
New Drugs in the Treatment of Schizophrenia – Clinical Aspects

Chair: K. Heinrich, Fed. Rep. of Germany, and K. M. Inanaga, Japan

---

TH.17.01 **Risperidone, a novel antipsychotic with thymostenic properties**
Y. Gelders, S. Heylen, G. Vanden Bussche, A. Reyntjens and P. Janssen, Belgium

TH.17.02 **Treatment of negative symptomes of schizophrenia not with drugs but with natural substances: L-DOPA and TRH**
K. S. Funatsu and K. Inanaga, Japan

TH.17.03 **Experimental comparison of remoxipride, clozapine and haloperidol in the treatment of acute schizophrenia**
E. Klieser, E. Lehmann and J. Tegeler, Fed. Rep. of Germany

TH.17.04 **Tiospirone, a novel antipsychotic agent**
S. Gershon, R. C. Shrotriya, D. S. Robinson and P. Owen, USA

TH.17.05 **Antipsychotics of the future: Medical needs and research strategies**
T. Lewander, Sweden

TH.17.06 **Examples for alternatives to the classical dopamine hypothesis**
B. Woggon, Switzerland

SYMPOSIUM
Mood Stabilizing Drugs – Clinical Aspects

Chair: R. H. Belmaker, Israel, and H. M. Emrich, Fed. Rep. of Germany

---

TH.18.01 **Carbamazepine-lithium combination: Clinical and laboratory effects**
R. M. Post and K. Kramlinger, USA

TH.18.02 **Stimulus intensity and the anticonvulsant properties of ECT**
H. A. Sackheim, D. P. Devanand, J. Prudic, I. Prohovnik and E. Maclin, USA

TH.18.03 **Characteristics of recurrencies and suicides or suicidal attempts during long-term lithium prophylaxis**
B. Müller-Oerlinghausen, Fed. Rep. of Germany

TH.18.04 **Double blind controlled studies on the therapeutic efficacy of carbamazepine in affective and schizophrenic patients**
T. Okuma, I. Yamashita, R. Takahashi, H. Itoh, M. Kurihara, S. Otsuki, S. Watanabe, K. Sarai, H. Hazama and K. M. Inanaga, Japan

TH.18.05 **Causes of relapse in bipolar affective disorder**
T. R. Silverstone and S. Romans-Clarkson, United Kingdom

TH.18.06 **Comparison of mood stabilizing efficacy of sodiumvalproate and carbamazepine in problem cases**
H. M. Emrich, Fed. Rep. of Germany

TH.18.07 **A clinical trial of demethylchlortetracycline as a lithium-like agent in excited psychosis**
R. H. Belmaker and G. Roitman, Israel

TH.18.08 **Antidepressants? Are they useful in the prophylaxis of unipolar depression?**
S. A. Montgomery, H Dufour, S. Brion, J. Gailledreau, X. Laqueille, G. Ferrey, P. Moron, N. Parant-Lucena, L. Singer, J. M. Danion, J. N. Beuzen and M. A. Pierredon, United Kingdom

SYMPOSIUM
AIDS

Chair: F. K. Goodwin, USA, and D. Naber, Fed. Rep. of Germany

---

TH.19.01 **The epidemiology of AIDS**
P. N. R. Heseltine, USA

TH.19.02 **Peptide T prevents GP 120-induced neuronal cell death in hippocampal cultures: Clinical implications**
D. Brenneman, J. M. Buzy, M. R. Ruff and C. B. Pert, USA

TH.19.03 **AIDS as a CNS disorder: Peptide T, VIP and HIV receptor**
J. M. Hill, D. Lazega, A. I. Kook, M. Harris, D. I. Lambie, P. L. Hallberg, J. B. O'Neill, M. R. Ruff and C. P. Pert, USA

TH.19.04 **Neuropsychiatry of AIDS: Clinical presentation and treatment research**
T. P. Bridge, L. J. Ingraham and F. K. Goodwin, USA

TH.19.05 **Human immunodefiency virus (HIV) neurobehavioural research issues**
F. K. Goodwin, T. P. Bridge, USA

TH.19.06 **Neuropsychological deficits in HIV infection**
D. Naber, D. Bove, A. Erfurth, A. Matuschke, C. Perro, I. Sadri, M. Schmauss and U. Schick, Fed. Rep. of Germany

SYMPOSIUM
Alcohol and Drug Abuse

Chair: G. L. Gessa, Italy, and L. Stein, USA

TH.20.01 **Serotonin and ethanol consumption**
Z. Amit, K. Gill and S.-O. Ogren, Canada

TH.20.02 **Evidence for an opioidergic molecular genetic determinant of alcohol ingesta behaviour**
K. Blum, USA

TH.20.03 **Ethanol catecholamines and cortisol: Functional studies in humans and animals**
D. J. Nutt, B. Adinoff, D. T. George, I. Mefford and M. Linnoila, USA

TH.20.04 **Effect of acute and chronic ethanol (ETH) on the activity of midbrain DA and non-DA neurons**
G. Mereu, Italy

TH.20.05 **Gamma-hydroxybutyricacid supresses ethanol consumption in alcohol-preferring rats**
F. Fadda, E. Mosca, G. Colombo and G. L. Gessa, Italy

SYMPOSIUM
Latest Methods in the Development of New Psychotropic Drugs

Chair: P. Janssen, Belgium, and D. C. U'Pritchard, USA

TH.21.01 **Serotonin (5-HT_2) dopaminergic interactions: Effects with ICI 169, 369 a selective 5-HT_2 antagonist**
A. I. Salama, J. M. Goldstein, B. A. Meiners, C. F. Saller, J. B. Malick, R. E. Giles and D. C. U'Pritchard, USA

TH.21.02 **The role of mixed dopamine-serotonin antagonists in extrapyramidal syndromes in cebus monkeys**
D. E. Casey, USA

TH.21.03 **Cortical glutamate dysfunction in schizophrenia**
J. F. W. Deakin, M. D. C. Simpson, A. C. Gilchrist, W. J. Skan and P. Slater, United Kingdom

TH.21.04 **A prevalence study and treatment study of ritanserin in dysthymic disorder**
D. Murphy and S. A. Checkley, United Kingdom

TH.21.05 **A human analogue of anxiety employing psychophysiological measures**
M. Wang, R. Hensman and J. F. W. Deakin, United Kingdom

SYMPOSIUM
Clinical Aspects of Neuropeptide Research

Chair: C. B. Nemeroff, USA, and S. Checkley, United Kingdom

TH.22.01 **Brain neuropeptides and their possible role in the etiology of depression**
C. B. Nemeroff, USA

TH.22.02 **The h-CRH stimulation test in psychiatry**
F. Holsboer, Fed. Rep. of Germany

TH.22.03 **Pro-opiomelanocortin related peptides in depression**
I. N. Ferrier, A. Leake, B. G. Charlton and H. G. Griffiths, United Kingdom

TH.22.04 **Endocrine responses to tricyclic antidepressants and peptides in depressive patients and healthy subjects**
G. Laakmann, A. Hinz, H. Neuhauser, O. A. Müller, U. Vorderholzer and M. Winkelmann, Fed. Rep. of Germany

TH.22.05 **Use of neuroendocrine testing in the medically ill as adjuncts in diagnosis of affective disorders**
D. L. Evans, USA

TH.22.06 **The TRH stimulation test in psychiatry**
C. M. Banki, M. Arató, G. Bissette and C. B. Nemeroff, Hungary

TH.22.07 **Alterations in neuropeptide systems in Alzheimer's disease**
G. Bissette and C. B. Nemeroff, USA

SYMPOSIUM

Plasma Amino Acids in Neuropsychiatry Disorders

Chair: M. A. Richardson and H. M. van Praag, USA

TH.23.01 **Availability of amino acids to the brain and its implications for transmitter amine function**
G. Curzon, United Kingdom

TH.23.02 **Effects of phenylalanine on catecholamine synthesis and mediated behaviours**
T. J. Maher, USA

TH.23.03 **Plasma phenylalanine/large neutral amino acid ratio as a marker for tardive dyskinesia vulnerability**
M. A. Richardson, R. Suckow, R. Whittaker, W. Boggiano, I. Sziraki, H. Kushner and A. Perumal, USA

TH.23.04 **Tyrosine in depression. Is specific activation of a particular monogamine a sufficient antidepressant measure?**
H. M. Praag, USA

TH.23.05 **Plasma amino acids as treatment predictors in depression**
S. E. Møller, Denmark

TH.23.06 **Decreased tyrosine transport in schizophrenic patients**
L. Bjerkenstedt, L. Hagenfeldt, F.-A. Wiesel and N. Wenizelos, Sweden

SYMPOSIUM

Light Therapy

Chair: N. E. Rosenthal, USA, and L. Wetterberg, Sweden

TH.24.01 **The vigilance-hypothesis: A model to explain effectivity of bright light (BL) treatment: Possible new indications**
M. Dietzel, I. Veit, L. Birsak and B. Saletu, Austria

TH.24.02 **Seasonality and the effects of light therapy in the general population**
S. Kasper, T. A. Wehr, S. L. B. Rogers and N. E. Rosenthal, USA

TH.24.03 **Nighttime melatonin in depressed patients: Effects of one hour light exposure and light therapy**
B. F. Kjellman, J. Beck-Friis, G. Borg, L. J. Petterborg, B.-E. Thalén, F. Undén and L. Wetterberg, Sweden

TH.24.04 **Wavelength phototherapy study of seasonal affective disorder**
J. P. Docherty, B. A. Welch, F. Frankel, A. F. Frank, E. Fierman and N. E. Rosenthal, USA

TH.24.05 **Light at night is as good as in the morning in sad patients**
A. Wirz-Justice, P. Graw, A. Jochum, B. Gisin, J. Arendt, M. Aldhous, K. Kräuchi and W. Pöldinger, Switzerland

TH.24.06 **Neurobiology of seasonal affective disorder and phototherapy**
N. E. Rosenthal, R. G. Skwerer, F. M. Jacobsen, C. C. Duncan, S. Kasper, P. M. Schulz, L. Tamarkin, P. Gaist, T. Hardin and T. A. Wehr, USA

SYMPOSIUM
Function and Modulation of Excitatory Amino Acid Receptors

Chair: E. Costa and C. W. Cotman, USA

FR.01.01 **Changes of kynurenic acid content in the rat brain during the development and aging processes, at different hours of the day and after the administration of precursors**
F. Moroni, V. Carla and P. Russi, Italy

FR.01.02 **Neuromodulation of the glutamate receptor: An electrophysiological study**
S. Vicini, M. Bertolino and E. Costa, USA

FR.01.03 **NMDA receptors transplanted into xenopus oocytes: Comparison to neuronal receptors and glycine requirement**
R. Dingledine, N. W. Kleckner and T. A. Verdoorn, USA

FR.01.04 **Expression of the NMDA/PCP receptor in oocytes**
M.V. L. Bennet, J. Lerma, L. Kushner and R. S. Zukin, USA

FR.01.05 **Neuronal death elicited by glutamate: Mechanism of action of its pharmacological inhibition**
E. Costa, H. Manev, H. Alho, M. Favaron, A. M. Szekely and A. Guidotti, USA

FR.01.06 **Excitatory amino acid receptors; anatomical organization and functional implications**
C. W. Cotman and D. Monagham, USA

SYMPOSIUM
Methodology and Evaluation of Psychotropic Drugs

Chair: O. Benkert, Fed. Rep. of Germany, and K. Rickels, USA

FR.02.01 **State of the art in evaluating antidepressants and anxiolytics**
K. Rickels, USA

FR.02.02 **Establishing the efficacy of new anti-psychotics**
S. R. Hirsch, United Kingdom

FR.02.03 **State of the art in evaluating nootropics**
T. H. Crook, USA

FR.02.04 **Placebo controlled studies in depression: Necessity and feasibility**
E. S. Paykel, United Kingdom

FR.02.05 **Design and ethics in controlled clinical trials**
H. Helmchen, Fed. Rep. of Germany

FR.02.06 **Assessment of treatment response: Rating scales**
W. Maier and P. Bech, Fed. Rep. of Germany

FR.02.07 **Biostatistical issues: Design and evaluation**
P. W. Lavori, USA

FR.02.08 **Are there new developments in planning clinical trials?**
O. Benkert, Fed. Rep. of Germany

SYMPOSIUM
Recent Developments in the Identification of Serotonin Receptor Subtypes

Chair: J. Leysen, Belgium, and H. Gozlan, France

FR.03.01 **Characteristics of central 5-HT_{1A} receptors**
H. Gozlan, S. El Mestikawy, M. B. Emerit and M. Hamon, France

FR.03.02 **5-HT_{1B} and 5-HT_{1D} receptors: Pharmacology, localization and second messengers**
D. Hoyer, Switzerland

FR.03.03 **Serotonin 5-HT_{1C} receptors: Pharmacology to cloning**
P. R. Hartig, USA

FR.03.04 **Regulation of 5-HT_2 receptors: Investigation in vivo and on cells in culture**
J. E. Leysen, P. J. Pauwels, P. F. M. Janssen, P. Van Gompel and D. Chaffoy de Courcelles, Belgium

FR.03.05 **Neuropeptide modulation of serotonin receptor function in CNS**
C. A. Marsden, K. C. F. Fone, J. V. Johnson, P. Shields and G. W. Bennett, United Kingdom

FR.03.06 **The classification of 5-HT_3 receptors**
M. B. Tyers, United Kingdom

SYMPOSIUM

The Depressed Out-Patient (Who are they and what are they treated for)

Chair: Y. Lecrubier, France, and J. L. Ayuso-Gutierrez, Spain

---

FR.04.01 **Clinical and psychological factors in the antidepressant response of depressive out-patients**
J. L. Ayuso-Gutierrez and L. Montejo Iglesias, Spain

FR.04.02 **Bipolar II disorder: Clinical, social and pharmacologic aspects**
H. S. Akiskal, USA

FR.04.03 **Personality disorders with recurrent suicidal behaviour and brief recurrent depression: Are they the same disorder?**
M. Green, S. A. Montgomery and D. B. Montgomery, United Kingdom

FR.04.04 **Which behavioural effects of psychotropic drugs in animals could be useful for the choice in depressive out-patients**
A. J. Puech, France

FR.04.05 **Recurrent brief depression: A new concept of mild depression**
J. Angst, Switzerland

FR.04.06 **The concept of thymasthenia, clinical and therapeutical arguments**
Y. Lecrubier, France

FR.04.07 **A protocol for the diagnostic evaluation and treatment follow-up of depressive states and equivalents in an out-patient population**
J.-P. Macher, M.-A. Crocq, F. Duval and C. Rebourg, France

Discussion including invited guests

SYMPOSIUM
Anorexia Nervosa and Bulimia

Chair: P. J. V. Beumont, Australia, and D. C. Jimerson, USA

FR.05.01 **Symptom severity and neurotransmitter studies in bulimia**
D. C. Jimerson, M. D. Lesem, W. H. Kaye and T. D. Brewerton, USA

FR.05.02 **The serotonergic system in anorexia nervosa and bulimia**
K. M. Pirke, Fed. Rep. of Germany

FR.05.03 **The role of drug treatments in anorexia and bulimia nervosa**
G. F. M. Russell, United Kingdom

FR.05.04 **Drug treatment for bulimia nervosa**
C. P. L. Freeman, United Kingdom

FR.05.05 **Fluoxetine versus placebo treatment of bulimia: A double-blind-study with in-patients**
M. M. Fichter, K. Leibl, W. Rief, M. Greitemeyer, E. Brunner and K. Giesemann, Fed. Rep. of Germany

Discussion

SYMPOSIUM
Psychological Research and Psychopharmacology

Chair: P. Netter, Fed. Rep. of Germany, and H. Weingartner, USA

FR.06.01 **Pharmacological strategies for exploring psychobiologically distinct cognitive systems**
H. J. Weingartner and O. M. Wolkowitz, USA

FR.06.02 **Serial stage models of information processing and site of drug action**
G. Debus and J. Fröhlich, Fed. Rep. of Germany

FR.06.03 **Cognitive models and cholinergic drugs**
J. M. Rusted and D. M. Warburton, United Kingdom

FR.06.04 **Drugs as research tools in the psychology of emotions**
W. Janke, Fed. Rep. of Germany

FR.06.05 **Development of drugs to treat appetite disorders**
J. E. Morley, USA

FR.06.06 **Symposium on psychological research in psychopharmacology discussion: Drugs as research tools in psychology, and vice versa**
H. Steinberg, United Kingdom

SYMPOSIUM
New Strategies for Research in ECT

Chair: T. G. Bolwig, Denmark, and M. Fink, USA

FR.09.01 **Neuroendocrines and ECT**
M. Fink, USA

FR.09.02 **Seizure threshold (kindling) theories**
H. A. Sackheim, USA

FR.09.03 Withdrawn

FR.09.04 **Changes in 5-HT_{1A} and $GABA_B$ receptor function following repeated ECS**
A. R. Green, United Kingdom

FR.09.05 **Neurotransmitter theories of electroconvulsive therapy (ECT): New insights from animal studies**
D. J. Nutt, C. H. Gleiter, A. Thiagarajan and J. Deckert, USA

FR.09.06 **Evidence of action of ECT**
V. Milstein and J. G. Small, USA

FR.09.07 **Repeated ECS and amygdala kindling**
T. G. Bolwig, Denmark

FR.09.08 **Studies on the prolactin response to ECT in depression**
C. N. Stefanis, Y. G. Papakostas, M. Markianos and G. N. Papadimitriou, Greece

SYMPOSIUM
Post-Marketing Surveillance of Psychotropic Drugs

Chair: H. Hippius, Fed. Rep. of Germany, and S. A. Montgomery, United Kingdom

---

FR.16.01 **Drug surveillance – quo vadis?**
H. Hippius, Fed. Rep. of Germany

FR.16.02 **Surveillance of toxicity of antidepressants in overdose**
S. A. Montgomery, United Kingdom

FR.16.03 **Assessment of drug utilization and adverse drug reactions in the Federal Republic of Germany**
B. Müller-Oerlinghausen, Fed. Rep. of Germany

FR.16.04 **Drug surveillance in psychiatric patients in the Federal Republic of Germany: The AMÜP-study**
R. Grohmann, L. G. Schmidt and E. Rüther, Fed. Rep. of Germany

FR.16.05 **Surveillance of adverse reactions of antidepressants**
B. E. Leonhard, Ireland

FR.16.06 **A general perspective of post-marketing surveillance**
D. G. Grahame-Smith, United Kingdom

SYMPOSIUM
Classification of Psychiatric Disorders and Response to Psychotropic Drugs

Chair: T. A. Ban, USA, and P. Berner, Austria

FR.17.01 **Pharmacotherapy and the classification of psychiatric disorders**
T. A. Ban, USA

FR.17.02 **Psychiatric nosology and the concept of mental disorders as receptor diseases**
O. Vinař, Czechoslovakia

FR.17.03 **Amisulpride vs fluphenazine – treatment in unproductive schizophrenics with negative symptoms: Importance of classification of so called deficiency**
P. Berner, J. Grünberger, B. Küfferle and A. Topitz, Austria

FR.17.04 **Subtypes of schizoaffective disorders and response to lithium prophylaxis**
M. Maj, Italy

FR.17.05 **Clinical factors predicting response to antidepressants**
O. Lingjaerde, Norway

FR.17.06 **Diagnostic determinants of the antidepressant response to tricyclics**
M. Philipp and W. Maier, Fed. Rep. of Germany

FR.17.07 **The relationship between diagnosis and treatment response in the anxiety and depressive disorders; some recent developments**
M. Roth, United Kingdom

FR.17.08 **Thymastenic patients and the transnosological effect of dopaminergic stimulation**
Y. Lecrubier, F. Aubin, A. J. Puech, C. Payan and P. Boyer, France

Concluding remarks
T. Ban, USA

SYMPOSIUM
Serotonin – Behavioural Disorders

Chair: D. Eccleston, United Kingdom, and R. P. Ebstein, Israel

FR.18.01 **The neurochemistry of suicide**
J. J. Mann, V. Arango, P. Marzuk, P. A. McBride, M. De Meo and D. J. Reis, USA

FR.18.02 **Serotonergic responsivity in obsessive compulsive disorder**
D. Murphy, United Kingdom

FR.18.03 **Role of serotonin in depression**
H. Y. Meltzer, USA

FR.18.04 **The antidepressant effect of serotonin uptake inhibitors**
A. Aberg-Wistedt, Sweden

FR.18.05 **Experimental treatments involving brain serotonin that reduce food intake**
S. Garratini, T. Mennini and R. Samanin, Italy

FR.18.06 **5-HT studies in personality disorders**
E. F. Coccaro, L. J. Siever, H. Klar, G. Maurer, R. C. Mohs and K. L. Davies, USA

FR.18.07 **Selective 5-HT uptake inhibitors in the treatment of depression**
S. A. Montgomery, United Kingdom

SYMPOSIUM
Psychopharmacology in Child Psychiatry

Chair: M. A. Riddle, USA, and G. Nissen, Fed. Rep. of Germany

FR.20.01 **The psychodrug therapy of aggressive behaviours in childhood depression: Report on 32 cases**
R. Cocchi, Italy

FR.20.02 **Treatment of the childhood obsessive compulsive disorder with clomipramine and desmethylimipramine: A double-blind crossover comparison**
J. L. Rapoport, H. L. Leonard and S. E. Swedo, USA

FR.20.03 **Molindone therapy for self-injurious behaviour**
B. G. Winsberg and J. A. Camp-Bruno, USA

FR.20.04 **Psychopharmacology in child psychiatry**
M. A. Riddle and G. Nissen, USA

FR.20.05 **Psychopharmacological therapy in children and adolescents – prejudice and reality**
T. Elliger, G.-E. Trott and G. Nissen, Fed. Rep. of Germany

FR.20.06 **Pervasive developmental disorders**
P. Ferrari, France

FR.20.07 **Attention deficit hyperactivity disorder**
R. Gittelman-Klein, USA

FR.20.08 **Anxiety disorders**
J. Simeon, Canada
Discussion
M. A. Riddle

SYMPOSIUM
The Effect of Psychoactive Drugs on Car Handling Ability

Chair: I. Hindmarch, United Kingdom, and W. Pöldinger, Switzerland

FR.21.01 **Alcohol car driving laboratory and "on the road" tests of performance**
G. A. Starmer, Australia

FR.21.02 **Assessment of drug-induced impairment of human skilled performance: Antihistamines on laboratory models**
M. J. Mattila and T. Seppälä, Finland

FR.21.03 **Driving fitness of patients taking psychoactive drugs**
U. Gerhard and V. Hobi, Switzerland

FR.21.04 **Use of computer assisted simulators to differentiate residual effects of hypnotics**
H. Laurell, Sweden

FR.21.05 **Epidemiological aspects of drugs and driving**
M. R. Möller, Fed. Rep. of Germany

FR.21.06 **Behavioural toxicity of antidepressants on aspects of skilled performance and car driving**
J. Moran and M. Linnoila, USA

FR.21.07 **Behavioural toxicity of antidepressants on aspects of skilled performance and car driving**
I. Hindmarch, United Kingdom

FR.21.08 **The fitness for driving of drug treated depressive and schizophrenic inpatients**
V. Hobi and W. Pöldinger, Switzerland

FR.21.09 **Residual effects of hypnotics on psychomotor function**
C. A. Alford, United Kingdom

PLENARY LECTURES

Chair: W. E. Bunney, USA

TU.15.01 **"Perception machines": Synthetic neural modeling and the design of recognition automata**
G. Edelman, USA

Chair: H. Hippius, Fed. Rep. of Germany

WE.15.01 **Homunculus in the age of biotechnology**
M. Eigen, Fed. Rep. of Germany

WE.15.02 **A view of the neuroscience and psychopharmacology of the major psychoses – present and future**
W. E. Bunney, USA

Chair: E. Costa, USA

TH.15.01 **Structural determinants of transmitter operated membrane channels**
B. Sakmann, Fed. Rep. of Germany

TH.15.02 **Future of psychopharmacology: Psychopharmacology and positron emission tomography**
G. C. Sedvall, Sweden

Chair: A. Coppen, United Kingdom

FR.15.01 **Perspectives on dopamine as a regulator of brain function**
A. Carlsson, Sweden

FR.15.02 **Improvement of the quality of sleep: A new goal in psychopharmacology**
P. Janssen, Belgium

FR.15.03 **Lithium is all right, but – about some misconceptions and some recent findings**
M. Schou, Denmark

Subject Index